Property of IV Services of America

CLINICAL IMMUNOLOGY

Jonathan Brostoff MA, DM (Oxon) DSc, FRCP, FRCPath
Reader in Clinical Immunology
Department of Immunology
University College & Middlesex School of Medicine
London, UK

Glenis K. Scadding MA, MD, MRCP
Consultant Rhinological Physician
Royal National Throat, Nose & Ear Hospital
Honorary Senior Lecturer
University College & Middlesex School of Medicine
London, UK

David K. Male MA, PhD
Senior Lecturer in Neuroimmunology
Department of Neuropathology
Institute of Psychiatry
London, UK

Ivan M. Roitt MA, DSc (Oxon), Hon MRCP (Lond), FRCPath, FRS
Professor & Head of Department of Immunology
University College & Middlesex School of Medicine
London, UK

Gower Medical Publishing • London • New York

J B Lippincott • Philadelphia

Distributed in USA and Canada by:
J B Lippincott Company
East Washington Square
Philadelphia, PA 19105
USA

Gower Medical Publishing
101 Fifth Avenue
New York, NY 10003
USA

Distributed in UK, Europe and rest of world by:
Gower Medical Publishing
Middlesex House
34–42 Cleveland Street
London W1P 5FB
UK

Distributed in Japan by:
Nankodo Company Ltd
42–6 Hongo 3-chome
Bunkyo-Ku
Tokyo 113
Japan

Slide Atlas
A slide atlas of Clinical Immunology, based on the contents of this book, is available. In the slide atlas format, the material is split into volumes, each of which is presented in a binder, together with numbered 35mm slides of each illustration. Further information can be obtained from:

Gower Medical Publishing
Middlesex House, 34-42 Cleveland Street
London W1P 5FB, UK

Gower Medical Publishing
101 Fifth Avenue, New York,
NY 10003, USA.

Project editor:	Michele Campbell
Design & illustration:	Anne-Marie Shine
	Catherine Duffy
	Jane Brown
Linework:	Marion Tasker
Production:	Susan Bishop
Index:	Anne MacCarthy
Publisher:	Fiona Foley

Library of Congress Cataloging-in-Publication Data
Clinical immunology/Jonathan Brostoff ... [et al.].
Includes bibliographical references and index.
ISBN 0-397-44563-6 (limp). — ISBN 0-397-44768-X (cased)
1. Clinical immunology. I. Brostoff, Jonathan.
[DNLM: 1. Allergy and Immunology. 2. Immunologic Diseases.
300 C64144]
QR182.C55 1991
616.07'9—dc20

British Library Cataloguing in Publication Data
Clinical Immunology
1. Medicine. Immunology
I. Brostoff, Jonathan
616.079

Typeset on Apple Macintosh®
CRC output by The Last Word.
Text set in Optima; legends and tables set in Univers.
Colour reproduction by Mandarin in Hong Kong.
Printed by Imago Services in Hong Kong.

© Copyright 1991 by Gower Medical Publishing, 34–42 Cleveland Street, London W1P 5FB, England. The right of Jonathan Brostoff, Glenis Scadding, David Male and Ivan Roitt to be identified as authors of this work has been asserted by them in accordance with the Copyright, Designs and Patents Act 1988. All rights reserved. No part of this publication may be reproduced, stored in a retrieval system or transmitted in any form or by any means electronic, mechanical, photocopying, recording or otherwise, without prior written permission of the publisher.

PREFACE

The explosion of information in Immunology in recent years has both enhanced our understanding of disease processes, and given us exciting tools with which to investigate an ever-increasing number of clinical conditions. This has, in turn led to the development of better diagnostic tests with refined reagents and treatment specifically targeted to the disease process.

The book is divided into sections: Introduction, Transplantation, Rheumatological Disorders, Organ-Based Disease, Hypersensitivity, Neoplasia, Immunodeficiency & Infection, Immune Intervention, and Immunological Tests. In the introductory chapter we have set the scene with an account of the mechanisms underlying the immune response, and hypersensitivity reactions are briefly outlined. In each of the succeeding chapters of the book we have identified the basic immunopathological features of each disease and then related this to the clinical features seen in the patient, looked at from both the diagnostic and therapeutic points of view. Lastly, there is a chapter on techniques which should amplify those outlined in the various clinical chapters.

We hope that this book will appeal to medical students concerned with the scientific basis of clinical immunology, to clinicians who wish to have a better understanding of immunological mechanisms in their speciality, and also to basic and applied scientists who wonder if information from in vitro and animal models sheds light on the human condition — as of course it does. We think the reader will find the book enjoyable.

JB, GKS, DKM, IMR
London 1991

USER GUIDE

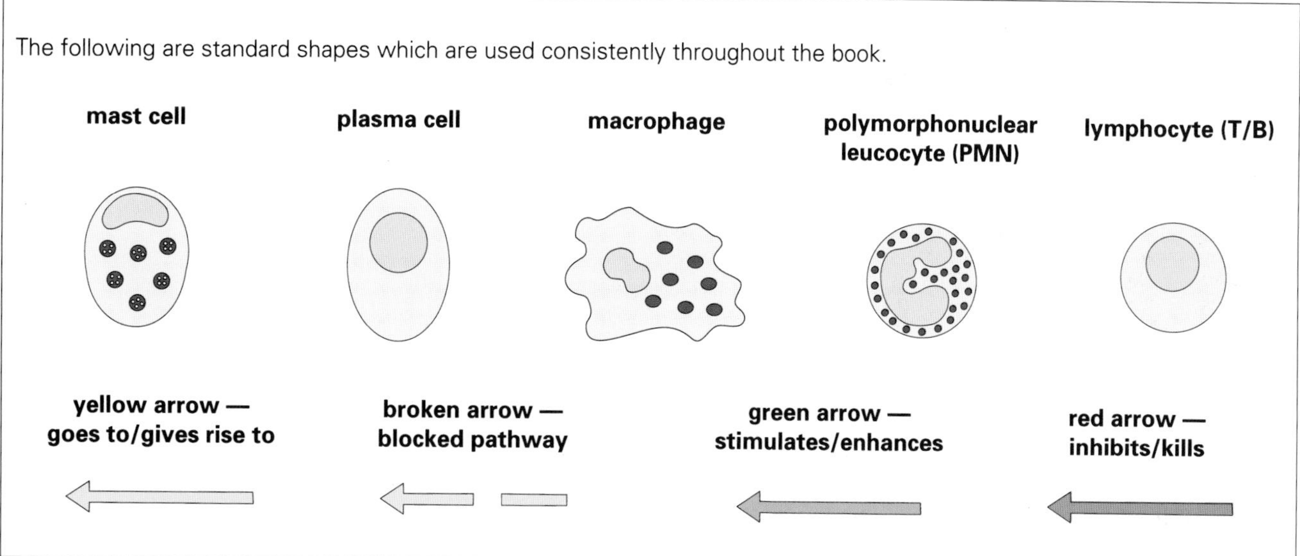

ACKNOWLEDGEMENTS

The tower of strength in seeing this book through to publication was Michele Campbell, who overcame all the problems with good humour, amazing efficiency and total unflappability.

The editors would also like to thank Anne-Marie Shine for her sterling work on the design and illustration of this book, with help from Catherine Duffy and Jane Brown. Claire Ginzler typed innumerable manuscripts and Charles Holmes produced excellent photographic material.

We are grateful to our many colleagues and friends who kindly lent us illustrated material. As always, Fiona Foley gave us continual support and encouragement.

JB, GKS, DKM, IMR
London 1991

CONTRIBUTORS

Dr A C Allison
Dept Immunology
Syntex Research Inc
Paolo Alto
California, USA

Professor R StC Barnetson
Professor of Dermatology
Dept Medicine
University of Sydney
Sydney, NSW, Australia

Professor J R Batchelor
Dept Immunology
Royal Postgraduate Medical School
Hammersmith Hospital
London, UK

Dr J Brostoff
Reader in Clinical Immunology
Department of Immunology
University College & Middlesex
School of Medicine
London, UK

Professor S J Challacombe
Dept Oral Medicine & Pathology
University of London
Guy's Hospital
London, UK

Professor R K Chandra
Memorial University of Newfoundland
Depts Pediatrics, Medicine & Biochemistry
Janeway Child Health Centre
St John's, Newfoundland, Canada

Dr S E Christmas
Dept Immunology
Paterson Institute for Cancer Research
Christie Hospital
Manchester, UK

Dr C H Dash
Director of Medical Affairs, UK Region
ER Squibb & Sons Ltd
Hounslow, UK

Professor D L Easty
Dept Ophthalmology
University of Bristol
Bristol Eye Hospital
Bristol, UK

Dr G T Fahy
Clinical Research Fellow in Cornea/
External Eye Disease
Dept Ophthalmology, University of Bristol
Bristol Eye Hospital
Bristol, UK

The late Professor H Festenstein
Dept Immunology
London Hospital Medical College
London, UK

Dr D J Gawkrodger
University Dept of Dermatology
Royal Hallamshire Hospital
Sheffield, UK

Professor M F Greaves
Leukaemia Research Fund Centre
at the Institute of Cancer Research
Chester Beatty Institute
London, UK

Dr A P Greening
Physician, Dept Respiratory Medicine
Northen General Hospital
Edinburgh, UK

Professor T J Hamblin
Consultant Haematologist
Dept Pathology
Royal Victoria Hospital
Bournemouth, UK

Professor AR Hayward
University of Colorado Health Sciences Center
Dept Pediatrics
Denver Colorado, USA

Dr D P Jewell
Consultant Gastroenterologist
Gastroenterology Unit
The Radcliffe Infirmary
Oxford, UK

Dr I Lampert
Dept Immunology
Royal Postgraduate Medical School
Hammersmith Hospital
London, UK

Professor W A Littler
Dept Cardiovascular Medicine
East Birmingham Hospital
Birmingham, UK

Dr P J Lowry
Consultant Physician
The Alexandra Hospital
Redditch, UK

Dr T Lund
Lecturer
Dept Immunology
University College & Middlesex School of
Medicine
London

Dr D K Male
Senior Lecturer in Neuroimmunology
Department of Neuropathology
Institute of Psychiatry
London, UK

Dr R Mirakian
Research Associate
Dept Immunology
University College & Middlesex Hospital
London, UK

Dr M Moore
Xenova Limited
Slough, UK

Dr A J Newman-Taylor
Consultant Physician
Brompton Hospital
London, UK

Professor J Newsom-Davis
Neurosciences Group
Institute for Molecular Medicine
John Radcliffe Hospital
Oxford, UK

Professor J R Pattison
Dean of the School of Medicine
& Faculty of Clinical Sciences
University College & Middlesex
School of Medicine

Dr A J Pinching
Senior Lecturer & Consultant Immunologist
Dept Immunology
St Mary's Hospital Medical School
London, UK

Professor JHL Playfair
Dept Immunology
University College & Middlesex
School of Medicine
London, UK

Professor I M Roitt
Head of Department of Immunology
University College & Middlesex
School of Medicine
London, UK

Dr D J Rowlands
Deputy Head
Dept Virology R & D
Wellcome Biotech
Beckenham, UK

Dr G K Scadding
Consultant Rhinological Physician
Royal National Throat, Nose & Ear Hospital
Honorary Senior Lecturer
University College & Middlesex
School of Medicine
London, UK

Dr M Snaith
Consultant in Rheumatology
Bloomsbury Rheumatology Unit
Arthur Stanley House
London, UK

Dr P Sweny
Senior Lecturer/Honorary Consultant
Dept Nephrology and Transplantation
The Royal Free Hospital
London, UK

Dr R A Thompson
Consultant Immunologist
Regional Dept Immunology
East Birmingham Hospital
Birmingham, UK

Dr P Venables
Senior Lecturer & Honorary Consultant
Physician
Institute of Rheumatology
London, UK

Professor A H Waters
Dept Haematology
St Bartholomew's Hospital
London, UK

Dr D White
Lecturer
Dept Surgery
University of Cambridge Clinical School
Addenbrook's Hospital
Cambridge, UK

Dr J Winer
Senior Registrar in Neurology
St Mary's Hospital
London, UK

CONTENTS

SECTION IV ORGAN-BASED DISEASE

1

Introduction to Immune Responses

IMMUNITY: INNATE AND ADAPTIVE

We are all exposed to a large variety of infectious microbial agents in our environment, including viruses, bacteria, fungi and parasites, and these can cause pathological damage if they multiply unchecked. The majority of infections in normal individuals are of limited duration and leave little damage because the individual's immune response combats the infection.

The two functional divisions of the immune system, the innate and adaptive systems, act in concert, with innate immunity forming the first line of defence. If these defences are breached the adaptive system is activated and produces a specific response to each infectious agent which normally eliminates the infection. The immune system then 'remembers' the infection which can lead to lifelong immunity, as in measles and diphtheria. Thus, the two key features of the adaptive response are specificity and memory. Both the innate and adaptive immune systems consist of a variety of cells and soluble factors which are distributed throughout the body. Both cells and soluble factors can act in both innate and adaptive responses.

FUNCTIONS OF THE ADAPTIVE IMMUNE SYSTEM

The function of the adaptive immune system is to recognize antigens on pathogenic micro-organisms, and to mount an appropriate immune response to eliminate the source of the antigen. Pathogens come in many different forms with a great diversity of different life-cycles, but the immune system must be able to respond to all of these challenges. Broadly speaking, there are two major types of immune response — those against intracellular pathogens, such as virus-infected cells, and those against extracellular micro-organisms. Of course, pathogens which infect cells must travel between them in the blood or tissue fluids, and therefore spend part of their life-cycle in the extracellular environment. The immune system has developed two ways of recognizing antigens: antibodies produced by B lymphocytes recognize extracellular antigens, while T lymphocytes recognize intracellular antigens, presented at the surface of cells of the body.

Another important distinction between the two arms of the immune system is that antibodies generally recognize intact antigens, while T cells can recognize only antigen fragments, which are presented to them associated with molecules encoded by the major histocompatibility complex (MHC molecules). This division corresponds roughly to the old-fashioned idea of humoral and cell-mediated immunity. Most effective immune responses involve both B and T cell mediated responses. For example T cells are required to destroy host cells infected with influenza virus, but antibody is essential to prevent the spread of the virus through the blood and re-infection of the individual.

FUNCTIONS OF ANTIBODIES

Antibodies are bi-functional molecules. One part (the Fab portion) is responsible for binding specifically to a particular antigen, while the Fc portion is capable of interacting with different cells of the immune system or the complement system. Antibodies recognize intact antigens, which may be free in solution (for example diphtheria toxin), associated with micro-organisms (for example surface antigens of bacteria) or may be molecules which are expressed intact on the surface of infected cells (for example influenza haemagglutinin). In some cases, antibody binding to particular antigens may be an important part of the immune defence. Examples include the antibody mediated neutralization of some toxins or the reduction of viral infectivity caused by antibodies binding to viral surface antigens involved in attachment to host cells.

More often, however, antibodies mediate their protective effects by acting as adapters, which cross-link the antigens to Fc receptors on host cells. Mononuclear phagocytes and neutrophils all express Fc receptors (FcR) which allow them to phagocytose antigen–antibody immune complexes for intracellular destruction. Antibodies can also sensitize cells or large parasites for attack by cytotoxic cells, expressing Fc receptors. This is called antibody-dependent cell-mediated cytotoxicity (ADCC). Eosinophils and large granular lymphocytes (LGLs) can engage their targets by this mechanism.

A final important role of antibody is in controlling the development of the inflammatory reaction. IgE antibodies bound to mast cells and basophils, via their Fc receptors, sensitize these cells, so that when they encounter the specific antigen they are triggered to release their inflammatory mediators. Also, in forming immune complexes antibody activates the complement system which generates a number of pro-inflammatory mediators. These functions are outlined in Fig. 1.1.

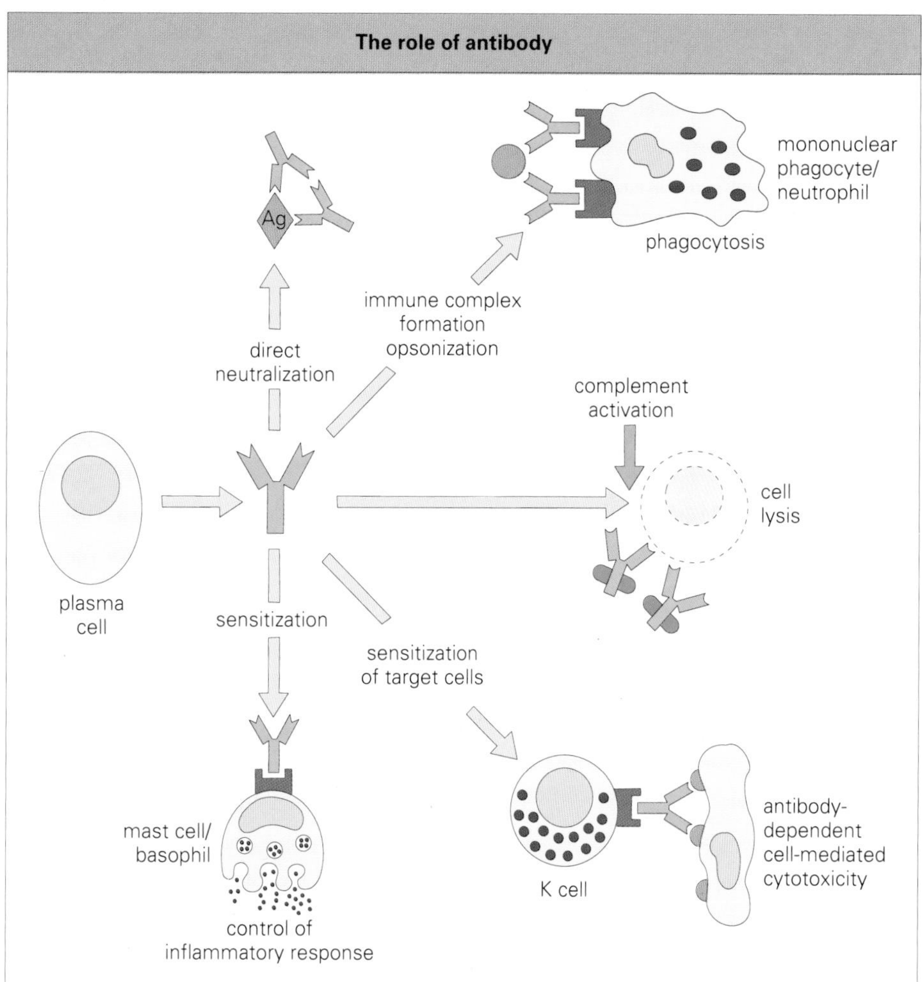

Fig. 1.1 The various ways in which antibody can act.

FUNCTIONS OF T CELLS

T cells recognize antigens originating from within other cells. There are two major types of T cell. $CD8^+$ T cells recognize antigen fragments associated with MHC class I molecules, while $CD4^+$ T cells recognize antigen associated with MHC class II molecules. These two subsets of T cell have essentially distinct functions.

The primary function of $CD8^+$ T cells is to recognize and kill virally infected cells. During the intracellular assembly of viruses, viral polypetides become associated with MHC class I molecules. These antigen–MHC complexes are transported to the cell surface for recognition by $CD8^+$ T cells. This is followed by T cell-mediated killing of the infected target cell.

$CD4^+$ T cells have a variety of functions in controlling immune responses, but they too recognize antigen fragments associated with MHC molecules. Antigen which is endocytosed by a group of cells called antigen presenting cells (APCs) can associate with MHC class II molecules, and be expressed at the surface of the APC for recognition by $CD4^+$ T cells. If these cells recognize antigen–MHC on a macrophage, they can release cytokines (soluble mediators of immunity) to activate the macrophage to destroy intracellular pathogens. If the T cell recognizes antigen–MHC on a B cell, they can release cytokines which activate the B cell to divide and differentiate. The T cells therefore help B cells to make antibody. $CD4^+$ T cells recognizing antigen–MHC on other cells of the body can also interact with them and activate them by releasing cytokines. The function of $CD4^+$ T cells is therefore in the control and development of immune responses.

It will be clear from the description above, that MHC class I and class II molecules are essential in the presentation of antigen to T cells. Moreover, MHC molecules vary structurally between individuals to a great extent, with different MHC molecules being more or less efficient at presenting each antigen. For this reason an individual's MHC haplotype determines the quality and quantity of an immune response that they can make to any particular antigen. Consequently MHC haplotype partly determines disease susceptibility in any condition where immune responses are involved. The functions of T cells are summarized in Fig. 1.2.

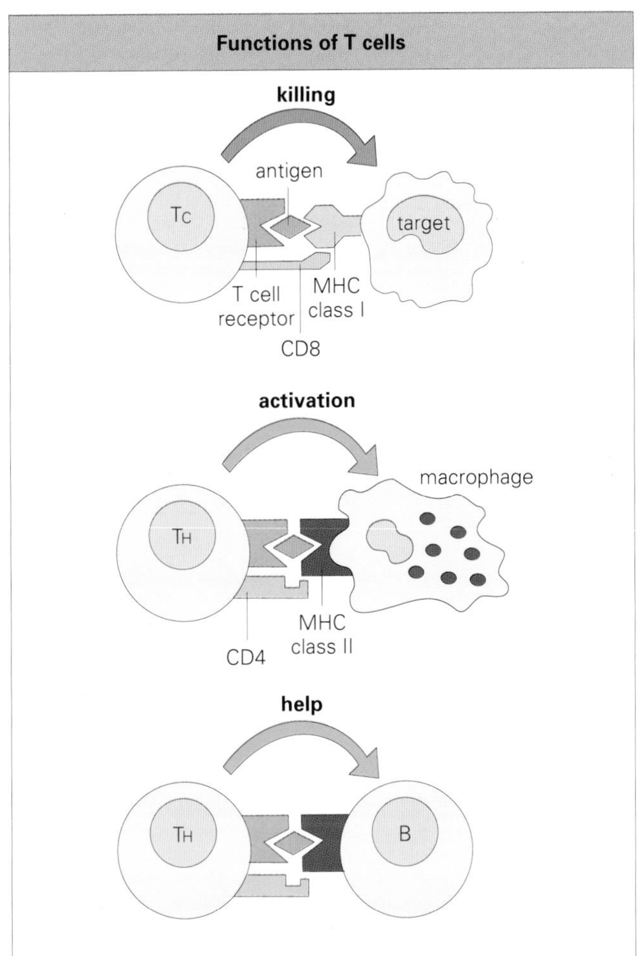

Fig. 1.2 The various functions of T cells include the killing of target cells through MHC class I, activation of APCs (macrophages) and help for B cell production of antibody through MHC class II.

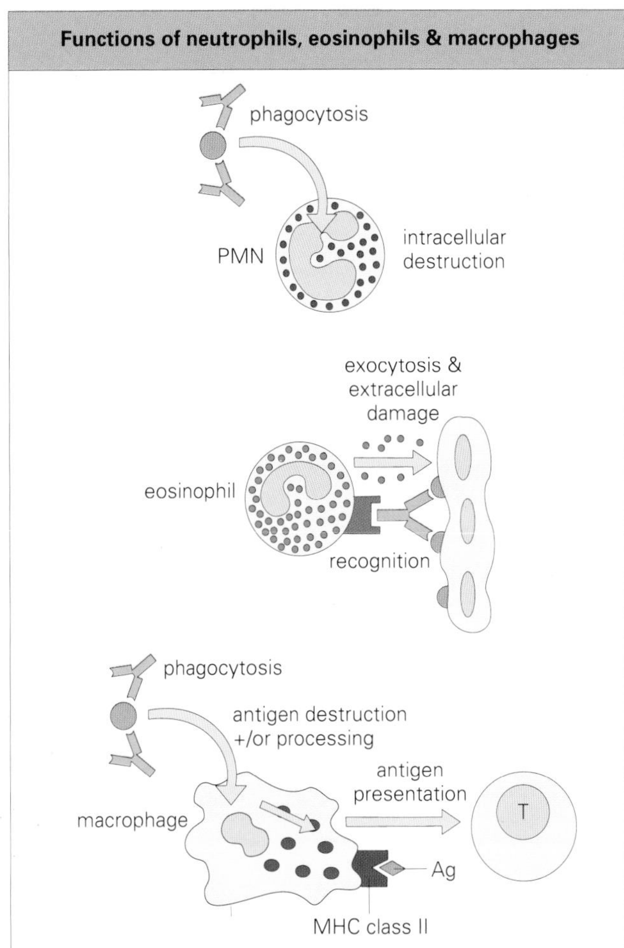

Fig. 1.3 Neutrophils and macrophages can phagocytose and destroy antigen intracellularly but antigen presentation is carried out by macrophages and other cells of this lineage. Eosinophil killing is guided by antibody and Fc receptor interaction and is effected extracellularly.

FUNCTION OF NEUTROPHILS, EOSINOPHILS AND MACROPHAGES

The primary function of this group of cells is to destroy antigens and pathogens. Neutrophils (PMNs) and macrophages can phagocytose antigens for intracellular destruction in their phagolysosomes. Destruction of endocytosed pathogens is brought about by reactive oxygen intermediates and their by-products, such as hypohalite, which are secreted into the phagolysosomes, along with other inhibitors of bacterial metabolism. Enzymes promote the degradation of phagocytosed immune complexes, micro-organisms and other antigens. In contrast to macrophages and neutrophils, eosinophils are only weakly phagocytic but they are important in damaging large pathogens (such as some intestinal worms) by releasing their granule contents to the exterior.

In all these cases the cells may recognize the target antigens via antibody binding to their Fc receptors or by complement molecules binding to receptors for activated C3. Macrophages and other mononuclear phagocytes are long-lived cells and they can also act as APCs, collecting antigen in the periphery, recirculating to secondary lymphoid tissues and presenting antigen fragments associated with MHC class II molecules to $CD4^+$ T cells. They may also be important in antigen presentation at sites of immune responses, where specialized APCs such as dendritic cells are less abundant. Macrophages also release a variety of cytokines, some of which are involved in cell activation, while others mediate cytotoxic damage to target cells (Fig. 1.3).

FUNCTIONS OF THE COMPLEMENT SYSTEM

Complement is one of the main mediators of inflammatory reactions, which can be activated either via antibody in immune complexes (classical pathway activation) or by

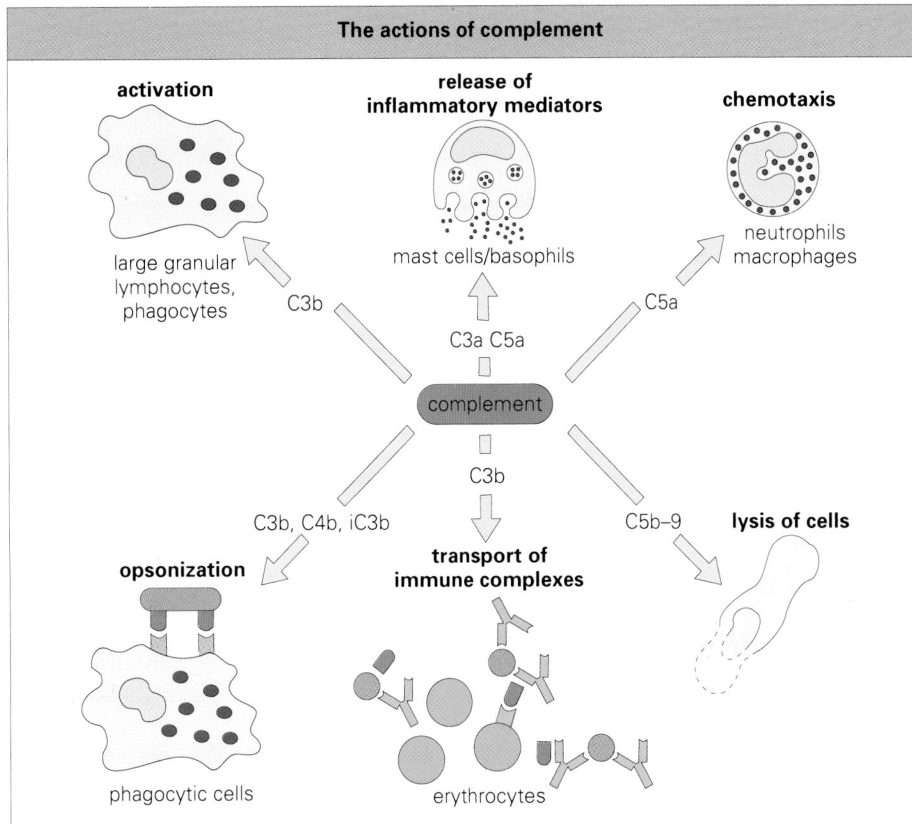

Fig. 1.4 In addition to cytotoxic activity, complement leads to degranulation of mast cells and basophils. It is also effective in opsonization of micro-organisms and transport of immune complexes.

an alternative pathway activated in the presence of certain microbial surfaces. It therefore mediates both adaptive and innate immunity. The central reaction of the complement cascade is the cleavage of C3 to form C3a and C3b. This can be initiated by either classical or alternative pathways, and it is the starting point of the lytic pathway.

Important functions of the complement system are illustrated in Fig. 1.4. Complement C3b, covalently deposited on particles, can opsonize them for phagocytosis by macrophages and neutrophils. Binding of C3b and inactivated C3b (iC3b) to receptors on large granular lymphocytes (LGLs), particularly when cross-linked to Fc receptors, initiates cellular activation. This is seen as increased microbicidal cytocidal activity, accompanied by a respiratory burst, the expression of new surface receptors and enhanced secretion of lysosomal enzymes. Erythrocytes (in man) can also take up immune complexes via bound C3b and transport them to the spleen and liver for transfer to phagocytic cells, and their ultimate destruction.

The small fragments, C3a and C5a, released during the activation of complement are called anaphylatoxins. They are important mediators of inflammation. Both of them can cause degranulation of mast cells with release of histamine, PAF and many other mediators which cause contraction of smooth muscle in vessel walls, and enhance permeability of small vessels. In addition, C5a is chemotactic for mononuclear phagocytes and neutrophils, and by its action on neutrophils it enhances capillary permeability.

The lytic pathway components (C5b–C9) are able to form pores of membrane attack complexes (MACs) on plasma membranes. This is important in damaging some bacteria, which have an outer membrane, such as *Neisseria*. However it is also important in immunopathology, since MACs can destroy incompatible red cells, or host cell tissue in autoimmune diseases, such as myasthenia gravis, where C9 is found on the damaged motor endplates.

INTRODUCTION TO IMMUNOPATHOLOGY

If one considers the essence of an immune response to be recognition and elimination of antigen, then it is clear that this can fail in one of three ways, and these form the basis of all immunopathological conditions. These areas are:

- failure of appropriate recognition leading to autoimmunity;
- failure to produce an adequate immune response seen as immunodeficiency;
- an overactive immune response, which produces more damage than it prevents.

The fundamental basis of the adaptive immune response is the ability to distinguish self molecules from non-self antigens and to mount an appropriate immune response to the antigens. Lymphocytes are initially generated which can recognize the complete repertoire of molecules, but

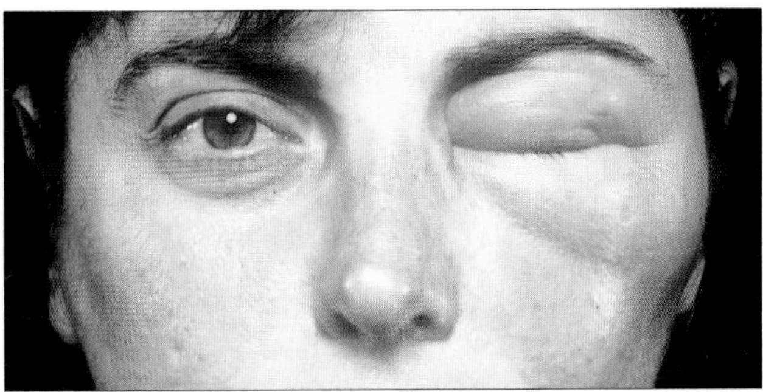

Fig. 1.5 Anaphylactic response to bee venom. This patient (a beekeeper) was stung on her face by a bee and the immediate hypersensitivity reaction appeared in minutes. She subsequently become hyposensitized by repeated stings and now shows no response when stung.

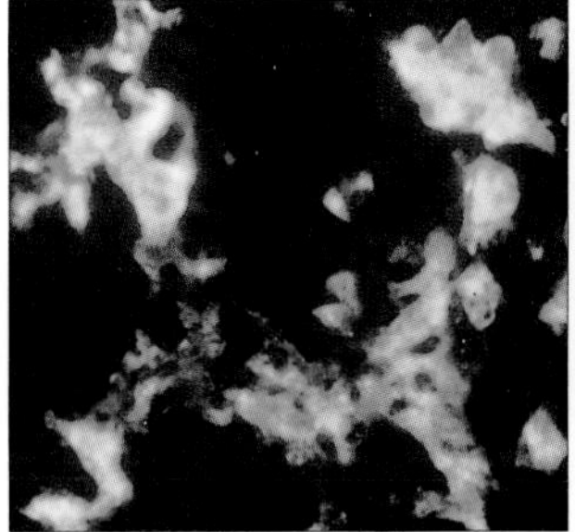

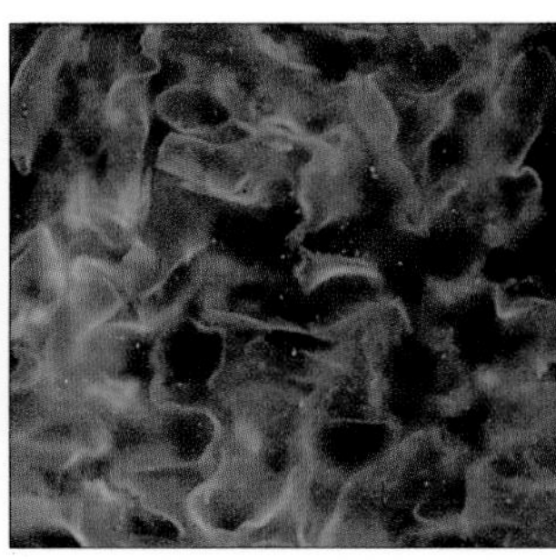

Fig. 1.6 Immunoglobulin deposition in the kidney: a comparison of type II and type III hypersensitivity. Left: a 'lumpy-bumpy' pattern is seen in the kidney in SLE due to formation of immune complexes, probably formed *in situ* in the glomerulus. Right: anti-basement membrane antibody (as in Goodpasture's syndrome) forms an even layer on the basement membrane.

those clones which recognize self are rendered anergic during development. In fact self-reactive clones are normally present in all individuals, although they are usually limited in their ability to recognize a small proportion of self molecules. Furthermore, autoimmune reactions occur in most individuals at some times, for example following certain infections. However it is only in a minority of cases that autoimmune reactions progress to autoimmune disease. This means that autoimmunity is controlled both at the stage of lymphocyte development and during the continued operation of the immune system. The basis of self-tolerance, autoimmunity and autoimmune disease will be discussed in chapter 4.

Immunodeficiency can be caused by failure of a variety of different elements of the immune system, but these are fundamentally due either to genetic defects or to acquired malfunctions. Examples of the former include severe combined immunodeficiency and Di George syndrome, while drug-induced aplastic anaemias and AIDS are examples of the latter. All of these deficiencies usually manifest as increased susceptibility to infection, although the precise pathogens involved depends on which element of the immune system is missing. There is a surprising amount of redundancy in the immune system, such that a deficiency in one arm of the system may be partly compensated by other immune defence mechanisms. However anything which compromises the ability of lymphocytes to recognize and react to antigen, or the ability of phagocytes to clear the antigens is usually serious. Immunodeficiency is discussed further in chapters 23 & 24.

HYPERSENSITIVITY

When an adaptive response occurs in an exaggerated or inappropriate form causing tissue damage, the term hypersensitivity is used. This response is not a general one but is characteristic of an individual, and is only manifest following second or subsequent contact with a particular antigen (allergen). The original classification by Coombs and Gell divided hypersensitivity into four types (Types I, II, III and IV) but from a clinical point of view they are rarely discrete and do not necessarily occur in isolation from each other. The first three types are mediated by antibody and the fourth is mediated by T cells and macrophages.

TYPE I

The essence of type I hypersensitivity is the immediacy of the reaction due to the interaction of antigen (allergen) with IgE sensitized mast cell and basophils. Following this triggering of the cells there is degranulation and a release of pharmacological mediators of inflammation leading to the clinical effects of allergy. These clinical effects can be shown in the skin or in target organs such as the nose and lung. Hay fever and extrinsic asthma are the most common atopic disorders. Anaphylactic reactions to venom (Fig. 1.5) can be very serious and are clear cut examples of type I hypersensitivity.

The triggering of IgE sensitized mast cells by allergen leads to immediate histamine release which produces a wheal and flare reaction in the skin which peaks at 15 minutes and clears by 1 hour unless a late phase response ensues.

TYPE II

Both type II and type III hypersensitivity are caused by IgG and IgM antibodies. The major difference is that the target antigen in type II is part of the surface of a specific cell or tissue whereas in type III hypersensitivity the antigen is soluble and the antigen–antibody complex can cause an inflammatory response wherever it is deposited. This is clearly seen in the kidney where immunoglobulin deposition is markedly different in type II compared with type III hypersensitivity (Fig. 1.6). Two other areas where type II reactions are notable are autoimmunity and transplantation.

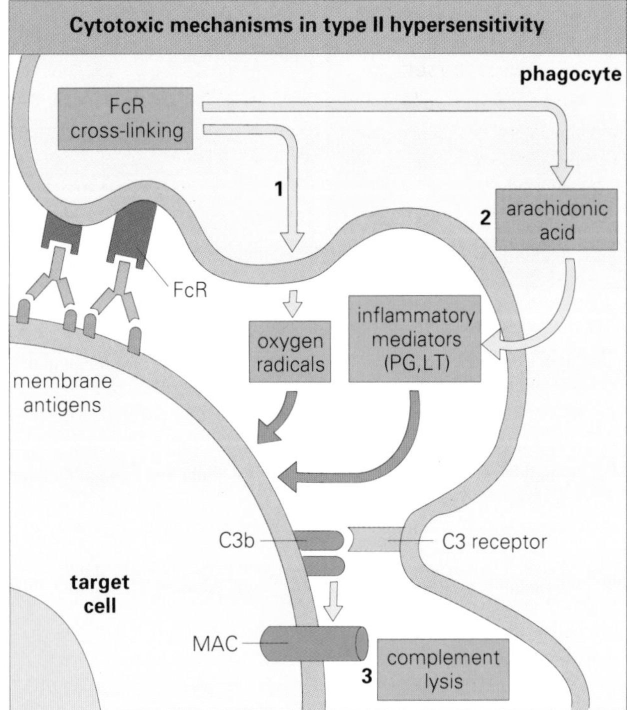

Fig. 1.7 Antibody bound to membrane antigen opsonizes them for phagocytes causing: (1) cross-linking of Fc receptors (FcR),activating the cell membrane to secrete oxygen radicals; (2) increased cell activation and release of arachidonic acid to produce prostaglandins (PG) and leukotrienes (LT); (3) after antibody attachment, C3b deposition occurs with lytic pathway activation.

Antibody bound to a surface antigen (Fig. 1.7) on the target cell allows phagocytes to be recruited through their Fc receptors. This then activates phagocyte membrane enzymes and cell function. Fixation of complement leads to further damage through assembly of the membrane attack complex (MAC) and activation of the lytic pathway. Some examples of type II hypersensitivity are haemolytic disease of the newborn, drug reactions and autoimmunity.

TYPE III

Diseases that are produced by immune complexes are those in which antigen persists without being eliminated, that is persisting infection, autoimmune disease or repeated exposure to extrinsic antigens, such as fungi in farmers' lung disease. The site of immune complex deposition is determined by various factors, such as the size of the complex, antibody affinity for the antigen, local blood flow and pre-existing inflammation. The complexes trigger a variety of inflammatory processes involving complement activation which can in turn lead to mast cell activation, platelet agglutination with formation of microthrombi and chemotaxis of neutrophils (Fig. 1.8). Skin testing in type III hypersensitivity leads to an Arthus reaction which has a delayed time course

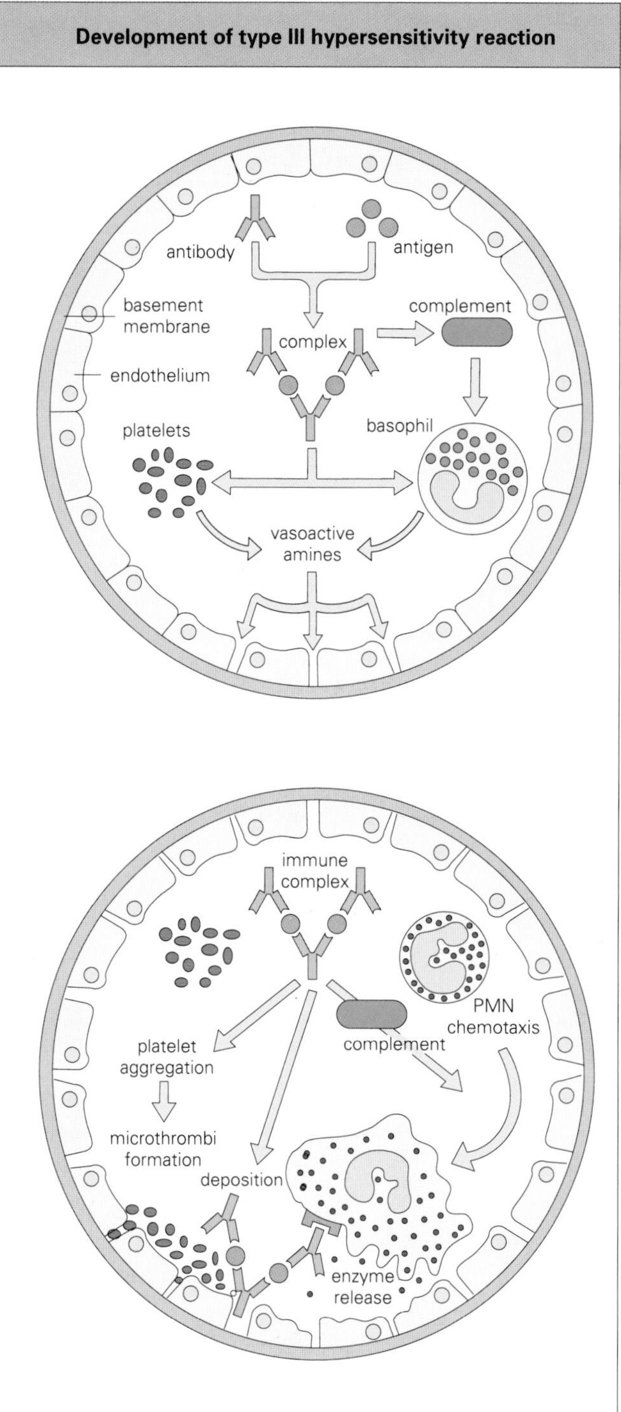

Fig. 1.8 Immune complexes (ICs) activate complement, releasing C3a and C5a which cause release of mediators from basophils and mast cells. They may also lead to platelet activation via their Fc receptors causing further release of histamine and eicosanoids, and inducing microthrombus formation. Mediators act on the vessel wall and, with C5a, activated neutrophils cause increased vascular permeability. ICs deposited on the vessel wall cause further deposition of complement, and hence chemotaxis and stimulation of phagocytic cells.

compared with type I IgE mediated reactions, although of earlier onset than type IV skin reactions (Fig. 1.9). The reaction starts at about 5 hours and continues for approximately 24 hours, with both complement activation and neutrophils being essential for a maximal response.

TYPE IV

In the original classification by Coombs and Gell, type IV or delayed type hypersensitivity included all those reactions which took more than 12 hours to develop. There are now several different types of immune reaction which can produce such a delayed response.

Type IV hypersensitivity is based on antigen–T cell interaction, which in turn recruits other cells to the site. The classical response in the skin is the tuberculin reaction or that of contact sensitivity. The time course of the reactions is more delayed than that of type I or III skin reactivity, reaching a peak 24–48 hours after application. This skin response is frequently used to test for sensitivity to micro-organisms following previous exposure, for example in tuberculosis.

Granulomatous hypersensitivity can follow on from the tuberculin reaction, and is clinically the most important form of delayed hypersensitivity causing many of the pathological effects in diseases which involve T cell mediated immunity (Fig.1.10). Contact hypersensitivity to occupational antigens such as nickel and chromate is also an important type IV reaction.

Cell-mediated immunity, as judged by skin tests, is affected by protein calorie malnutrition, advanced age and drugs such as corticosteroids.

Conclusion

A clear knowledge of the various mechanisms described above will help in the understanding of the diseases described in the following chapters.

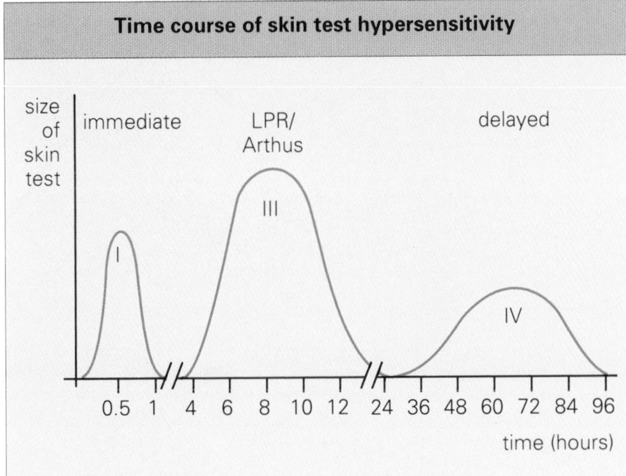

Fig. 1.9 The three main types of hypersensitivity, as shown in the skin reaction, are distinguished by the appearance and timing of the response. The timing of the Arthus reaction and the late phase response (LPR) are similar and are differentiated by the clinical picture and serological response.

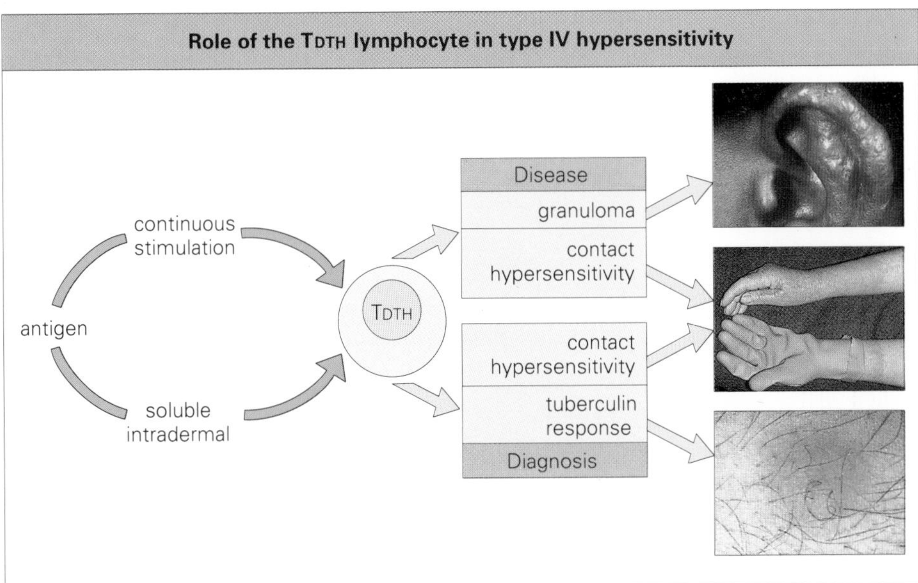

Fig. 1.10 The tuberculin skin reaction (lower; courtesy of Professor JHL Playfair) is the classical diagnostic test for cell-mediated immunity in tuberculosis. If there is continuous antigenic stimulation instead of a single injection of soluble antigen, a granulomatous reaction (upper; courtesy of Dr A du Vivier) or contact hypersensitivity (middle; courtesy of Dr D Sharvill) follows. This can also occur if the macrophages cannot destroy the antigen.

FURTHER READING

1.8 Roitt IM, Brostoff J, Male DM, eds. *Immunology (2E)*. London: Gower Medical Publishing; Edinburgh: Churchill Livingstone, 1989.

2

HLA and Disease

INTRODUCTION

The discovery of associations between certain diseases and the major histocompatibility complex (MHC) represents one of the most important advances in clinical medicine in the last two decades; it also provides a firm foundation for understanding the aetiology of a range of hitherto perplexing diseases ranging from multiple sclerosis to rheumatoid arthritis.

HUMAN LEUCOCYTE ANTIGENS (HLA)

The human MHC is known as the HLA (human leucocyte antigen) locus and is located on chromosome 6 (Fig. 2.1) There are at least four blocks of genes within the complex:

- MHC class I genes, which are expressed on all nucleated cells.
- MHC class II genes, expressed on cells which may present antigens to $CD4^+$ T lymphocytes.
- MHC class III genes, which include the complement components C4, C2 and factor B, and the isoenzymes of 21-hydroxylase. Recently a number of additional genes have been found within this region.
- MHC class IV genes, which encode molecules with a similar structure to class I, but with restricted distribution. They are thought to act as differentiation antigens during embryogenesis.

Disease association

The first clue to indicate the important role of the MHC in the pathogenesis of disease was the discovery that in mice, the MHC-linked genes controlled resistance to viral leukaemogenesis and specific immune response. However, investigations of the relationship between HLA and human malignant diseases showed there to be only weak correlations. More recently, a highly significant association has been found between HLA–Bw46 and nasopharyngeal carcinoma, a condition almost wholly restricted to the Chinese. Although links with carcinomas are uncommon, there are striking associations of particular HLA haplotypes with other diseases, particularly those with a suspected or presumed autoimmune aetiology; the most remarkable example is ankylosing spondylitis.

HLA MOLECULES

Class I

The original classical HLA tissue types are now known as HLA class I molecules. Each class I molecule is heterodimeric, consisting of a 43 kDa chain encoded in the MHC region non-covalently associated with a molecule of β_2-microglobulin (12 kDa) which is encoded outside the HLA region on chromosome 15 (Fig. 2.2). The α chain is highly polymorphic and each tissue type has a slightly different configuration which can be identified by specific antibodies. In contrast, the β_2-microglobulin polypeptide is monomorphic.

The MHC-encoded α chain consists of an extracellular part divided into three domains, a transmembrane portion and a short cytoplasmic section, the size of which can vary slightly. The N-terminal (α_1) domain contains an attachment site for a carbohydrate side chain, and the second (α_2) and third (α_3) domains are stabilized by intrachain disulphide bonds. The whole structure is stabilized by association with the β_2-microglobulin which is folded into a single extracellular domain.

The genes coding for the class I antigens consist of seven exons, or translated regions, interrupted by non–coding introns. Exons II, III, and IV contain the sequences for the three external domains, exon V codes for the transmembrane segment and exons VI and part of VII encode the cytoplasmic tail. The majority of the polymorphism in

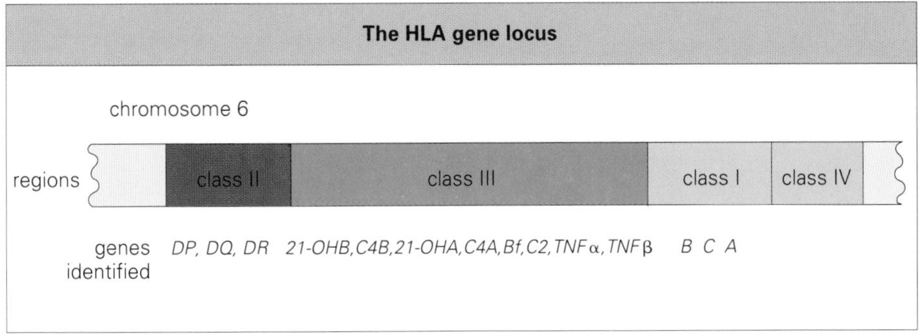

Fig. 2.1 The classical tissue transplantation antigens are class I molecules encoded in the A, B and C loci. The HLA-D region encodes class II molecules. The class III region contains genes for miscellaneous enzymes, complement components and TNF, while the class IV region contains genes for molecules thought to be expressed during development.

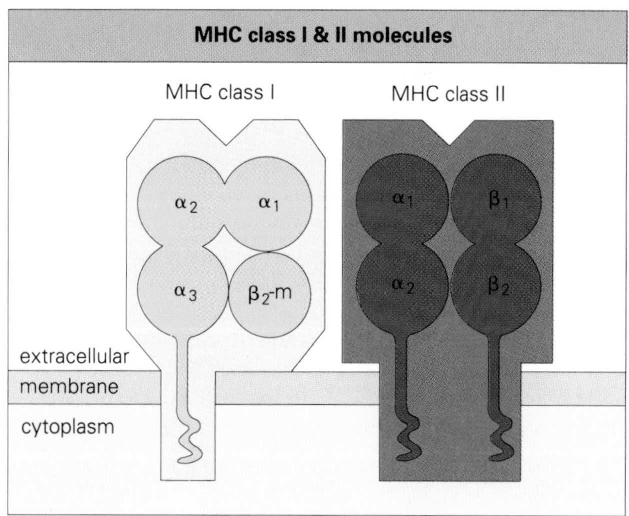

Fig. 2.2 Class I molecules consist of an α chain encoded by either the A, B or C locus, associated with β_2-microglobulin (β_2-m). Class II molecules, encoded by the D region, have two MHC-encoded polypeptides, α and β. Both molecules have four extracellular domains, named as indicated.

class I molecules is confined to the α_1 and α_2 domains, which together form a site that can bind antigenic peptides (Fig. 2.3) and present them to $CD8^+$ T lymphocytes.

Class II

The second group of HLA tissue types are known as class II antigens. These were first discovered when lymphocytes from unrelated individuals were cultured together; when tissue types differed, the antigens would stimulate T cell proliferation.

Class II molecules are glycoproteins consisting of two chains — an α chain of 31–35 kDa and a β chain of 27–30 kDa. Like class I, class II molecules have four external domains, but in this case the α and β chains each have two domains, a transmembrane segment and an intracytoplasmic tail. The two chains are non-covalently associated. The genes coding for the α chain contain five exons, of which exons II and III are mainly responsible for encoding each of the two external domains, and exon IV codes the sequence for the transmembrane and cytoplasmic segments. The β genes contain six exons, of which exons II and III are mainly responsible for encoding the extracellular domains. Exon IV encodes the sequence for

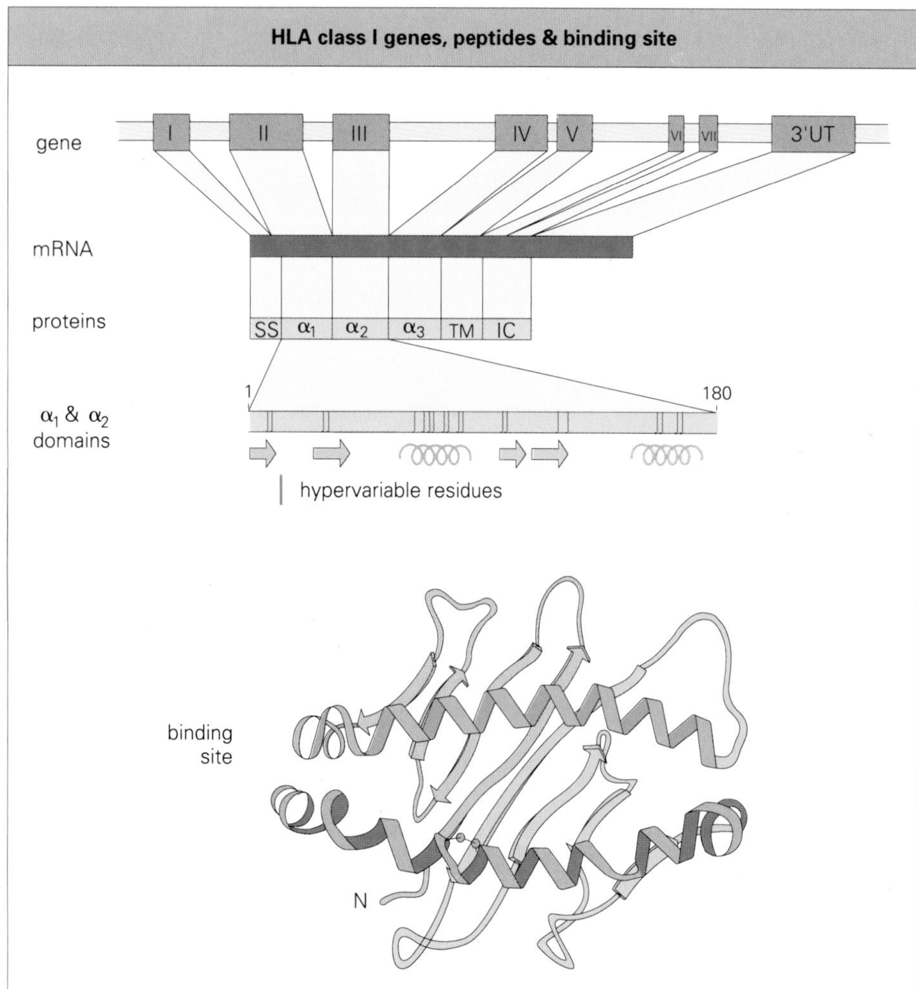

Fig. 2.3 Seven exons code for the signal sequence (SS), three external domains (α_1, α_2, α_3), the transmembrane segment (TM) and the intracytoplasmic tail (IC). 3'UT= untranslated region. The first and second external domains are organized into a β-pleated sheet forming a floor, and two α helices which form the walls of a groove into which the antigen peptides can bind.

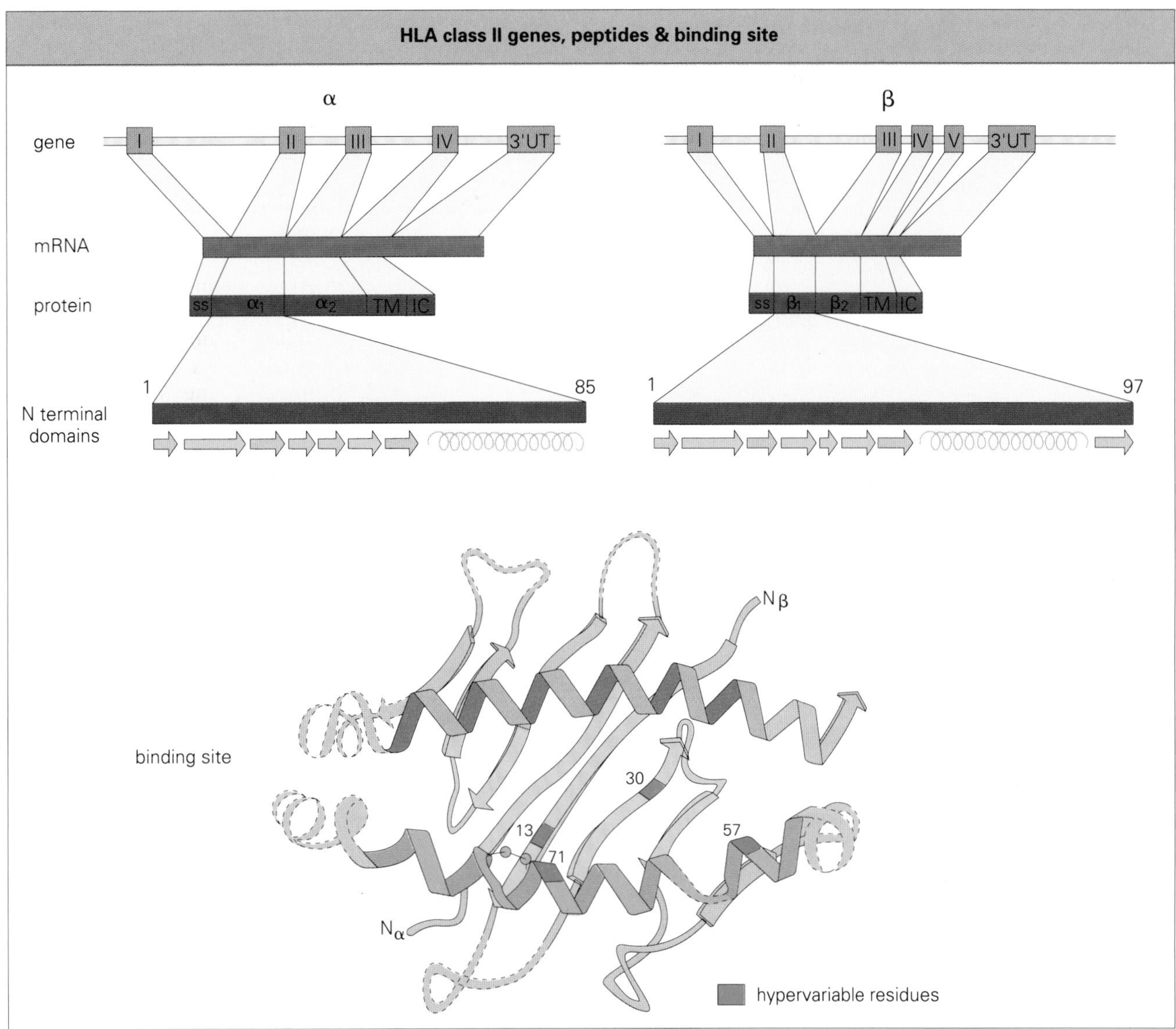

Fig. 2.4 In the α chain the transmembrane and cytoplasmic segments are contained within a single exon, whereas in the β chain the transmembrane segment is contained in a separate exon, and the cytoplasmic region is encoded by exon V. In DR chains, many of the polymorphic sites are in the β-pleated sheet. Residues 13 and 30 seem highly polymorphic. In addition, the amino acids of the α helix facing the inside of the groove are polymorphic, particularly residues 57 and 71. In DQ, residues 26, 30 and 37 in the β-pleated sheet and 57 and 71 in the α helix seem to be most polymorphic, although other residues forming part of the antigen binding site also show polymorphism.

the transmembrane segment, and exon V the cytoplasmic sequences. The polymorphic residues are primarily confined to the two N-terminal domains which are thought to form a binding site for the antigen to be presented to $CD4^+$ T cells (Fig. 2.4).

The postulated structure of the antigen binding site is based on the crystal structure of class I molecules. The first half of domain 1 is organized into a β-pleated sheet forming the floor of the binding site and the second half is an α helix which forms the walls of the antigen binding groove.

Unlike class I molecules, class II surface antigens have a restricted tissue distribution. They are expressed mainly on B cells, monocytes and leucocytic dendritic cells. However, many other cell types may be induced to express class II when stimulated by the cytokine interferon-γ (IFNγ) which is released by activated T cells.

HLA LOCUS

Class I

There are three loci, or genes, encoding class I molecules in the HLA region, termed HLA-A, HLA-B and HLA-C. Class I antigens are all defined by serological reactions and typing is performed using standard serological techniques (Fig. 2.5). The antibodies which recognize HLA molecules may bind uniquely to a particular molecule from a single locus, or they may bind to a group of molecules which share some common structures. As new typing antibodies become available, some specificities are found to consist of different subtypes. When this occurs, the original haplotype is said to be split.

There are at least 24 different types of HLA-A molecules, which may be grouped into six broad specificities. HLA-A9 is split into two subtypes, HLA-A10 into four, HLA-A28 into two and HLA-Aw19 into six. In addition, four subtypes of HLA-A2 have been identified by isoelectric focusing (see Appendix 2.1). As the nucleotide or amino acid sequences become available, many of the serological specificities (alleles) are found to consist of families of closely related alleles differing from each other by only one or two amino acids. International guidelines have been laid down for the nomenclature of genes and alleles of class I and class II based on nucleotide or amino acid sequencing. So far, allele names are based on the translated amino acid sequence (Fig. 2.6).

Class II

There are at least three class II regions: HLA-DP, HLA-DQ and HLA-DR (Fig. 2.7). The term DR was originally used to describe the HLA tissue types detected by antibody testing, which approximate to those lymphocyte activating determinants (LADs) assigned by their ability to stimulate T cell proliferation in mixed lymphocyte reactions (MLR) (Fig. 2.8). The LADs were originally termed alleles of the HLA-D locus, and the HLA-DR specificities were related to the particular HLA-D allele. Thus, antibodies which identified HLA-DR4 recognized the HLA-Dw4 allele identified in MLR.

HLA-DR subregion. In this subregion there is only one gene for a class II α chain which is not polymorphic, and 1–4 genes for β chains which are polymorphic, the number depending on the individual's haplotype. For example, the haplotype DR1 has only one β chain (DR-β1), whereas there are four β chain genes in the DR7 haplotype.

The LADs of the HLA-DR subregion belong to an independently segregated series known as the HLA-D(Dw) types. For example, HLA-DR is associated with D(Dw4) *[DRB1*0401]*, D(Dw10)*[DRB1*0402]*, D(Dw14)*[DRB1*0404]* in Caucasians and with D(Dw15)*[DRB1*0405]* and D(DwDKT2)[DRB1*0406] in Mongoloids. It is doubtful whether it will ever be possible to obtain antibodies (i.e. DR specificities) which uniquely correspond to all individual D(Dw) types. Since the D(Dw) determinants activate the large subpopulation of helper T cells, they are critical in graft-versus-host reactions, in bone marrow transplantation, and also act as restriction elements in certain autoimmune diseases.

HLA-DQ subregion. This subregion includes two α chain and two β chain genes, although only one α/β pair (DQA1/DQB1) encode the DQ specificities. The alternative pairs, known as DXA, DXB or DQA2, DQB2, whilst clearly polymorphic at the DNA level, constitute essential components of certain DR4 and DR3 haplotypes and are strongly associated with insulin-dependent diabetes mellitus in British Caucasians. Although the DQ determinants also activate subpopulations of T cells in the MLC, the reactions are relatively weak and do not contribute to the D(Dw) assignment. The biological role of the HLA-DQ specificities seems to be different from those of HLA-DR, in that they appear to be involved in the control of certain suppressor systems. In addition, DQ molecules appear to

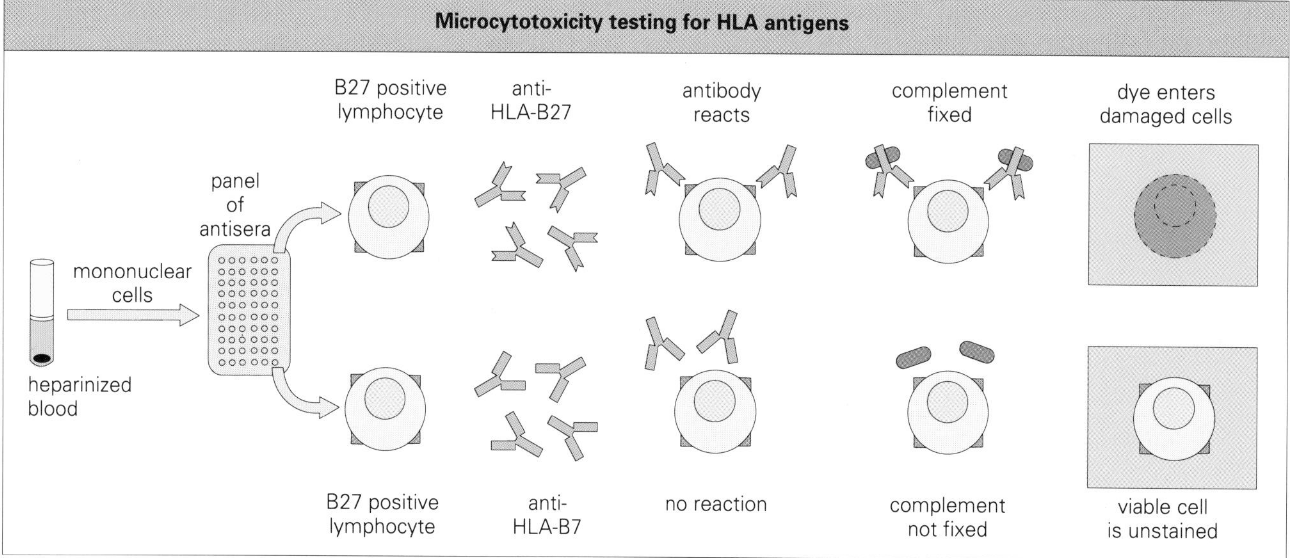

Fig. 2.5 Mononuclear cells (obtained by Ficoll-Hypaque gradient centrifugation on heparinized blood) are tested against a panel of anti-HLA class I antibodies. HLA-B27 positive cells will bind anti-B27 antibodies, and the complex fixes complement. The damaged cells will allow eosin to enter, and appear red under phase contrast microscopy.

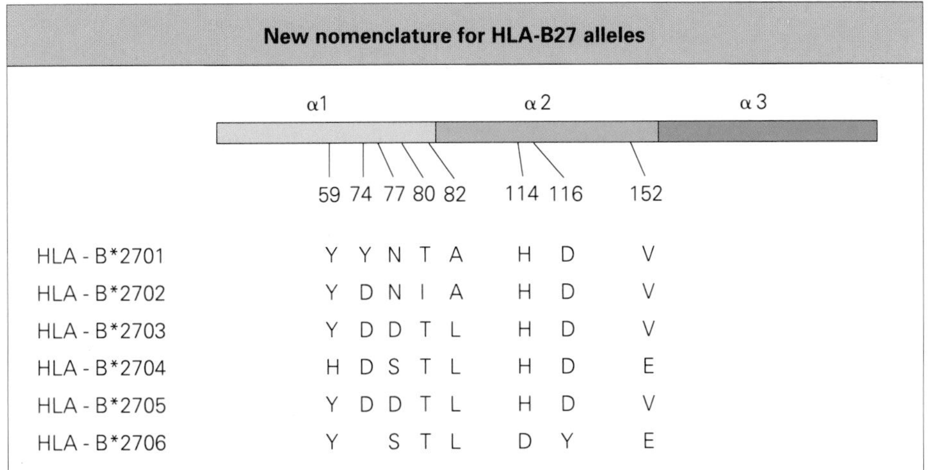

New nomenclature for HLA-B27 alleles
α1
α2
α3
59 74 77 80 82
114 116
152
HLA - B*2701 Y Y N T A H D V
HLA - B*2702 Y D N I A H D V
HLA - B*2703 Y D D T L H D V
HLA - B*2704 H D S T L H D E
HLA - B*2705 Y D D T L H D V
HLA - B*2706 Y S T L D Y E

Fig. 2.6 According to the new nomenclature the gene name is followed by an asterisk, and then a four digit number. The first two numbers describe the most closely associated serological specificity and the other two complete the allelic number.

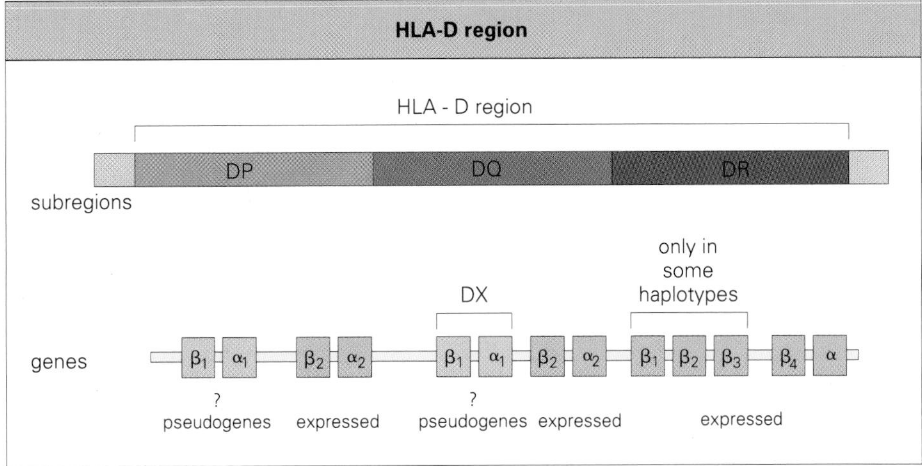

Fig. 2.7 The DP and DQ regions each have two sets of α and β genes, although it is not certain that both sets are expressed. One set of the DQ region is also called DX. The DR region has one α chain and one or more β chains, depending on the haplotype. Several other pseudogenes have been omitted from this diagram for simplicity.

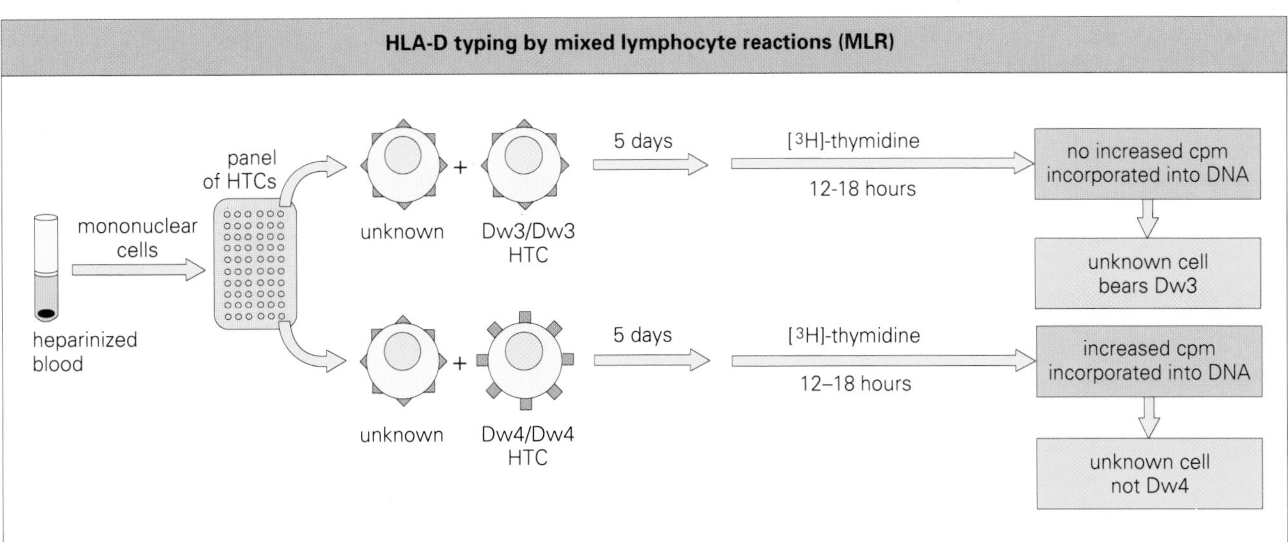

Fig. 2.8 Mononuclear cells (separated by Ficoll-Hypaque gradient centrifugation of heparinized blood) are added to a panel of mitomycin-treated homozygous typing cells (HTCs) and incubated. Cells which recognize an HTC as foreign are stimulated and proliferate; these are detected because of their increased incorporation of [^{3}H]-thymidine. In this case the unknown cell is Dw3 positive, Dw4 negative.

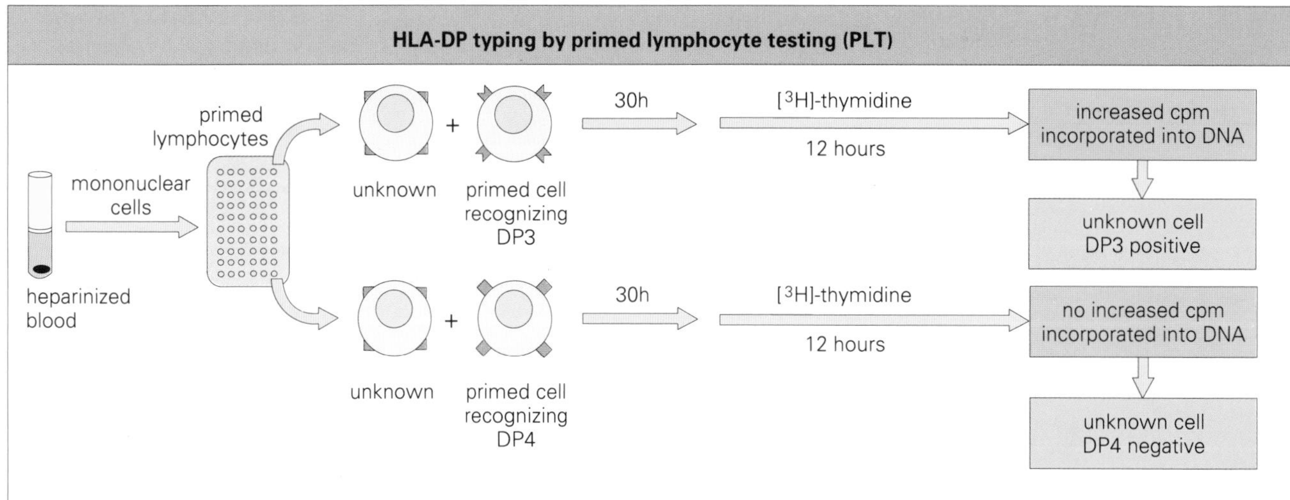

Fig. 2.9 Mononuclear cells (separated by Ficoll-Hypaque gradient centrifugation of heparinized blood) are treated with mitomycin, and tested against a panel of lymphocytes primed to recognize DP antigens. Primed cells which recognize a particular DP specificity on the unknown cell are stimulated and proliferation is detected by increased [^{3}H]-thymidine uptake. This example shows a cell which is DP3 positive, DP4 negative.

be able to induce a subset of potentially cytotoxic $CD4^+$ T cells. If DQ needs to be present on target cells to generate Tc cells, then the selective absence of this antigen on acute myeloid leukaemia cells and certain acute lymphoid leukaemia cells may impair surveillence of these and other malignancies.

HLA-DP determinants. These were originally discovered through primed lymphocyte typing (PLT) (Fig. 2.9). In this technique, T cells from two individuals identical for HLA-DR and HLA-D(Dw) are co-cultured in a mixed lymphocyte culture (MLC). These cells should not recognize each other, but when they differ at HLA-DP, primed DP-specific T cells are generated. These are then detected by their ability to mount a secondary response when restimulated with the same DP haplotype molecules.

Appropriate T cell clones have now been developed which can recognize DP specificities and these are used as typing reagents. Four DP genes have been identified — two α and two β. One α/β pair is definitively expressed but it is still debated whether the genes of the other pair are expressed or are pseudogenes. A monoclonal antibody (B7/21) reacts specifically with DP determinants and blocks proliferation following DP activation. Meanwhile, the search continues for antibodies which recognize the six known HLA-DP alleles, and some progress has been made in identifying them by DNA typing techniques.

HLA-linked complement loci. These also display polymorphism which can be distinguished biochemically using isoelectric focusing gel electrophoresis. There are two distinct genetic loci for C4 (C4A and C4B) with different numbers of allelic forms (Fig. 2.10). Molecular cloning of the region between the complement genes and the HLA-B locus has so far identified at least 19 new genes, including two for the 70 kDa heat shock protein family HSP70 (HSP70-1 and HSP70-2) and genes for the cytokines TNFα and TNFβ (Fig. 2.11). The functions of the additional genes have yet to be identified; although some seem to be expressed in a restricted number of cell lines, the mRNA of most are present in a variety of different cell types.

Common alleles of the HLA-linked complement loci

BF	C2	C4A	C4B
BF*F BF*S BF*F1 BF*S1	C2*C C2*A C2*00	C4A*1 C4A*2 C4A*3 C4A*4 C4A*5 C4A*6 C4A*7 C4A*00	C4B*1 C4B*2 C4B*3 C4B*00

Fig. 2.10 Allelic forms of complement genes.

DNA TYPING TECHNIQUES

Restriction fragment length polymorphism (RFLP)

The conventional way to determine HLA specificities is still based on immunological methods. The cloning of MHC genes allows tissue typing using restriction fragment length polymorphism (RFLP) (Fig. 2.12) to be included in the list of techniques that can be used to further subdivide particular MHC class II molecules. This technique is particularly useful for HLA-DP typing but can also be used

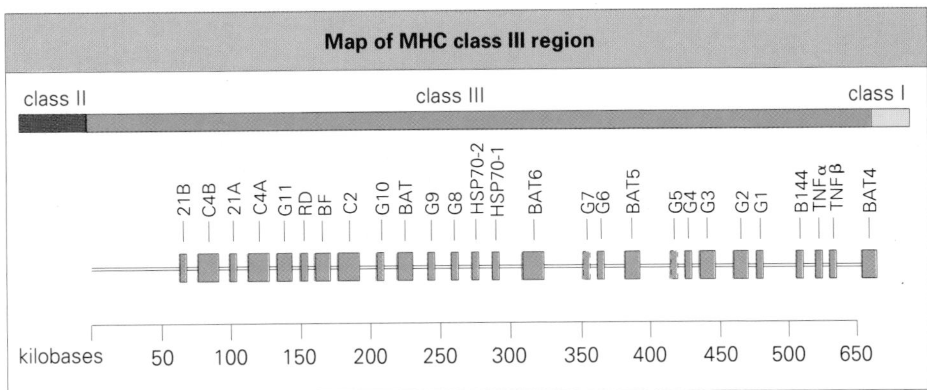

Fig. 2.11 There is no mutually agreed nomenclature of these new genes. Those used in this figure, suggested by Sargent *et al.* (1989) *EMBO J.* **8**, 2305, are most often used. The BAT (HLA-B-associated transcripts) nomenclature is used by Spies *et al.* (1989) *PNAS*, **86**, 8955. G=unknown; B144 is a B cell specific gene of as yet unknown function.

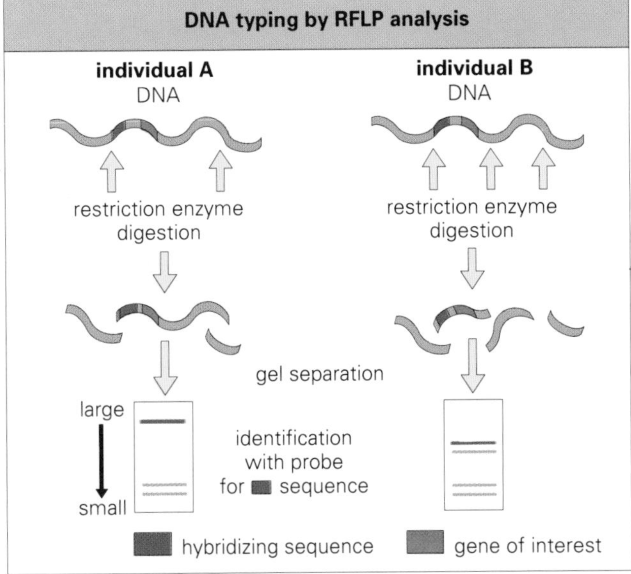

Fig. 2.12 DNA from two individuals containing a particular gene of interest and a sequence which will hybridize to a radioactive probe is digested with a restriction enzyme. A polymorphism in the sequences in A and B means that they have different numbers of restriction enzyme sites. The DNA is separated by size on agarose gels and probed with labelled DNA recognizing the hybridizing sequence. In A this binds to a large fragment, but in B it recognizes a medium-sized fragment. For clarity, only the DNA of the relevant gene segment is shown. In practice this would be one of hundreds of fragments produced by digestion of the entire genome.

for HLA-DR haplotyping because the RFLP patterns are different for each HLA-DR tissue type.

Polymerase chain reaction (PCR)

Recently the polymerase chain reaction (PCR) has been used to analyse and characterize HLA class II subtypes. It is a powerful technique that allows rapid amplification of specific segments of the genome (Fig. 2.13). When combined with DNA sequencing, RFLP analysis or hybridization to oligonucleotides specific for the different alleles, this technique has proved to be extremely useful in the identification of HLA types.

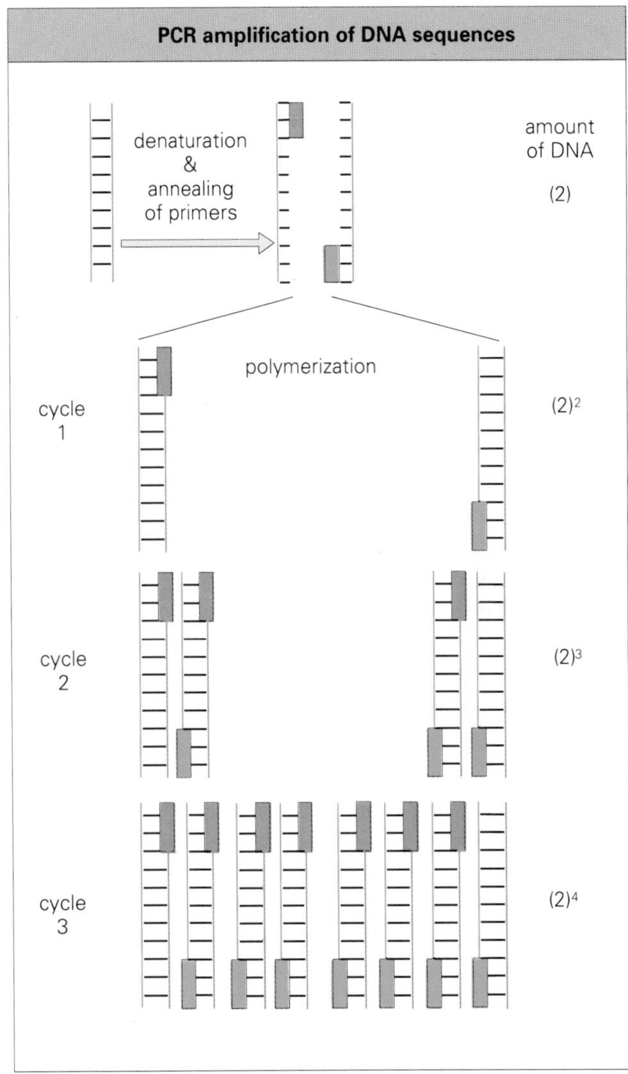

Fig. 2.13 Two synthetic oligonucleotides, unique but complementary to sequences flanking the desired DNA segment, are hybridized to denatured DNA strands and act as primers for DNA-dependent DNA synthesis. The end products are then heat denatured for a new cycle, giving rise to twice as many DNA templates for the DNA synthesis. After repeating the cycle 20–60 times, the desired fragment can be amplified up to 10^{12} times.

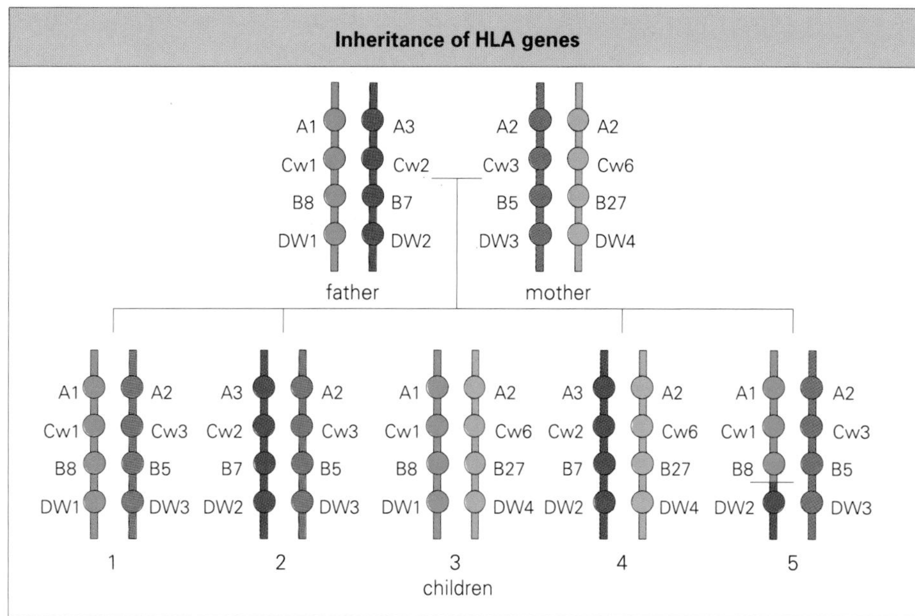

Fig. 2.14 Each member of the family will inherit a paternal and a maternal chromosome, and the MHC genes on both chromosomes will be expressed on the cell surface. Four different combinations of the parental haplotypes can be present in the children, as illustrated for children 1–4. Child 5 has a new haplotype created by a recombination event between HLA-B and HLA-D on the father's chromosome.

HLA-B locus gene frequencies (%)

Allele	European caucasoids (228)	African blacks (102)	Japanese (195)
B5	5.9	3.0	20.9
B7	10.4	7.3	7.1
B8	9.2	7.1	0.2
B12	16.6	12.7	6.5
B13	3.2	1.5	0.8
B14	2.4	3.6	0.5
B18	6.2	2.0	—
B27	4.6	—	0.3
B15	4.8	3.0	9.3
Bw38] Bw16	2.0	—	1.8
Bw39] Bw16	3.5	1.5	4.7
B17	5.7	16.1	0.6
Bw21	2.2	1.5	1.5
Bw22	3.6	—	6.5
Bw35	9.9	7.2	9.4
B37	1.1	—	0.8
B40	8.1	2.0	21.8
Bw41	1.2	1.5	—
Bw42	—	12.3	—
blank	2.4	17.9	7.6

Fig. 2.15 Population differences in HLA haplotypes.

HAPLOTYPES

The MHC region spans only approximately 3000 kilobase pairs (kbp) on chromosome 6, which means that the combination of HLA loci are usually inherited as a unit. The unit on each chromosome is referred to as the haplotype, and these are inherited in a Mendelian manner (Fig. 2.14). The likelihood of a recombination event between the parental chromosomes within the MHC region is dependent on the size of the MHC region and is about 1%.

There is a substantial difference in the frequency of the main alleles at each of the HLA loci, and in some cases considerable variations between different populations (Fig. 2.15). HLA-A2 is present at a relatively high frequency (27%) in all populations, however HLA-A1 and HLA-A3 are present in most ethnic groups but absent in the Japanese. In African blacks, A11 is absent, whereas HLA-Aw43 and -Aw42 are present and seem to be specific for that one ethnic population.

Linkage disequilibrium

Population associations between different HLA loci occur if there is a tendency for these alleles to occur more frequently together on the same chromosome or haplotype than expected by chance. These associations are known as linkage disequilibrium which can be measured quantitatively as the difference (Δ) between the observed and expected frequency (Fig. 2.16). These associations vary in different populations. They are particularly important in helping to evaluate the fine structure of the HLA complex. For example, in Caucasians the HLA-DQw1 antigen is associated with HLA-DR1, -DR2, and -DR6 but not with HLA-DR5, whereas in blacks it is often associated with HLA-DR5, indicating that the HLA-DQ determinants are separated from those of HLA-DR.

HLA AND DISEASE

STATISTICAL CONSIDERATIONS

There are several statistical pitfalls which may arise when trying to relate HLA haplotypes with disease. Thus, many weak associations are suspected because the probability of finding associations solely by chance (1 for every 20 comparisons made at $p = 0.05$) has not been considered. Failure to correct for the number of comparisons has led to several reports of falsely significant associations. The correction is made by multiplying each p value by the number of comparisons made. Hence the correct value for an initial p value of 0.05 when typing for 20 antigens is 1, which is clearly not significant. The method for assessing a disease association is shown in Fig. 2.17.

Relative risk

This is defined as the risk of developing a disease when an antigen is present, relative to the risk when it is lacking. This holds only for diseases with a low frequency in the population. A relative risk higher than 1 is found when the antigen is more frequent in the patients than in the controls (Fig. 2.18), whereas a risk of less than 1 reflects negative association or protection.

Single or multiple studies

Two types of assessment may be undertaken: one relating to a single study in which a negative or positive association between a disease and an HLA molecule has occurred, and the second using data from several studies. In the latter case, the results may be heterogeneous due to

Linkage disequilibrium		
alleles		Δ/1000
A1	B8	57.2
Aw23	B12	17.6
A29	B12	27.6
B12	Cw5	40.2
B15	Cw3	28.3
B27	Cw2	22.6
B7	DRw2	37.6
B8	DRw3	62.3

Fig. 2.16 If the value for Δ/1000 is 0, there is no linkage disequilibrium.

Method of establishing disease association

		HLA haplotype		
		Present	Absent	Total
Disease	+	a	b	$n_3(a+b)$
	—	c	d	$n_4(c+d)$
	Total number	$n_1(a+c)$	$n_2(b+d)$	N

$$\text{relative risk} = \frac{a \times d}{b \times c}$$

$$X_1^2 = \frac{(ad - bc)^2 N}{(n_1)(n_2)(n_3)(n_4)}$$

Fig. 2.17 A contingency table is prepared (top) in which the numbers of people with the disease (n_3) and the numbers with (a) and without (b) the particular haplotype are determined. Likewise for those without the disease (n_4) the number with (c) and without (d) the haplotype is measured. The formula beneath gives the estimate of relative risk, in which RR >1 shows an increased risk and RR <1 a decreased risk. To determine whether this is significant a X^2 value is determined for the appropriate number of degrees of freedom (n-1).

Disease associations with HLA antigens		
Disorders	Antigen	Relative risk
Rheumatological disorders		
rheumatoid arthritis	Dw4	4.2
	DR4	5.8
juvenile rheumatoid arthritis	B27	4.5
ankylosing spondylitis	B27	90.0
reactive arthropathies:		
Reiter's disease	B27	33.0
post-salmonella arthritis	B27	17.6
post-shigella arthritis	B27	20.7
Endocrine disorders		
Graves' disease	B8	2.3
	Dw3	3.6
	DR3	3.5
Hashimoto's disease	DR3	2.6
juvenile onset diabetes	B8	2.6
	DR3	5.7
	DR4	2.8
Neurological disorders		
myasthenia gravis (early onset disease in females)	B8	12.7
multiple sclerosis	B7	1.8
	Dw2	4.05
	DR2	4.8
	Dw3	2.7
Dermatological disorders		
psoriasis vulgaris	B37	6.4
	B17	4.7
	B13	4.7
	Cw6	13.3
dermatitis herpetiformis	B8	8.7
	Dw3	13.5
	DR3	56.4
pemphigus:		
Caucasian	A10	2.8
Japanese	A10	6.0
Renal disorders		
Goodpasture's syndrome	DR2	13.1
Berger's disease	Bw35	2.5
Gastrointestinal & hepatic disorders		
chronic active autoimmune hepatitis	B8	9.0
	DR3	13.9
coeliac disease	B8	8.3
	Dw3	10.9
idiopathic haemochromatosis	A3	8.2
	B7	3.0
	B14	4.7

Fig. 2.18 Relative risk.

different diagnostic criteria and definitions of antigens, as well as true differences in the risk due to genetic or environmental factors. In these circumstances the X^2 test is carried out with n-1 degrees of freedom, where n is the number of separate studies.

HOW HLA MOLECULES INFLUENCE DISEASE

HLA molecules act as receptors for foreign antigens and present them to CD4$^+$ T cells in the case of HLA class II antigens, and CD8$^+$ T cells in the case of MHC class I antigens (Fig. 2.19). There are several ways in which the HLA system can alter the immune response of the organism to microbial invaders, neoplasia and to self:

- quantitative variation in HLA molecules;
- variation in expression of HLA molecules;
- variation in HLA pattern in different populations.

Quantitative variation in HLA molecules

The generation and effector function of Tc cells depends on adequate representation of MHC class I antigens on the activated T cell as well as target tissue. This applies to tumours which have been initiated by oncogenic viruses. For example, cells of Burkitt's lymphoma are not a good target for cells, while EBV-transformed B cells are easily killed. The Burkitt's lines (studied by Georg Klein) seem to require expression of HLA-A11 for T cell cytotoxicity. All the Burkitt's lymphoma lines tested by Klein and his colleagues showed a very low expression of this restriction element.

The oncogenicity of cells infected with adenovirus 12, but not adenovirus 5, is caused by selective switching off of the surface expression of HLA class I genes by gene products of adenovirus 12 (Fig. 2.20). A considerable amount of clinical data concerning the relevance of MHC molecules in human tumours has also been reported. HLA-DQ molecules are also selectively absent from acute myeloid leukaemias and some acute lymphatic leukaemias. The influence of this deletion has not yet been established, but since HLA-DQ is a modulator of the immune response and is important in the generation of killer T cells, the absence of HLA-DQ may facilitate tumour growth.

Variations in expression of HLA molecules

Relevance to infection. Specific HLA class I alleles have been shown to be important in the control of influenza by acting as restriction elements in the elimination of virus-infected cells by cytotoxic T cells. Particular specificities, especially HLA-B27 and HLA-A2 are necessary for the elimination of a specific influenza virus. Subjects with

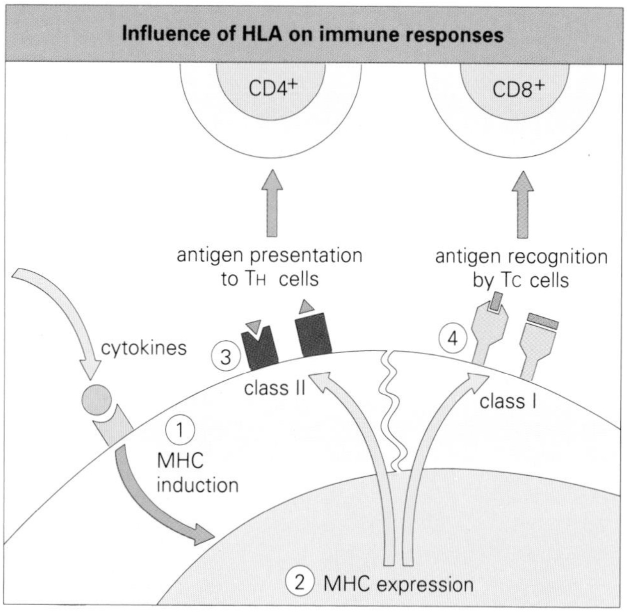

Fig. 2.19 HLA haplotype can influence the immune response in several ways: 1) HLA genes are induced by cytokines and the controlling sequences which determine induction may vary; (2) the static levels of expression on different tissues is genetically determined; 3) MHC molecules of different haplotypes can present antigen in different ways depending on their structure and antigen-binding sites — this will determine how CD4$^+$ cells (predominantly TH) are stimulated; 4) the structure of class I molecules will determine how they interact with and present antigen to CD8$^+$ cells (predominantly Tc).

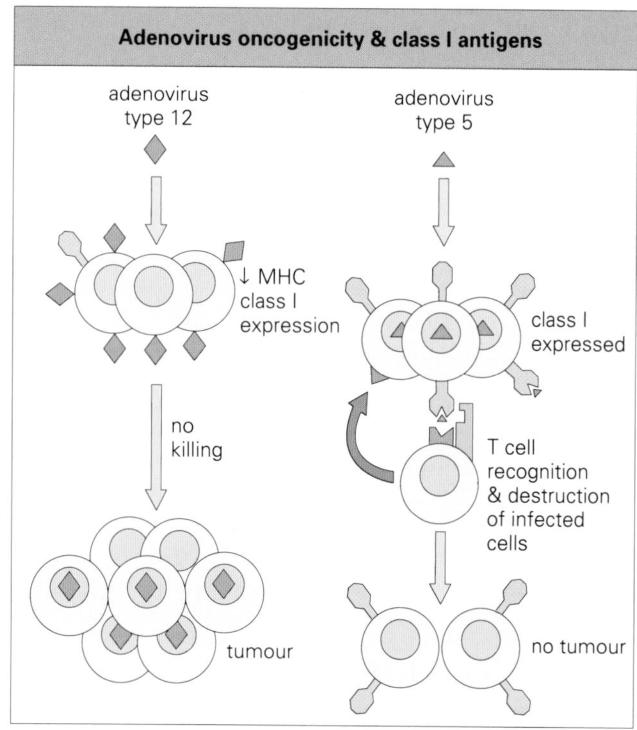

Fig. 2.20 Adenovirus 12 causes decreased expression of HLA class I molecules on the surface of infected cells, which are then not recognized by Tc cells, and cell proliferation results. Adenovirus 5 infection does not affect class I expression, and tumour growth is prevented by T cell recognition and destruction of the infected cells.

these antigens can control the infection whilst those lacking them are unable to do so.

Typhoid. When Dutch immigrants arrived in Surinam, 50% of the immigrant population succumbed to typhoid fever. When the survivors were tissue typed the HLA-B7, DR2 haplotype was significantly reduced, while haplotypes including HLA-DR4, -DR7, -DRw8 and -DRw13 were significantly increased. RFLP analysis of the latter four haplotypes showed a common DRb fragment, suggesting the existence of a relevant common epitope or gene corresponding to this fragment or in disequilibrium with it. The molecule specified by this gene appears to confer resistance to typhoid. The HLA-B7, DR2 haplotype may include a susceptibility factor.

An explanation for these cases may be that the respective HLA antigens contain an amino acid sequence dictating a particular conformation of the antigen binding site, which would either bind the foreign antigen better and thus facilitate a cytotoxic clearing of the infection, or not bind the infectious antigen at all, thus acting as a restriction element.

Population genetics and HLA

Climatic and environmental circumstances determine which micro-organisms are prevalent in particular areas; these changes are especially relevant as one moves north to south and vice versa. Therefore different HLA haplotypes in different environments will help to protect neonatal populations from fatal infectious diseases, and individuals with non-resistant haplotypes will not survive. This could partly explain why there are substantial differences in the HLA pattern in different populations.

Haplotype association with disease. As indicated above, certain haplotypes are associated with susceptibility to disease and others are associated with resistance. The main objective would be to try and identify a particular molecule within the haplotype which is the resistance or susceptibility factor for that disease. In some cases one may be able to identify a particular sequence on the molecule which constitutes the relevant factor. Most investigations in this area have not yet produced a satisfactory answer because the particular component of the haplotype is usually not completely correlated with a particular (for example, MHC class II) specificity. In different populations the correlation with a particular specificity seen in the original population is not found. This could be explained if the particular specificity were in linkage disequilibrium with the relevant molecule which has not yet been identified or if a critical amino acid sequence on the HLA molecule were not yet recognized directly by the allotyping reagents, but became associated by random recombination mechanisms with different HLA specificities in different populations, or even within a population. In the latter case, one would be concerned with those amino acid residues making contact with the processed peptide antigen rather than the T cell receptor, and which did not form part of the structure recognized by alloantibodies or alloreactive T cells used for tissue typing. Possible examples are afforded by the Surinam Dutch immigrants described above, and the heterogeneous association with HLA-DR seen in rheumatoid arthritis patients in different ethnic populations discussed below. The identification of all genes in the MHC region following cloning of the region may provide the answers.

Another possibility is that different components of the haplotypes supplement each other with respect to function. Other possibilities involving apparently partial correlation with HLA specificities could be explained by multiple genes including HLA but also by failure of adequate clonal deletion of autoreactive T cell clones.

Pathogenesis of autoimmune diseases. Two of the multifactorial factors underlying the pathogenesis of autoimmune diseases may be HLA-related. If an infectious agent such as a virus is involved, resistance or susceptibility to this agent may be related to particular MHC alleles. This would explain why, for example, the antigens associated with insulin-dependent diabetes mellitus (IDDM) in Britain (HLA-DR3, -DR4) and in China (HLA-DR9) are different. The same is likely to be true for Graves' disease, multiple sclerosis and other autoimmune diseases. These haplotypes may provide the relevant restriction elements for cytotoxicity and for effective antigen presentation for the elimination of virally-infected cells. Secondly, the presentation to autoreactive T cells of peptides derived from self-proteins, or from proteins associated with the infection which cross-react with self and may 'break tolerance', may be strongly influenced by the polymorphic MHC variant. Furthermore, if it should prove to be the case that there are ethnic variations in the structure of certain autoantigens, this would provide a further factor influencing HLA involvement in different populations.

HLA-(A1,B8,DR3) haplotype in Caucasians

The most frequent extended haplotype in British Caucasians (and in Scandinavian and Dutch) is HLA-(A1, B8, DR3). It is also the most frequently encountered haplotype in many autoimmune diseases including dermatitis herpetiformis, myasthenia gravis, chronic active hepatitis, sicca syndrome and coeliac disease. In addition to being associated with autoimmune diseases, HLA-B8 is also linked with a heightened immune responsiveness or reactivity. For example, HLA-B8 recipients reject kidney allografts more readily than non-HLA-B8 recipients. The HLA-B8 associated hyper-reactive immune response could be controlled by HLA-B8 or by a 'high responder' gene(s) in linkage disequilibrium with HLA-B8. The 'high responder' effect could be due to:

- hyper-reactivity against self, as in autoimmune diseases;
- hyper-reactivity influencing the course of a disease. (HLA-B8 positive patients with Hodgkin's disease or lymphocytic leukaemia have a better prognosis than those negative for HLA-B8);

- hyper-reactivity influencing the survival of allografted tissue;
- heightened reactivity against normal food products, as in gluten enteropathy (coeliac disease);
- heightened reactivity agianst microbially damaged tissue, as in diabetes.

HLA and insulin dependent diabetes mellitus

Caucasians. Insulin dependent diabetes mellitus (IDDM) in Caucasians is strongly associated with HLA-DR3 and -DR4 whereas other HLA-DR specificities, notably HLA-DR2, show a protective association. Haplotypes that share HLA-DR3/DR4 specificities differ considerably with respect to HLA-DQ genes. RFLP analysis and DNA sequencing of the HLA-DQ genes have shown that DQB1 allele DQ3.2*[DQB1*0302]* identifies the IDDM association for these two haplotypes. Further analysis of associations between HLA-DQ genes and IDDM suggests that the amino acid in position 57 of the DQ gene encoded protein may be responsible for the HLA association with IDDM. The presence of aspartic acid in this position has a strong negative association with IDDM, whereas a neutral amino acid (alanine, valine or serine) appears to determine positive or neutral association with the disease (Fig. 2.21). However, recent analysis suggests that neither HLA-DQ nor HLA-DR are individually responsible for maximum susceptibility to IDDM, but that both DR-(HLA-Dw4*[DRB1*0401]* and -Dw10*[DRB1*0402]*) and DQ-(HLA-DQ3.2*[DRB1*0302]*, which is non-asp 57) are needed. This points to the possibility that either the MHC class II genes are responsible for the MHC susceptibility to IDDM or that HLA-(Dw4, Dw10, DQ3.2) are in linkage disequilibrium with a gene yet to be identified which controls the disease predisposition.

Other racial groups show different associations between HLA and IDDM. In blacks, HLA-DR7 is positively associated with IDDM whereas this allele in whites shows neutral association. The HLA-DR7 in blacks is in linkage disequilibrium with the A3*[DQA1*0301]* allele in the DQA1 locus but not with the A2*[DQA1*0201]* allele found in whites, suggesting that A3 may in part determine the susceptibility.

HLA and rheumatoid arthritis

Rheumatoid arthritis (RA) has been strongly associated with HLA-DR4 (Dw4*[DRB1*0401]* and Dw14 *[DRB1*1401/*1402]*) and -DR1 in most Caucasians, including most Europeans, North Americans, Venezuelans and Australians. One exception is in Greeks, in whom there is no HLA-DR antigen association with RA. Non-white RA patients also have a heterogeneous association with HLA-DR; Japanese RA patients have a strong association with HLA-DR4 and HLA-Dw15*[DRB1*1501/1502]*. Whilst North American Blacks have an HLA-DR4 association with RA, Nigerian RA patients do not; this association is also absent in Thai RA patients. So far sequence analysis of HLA-DR genes in the RA susceptible haplotypes suggests that the genes, irrespective of different serological specificities, share the sequences of the third diversity region from amino acid residue 67 to 73. This may suggest that the RA susceptibility is dependent on a particular MHC class II conformation and may result from recognition of a critical processed peptide.

RFLP analysis of the HLA-DQ and HLA-DP regions in RA patients suggests that there is no influence of either HLA-DQ or HLA-DP genes in the susceptibility haplotype.

Association of HLA-DQ$_\beta$ with insulin-dependent diabetes mellitus			
DR	**DQ**	**IDDM association**	**Residue 57**
1	w5	positive	Val
2	w6	negative	Asp
2	w1.12	neutral/negative	Asp
2	w1.AZH	positive	Ser
3	w2	positive	Ala
4	w7	neutral/negative	Asp
4	w8	positive	Ala
5	w7	neutral/negative	Asp
6(w13)	w1.18	neutral/negative	Asp
6(w13)	w1.19	positive	Val
6(w14)	w1.9	neutral/negative	Asp
7	w2	neutral	Ala
8	w4	neutral	Asp
9	w9	neutral	Asp

Fig. 2.21 Association of HLA-DQβ with insulin-dependent diabetes mellitus.

HLA-B27 associated diseases

There is a striking association between ankylosing spondylitis (AS) and HLA-B27, with more than 90% of AS sufferers being HLA-B27 positive. AS is inherited as a Mendelian dominant trait with 70% penetrance in males and 10% in females. However, several factors are probably involved in the pathogenesis of the disease and HLA-B27 may be associated with only one of these. Thus, not all individuals with AS are HLA-B27 positive and only 8% of HLA-B27 males and 1% of females develop the disease. The association with HLA-B27 is stressed by ethnic studies. In American Indians, in whom the incidence of HLA-B27 is very high, the incidence of AS is also very high (10%); in blacks, HLA-B27 is nearly absent, and AS is diagnosed in only a few individuals. Similarly, most Japanese patients suffering from AS are HLA-B27 positive, even though the incidence of this MHC specificity is very low.

Although several allelic forms of HLA-B27 exist (see Fig. 2.6), no studies have so far suggested a preferential association between AS and any of the B27 alleles. Neither RFLP nor DNA sequence analysis have shown any difference between HLA-B27 alleles from AS patients and disease-free normals. Like other HLA-B27 associated disease, AS has an obvious infectious history, with *Klebsiella* infection preceding the arthritis although a causal link is still contentious.

Arthritis following Reiter's syndrome. Reiter's syndrome is a joint disease associated with gonococcal or non-specific urethritis. When urethritis occurs in an individual who is HLA-B27 positive, that person is 40–100 times more likely to develop arthritis than somebody who is B27 negative. Of all patients suffering from acute arthritis following urethritis, 75% are HLA-B27 positive, while 98–99% of persons having urethritis do not develop the rheumatic symptoms of Reiter's disease.

Molecular mimicry. While many people are infected with gonococci, *Shigella, Klebsiella, Yersinia* and other organisms, joint disease occurs with particular frequency in those who are HLA-B27 positive. Sequence analysis of HLA-B27 has identified a cysteine at position 67 in all allelic forms and it has been suggested that this amino acid may establish covalent bonds with antigens and thus form extremely stable complexes with peptides or other molecules found in the antigen binding site. The cysteine is very close to a lysine and an asparagine in positions 70 and 97 respectively, which are not found in other HLA-B sequences, and these three amino acids may form a specific antigen binding site. An alternative mechanism based on antigenic mimicry has been proposed (Fig. 2.22) following the observation that the protein nitrogenase of *Klebsiella pneumoniae* and HLA-B27 share six consecutive amino acid residues. Cross staining and cross absorption studies show substantial similarity between surface antigens of *Klebsiella pneumoniae* and B27.

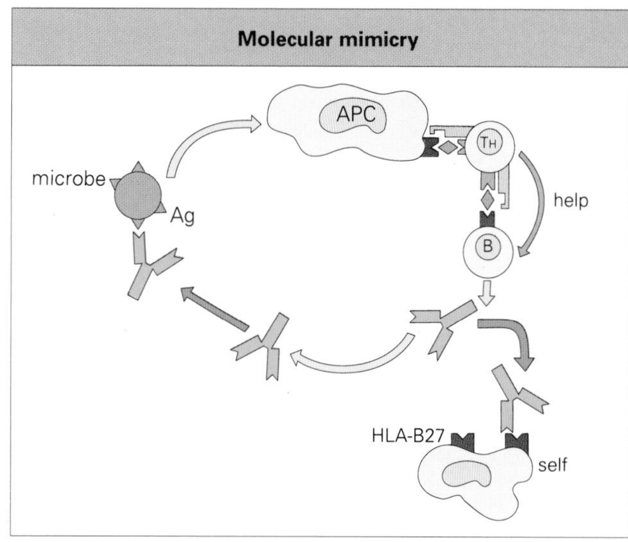

Fig. 2.22 This theory proposes that the micro-organism displays surface antigen which is very similar in structure to a particular HLA molecule (e. g. B27). TH cells recognize processed microbial antigen and stimulate B cells to produce antibodies which react with the intact antigen on the micro-organism, and therefore also bind to the HLA molecule. Alternatively, the TH cells may themselves be effectors which recognize processed B27 on the cell surface.

FURTHER READING

Benjamin R, Parham P. Guilt by association: HLA-B27 and ankylosing spondylitis. *Immunol Today* 1990;**11:**137–142.

Björkman PL, *et al.* The foreign antigen binding site and T-cell recognition regions of class I histocompatibility antigens. *Nature* 1987;**329**:512–518.

Björkman PL *et al.* Structure of the human class I histocompatibility antigens. *Nature* 1987;**329**:506–512.

Bodmer JG, Marsh SGE, Albert E. Nomenclature for factors of the HLA system, 1989. *Immunol Today* 1989;**11**:3–10.

Brown JH *et al.* A hypothetical model of the foreign antigen binding site of class II histocompatibility molecules. *Nature* 1988; **332**:845–850.

Dupont Bo, ed. *Immunobiology of HLA. I: Histocompatibility testing.* Berlin, Heidelberg: Springer-Verlag, 1987.

Thomson G *et al.* Genetic heterogeneity, modes of inheritance and risk estimates for a joint study of caucasians with insulin-dependent diabetes mellitus. *Amer J Hum Genetics* 1988; **43**:799–816.

Zamvil SS, Steinman L. The T lymphocytes in experimental allergic encephalomyelitis. *Ann Rev Immunol* 1990;**8**:579–621.

Recognized HLA specificities

A	B	C	D*	DR	DQ	DP
A1	B5	Cw1	Dw1	DR1	DQw1	DPw1
A2	B7	Cw2	Dw2	DR2	DQw2	DPw2
A3	B8	Cw3	Dw3	DR3	DQw3	DPw3
A9	B12	Cw4	Dw4	DR4	DQw4	DPw4
A10	B13	Cw5	Dw5	DR5	DQw5(w1)	DPw5
A11	B14	Cw6	Dw6	DRw6	DQw6(w1)	DPw6
Aw19	B15	Cw7	Dw7	DR7	DQw7(w3)	
A23(9)	B16	Cw8	Dw8	DRw8	DQw8(w3)	
A24(9)	B17	Cw9(w3)	Dw9	DR9	DQw9(w3)	
A25(10)	B18	Cw10(w3)	Dw10	DRw10		
A26(10)	B21	Cw11	Dw11(w7)	DRw11(5)		
A28	Bw22		Dw12	DRw12(5)		
A29(w19)	B27		Dw13	DRw13(w6)		
A30(w19)	B35		Dw14	DRw14(w6)		
A31(w19)	B37		Dw15	DRw15(2)		
A32(w19)	B38(16)		Dw16	DRw16(2)		
Aw33(w19)	B39(16)		Dw17(w7)	DRw17(3)		
Aw34(10)	B40		Dw18(w6)	DRw18(3)		
Aw36	Bw41		Dw19(w6)			
Aw43	Bw42		Dw20	DRw52		
Aw66(10)	B44(12)		Dw21			
Aw68(28)	B45(12)		Dw22	DRw53		
Aw69(28)	Bw46		Dw23			
Aw74(w19)	Bw47		Dw24			
	Bw48		Dw25			
	B49(21)		Dw26			
	Bw50(21)					
	B51(5)					
	Bw52(5)					
	Bw53					
	Bw54(w22)					
	Bw55(w22)					
	Bw56(w22)					
	Bw57(17)					
	Bw58(17)					
	Bw59					
	Bw60(40)					
	Bw61(40)					
	Bw63(15)					
	Bw64(14)					
	Bw65(14)					
	Bw67					
	Bw70					
	Bw71(w70)					
	Bw72(w70)					
	Bw73					
	Bw75(15)					
	Bw76(15)					
	Bw77(15)					
	Bw4					
	Bw6					

The following specificities are generally agreed inclusions of HLA–B specificities Bw4 and Bw6

Bw4: B5, B13, B17, B27, B37, B38(16), B44(12), Bw47, B49(21), B51(5), Bw52(5), Bw53, Bw57(17), Bw58(17), Bw59, Bw63(15), Bw77(15)

Bw6: B7, B8, B14, B18, Bw22, B35, B39(16), B40, Bw41, Bw42, B45(12), Bw46, Bw48, Bw50(21), Bw54(w22), Bw55(w22), Bw56(w22), Bw60(40) Bw64(14), Bw67, Bw70, Bw71(w70), Bw73, Bw75(15), Bw76(15)

The following specificities are generally agreed to be associated with DRw52 and DRw53:

DRw52: DR3, DR5, DRw6, DRw8, DRw11(5), DRw12(5), DRw13(w6), DRw14(w6), DRw17(3), DRw18(3),

DRw53: DR4, DR7, DR9

* T cell defined

Appendix 2.1 Courtesy of Bodmer W F *et al.* (1987) Nomenclature for factors of the HLA system. In: Dupont B (Ed.) *Immunobiology of HLA* (Volume I) New York: Springer–Verlag; 1989.

3

Transplantation

INTRODUCTION

Fifty years have elapsed since the first transplantation antigen was discovered in inbred mice, and its effect was demonstrated on the survival of an incompatible tumour graft. Since then transplantation biology has grown into an enormous subject, particularly because of its successful clinical applications. Only those types of allograft which have reached a high level of success will be discussed. An understanding of the principles of the human major histocompatibility complex (MHC), the human leucocyte antigen (HLA) system, is useful and can be found in chapter 2.

KIDNEY TRANSPLANTATION

Renal transplantation is employed for end-stage renal disease, irrespective of cause. Although factors such as age and general condition limit the number of suitable patients, and the availability of donors and medical facilities limit the number of operations, approximately 21,000 kidney grafts were performed in 1986.

The main immunological factors affecting the survival of kidney allografts are listed in Fig. 3.1.

GENETIC SIMILARITY OF DONOR AND RECIPIENT

Living related donors

Live donors are normally first degree blood relatives, and very occasionally will be the identical twin of the recipient. In the latter circumstance the donor tissue is compatible at all histocompatibility loci. More often however, the donor is a parent or sibling whose tissues are partially compatible with those of the prospective recipient. Before considering any immunological aspects, the transplant team will obviously restrict their choice of potential donors to those who are in good health, and are suitable on ethical and medical grounds.

From the immunological standpoint, the first question to consider is whether the potential donor is compatible for the ABO blood group system, as there is a high risk of hyperacute graft rejection of ABO-incompatible kidneys. The number of HLA haplotypes shared by any prospective donor and the recipient must then be ascertained. Graft survival rates of more than 90% are obtainable at 1 year if the donor and recipient are HLA-identical siblings. If only one haplotype is shared, graft survival rates of approximately 85% are expected. Most transplant teams working in areas with an active cadaveric donor programme would avoid using a living related donor who did not share at least one haplotype. However, in areas where such programmes are not well developed, some teams have concluded that graft survival figures of more than 80% at one year can be obtained, provided the management of rejection episodes is aggressively implemented.

Cadaveric donors

It is obviously desirable to avoid using a living donor, if a satisfactory graft can be obtained from a cadaver. However, because of the great polymorphism of the HLA system and the fact that cadaveric donors are not related to the recipient, there is little likelihood of any random donor and recipient matching for HLA. Therefore a variety of co-operative agencies (national and international) have been formed, which ensure that prospective recipients and potential cadaver donors are HLA typed; cadaver kidneys are then offered to the recipients who are the closest HLA match and compatible for ABO.

HLA matching

The main barrier to successful transplantation is the recipient's immune response against the antigens of the MHC expressed in the allograft. Responses against minor system antigens are much weaker, and are readily controlled by

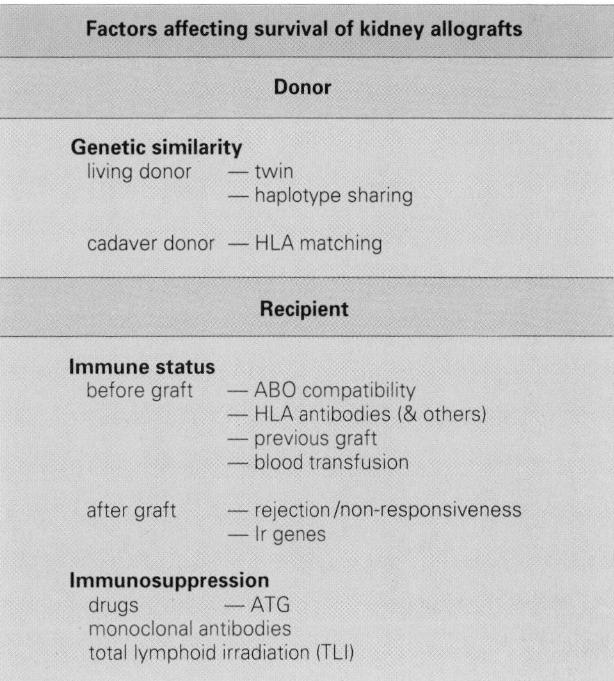
Factors affecting survival of kidney allografts

Donor

Genetic similarity
living donor — twin
— haplotype sharing

cadaver donor — HLA matching

Recipient

Immune status
before graft — ABO compatibility
— HLA antibodies (& others)
— previous graft
— blood transfusion

after graft — rejection/non-responsiveness
— Ir genes

Immunosuppression
drugs — ATG
monoclonal antibodies
total lymphoid irradiation (TLI)

Fig. 3.1 Immunological factors affecting kidney allograft survival.

immunosuppression. When kidney allografting became a clinical procedure, it was assumed by many that unless donor and recipient matched for HLA, the graft would inexorably be rejected, even in the face of immunosuppressive treatment. This expectation proved to be wrong, and many kidney transplants documented as HLA incompatible have functioned satisfactorily for prolonged periods. This experience has led to a long and continuing debate on the value of HLA matching in cadaveric kidney transplantation.

Mismatched transplants. Numerous studies have been directed at resolving this question. Most of the early ones are difficult to evaluate because the HLA system was so incompletely explored. Even now there is much biochemical and cellular immunological data which show that HLA polymorphism is greater than that recognized by conventional serological methods currently in use. Despite this, however, there is strong evidence that HLA matching has a statistically significant beneficial effect on the survival of cadaveric kidney grafts. The largest body of data (10,866 cadaveric first grafts performed at 239 participating centres) has been collected and analysed by Opelz and colleagues. The data showed that matching for HLA-B and -DR antigens leads to a statistically significant improvement in graft survival (Fig. 3.2); it is important to note that this cohort of patients had been immunosuppressed with cyclosporin. Matching for HLA-A did not produce any significant further gain.

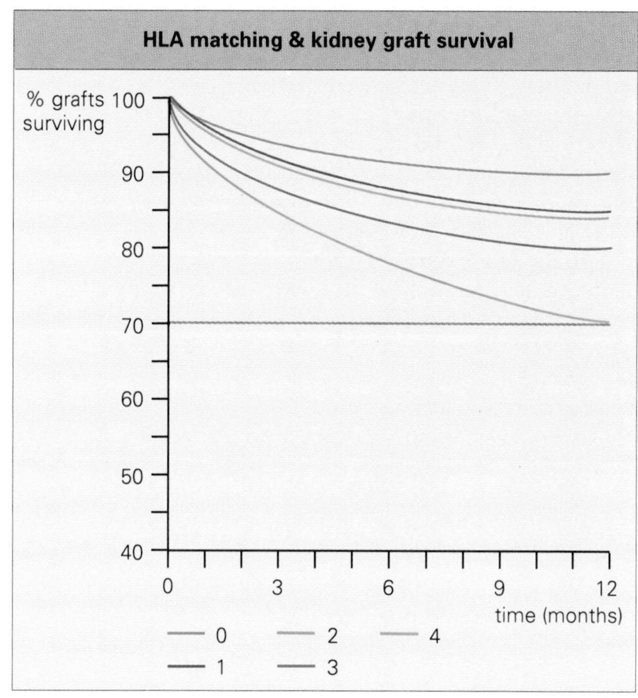

Fig. 3.2 The effect of matching for HLA-B plus DR in cadaver kidney transplant patients treated with cyclosporin. The curves show survival rates of grafts incompatible for 0 to 4 HLA-B plus DR antigens. Modified from Opelz, G (1987).

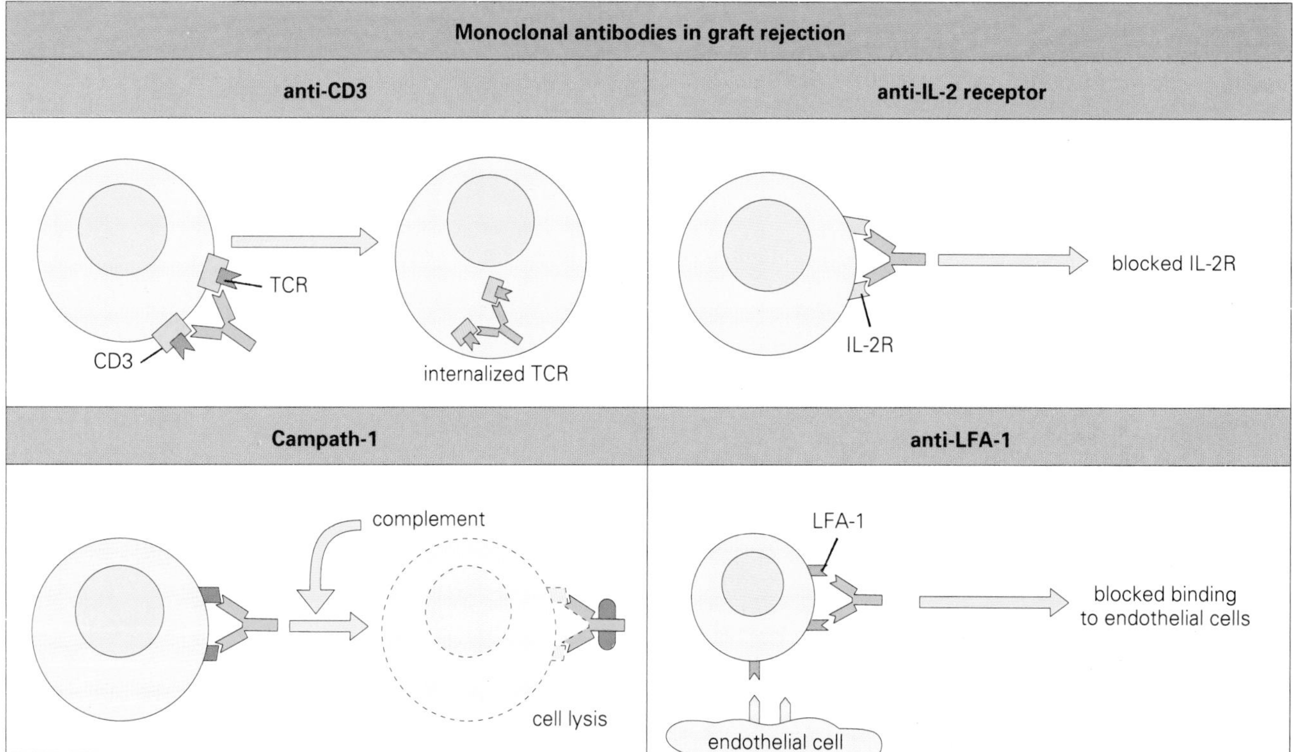

3.2 **Fig. 3.3** Some examples of monoclonal antibodies used to prevent graft rejection.

Benefits of matching. Although this evidence shows that significant benefits can be obtained by matching for HLA, the difference in graft survival rates between the worst and best matched groups is just less than 20% at one year; 88% of grafts with no mismatched HLA-B and -DR antigens were functioning then, compared with 71% of those with four mismatched antigens. What remains to be determined is the amount of benefit after a longer follow-up period, not only in the crude terms of graft survival, but also in the frequency of toxic complications of immunosuppression.

It is clear that the deleterious effect of HLA incompatibility can, to some extent, be avoided by skilfully managed immunosuppression, and it is also true that immunosuppressive regimens are undergoing changes. However, it does seem sensible to maintain a policy of HLA matching donor and recipient whenever feasible.

IMMUNOSUPPRESSIVE REGIMEN

Immunosuppression is discussed in more detail in chapter 27.

Chemical suppression

The search for an optimum drug regimen continues, with most centres using cyclosporin as one component in their regimen. There is no doubt that the introduction of this drug is one of the factors responsible for the improved results of kidney transplantation seen in the 1980s. Early experience using high dose levels suggested that cyclosporin was dangerous when used with other immunosuppressive drugs. However, with lower doses, multiple therapy regimens (combinations of cyclosporin, azathioprine, steroids, and anti-thymocyte globulin) can be safe and extremely effective.

Antibody-mediated suppression

Anti-thymocyte globulin (ATG), employed by some centres, is chiefly used for treatment of acute rejection episodes. Different preparations vary in their efficacy but some are undoubtedly useful. Patients should be skin tested for hypersensitivity to the foreign horse or rabbit protein beforehand, and sensitive patients should not be treated with ATG.

Monoclonal antibodies against T lymphocytes, or subpopulations of T cells thought to be involved in graft rejection are being investigated (Fig. 3.3). At present it is too early to reach firm conclusions about their clinical value. Two types of treatment schedules have usually been tried. In the 'prophylactic' schedule, the monoclonal antibody is given for 2–3 weeks, starting at the time of transplantation. The alternative protocol is one in which the monoclonal antibody is given to treat rejection episodes. Anti-CD3, which *in vitro* causes cross-linking of the CD3 complex and subsequent internalization of both the CD3 complex and the T cell antigen receptor (TCR), has been found to have a significant effect when used for treating acute rejection episodes, but is of no benefit when used in a 'prophylactic' schedule.

Recently, promising clinical results have been found in transplant patients treated with a monoclonal antibody against the IL-2 receptor, an antibody which has the theoretical advantage of binding with high affinity to activated T cells. Other antibodies under investigation make use of different strategies. Campath-1, a rat monoclonal antibody against peripheral lymphocytes, fixes human complement and lyses its target cells *in vivo*; anti-LFA-1 can block intercellular adherence and lymphocyte adhesion to vascular endothelium; toxin conjugated monoclonal antibodies kill only the cells to which they bind.

Systematic clinical trials are needed to evaluate these monoclonal antibodies. Their major drawback is that the foreign immunoglobulin provokes an antibody response which can not only give rise to hypersensitivity reactions, including serum sickness, but also accelerates elimination of the monoclonal antibody, thus reducing its therapeutic activity. This may be overcome by the use of hybrid monoclonals which consist of a foreign (usually mouse) Fab portion with a human Fc portion (see chapter 20).

Total lymphoid irradiation (TLI)

This is a method of X-irradiation originally developed for treatment of Hodgkin's disease, in which repeated small doses of X-rays are delivered to an inverted Y area (Fig. 3.4). It induces a profound and long-lasting immunosuppression with minimum side-effects. It has been successful as a form of immunosuppression for kidney allografting, but at present remains less widely used than drug therapy.

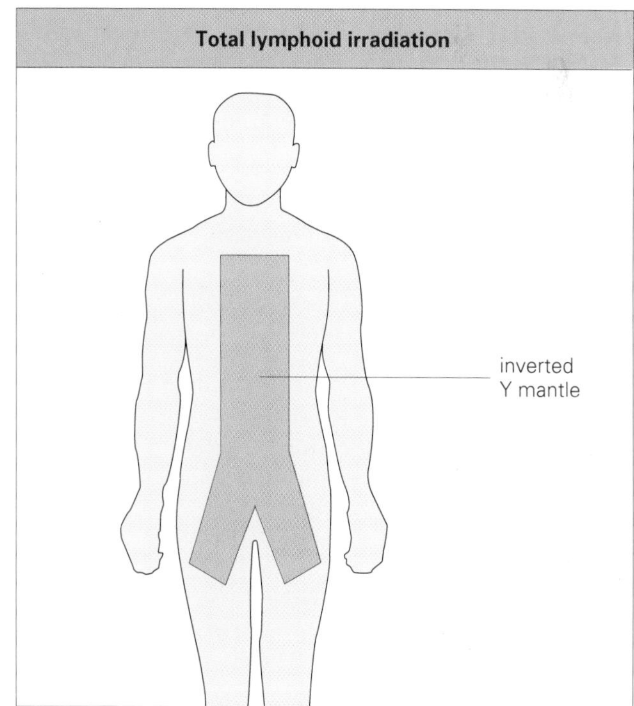

Fig. 3.4 Total lymphoid irradiation. Radiation is administered to an area shaped like an inverted Y, which includes the mediastinal, paravertebral and inguinal lymph nodes.

IMMUNOLOGICAL STATUS OF RECIPIENT

The ABO blood group system

Most centres have always followed the rules of blood transfusion, avoiding an ABO system incompatibility because early studies showed that transgressing an ABO barrier could lead to immediate graft failure. It is posssible to avoid graft failure, at least in some cases, by strenuous plasma exchange (see chapter 29), but there is little information on long term results.

The HLA system

Whether or not a patient is already sensitized against the HLA antigens present on a kidney at the time of its transplantation is a critical factor affecting graft survival. There is no generally agreed method available for measuring pre-existing cellular immunity so the level of sensitization is inferred, partly from the previous transplantation history of a patient, and partly from the results of screening the patient's serum for antibodies.

Lymphocytotoxic antibodies. All transplant units screen their prospective recipients' sera for antibodies approximately every three months. If a lymphocytotoxic antibody is found, attempts are made to identify its specificity. Four types of reactivity have been described (Fig. 3.5). Very frequently, the patient's serum contains mixtures of the various antibodies and the analysis becomes difficult.

*Antibodies against class I.*If a patient with antibodies against class I HLA antigens receives a kidney transplant expressing those same antigens, there is a high risk of hyperacute graft rejection (HR) (Fig. 3.6). Thus, serum screening warns the transplant team which patients are at risk. In addition, all sera of prospective recipients are cross matched with the lymphocytes of a donor before a transplant operation, to ensure by direct testing that a recipient does not have antibodies against the donor's HLA class I antigens. If a positive result is obtained, the transplant should not proceed and an alternative recipient should be selected. However, anti-class I antibody titres may decline over a period of time. It has been shown that if the current serum sample gives a negative cross match, but a previous sample is positive with the lymphocytes of a prospective donor, transplantation can be performed without incurring the risk of HR or early graft failure. Further experience is required to determine whether this unexpected observation is true in all circumstances. With a second graft, many transplant units still prefer to avoid the antigenic incompatibility that was involved in a first graft which subsequently suffered rejection.

Antibodies against class II. Although antibodies against HLA class II antigens do not appear to cause HR, their presence suggests that a patient may have been previously immunized by blood transfusion, an earlier graft, or a pregnancy, and may be at risk of accelerated rejection. Transplant units vary in their policy when faced with this problem, some proceeding with the transplant, while others do not.

Lymphocyte autoantibodies. The presence of these autoantibodies is suspected when the serum reacts with most or all of the lymphocyte panel used in the screening exercise. The antibody is usually IgM, and can be absorbed by cell lines such as K562, which do not express HLA. The critical test is to determine whether the serum is cytotoxic for the patient's own lymphocytes *in vitro* with rabbit complement. Presumably the autoantibody has low affinity for autologous lymphocytes *in vivo,* otherwise it

Antibodies & kidney grafts			
Antigen system	**Antibody presence**	**Effect of antibody on graft**	**Clinical policy**
ABO	naturally occurring	immediate rejection	ensure ABO compatibility
HLA	result of previous graft, transfusion, or pregnancy	class I: hyperacute or accelerated rejection	positive cross match of serum with donor lymphocytes absolute contraindication for graft
		class II: not associated with hyperacute rejection	screen sera & distinguish from other antibodies
autoantigens on T & B cells	found after virus infections & in SLE	no damaging effects	not a contraindication for grafting; distinguish from other antibodies
monocyte/ endothelial cell antigens	found after previous grafts	associated with hyperacute rejection	antibodies not well defined; not routinely screened

Fig. 3.5 Antibodies may be specific for HLA class I or II antigens, or they may react with an undefined autoantigen (present on B and T lymphocytes). Alternatively, they may react with a partially characterized system of polymorphic antigens present on monocytes and endothelial cells.

would be difficult to explain a positive result in this test. It is important to distinguish this autoantibody from alloantibodies since it is not associated with HR. Thus if no other antibody is present, a positive crossmatch test due to anti-lymphocyte autoantibody is not a contraindication to transplantation.

Monocyte and endothelial cell antibodies. Less is known about the antibody which reacts with monocytes and endothelial cells. It has been reported as a poor prognostic sign if found during an episode of graft rejection. However, virtually all examples have been found in sera which also contain HLA antibodies, and it is therefore uncertain which clinical effects are caused by anti-monocyte and endothelial cell antibodies.

Blood transfusion

Severe anaemia is common in end-stage renal disease and, until the recent introduction of recombinant erythropoietin therapy, was either endured by the patient or treated by transfusions. At one time, it was assumed that transfusion should be avoided for fear of inducing HLA antibodies, thereby jeopardizing the success of any subsequent transplant. However, both experimental and clinical experience have shown that blood transfusions may alter the host's cellular response so that there is a marked reduction in the rejection process. Unfortunately the mechanisms of this effect are only partially understood. Thus the optimum transfusion protocol — one that induces a diminished rejection response without provoking synthesis of HLA antibodies which cause hyperacute rejection — remains uncertain.

The multi-centre study of Opelz showed that the highest graft survival rates occurred in patients given 6–10 units of blood before transplantation; however 2–5 units also produced a significant benefit (Fig. 3.7). In the most recent follow-up of this study, there appears to be a decreasing beneficial influence of blood transfusion, the reason for which is unknown. It is therefore necessary to reserve judgement on the place of blood transfusion in pre-transplant practice at present.

Second and subsequent kidney grafts

Patients who have already lost a first graft can be successfully re-transplanted, but the fate of the second graft depends on the state of immunity induced by the first graft. If the first graft is rejected during the first six months after transplantation, there is a higher risk of failure of the

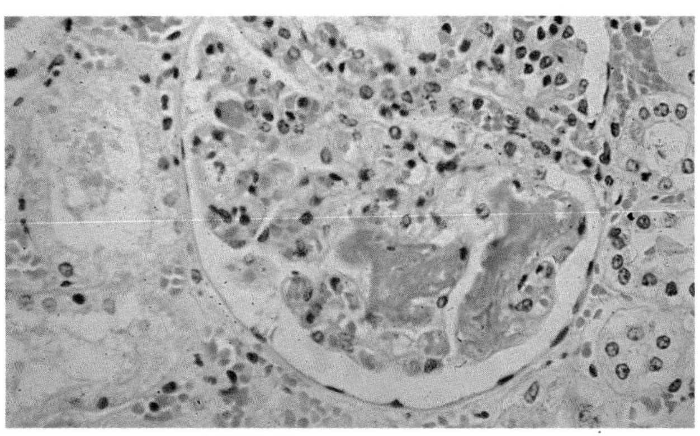

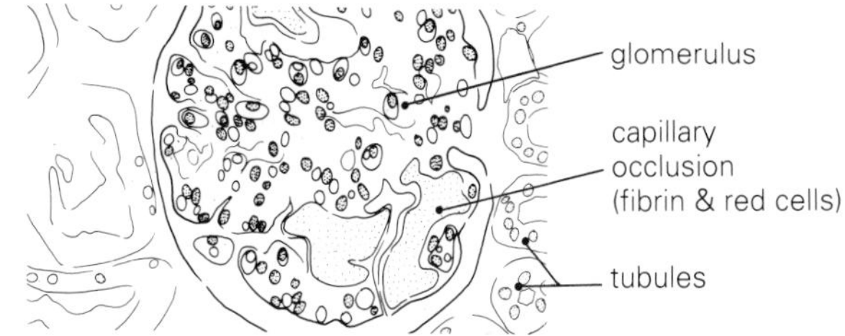

Fig. 3.6 Hyperacute graft rejection, showing characteristic histological appearance of glomerular capillary thrombosis. Courtesy of Professors M R Garavoy, F Vincenti, W J C Amend & N J Feduska.

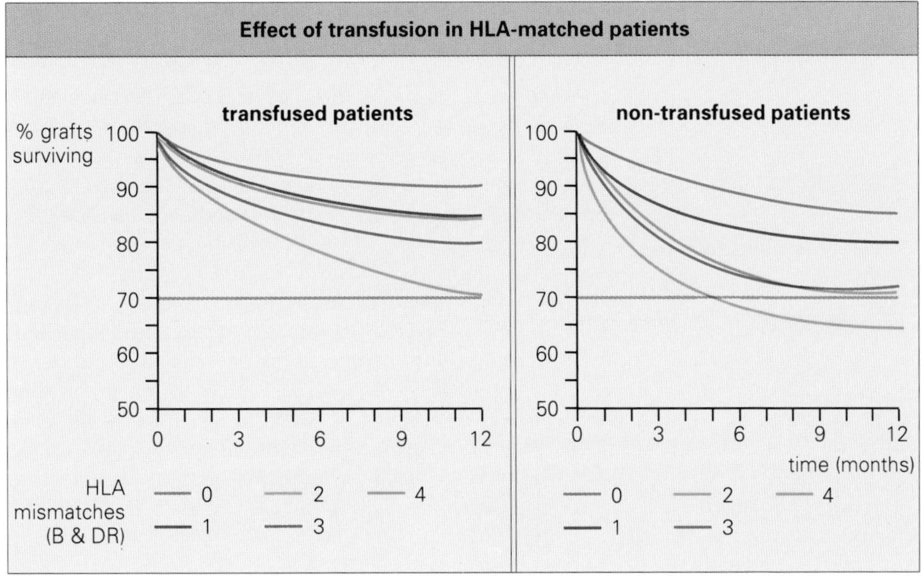

Fig. 3.7 Patients given blood transfusion prior to transplantation (left) showed better graft survival rates than those who were not transfused (right). Modified from Opelz, G (1987).

Monitoring renal allograft rejection
clinical signs — fever, malaise, hypertension
biochemical tests of renal function
presence of HLA antibodies in serum
proliferation and/or cytotoxicity of patient's lymphocytes after donor cell stimulation
histology — mononuclear cell infiltration
immunohistology — ↑class II antigens on renal cortical cells

Fig. 3.8 Proliferation/cytotoxicity of the patient's lymphocytes may be stimulated by cells from the donor using third party cells as controls.

Appearance of antibodies & graft survival				
No. of patients	**Antibodies present**		**Graft survival (%)**	
	before transplant	**after transplant**	**1 year**	**5 years**
5	+	–	100	100
171	–	–	81	76
27	+	+	70	67
63	–	+	48	12

Fig. 3.9 The disappearance of antibodies after transplantation is associated with an excellent prognosis, but the appearance of antibodies for the first time after transplantation correlates with a very high failure rate. Modified from Martin *et al.* (1987).

second graft than if the first graft functioned for longer than six months. A frequent consequence of loss of a first graft through rejection is the development of widely reactive HLA antibodies. This limits the number of potential donors whose cells will give a negative result when tested in the direct cross match with the recipient's serum. In difficult cases, the wide reactivity of a serum prevents the patient from receiving anything other than a very well matched kidney.

The management of highly sensitized patients with widely reactive HLA antibodies is one of the most intractable clinical problems confronting transplant units. The majority of such patients are those in whom the first graft has been rejected, and only a minority have been sensitized entirely by multiple blood transfusions. One strategy, as yet of uncertain value, is multiple plasma exchange combined with immunosuppression in an attempt to remove the antibodies and to prevent their resynthesis (see chapter 29). However, this approach cannot be used for large numbers of patients and most are doomed to remain on dialysis.

IMMUNE STATUS OF RECIPIENT AFTER TRANSPLANTATION

After transplantation, two immunological processes start to occur:

- the rejection response, which, if unchecked, can lead to graft destruction;
- the development of non-responsiveness to the allograft.

Rejection response

Rejection responses vary in strength between different patients, and the primary clinical task after transplantation is to manage the immunosuppression, which should protect the graft without endangering the patient's life by infections or other causes. Usually, rejection is diagnosed because of deterioration of graft function and systemic signs (Fig. 3.8). Early diagnosis of rejection and its management by judicious increase of immunosuppression requires skill and experience. It would obviously be useful if a patient's immune function could be monitored by *in vitro* tests. Most of the early methods measuring the activity of the patient's T cells are too time consuming. However, very recently the fluctuations in soluble IL-2 receptor levels have been found to correlate with episodes of rejection and infection. Clinical and biochemical features still remain an important guide to graft function.

Immune response. The presence of HLA antibodies, and when they appear or disappear can provide some prognostic guidance (Fig. 3.9). Monitoring the proliferative or cytotoxic properties of a patient's lymphocytes after stimulation with cells from the graft donor or third party controls can provide interesting data, but the techniques are too slow and complex for routine use.

Histological assessment of mononuclear cell infiltration in biopsy material is useful, but variation in infiltration in different parts of the same kidney, and the effects of nephrotoxic drugs can make interpretation difficult. Immunohistological studies on the specific sub-populations of T cells detected with anti-CD4 or -CD8 monoclonal antibodies, either in the graft or in blood, have not provided reliable indices of rejection.

Expression of HLA molecules. Rejection can be indirectly assessed by visualizing the level of expression of HLA molecules using monoclonal antibodies specific for the non-variant epitopes present on class I or II antigens. In a normal kidney, HLA class II molecules are detectable on mononuclear cells within blood vessels, on some vascular endothelium, and on interstitial macrophages and dendritic cells, but not on renal tubular cells. Class I molecules are expressed by all nucleated cells of the kidney. During the course of an immune response, activated mononuclear cells secrete IFNγ and other cytokines which induce the increased expression of both class I and II molecules. Under these circumstances, class II molecules can be detected on many renal cortical tubular cells. This feature has been used as a marker for rejection responses but it should be interpreted with caution for the following reasons:

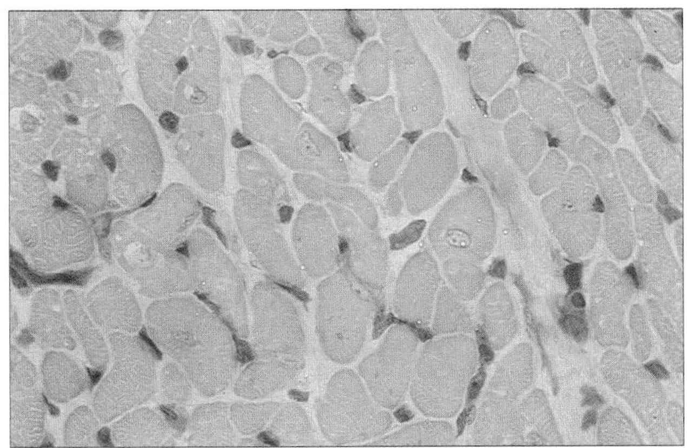

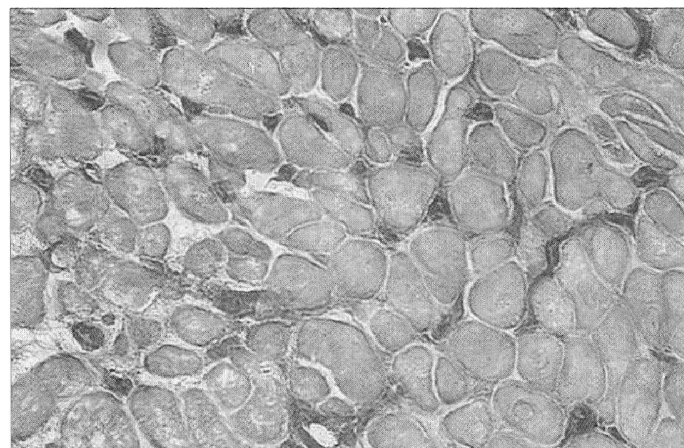

Fig. 3.10 HLA class I expression in myocardium. Left: normal myocardium from the donor heart shows minimal class I expression. Right: class I expression is greatly increased in the myocardium during rejection. In both cases, 6mm cryostat sections were labelled with monoclonal antibody w6132 (directed against class I), stained with peroxidase and counterstained with H & E. Courtesy of Dr M Rose.

- the rate at which class II expression disappears after successful treatment of a rejection episode varies in individual patients, and if there is a previous history of rejection, it may not be clear whether the induced expression is a recent or old event;
- the possible influence of infection must also be considered;
- studies in animal models suggest that induced expression of class II antigens occurs even in recipients who develop non-responsiveness to a kidney allograft.

Specific immune unresponsiveness

The induction of specific unresponsiveness to allografts still represents the most outstanding challenge to our understanding of a recipient's immune response. There is ample evidence with vascularized organ allografts of experimental animals that unresponsiveness develops in a cumulative manner after transplantation, provided that destruction of the allograft is prevented by immunosuppressive drugs or other means. The reasons for this are not entirely clear, but include the fact that the graft becomes less immunogenic because of the loss of its passenger leucocytes, of which the dendritic cells appear to be the most powerful stimulus. Furthermore, specific suppressor T lymphocytes are induced; how these cells prevent graft destruction remains unknown. It is of course unproven that the same immunological phenomenon occurs in successful human kidney transplants, but it is difficult to explain in any other way the well known clinical observation that the frequency of rejection episodes is highest during the first 3–6 months after transplantation and falls afterwards. The requirements for immunosuppression follow the same pattern, and in rare instances patients have stopped immunosuppressive therapy entirely without subsequent rejection of the graft.

It is also clear from experiments on rats that immune responses to allogeneic tissues are under the control of MHC region immune response genes; it seems probable that the same principle also applies to human grafts. Unfortunately there is no method currently available which allows us to predict the strength of immune responsiveness in any given donor-recipient combination.

HEART TRANSPLANTATION

Heart and heart-lung allotransplantation in centres with experience has reached the position where graft survival is now approximately 80% at one year. There are numerous non-immunological reasons for this considerable achievement, but improved immunosuppression with cyclosporin is one of the more important immunological factors. Because no artificial support system is available to maintain the circulation beyond a few hours, early diagnosis of rejection and institution of appropriate therapy is vital. If rejection is suspected on clinical grounds and the appearance of electrocardiographic changes, confirmation of the diagnosis can be made by immunohistological studies of endomyocardial biopsy. This shows a characteristic increase in HLA class I expression (Fig. 3.10), which is synthesized and expressed by myocardial cells at an early stage of rejection. Oedema, the appearance of infiltrating mononuclear cells, and induced expression of HLA class II antigen occur later.

HLA MATCHING BEFORE TRANSPLANTATION

Recent studies have shown that matching of donor and recipient for HLA-DR has a significant beneficial influence on graft survival in cardiac transplantation. However, without an artificial heart capable of supporting a patient for at least several weeks, there is little or no opportunity to delay the transplant until a well matched donor organ becomes available. At present, HLA antibodies in the serum of a patient at the time of cardiac transplantation is not thought to be a contraindication to grafting.

LIVER TRANSPLANTATION

Like heart and heart-lung transplantation, the results of liver transplantation have also improved markedly during the past 8–10 years. This is partly due to the solution of the many formidable surgical and physiological problems associated with the operation. In addition, the more effective immunosuppression achieved with cyclosporin after transplantation has played a significant part. One year graft survival rates of over 70% are currently reported by many centres.

IMMUNOGENICITY OF LIVER

The liver is of particular interest because it is less immunogenic than other organ allografts. One effect of this phenomenon is a great variation in the fate of liver grafts in experimental animals not treated with immunosuppressive drugs. This work on animal models has shown that some donor-recipient combinations suffer acute graft rejection, some have chronic rejection, but others accept the liver allografts indefinitely, merely sustaining a transient rejection response.

The cause of the feeble immunogenicity of the liver and its tendency to be accepted is not understood. As mentioned earlier, the strength of alloimmune responses in experimental animals is controlled by MHC genes, which presumably also exert a significant effect in human liver allografting. Certainly some grafts do undergo acute rejection despite immunosuppressive therapy.

HLA MATCHING BEFORE TRANSPLANTATION

Matching donor and recipient for HLA is an impracticable strategy, given the clinical circumstances of liver allografting and the lack of an artificial liver support system. Furthermore, there is no evidence that matching is beneficial.

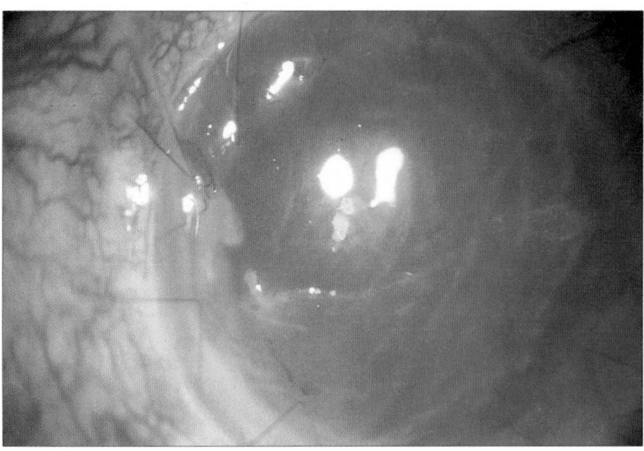

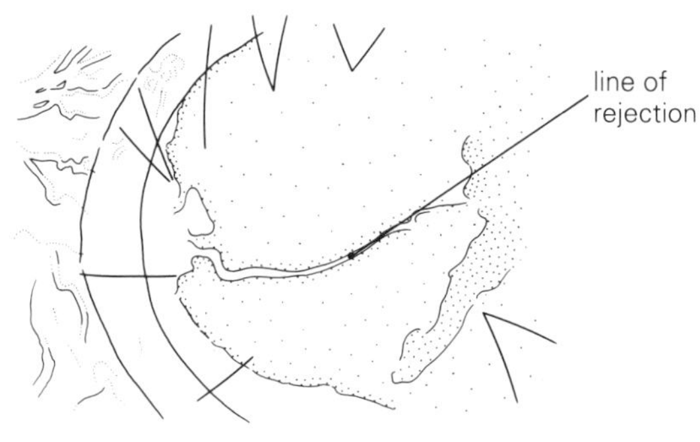

Fig. 3.11 Epithelial rejection of corneal graft. Note the wavy rejection line running almost horizontally. Courtesy of Mr T A Casey.

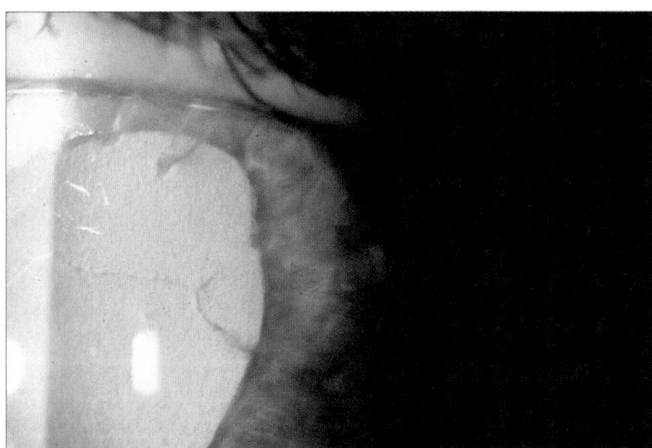

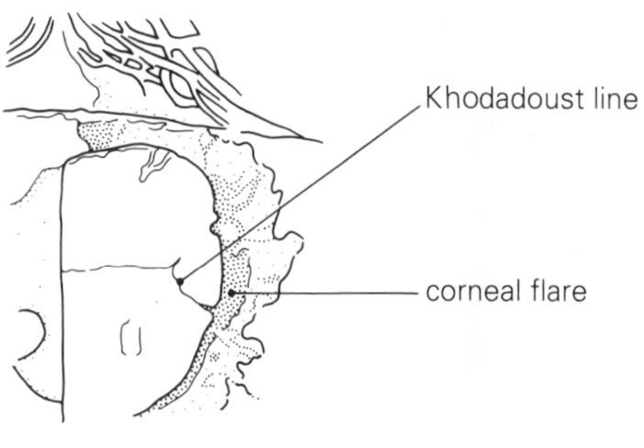

Fig. 3.12 Early rejection of corneal endothelium seen by slit lamp microscopy. Note the corneal 'flare' and Khodadoust line. Courtesy of Mr T A Casey.

Unlike kidney grafts, a positive cross-match of the patient's serum with donor lymphocytes (due to the presence of anti-HLA class I antibodies) is not considered a contraindication to liver grafting; hyperacute graft rejection does not seem to occur in these circumstances. More recently, a form of rejection preferentially destroying biliary epithelium — the vanishing bile duct syndrome — has been described in patients with positive cross matches at transplantation due to antibodies against HLA class I antigens.

The differential diagnosis of graft rejection can be very difficult after liver transplantation. Immunohistological study of graft biopsy material can provide useful information. Class I HLA antigen expression on normal hepatocytes is weak or absent, but increases after transplantation and becomes further enhanced in graft rejection. Class II antigen expression by hepatocytes occurs during severe rejection and viral infections.

CORNEAL TRANSPLANTATION

For many years it was thought that the cornea was an immunologically privileged site, and that the small amount of foreign tissue in the graft could not provoke an immune response. Neither of these ideas is correct. Corneal grafts, like others, are subject to rejection.

EXPRESSION OF HLA MOLECULES

HLA-A and -B are expressed by all cells in the cornea, although the density is low on endothelial cells. In normal corneas, there are no capillaries and thus no vascular endothelial cells, which in man express HLA-DR; a few DR-positive dendritic cells can be found in the periphery of the cornea.

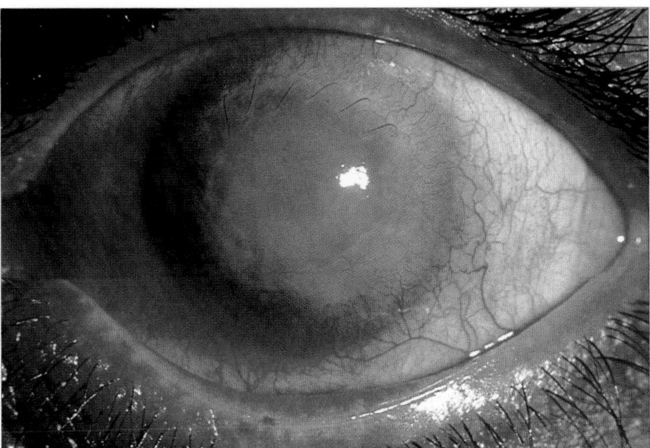

Fig. 3.13 Corneal graft showing rejection of endothelium, which appears typically cloudy. Courtesy of Mr T A Casey.

REJECTION

Unless anti-rejection therapy (local steroid drops) is used, 80% of grafts would be rejected. Normally this therapy is highly effective, and rejection does not become clinically apparent. However, grafts transplanted into corneas which have become vascularized, as a result of a chemical burn or chronic viral infections, are at high risk of rejection. Different clinical forms of rejection, which can be seen through the slit lamp microscope, have been described. Epithelial rejection (Fig. 3.11) appears as a wavy, superficial line that sweeps across the cornea. Clinically, this is the least dangerous form because new epithelium from the corneal periphery (recipient type) proliferates and replaces the graft epithelium. Stromal rejection is not seen in clinical practice.

Rejection affecting the endothelium is a serious event. One function of endothelium is to pump excess water from the cornea, maintaining its clarity. In adult life, endothelial cells do not proliferate, and any loss through rejection is not replaced. The earliest sign is an increase in lymphocytes in the aqueous humour, seen as a 'flare' by slit lamp microscopy (Fig. 3.12). Later, lymphocytes adhere to endothelium in a visible line — the Khodadoust line — and the overlying cornea becomes cloudy (Fig. 3.13).

As in the case of other types of allograft, rejection of corneal grafts occurs most frequently during the first 3–6 months (Fig. 3.14) but late rejections, even after intervals of 17 years, have been observed.

HLA MATCHING

A number of studies have demonstrated that donor-recipient matching for HLA-A and -B antigens is beneficial in high risk cases, for example when the recipient's corneas are vascularized. The incidence of graft failure through rejection can be reduced by approximately 20% in such cases. The value of matching for HLA-DR antigens is still under investigation, and firm conclusions have not yet been reached.

CROSS MATCHING

Antibodies against HLA are found less frequently in the sera of patients waiting for corneal grafts than in prospective recipients for kidney grafts. It has been observed that a positive cross match between the recipient's serum and the donor's lymphocytes is not necessarily associated with rejection, but more studies are needed.

IMMUNOSUPPRESSION

Topical and sub-conjunctival steroids have been the traditional form of anti-rejection therapy. Topical cyclosporin in drop form has not been successful, but systemic treat-

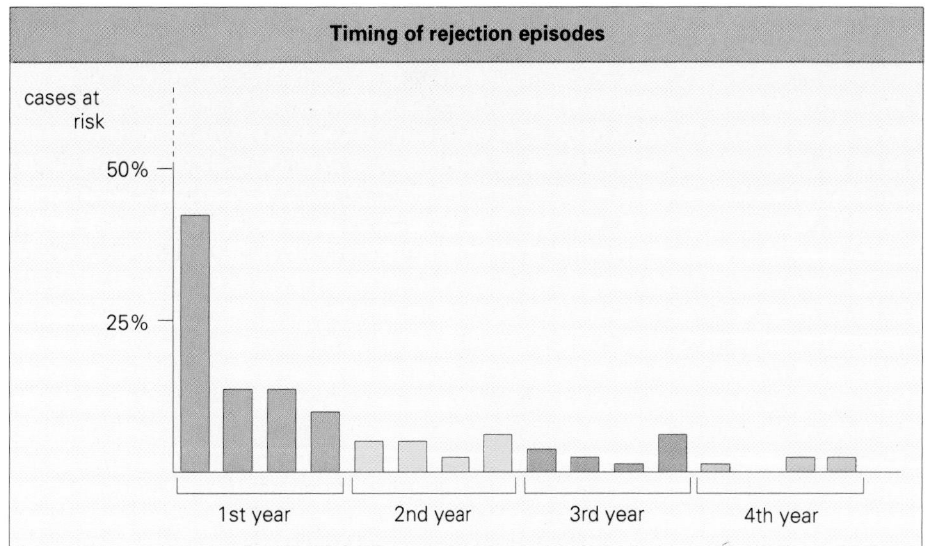

Fig. 3.14 As with other types of allograft, corneal rejection most frequently occurs 3–6 months after transplantation. Courtesy of Mr T A Casey.

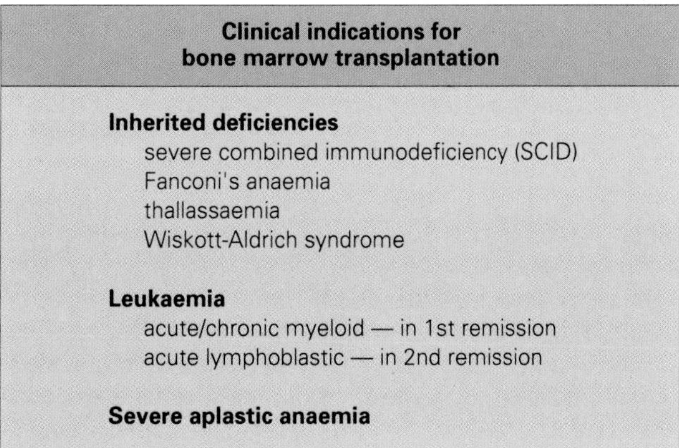

Clinical indications for bone marrow transplantation

Inherited deficiencies
severe combined immunodeficiency (SCID)
Fanconi's anaemia
thallassaemia
Wiskott-Aldrich syndrome

Leukaemia
acute/chronic myeloid — in 1st remission
acute lymphoblastic — in 2nd remission

Severe aplastic anaemia

Fig. 3.15 In aplastic anaemia, 70–80% of transplanted patients show long term survival, in other words are cured. In patients with leukaemia, provided transplantation is undertaken at an early stage of the disease, long term survival of approximately 50% of patients is expected. In contrast, only about 10% of patients grafted at later stages show long term survival.

ment with this drug in low dosage is being evaluated in patients at very high risk of graft rejection.

BONE MARROW TRANSPLANTATION

The clinical indications for bone marrow transplantation are outlined in Fig. 3.15.

MATCHING FOR BONE MARROW TRANSPLANTATION

Because bone marrow contains some immunologically competent lymphocytes as well as marrow stem cells, transplantation can give rise to graft-versus-host disease (GVHD) as well as the usual host-versus-graft (HVG) response. In order to reduce both of these to clinically manageable levels, transplantation is limited in most cases to donor-recipient pairs who are HLA-identical siblings. These are identified by conventional HLA serology, and confirmed by demonstrating non-reactivity in mutual one-way mixed lymphocyte cultures, performed with appropriate positive and negative controls.

Recently, attempts have been made to extend bone marrow transplantation to patients who do not have an HLA-identical sibling donor available. Two types of donors are being investigated:

- family members who share one haplotype with the recipient, and some (but not all) antigens on the other haplotype;
- unrelated subjects, selected from a volunteer panel who are HLA-identical.

It is too early to draw firm conclusions about the value of these categories of donors, but it does appear that some can be successful despite a higher frequency and severity of GVHD. In unrelated donors it is crucial to have very precise HLA typing and it seems probable that the use of southern blotting to discriminate between the different HLA polymorphisms will facilitate this.

ABO incompatibility

If the only available HLA-identical donor is ABO incompatible, it is necessary to remove the donor's red cells from the marrow before it is administered to the recipient. Although stem cells do not express A or B antigens the large number of mature red cells in the marrow inoculum can give rise to a severe haemolytic episode. Provided this precaution is taken, ABO incompatibility is not a serious problem in bone marrow transplantation, unlike solid organ transplantation.

Causes of failure of bone marrow to engraft
insufficient numbers of stem cells grafted
unappreciated HLA disparity between donor & recipient
inadequate immunosuppression of host
T cell depletion of donor marrow
sensitization of recipient before transplantation to non-MHC antigens on donor marrow
drug toxicity & viral infection

Fig. 3.16 Causes of failure of bone marrow to engraft.

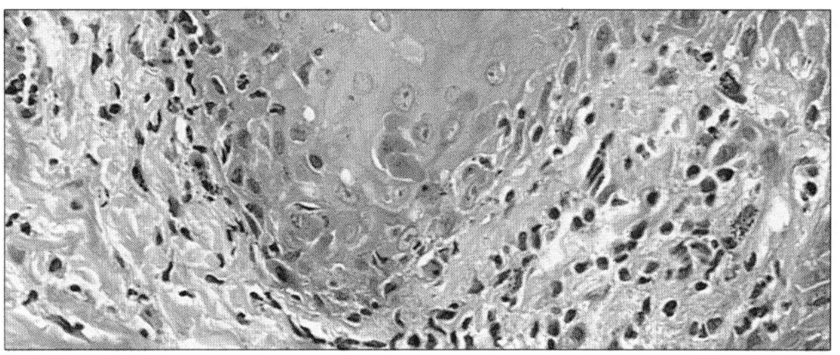

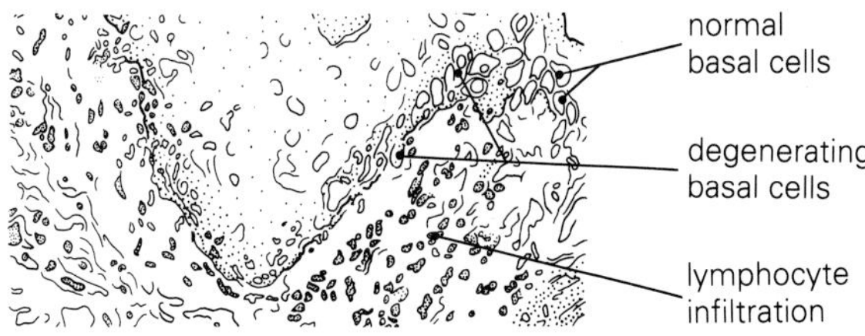

Fig. 3.17 Acute GVHD of skin. Note the vacuolar degeneration of basal keratinocytes with moderate lymphocyte infiltration. H & E stain.

Conditioning for transplantation

This is undertaken for several reasons;

- in patients with leukaemia, conditioning is given to ablate the tumour cells;
- it is used in all patients to suppress the HVG immune response;
- it prepares the marrow environment to accept a graft.

Most conditioning regimens consist of high dose chemotherapy combined with total body irradiation, given before transplantation. Irradiation can be omitted from the regimen for patients with non-malignant diseases. After transplantation, if the marrow has not been depleted of T cells, cyclosporin is given with or without methotrexate to prevent the development of GVHD. If GVHD does ensue, pulse doses of methyl-prednisolone are given, and the immunosuppressive therapy is increased.

Marrow engraftment

Marrow is obtained by multiple aspirations from the posterior iliac crests. Ordinarily, the only processing required is passage through a sieve screen to remove particulate material before the marrow cells are infused intravenously. The dose of nucleated viable cells given is 2–4 x 10^8/kg body weight of the recipient. Early signs of engraftment are generally seen 2–3 weeks after transplantation, but can be delayed up to 4–5 weeks in rare instances.

To avoid GVHD, many centres have adopted a strategy of depleting donor marrow of T lymphocytes. The methods used include removal of the unwanted T cells by lectins, or by magnetic beads coated with monoclonal antibodies (see chapter 20), or lysis of the T cells with monoclonal antibodies which spare the marrow stem cells. These methods can undoubtedly reduce the incidence of GVHD, but are associated with higher frequencies of failure to engraft (Fig. 3.16), and a higher relapse rate of leukaemia. The optimum treatment protocols remain to be established.

Acute GVHD

Although it is clear that acute GVHD is initiated by T lymphocytes of the graft reacting against the foreign histocompatibility antigens of the recipient, our understanding of the immunopathogenic events at the molecular level remains incomplete.

When it does occur, GVHD usually makes its clinical appearance within the first four weeks after transplantation. The syndrome is classified by severity into four grades depending on the.damage to the skin, liver and gastrointestinal tract, which bear the brunt of the immunological attack. Figs 3.17–3.19 illustrate the histological appearance of severe acute GVHD of the skin and colon.

Uncomplicated GVHD is treated by increasing the immunosuppressive therapy. However, in many cases the disease is complicated by accompanying infections, and diagnosis and management require much clinical skill and experience. Biopsy of the affected tissues can provide helpful information. Typically, there is class II HLA antigen expression by keratinocytes in the basal layer of the epidermis, and by biliary epithelium in the liver.

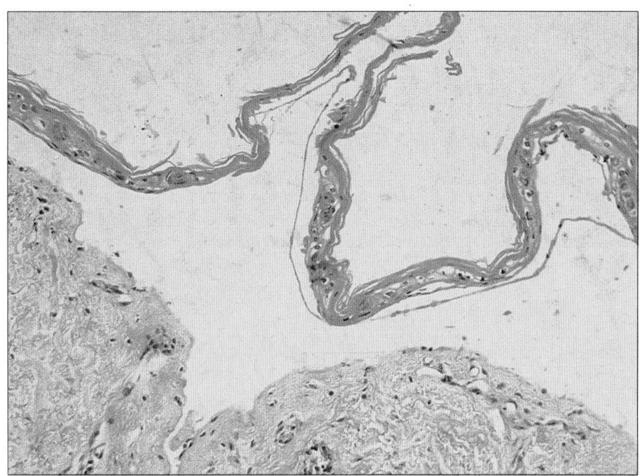

Fig. 3.18 Acute GVHD of skin. In this case the lesion resembles toxic epidermal necrolysis.

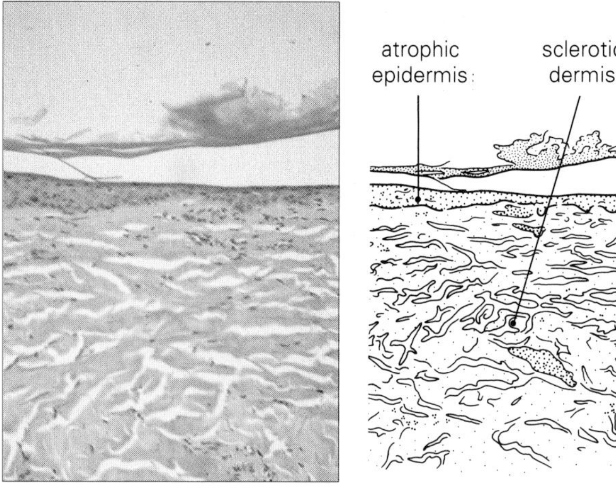

Fig. 3.20 Chronic GVHD of skin. The dermis is markedly sclerotic, with an appearance resembling scleroderma.

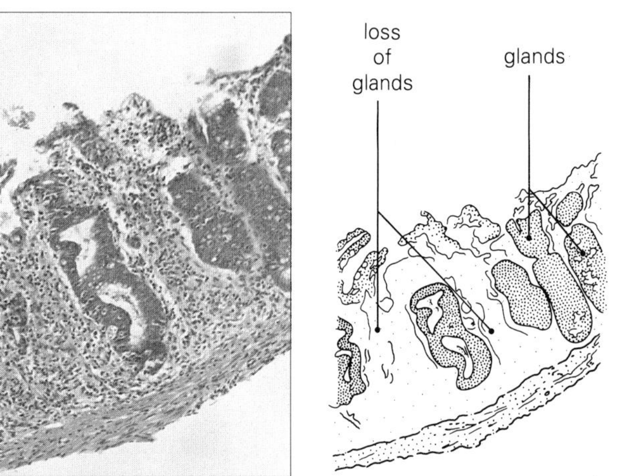

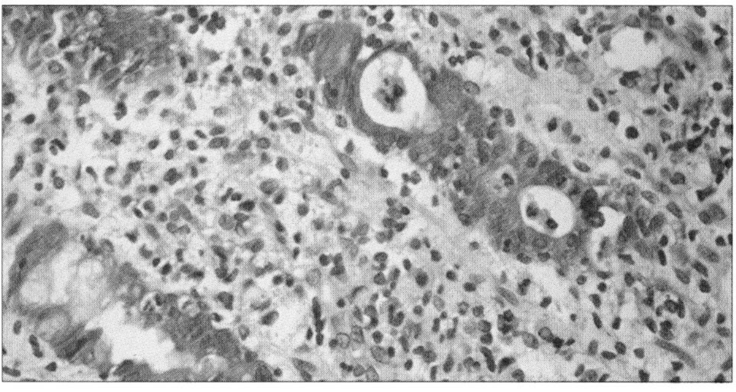

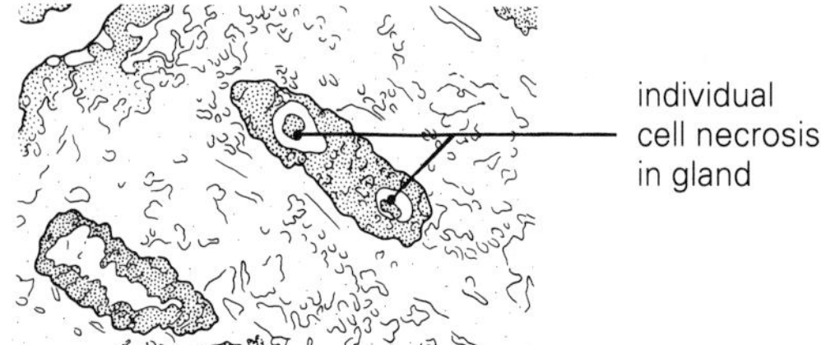

Fig. 3.19 Acute GVHD of colon. Upper: irregular loss of glands. Lower: note the pattern of single cell death involving glandular structures.

Chronic GVHD

This has been arbitrarily defined as GVHD present at 100 days or more after transplantation. It generally follows the acute form, but 20–30% of cases arise *de novo*. The clinical features are rather different to the acute form and it is classified merely as localized or generalized. The main features resemble those of Sjögren's syndrome, scleroderma (Fig. 3.20), primary biliary cirrhosis or chronic active autoimmune hepatitis. Polymyositis and skin lesions similar to lichen planus may also be seen, and a wide variety of autoantibodies may be found in the patient's sera. The different clinical picture of chronic GVHD suggests that the mechanisms of tissue damage are different to those of the acute form of disease. There is, however, no agreement on the mechanisms involved.

Opportunistic infections

As with all immunosuppressed patients, opportunistic infections are a serious hazard. In addition to the immunosuppressive effects of the conditioning and post-transplant therapy, GVHD itself causes further immunosuppression. In practice, the most frequent and serious infections are with Herpes simplex, cytomegalovirus, and varicella-zoster. In many cases these infections are due to reactivation of an already present virus. The time at which the infection appears tends to be characteristic for the different viruses:

- Herpes simplex infections are usually seen in the first month after transplantation;
- cytomegalovirus infections tend to occur later;
- varicella-zoster reactivation occurs at 4–6 months after transplantation.

Acyclovir treatment successfully controls most Herpes simplex and varicella-zoster infections, but cytomegalovirus infections remain difficult problems to manage.

RESULTS OF BONE MARROW TRANSPLANTATION

The majority of bone marrow transplants engraft satisfactorily. Normal blood counts are expected in 2–3 months, but marrow cellularity remains reduced for up to 2–3 years. There is also considerable delay before normal immune responsiveness has been reconstituted.

Long term survival of transplanted patients depends on four interrelated factors:

- whether the marrow shows stable engraftment;
- the severity of GVHD;
- the development of severe infections;
- whether the leukaemia relapses, in the case of leukaemic patients.

For patients with aplastic anaemia and a suitable HLA-identical sibling donor, bone marrow transplantation is the treatment of choice.

FURTHER READING

Casey TA, Mayer D. *Corneal grafting. Principles and practice.* Philadelphia: Saunders, 1985.

Hayry P, Koskimies S, eds. Proceedings of the XIth International Congress of the Transplantation Society. *Transplantation Proc* 1987; **19**.

Morris PJ. *Kidney transplantation. Principles and practice* (2E). Orlando: Grune and Stratton, 1984.

Martin P, Hansen JA, Storb R, Thomas ED. Human marrow transplantation: An immunological perspective. *Adv Immunol* 1987;**40**,379–438.

4

Autoimmune Diseases: A General Introduction

SELF TOLERANCE

Lymphocytes recognize foreign antigens through complementariness in shape between the lymphocyte receptor and a foreign molecule. Since the building blocks used to form microbial and host molecules are essentially the same, it is the assembled shapes of self and non-self molecules which have to be discriminated by the immune system if potentially disastrous autoreactivity is to be avoided. The immune system has therefore evolved such tolerance mechanisms which make it unresponsive to self antigens. Self tolerance operates through several different mechanisms. Since each lymphocyte requires a single antigen, all that is required for the induction of self tolerance is a mechanism which functionally deletes those cells which react with self and leaves the remainder of the repertoire untouched.

Tolerance resulting from early clonal deletion

In the early stages of lymphocyte development within the primary organs (the thymus for T cells and the bone marrow for B cells) contact with self molecules usually leads to deletion of those clones which recognize the self antigen (Fig. 4.1). Evidence for physical deletion of self-reactive T cells has come from many experiments. For example in male mice carrying a transgene which encodes a T cell receptor specific for the male HY antigen, (present on every cell in the male body) the thymus does not bear any lymphocytes which express this receptor for self-HY. In contrast, the females which lack HY have large numbers of cells with these receptors in their thymuses.

Tolerance due to clonal anergy

Mature lymphocytes which leave the primary organs can become tolerized to self molecules in the periphery, particularly when they are not present on conventional antigen presenting cells. This is termed clonal anergy because the cells become unresponsive but can still be demonstrated in the circulation and lymphoid tissue. Evidence for the induction of clonal anergy is provided in transgenic animals expressing the class II MHC molecule, I-E, on the β cells of the pancreas but not other cells. These animals are tolerant to I-E. Even though the I-E molecule did not appear in the thymus to delete the self-reactive T cells, it was still able to induce unresponsiveness when acting in the periphery.

Tolerance caused by lack of communication

Clearly, if the self molecule cannot contact T cells, there can be no response. Molecules like the lens protein of the eye and myelin basic protein in the brain are anatomically

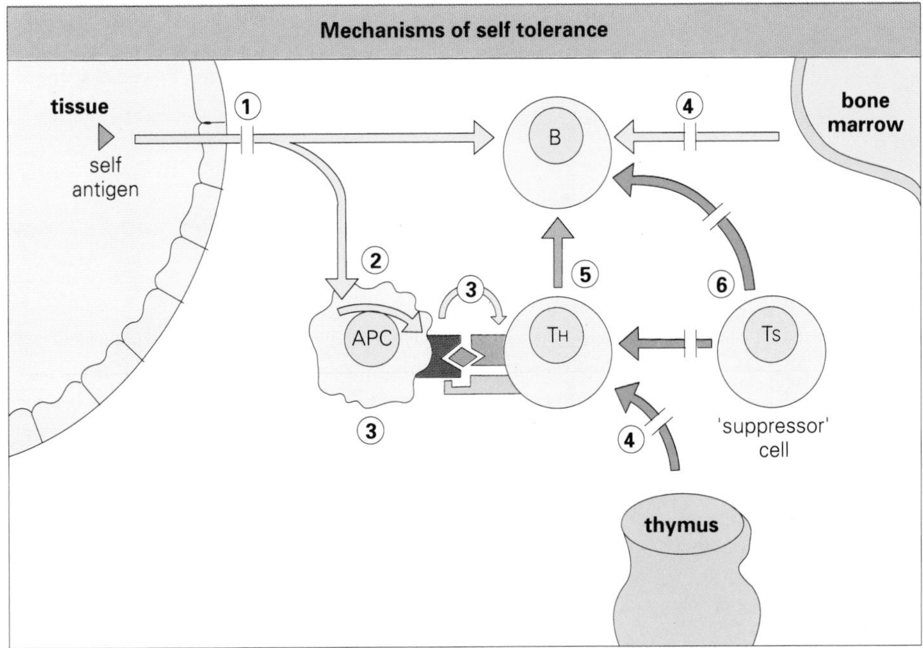

Fig. 4.1 Tolerance to self molecules may be due to a combination of mechanisms: 1) many antigens are confined to tissues and do not contact lymphocytes in sufficient quantity; 2) an absence of functional APCs will prevent presentation to T cells; 3) failure to express MHC class II prevents presentation, while lack of costimulation signals may render T cells anergic; 4) autoreactive T or B cells may be deleted during development in the tissues and bone marrow; 5) failure of cells to communicate effectively can limit immune reaction; 6) T cell (or B cell or macrophage) suppressor activity can control an inappropriate immune response. Absence of such control can lead to persistence of the autoimmune response.

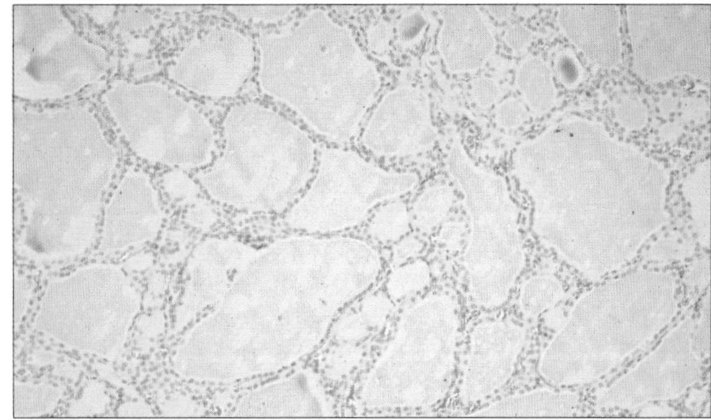

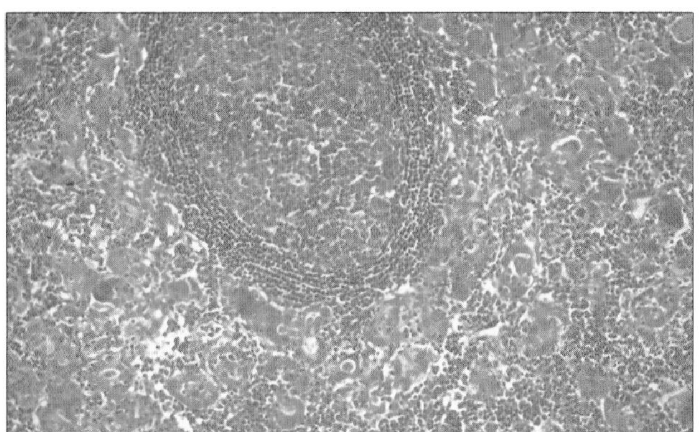

Fig. 4.2 Histological changes in Hashimoto's thyroiditis. Upper: normal thyroid showing the follicular cells lining the colloid space into which they secret thyroglobulin, which is broken down on demand to provide thyroid hormones. Lower: Hashimoto gland in which the normal architecture is virtually destroyed and replaced by invading cells which consist essentially of lymphocytes, macrophages and plasma cells.

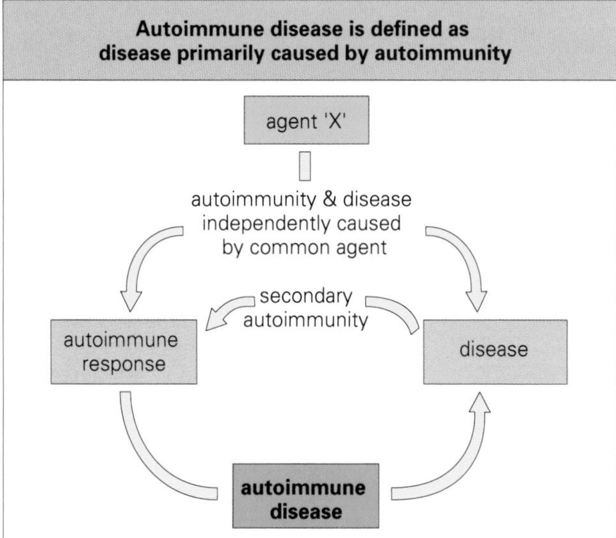

Fig. 4.3 Autoimmune disease is defined as disease primarily caused by autoimmunity, as distinct from a disease in which an agent causes disease and a separate autoimmune response.

isolated and virtually precluded from contact with lymphocytes, except perhaps for minute amounts of breakdown metabolic products which leak out and may be taken up by antigen presenting cells, but concentrations are usually below that required to trigger naive T cells.

Molecules restricted to particular organs which come into contact with circulating lymphocytes usually cannot be recognized because although they are not present in the thymus to cause clonal deletion of their self-reacting lymphocyte counterparts, the organs in which they appear do not normally express MHC class II. Also, as a consequence, there is no opportunity for tolerization of T-helpers in the periphery.

T suppressor cells and tolerance

For many years it was proposed that T suppressor (Ts) cells could induce self tolerance, and autoimmunity could result from a lack of T suppressor cell activity. However the nature and even the separate existence of such cells has become controversial. The suppressive activity seen in immune responses is now often ascribed to a combination of possible interactions, including:

- a change in the mode of the immune response, from cell-mediated to antibody-mediated immunity (or vice versa), due to the production of different sets of cytokines by different T cell populations;
- absorption of essential cytokines by the suppressor cells, thus preventing the division of other lymphocytes;
- release of non-specific immunosuppressive molecules such as prostaglandins or ACTH (which induces corticosteroids);
- specific cytostatic activity of the suppressor cells on the autoreactive cells;
- induction of anergy in the autoreactive population caused by stimulating cells giving only a partial activation signal.

In animal models of acute autoimmunity, such as EAE, there is evidence that the first of these mechanisms is active. Similarly if autoimmunity is induced in a normal animal with a cross-reacting antigen, a form of T cell mediated suppression develops. These results suggest that suppression mediated by T cells may be important in control of autoreactivity, even though the precise identity of the effector population is still uncertain.

THE CONCEPT OF AUTOIMMUNE DISEASE

In all instances of self tolerance which do not involve clonal deletion or constitutional absence of self-reactive receptors, potentially self-reactive cells exist in the body. All mechanisms have a risk of breakdown and these mechanisms for self tolerance are no exception. Thus, a number of diseases have been identified in which there is copious production of autoantibodies and autoreactive T cells. One of the earliest examples of a breakdown in these mechanisms giving rise to autoimmune disease was Hashimoto's thyroiditis, in which changes in the thyroid gland were associated with the presence of autoantibodies specific for the thyroid itself. The gland is infiltrated, sometimes to an extraordinary extent, with inflammatory lymphoid cells which leads to widespread breakdown of the natural follicular architecture (Fig. 4.2). There are now a very large number of different disorders associated with autoimmunity.

However, the association between an autoimmune response and the manifestations of a given disease do not necessarily imply a causal relationship between them. For example, an independent agent such as a virus might independently provoke an autoimmune response and the lesions of the disease (Fig. 4.3). Alternatively, the disease process itself may cause release of self molecules or changes in them which provoke an autoantibody response secondarily. It is only when the autoimmune process itself appears to be primarily responsible for producing the disease, that we speak of an autoimmune disease as such.

THE SPECTRUM OF AUTOIMMUNE DISEASE

Diseases associated with autoimmune phenomena tend to distribute themselves within a spectrum. At one pole, typified by Hashimoto's thyroiditis, the antibodies and the invasive destructive lesion are directed against just one organ in the body. At the other end of the spectrum, typified by systemic lupus erythematosus (SLE) the antibodies are directed to antigens, which are widespread throughout the body and the characteristic lesions of the disease are also widely disseminated. Thus we speak of organ-specific and non-organ-specific (or sometimes systemic) autoimmune diseases; in Fig. 4.4 the diseases are classified according to where they lie within this spectrum.

The common target organs in organ-specific disease include the thyroid, adrenal glands, stomach and pancreas. The non-organ-specific diseases, which include the so-called rheumatological disorders, involve skin, kidney, joints and muscle (Fig. 4.5).

Interestingly, there are remarkable overlaps at each end of the spectrum. For example, thyroid antibodies occur with a high frequency in patients with pernicious anaemia who have gastric autoimmunity, and these patients have a higher incidence of thyroid autoimmune disease than the normal population. Similarly, patients with thyroid autoimmunity have a high incidence of gastric autoantibodies and, to a lesser extent, the clinical disease itself, pernicious anaemia.

The cluster of rheumatological disorders at the non-organ-specific end of the spectrum also shows considerable overlap and features of rheumatoid arthritis, for example, are often associated with the clinical picture of SLE.

In non-organ-specific disease, immune complexes formed with the antigens involved are deposited systemically, particularly in the kidney, joints and skin, so giving rise to the more disseminated features of the disease. In contrast, overlap between diseases at the two ends of the

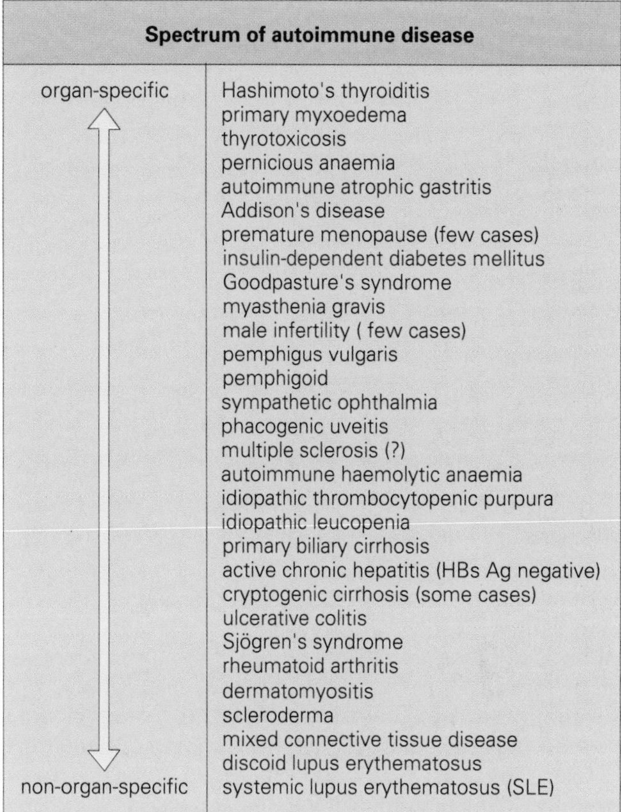

Spectrum of autoimmune disease	
organ-specific	Hashimoto's thyroiditis primary myxoedema thyrotoxicosis pernicious anaemia autoimmune atrophic gastritis Addison's disease premature menopause (few cases) insulin-dependent diabetes mellitus Goodpasture's syndrome myasthenia gravis male infertility (few cases) pemphigus vulgaris pemphigoid sympathetic ophthalmia phacogenic uveitis multiple sclerosis (?) autoimmune haemolytic anaemia idiopathic thrombocytopenic purpura idiopathic leucopenia primary biliary cirrhosis active chronic hepatitis (HBs Ag negative) cryptogenic cirrhosis (some cases) ulcerative colitis Sjögren's syndrome rheumatoid arthritis dermatomyositis scleroderma mixed connective tissue disease discoid lupus erythematosus systemic lupus erythematosus (SLE)
non-organ-specific	

Fig. 4.4 Autoimmune diseases may be classified as organ-specific or non-organ-specific depending on whether the response is primarily against either antigens localized to particular organs, or widespread antigens.

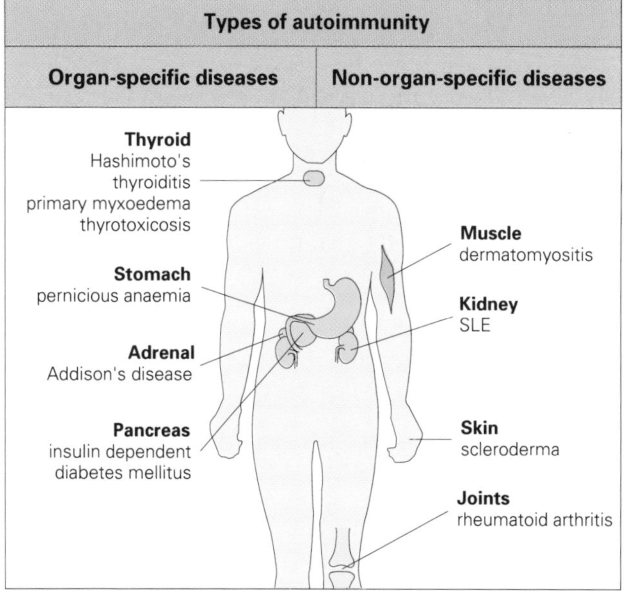

Fig. 4.5 Two types of autoimmune diseases — organ-specific and non-organ-specific. Although the non-organ-specific diseases produce symptoms in different organs, particular organs are more markedly affected by particular diseases.

Comparison of organ-specific & non-organ-specific disorders		
	organ-specific	**non-organ-specific**
antigen	esssentially localized to given organ	widespread throughout the body
lesions	antigen in organ is target for immunological attack	complexes deposit systemically particularly in kidneys, joints & skin
overlap	with other organ-specific antibodies & diseases	with other non-organ-specific antibodies & diseases

Fig. 4.6 Comparison of organ-specific and non-organ-specific disorders.

spectrum is relatively rare, and cases in which thyroiditis and SLE occur together are extremely unusual. In organ-specific diseases, lesions are restricted because the antigen in the organ acts as a target for immunological attack.

The mechanisms by which immunopathological damage occur in autoimmunity vary depending on where the disease lies in the spectrum. Where the antigen is localized in a particular organ, type II hypersensitivity and cell-mediated reactions are most important. In non-organ-specific autoimmunity, immune complex deposition at sites of filtration is also relevant. The features of organ-specific and non-organ-specific disorders are compared in Fig. 4.6.

AETIOLOGY

We have already discussed how self tolerance prevents potential autoantigens and their corresponding lymphocytes from interacting. Fig. 4.7 outlines possible ways in which these normal controls on autoreactivity may be bypassed. One method is by directly bypassing these regulatory processes which hold down the responsiveness of autoreactive T helper (TH) cells.

T suppressor activity

These controls include different types of Ts cells, which go to make up a rather ill-defined complex of Ts activity. It has been postulated that defects in perhaps more than one type of suppressor cell may be important for the development of an autoimmune response. It is interesting to note that studies on the clinically unaffected relatives of patients with SLE have shown that these individuals share with the patients themselves a defect in the generation of non-specific Ts cells, suggesting first that the defect is not a consequence of the disease, and secondly that it is unable to cause SLE by itself. This is consistent with the previous discussion, suggesting that several factors may be implicated in the causation of autoimmune disease.

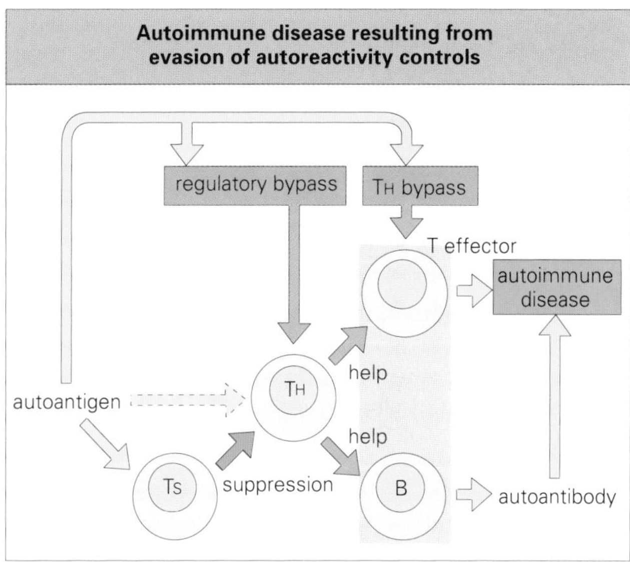

Fig. 4.7 Self-reactive B cells, effector T cells and autoantigens are all normally present but TH cells capable of inducing an autoimmune response are functionally absent, due either to clonal abortion or anergy, or to the action of Ts cells (Ts antigen-, idiotype-, or non-specific), or to a failure of adequate autoantigen presentation. Thus the self-reactive T and B cells are not activated. (Idiotype-specific Ts cells may also act directly on B cells). Autoimmunity may arise by a regulatory bypass which either causes direct activation of the TH cell or, by activating another cell, the T contrasuppressor (Tcs), renders the TH cell resistant to suppression. The existence of contrasuppressors is equivocal. Autoantigen could also bypass the TH cell to stimulate directly T effectors and B cells, particularly if presented correctly and in adequate concentration.

'Immunological silence'

Most cells do not normally express MHC class II molecules and so cannot present antigens to $CD4^+$ T cells which are essential for the induction of autoimmunity. One can then propose that if cells are induced to express MHC class II, they could present self antigens and stimulate autoimmunity. It was therefore exciting when cells in thyrotoxic thyroiditis were found to be actively synthesizing MHC class II molecules, and so might act as antigen presenters (Fig. 4.8).

Subsequently it has been shown that many cell types can be induced to express class II molecules following stimulation with interferon-γ. It is still not certain, however, whether these cells can actually initiate an autoimmune response, since they may not provide the T cells with the necessary costimulatory signals or cytokines. Thus, we do not yet know whether MHC class II expression is a cause or a consequence of autoimmune reactions in tissues, or indeed whether it has any functional significance.

Cross-reacting antigens

Another way to break self tolerance occurs if T cells are stimulated by a cross-reacting microbial antigen which

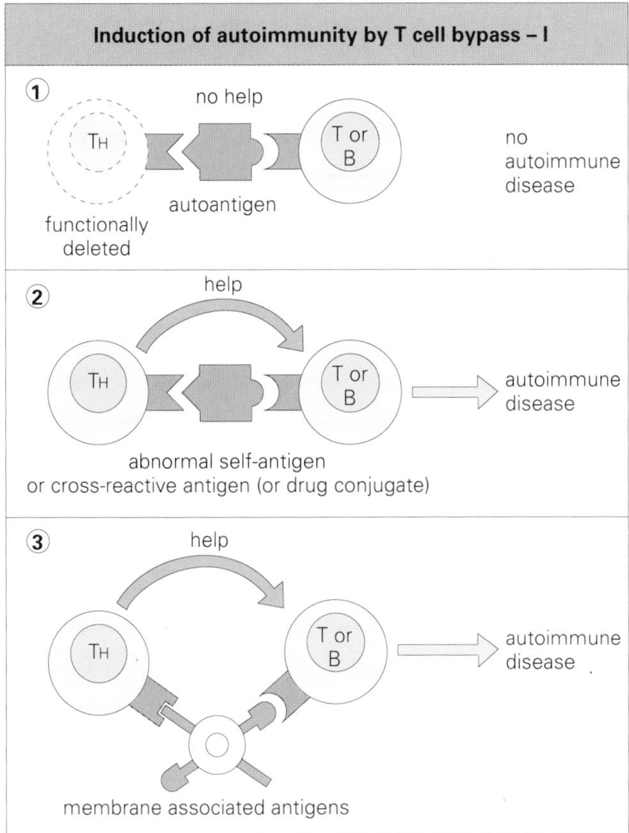

Fig. 4.8 Normally autoimmune disease does not occur since T cells reacting with autoantigen are functionally deleted or suppressed (1). In the presence of a cross-reacting antigen, a new population of TH cells reacting with a foreign carrier determinant can supply help (2). The binding of a drug to self-antigen may also act as the carrier determinant recognized by the TH cells. Another possibility is that the autoantigen can be structurally altered through abnormalities in synthesis or processing. The new carrier determinant can either be on a molecule which also bears the autoantigenic determinant (as in 2), or it can be on a different molecule associated with the autoantigen on a cell membrane (3).

has peptide sequences in common with the autoantigen, to which it reacts with high avidity. Since primed cells have a higher avidity for peptide on antigen presenting cells (because of their high surface expression of accessory molecules such as LFA-1 and CD2), it is conceivable that the primed autoreactive T cells could now be chronically stimulated by available autoantigen. Interest is also focused on the possibility that anergic T cells might be converted to the responsive state, perhaps by local high concentrations of cytokines released during a particularly vicious inflammatory response to some infectious agent.

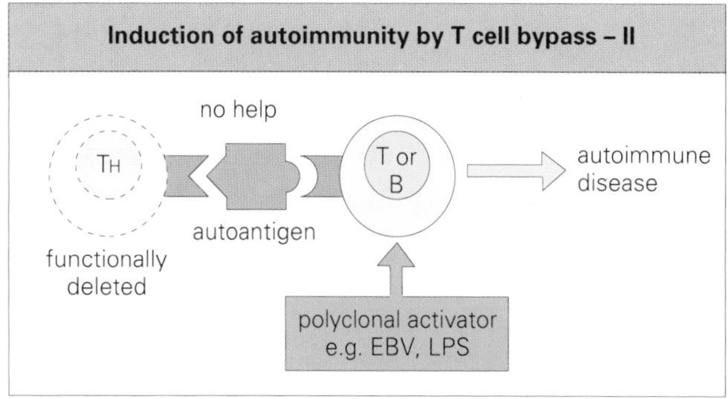

Fig. 4.9 Self-reactive cells can be stimulated directly by polyclonal activators, for example Epstein-Barr virus or bacterial lipopolysaccharides.

T helper cell bypass

Particular interest was aroused by the suggestions of Allison and Weigle that a TH cell bypass mechanism might operate. They argued that since the unresponsiveness of the final effector T and B cells could be a consequence of suppression or tolerization of the autoantigen-specific TH cells (inducer T cells), any circumstances leading to the circumvention of these tolerant T cells would lead directly to the triggering of effector lymphocytes. A number of different ways in which this could be achieved are outlined in Figs. 4.8 & 4.9. For simplicity, these diagrams show T and B cells interacting via antigen bridges, although in reality the T cell would probably recognize processed antigen on the B cell surface.

A disease in which this mechanism operates is rheumatic fever, where autoantibodies to heart can be detected. This condition occurs in a small proportion of individuals several weeks after a streptococcal infection of the throat. Carbohydrate antigens on the streptococcal surface cross-react with an antigen on heart valves, so the infection may bypass T cell self tolerance to heart valve antigens. Pertinent to Fig. 4.9 is the intriguing recent discovery that IgG in patients with rheumatoid arthritis shows defective addition of galactose to the Fc region oligosaccharides. This gives added impetus to the view that abnormal sensitization to IgG in rheumatoid arthritis is a major contributing factor to the chronic synovial inflammatory process.

Fig. 4.10 shows experiments in which rat red cells can induce autoantibodies to self-erythrocytes in mice as an example of 'tolerance breaking' by cross-reacting antigen. Whereas normal mice switch off autoantibody production after a few weeks, (probably through the action of suppressors) animal strains which are prone to autoimmunity (NZB), or have poorly developed suppressors (SJL) do not. This raises the important point that development of autoreactivity, development of disease and recovery are distinct and are controlled by many factors.

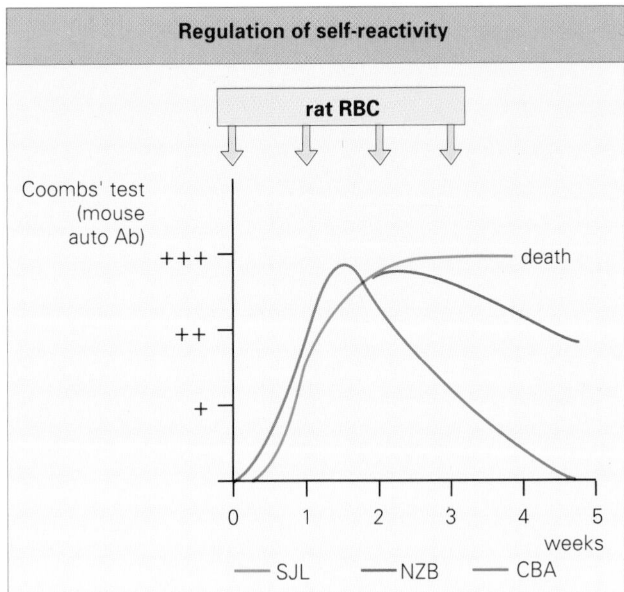

Fig. 4.10 When CBA mice are injected with rat red cells, autoantibodies are produced by this cross-reacting antigen. These coat the host erythrocytes and are detected by the Coombs' test. The SJL strain, in which suppressor activity declines rapidly with age, is unable to regulate the autoimmune response and develops particularly severe disease. The response is also prolonged in the autoimmune NZB strain Modified from Cooke & Hutchings.

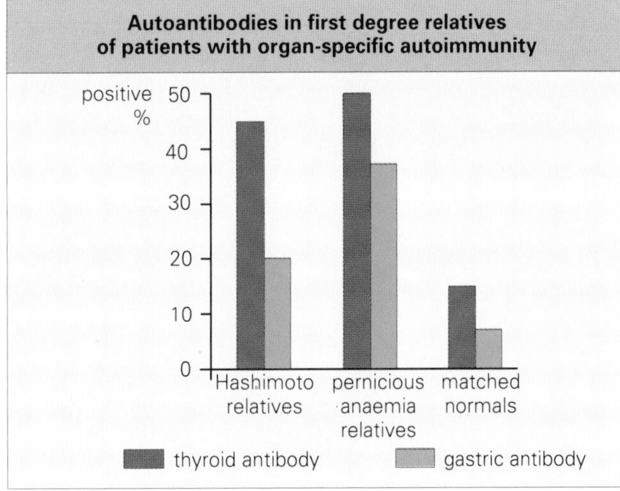

Fig. 4.12 Thyroid and stomach antibodies in first degree relatives of patients with Hashimoto's disease or pernicious anaemia. A remarkably high proportion of the first degree relatives of patients with Hashimoto's disease have thyroid autoantibodies and to a lesser degree, parietal cell (gastric) autoantibodies. The relatives of patients with pernicious anaemia also have a very high incidence of thyroid autoimmunity, indicative of a predisposition to develop organ-specific autoantibodies; the percentage with gastric autoantibodies is also high, even when compared with the Hashimoto relatives, suggesting an inherent bias of the immune system for reactivity against particular organs.

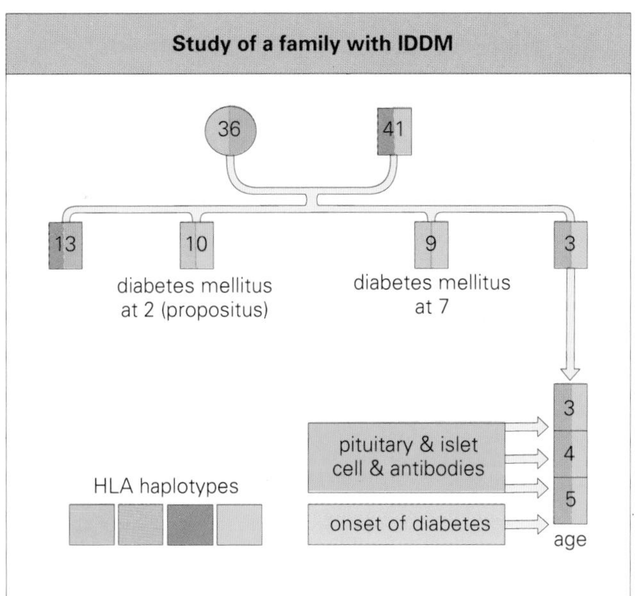

Fig. 4.11 Study of a family with insulin dependent diabetes mellitus. The sibling sharing a haplotype with the propositus and having complement fixing islet cell antibodies became diabetic 3 years after the study had begun.

AUTOIMMUNE DISEASES ARE MULTIFACTORIAL

There is an undoubted familial incidence of autoimmunity, a striking example of which is shown in Fig. 4.11. This familial incidence has a strong genetic component, as may be seen from studies of identical and non-identical twins, and from the association of, for example, thyroid autoantibodies with abnormalities of the X chromosome.

Just as there is an overlap between organ-specific disorders in given individuals, so the tendency to develop autoimmunity within families shows a bias towards organ-specific autoimmunity (Fig. 4.12). In addition to this predisposition to develop organ-specific antibodies, it is clear that other genetically controlled factors tend to select the organ which will be mainly affected. It is interesting to note that, although relatives of Hashimoto patients have a higher than expected incidence and titre of thyroid autoantibodies and that the same is seen in relatives of patients with pernicious anaemia, the latter are distinguished by having a far higher frequency of gastric autoantibodies; this suggests that the stomach is being differentially selected as the target organ within this group.

Genetic factors

Further evidence for the operation of genetic factors in the development of autoimmune disease comes from their tendency to be associated with particular HLA specificities (Fig. 4.13). The haplotype B8, DR3 is particularly common in the organ-specific diseases.Rheumatoid arthritis showed no HLA associations when only the specificities

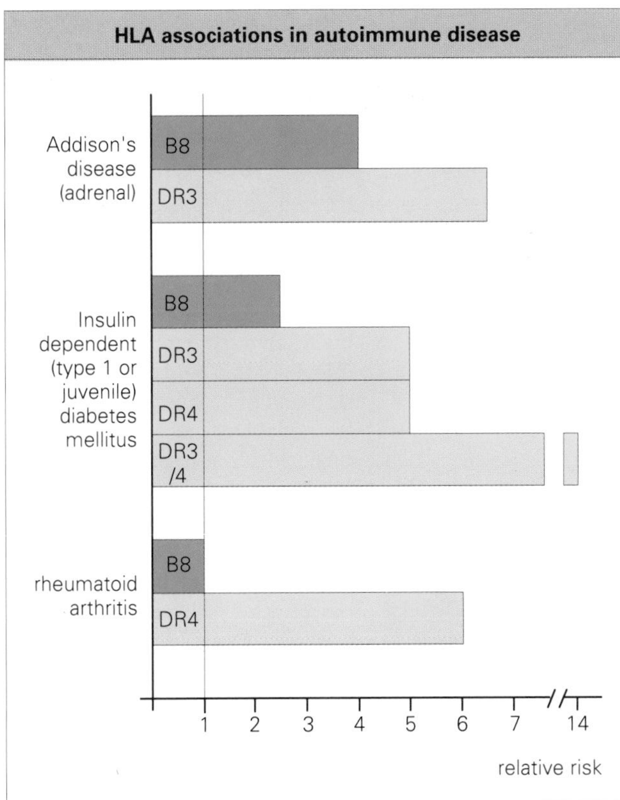

Fig. 4.13 The relative risk is a measure of the increased chance of contracting the disease for individuals bearing the antigen relative to those lacking it. Virtually all autoimmune diseases studied show an association with some HLA specificity. The greater relative risk for Addison's disease associated with DR3 as compared with B8 suggests that DR3 is closer to, if not identical with, the 'disease susceptibility gene'. In this case B8 has a relative risk greater than 1 because it is known to occur together with DR3 more often than expected by chance, a phenomenon termed linkage disequilibrium.

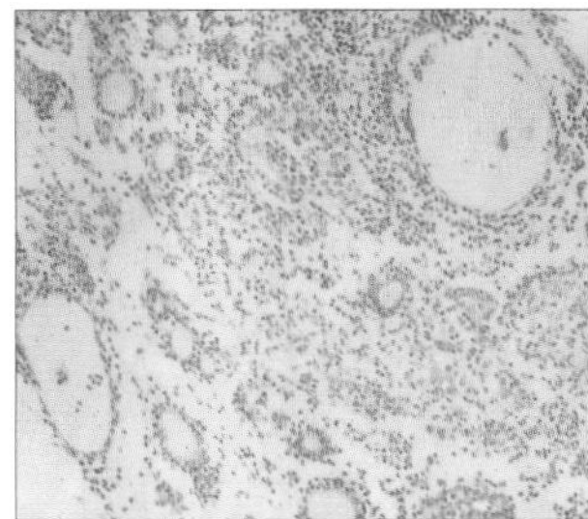

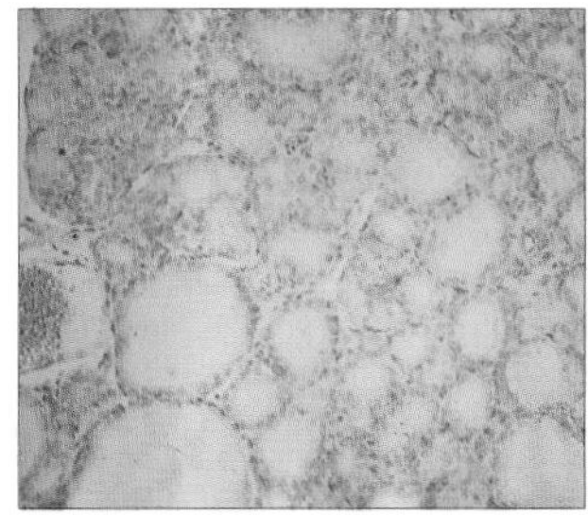

Fig. 4.14 The histological appearance of experimental autoallergic thyroiditis. Left: section from a thyroglobulin-injected animal. There is gross destruction of the follicular architecture with extensive invasion by mononuclear inflammatory cells, associated with distended blood vessels, oedema and fibrosis. H&E stain, x200. Right: control section. H & E stain, x 110.

at the A and B loci were studied, but it has now been shown to be associated with HLA-DR4; individuals with this tissue type have a higher chance of developing the disease. Of note is the finding that in the organ-specific disease, insulin dependent or type 1 diabetes mellitus, heterozygotes for DR3 and DR4 have a greatly increased risk of developing the disease, supporting the concept of multiple genetic factors. These observations indicate that specific MHC molecules are involved in presenting particular autoantigens.

In addition to MHC molecules, there are a variety of less well defined genetic factors predisposing to autoimmune disease. These include genes involved in immunoregulation, for example those controlling responses to cytokines, and those involved in corticosteroid production. Levels of plasma enzyme inhibitors and pro-inflammatory mediators may affect the development of the immune-mediated damage. Also local factors within affected tissues can partly control the access of the autoreactive leucocytes to the target organs.

Environmental factors

It is more difficult to pinpoint the influence of environmental factors. In certain instances, such as Goodpasture's syndrome, it has emerged that individuals with the HLA-DR2 allele may develop the disease when exposed to organic vapours such as those occurring in dry-cleaning units. Examples have been reported of abnormalities seen in patients with autoimmune disease occurring in their spouses even though they do not develop frank autoimmune disease, suggesting again that more than one abnormality is required before there is a complete breakdown leading to the development of autoimmune disorder. There are also examples in which infection with particular micro-organisms has appeared to provoke autoimmune disease.

EVIDENCE THAT AUTOIMMUNITY CAN CAUSE DISEASE

EVIDENCE FROM EXPERIMENTAL AUTOIMMUNITY

If autoimmunity is responsible for lesions of a given disease, then deliberate induction of autoimmunity in an experimental animal should lead to the production of the lesions. In fact, it is possible to provoke certain organ-specific diseases in experimental animals by injecting the causative antigen with Complete Freund's Adjuvant (CFA) — thyroglobulin can induce an inflammatory disease of the thyroid while myelin basic protein can cause encephalomyelitis. Strict organ specificity may be seen, since the lesions are confined in both cases to the organ or organ system in which the antigen used for immunization is located. In the case of the thyroglobulin-injected animals, not only are thyroid autoantibodies produced, but the gland becomes infiltrated with mononuclear cells and the acinar architecture crumbles under their influence (Fig. 4.14). Although not identical in every respect with

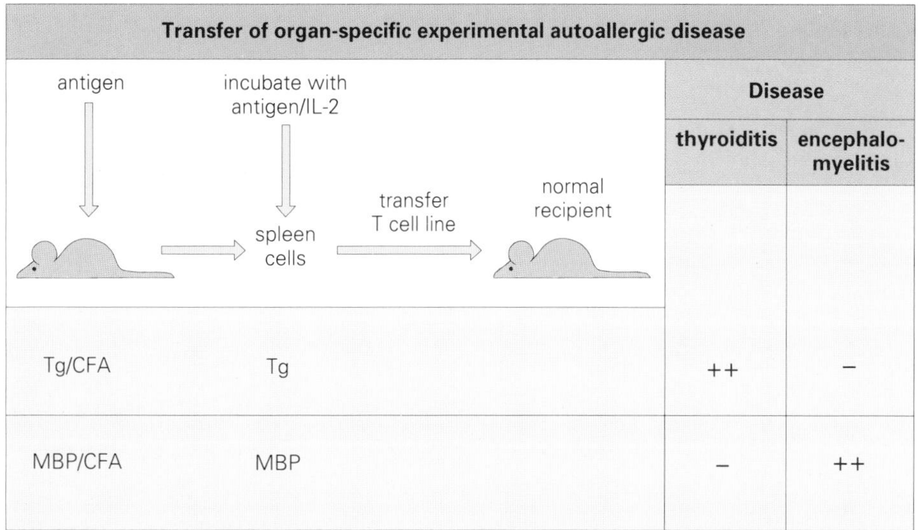

Fig. 4.15 Transfer of organ-specific experimental autoallergic disease by $CD4^+$ T cell lines or clones obtained by stimulating sensitized spleen cells alternately with antigen and IL-2 *in vitro*. Tg specific T cells induce histological inflammation of the thyroid but no encephalomyelitis in histocompatible recipients; MBP-specific T cells likewise produce lesions in the brain and not the thyroid. The effects of transfer can be blocked by treatment of the T cell line or the normal recipient with anti-CD4 monoclonals. Tg = thyroglobulin; MBP = myelin basic protein; CFA = Complete Freund's Adjuvant.

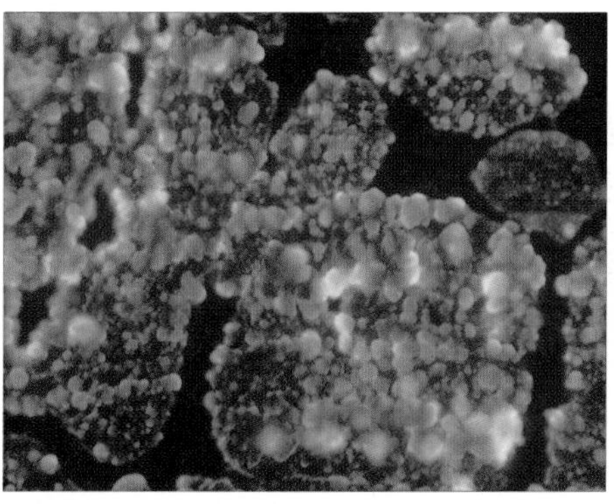

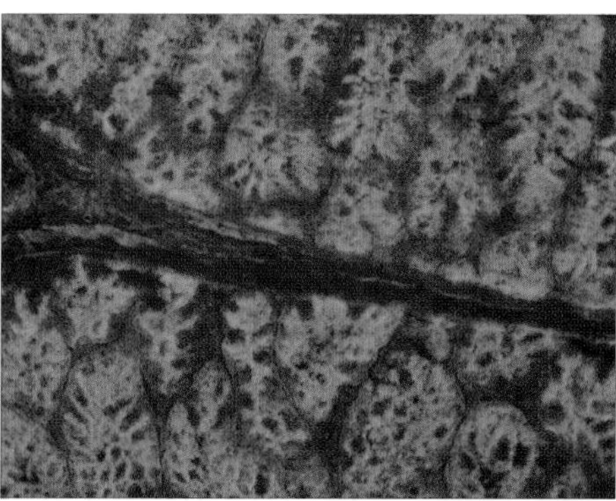

Fig. 4.16 Autoantibodies in OS chickens. Left: fluorescent staining of a fixed thyroid section showing reaction in the colloid. Right: approximately 15% of the birds have serum antibodies which stain the chicken stomach (proventriculus), giving the characteristic pattern shown. This pattern is also seen if human sera containing parietal cell antibodies are tested against this organ.

Hashimoto's disease, the thyroiditis produced bears a remarkable overall similarity to the human condition.

Strain susceptibility to autoimmune diseases

The ability to induce these experimental autoimmune diseases depends on the strain of animal used. For example, it is found that the susceptibility of rats and mice to myelin basic protein-induced encephalomyelitis depends on a small number of gene loci, of which the most important are MHC class II genes. It is also possible to induce autoallergic encephalomyelitis in susceptible strains by injecting myelin basic protein-specific T cell lines. These lines are $CD4^+$ and it has been found that induction of the disease can be blocked by treating the recipients with antibody to CD4, just before the expected time of disease onset. Similar findings are obtained in thyroglobulin induced experimental autoallergic thyroiditis (Fig. 4.15). The results indicate the importance of class II restricted autoreactive T cells in the development of these conditions, and emphasize the role of the MHC.

Antibody mediated disease

In some experimental models, antibody rather than T cells can be shown to be the principal effectors of disease. Thus, polyclonal antibodies to acetylcholine receptors will produce the muscle weakness characteristic of experimental myasthenia gravis, which is normally induced by immunization with the antigen in Complete Freund's Adjuvant. Similarly, Goodpasture's glomerulonephritis can be provoked in normal cases with the introduction of antibodies to glomerular basement membrane.

Spontaneous autoimmune disease

There is much to learn from spontaneous examples of autoimmune disease in animals. One well-established example is the Obese strain (OS) chicken in which thyroid autoantibodies occur spontaneously and the thyroid undergoes progressive destruction associated with a chronic inflammatory lesion. The sera of these animals contain anti-thyroglobulin autoantibodies. Furthermore, approximately 15% of the sera react with the proventriculus (stomach) of the normal chicken giving a pattern similar to that obtained when the test is carried out with sera from patients with pernicious anaemia who have parietal cell autoantibodies (Fig. 4.16). This example parallels spontaneous human autoimmune thyroid disease in terms of the lesion in the gland, the production of antibodies to different components in the thyroid, and the overlap with gastric autoimmunity. When the immunological status of these animals is altered, quite dramatic effects on the

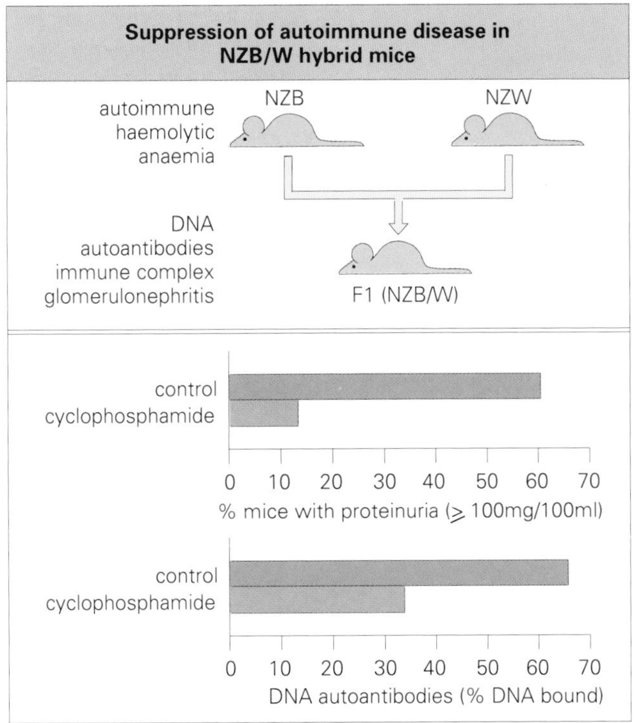

Fig. 4.17 The New Zealand Black (NZB) spontaneously develops autoimmune haemolytic anaemia and when crossed with the New Zealand White (NZW) strain, the F1 develops DNA autoantibodies and immune complex glomerulonephritis like patients with SLE. Immunosuppression with cyclophosphamide (an anti-mitotic agent) considerably reduces the severity of the glomerulonephritis and the amount of DNA autoantibodies, showing the relevance of the immune processes to the generation of the disease.

outcome of the disease are seen. For example, if the bursa of Fabricius is removed soon after hatching, the severity of the thyroiditis is greatly diminished, indicating a role for antibody in the pathogenesis of the disease. Paradoxically, removal of the thymus at birth appears to exacerbate the lesion, suggesting that the thymus exerts a controlling effect on the outcome of the disease.

Murine SLE. Another fascinating animal is the hybrid of the New Zealand Black and White strains of mice, providing a spontaneous model of murine SLE in which immune complex glomerulonephritis and anti-DNA antibodies are major features. What is particularly relevant to our argument is that measures which suppress the immune response in these animals, for example the drug cyclophosphamide, likewise suppress the development of disease and prolong the survival of these mice (Fig. 4.17).

EVIDENCE FROM HUMAN DISEASE

In investigating human autoimmunity, it is of course more difficult to carry out direct experiments, but there is a great deal of evidence which favours the view that the autoantibodies are of importance in the pathogenesis. A number of diseases have been recognized in which there are autoantibodies to hormone receptors which may actually mimic the function of the normal hormone concerned.

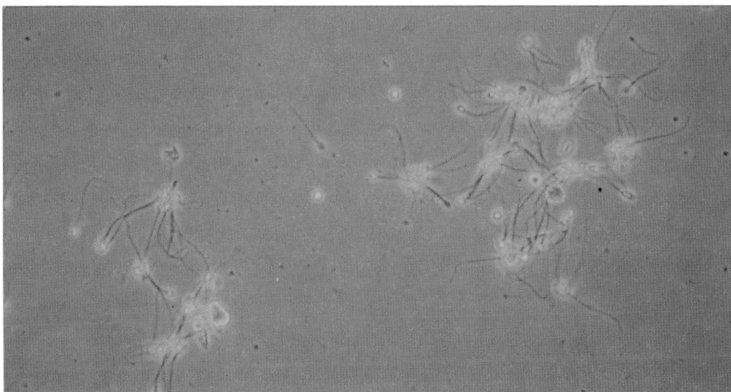

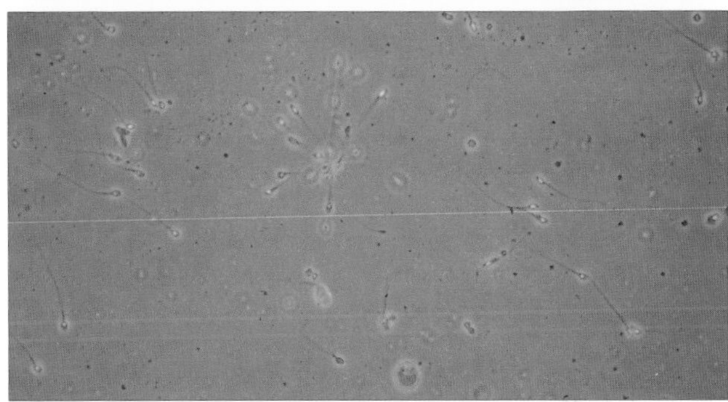

Fig. 4.18 Sperm agglutination. The presence of sperm autoagglutinins produces either head-to-head (upper) or tail-to-tail (lower) agglutination.

Thyrotoxicosis

Thyrotoxicosis was the first disorder in which anti-receptor antibodies were clearly recognized. The phenomenon of neonatal thyrotoxicosis provides us with a 'natural' passive transfer study in which the IgG antibodies from the mother can cross the placenta; if these antibodies are capable of acting *in vivo*, they should stimulate the thyroid of the baby. Indeed, many babies born to thyrotoxic mothers have thyroid hyperactivity. As might be expected, the overactivity of the thyroid spontaneously resolves as the maternally derived thyroid stimulating IgG is catabolized in the baby over several weeks.

Neonatal myasthenia gravis

A similar phenomenon has been observed in neonatal myasthenia gravis, where antibodies to acetylcholine receptors cross the placenta into the fetus and cause transient muscle weakness, due in this case to destruction of the receptors.

Male infertility

Yet another example of disease due to autoantibodies is seen in rare cases of male infertility where antibodies to spermatozoa lead to clumping of spermatozoa, either by their heads or by their tails, (Fig. 4.18).

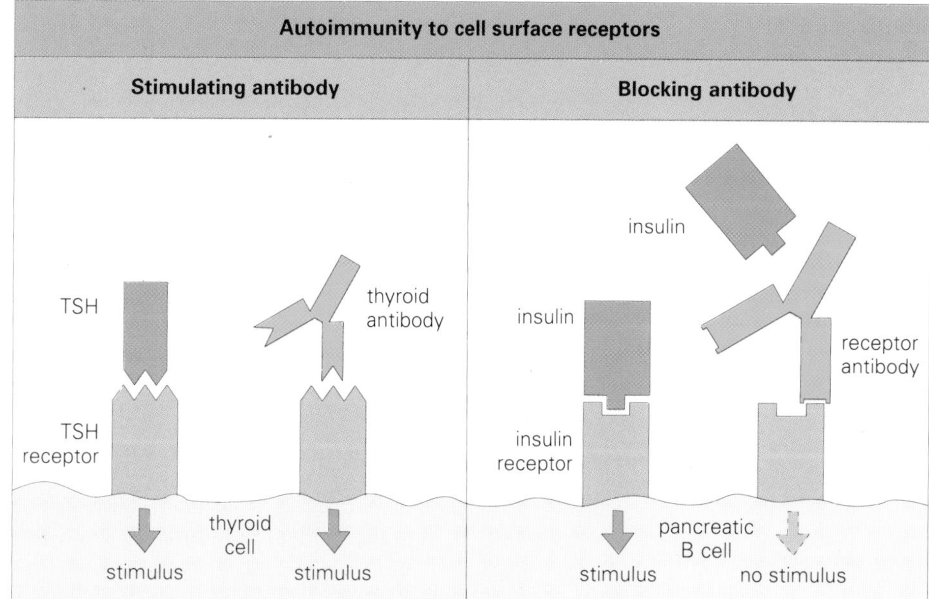

Fig. 4.19 The thyroid cell is stimulated when its receptors for thyroid stimulating hormone (TSH) from the pituitary, bind the hormone. Antibody to the TSH receptor present in the serum of a patient with thyrotoxicosis (Graves' or Basedow's disease) combines with the receptor in a similar fashion to pituitary TSH, thereby delivering a comparable stimulus to the thyroid cell. Antibody to receptors can also block the action of the hormone, as in the insulin resistance of patients with acanthosis nigricans.

Glomerular basement membrane antibodies

In Goodpasture's syndrome, antibodies to the glomerular capillary basement membrane are bound to the kidney *in vivo*. These antibodies were eluted from the kidney of a patient who had died of this disease and transferred to a primate whose renal antigens are similar to those of the human. The injected antibodies localized on the glomerular basement membrane, and the injected monkey subsequently died of glomerulonephritis.

Other autoantibodies

Rarely, autoantibodies to insulin and to β-adrenergic receptors can be found, the latter occurring in a minority of patients with bronchial asthma. These directly block the binding of hormone to its receptor but are not capable of mimicking hormone action unlike the situation in thyrotoxicosis (Fig. 4.19).

The role of antibodies to intrinsic factor in blocking vitamin B_{12} absorption in patients with pernicious anaemia will be discussed in more detail in chapter 10.

Demonstration of cause of disease

Classically, one demonstrates the role of a particular disease-causing entity by transferring it from man to another host to reinduce the original disease (Koch's postulates). Although this is possible for autoantibodies, as shown above, it is not possible to do this with autoreactive T cells since it is not possible to transfer T cells from man to other species. However, the importance of T cells can be inferred from the association of particular MHC haplotypes with autoimmune disease. Also, $CD4^+$ T cells are usually the first lymphocytes to be seen infiltrating sites of tissue damage in organ-specific autoimmune diseases. Furthermore many autoantigens are T-dependent and so the presence of autoantibody implies that autoreactive T cells are also present (except in cases of T cell bypass).

DIAGNOSTIC AND PROGNOSTIC ASPECTS

Whatever the relationship of autoantibodies to the disease process, they undeniably provide valuable markers which can be exploited for diagnostic purposes. In the clinical immunology laboratory of today, tests for a wide range of different autoantibodies are carried out with this end in view. A particularly good example is the test for mitochondrial antibodies for diagnosing primary biliary cirrhosis (see chapter 10). The need for exploratory laparotomy, which was previously necessary to obtain this diagnosis and was often hazardous because of the age and condition of the patients concerned, is consequently avoided.

Autoantibodies may also have a predictive value (see Fig. 4.11). In this example, a child related to siblings with insulin dependent diabetes mellitus shared an HLA haplotype with them, developed complement fixing antibodies to the islet cells of the pancreas, and within three years after the study had begun had become frankly diabetic. This illustrates the predictive value of these antibodies and the time lag before the disease becomes overt.

TREATMENT

Metabolic control. Conventionally, in organ-specific disorders, the lesion can often be corrected by metabolic control. For example, in hypothyroidism the lack of thyroid hormone can be controlled by administration of thyroxine, while in thyrotoxicosis, anti-thyroid drugs are normally prescribed. In pernicious anaemia, metabolic correction is achieved by injection of depot vitamin B_{12}, and in myasthenia gravis, by adminstration of cholinesterase inhibitors.

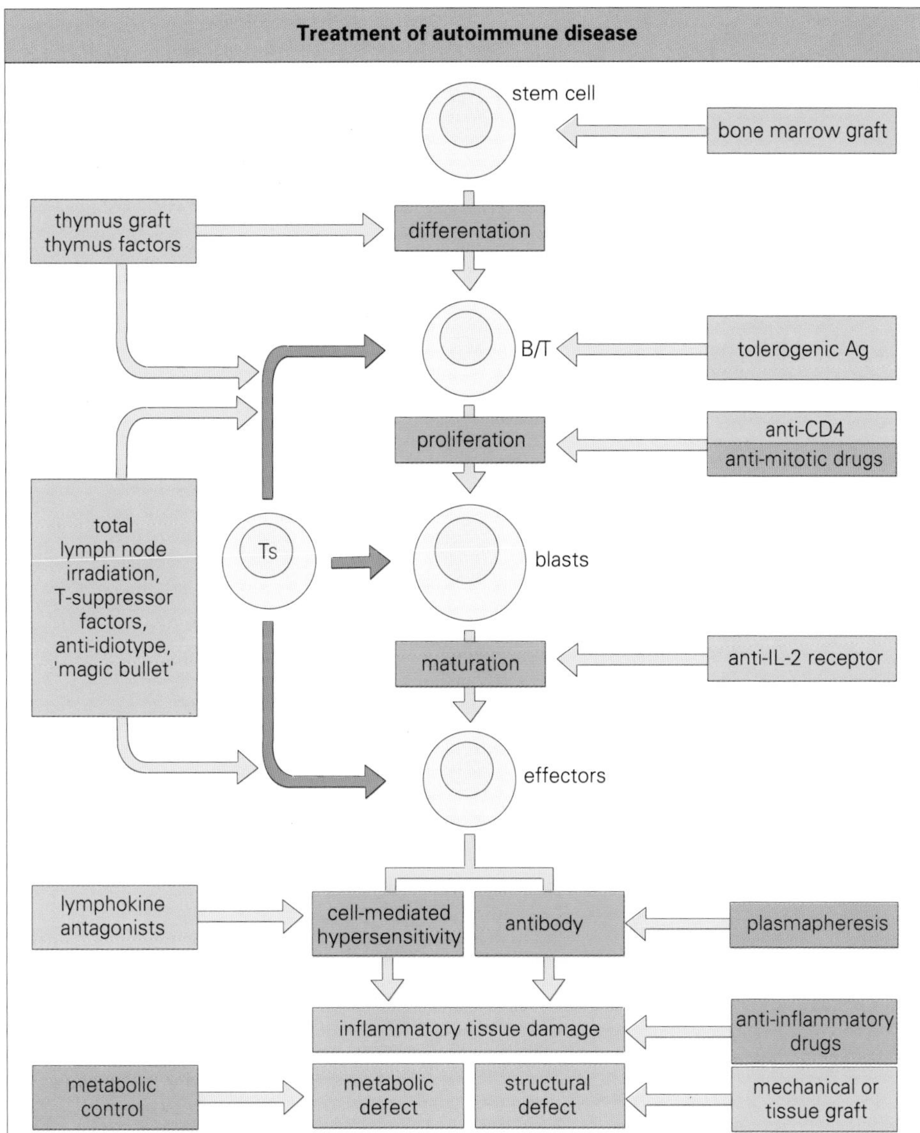

Fig. 4.20 Current treatments for arresting the pathological developments in autoimmune disease are shown in mauve, and those that may become feasible, in turquoise. For example, anti-mitotic drugs are given in severe cases of systemic lupus erythematosus or chronic active hepatitis. Organ-specific disorders which lead to a metabolic defect, for example primary myxoedema or pernicious anaemia, can usually be treated by supplying the defective component; in these examples, thyroid hormone and depot vitamin B_{12}. Where a live graft becomes necessary, the immunosuppressive therapy used may protect the tissue from autoimmune damage.

Grafts. Where function is lost and cannot be substituted by hormones, as may occur in lupus nephritis or chronic rheumatoid arthritis, mechanical or tissue grafts may be appropriate, although in the case of tissue grafts, protection from the immunological processes which originally necessitated the transplant may be required.

Immunosuppressive drugs. Conventional immunosuppressive therapy with anti-mitotic drugs may be employed to damp down the immune response, but because of the dangers involved, this tends to be used only in life-threatening disorders such as myasthenia gravis, SLE and dermatomyositis. The potential of cyclosporin and possible derivatives in the therapy of autoimmune disease has yet to be fully realized, but quite dramatic results have been reported in the treatment of type I diabetes mellitus. Anti-inflammatory drugs are, of course, prescribed for rheumatoid disease.

Immunological manipulation. As we understand more about the precise defects in different autoimmune diseases and learn how to manipulate the immunological status of the patient, a number of the less well established approaches may become practical (Fig. 4.20). In particular, the successful treatment of experimental autoimmune disease by 'vaccination' with antigen-specific T cell clones suggests that elimination of clones of potentially autoreactive cells with a particular type of T cell receptor could prove to be promising approach. The ability of anti-CD4 to make anergic T cells which are undergoing stimulation by antigen provides the basis for yet another potentially successful strategy, and encourages the view that autoimmune disease will ultimately prove vulnerable to our attempts at control.

FURTHER READING

McGregor AM, ed. *Immunology of endocrine diseases.* Lancaster: MTP Press, 1986.

Morrow J, Isenberg DA. *Autoimmune rheumatic disease.* Oxford: Blackwell Scientific Publications, 1987.

Schoenfeld Y, Isenberg DA. *The mosaic of autoimmunity: the factors associated with autoimmune disease.* Amsterdam: Elsevier, 1989.

Thompson RA, series ed. *Recent advances in clinical immunology.* Edinburgh: Churchill-Livingstone.

5

Rheumatoid Arthritis & Other Joint Diseases

RHEUMATOID ARTHRITIS

CLINICAL AND PATHOLOGICAL FEATURES

Rheumatoid arthritis (RA) is an inflammatory disease of the synovium which results in erosion, deformity and destruction of joints (Fig. 5.1). It occurs predominantly in women (with a male to female ratio of 1:3) in young adult life or middle age, although it has been recorded in people of all ages. The prevalence has been estimated to be around 1–3% of the population.

The disease characteristically starts in the small joints of the hands and feet, the metacarpophalangeal (knuckle) joints often being the first to be affected. In the early stages of the disease the main symptoms are of pain and swelling of the affected joints (Fig. 5.2) associated with restricted movement, particularly after periods of immobility; this leads to the characteristic symptom of early morning stiffness. Involvement of other more proximal joints then follows, usually with symmetrical distribution. Although disease in the spine is frequent in post-mortem studies it rarely gives rise to clinical symptoms, except when erosion of the upper odontoid peg in the cervical spine leads to dislocation of the neck and spinal cord compression.

Inflammation of the joints is associated with a villous hypertrophy of the synovial membrane (Fig. 5.3), which

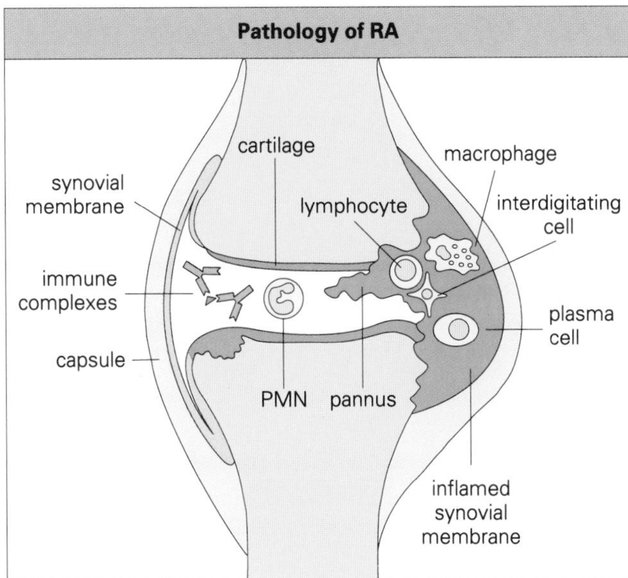

Fig. 5.1 In rheumatoid arthritis an inflammatory infiltrate is found in the synovial membrane which hypertrophies, covering and eventually eroding the synovial cartilage and bone. Immune complexes and polymorphonuclear leucocytes are detectable in the joint space.

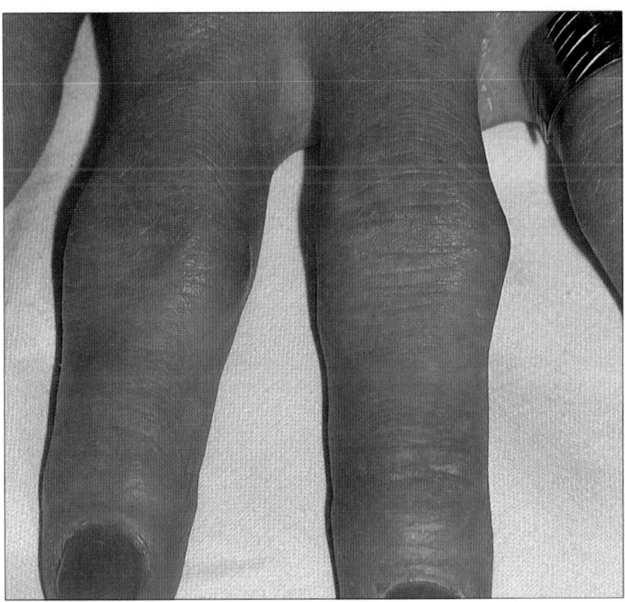

Fig. 5.2 Patient with early RA. At this stage there is swelling and tenderness of the metacarpophalangeal (MCP) joints and the proximal interphalangeal joints.

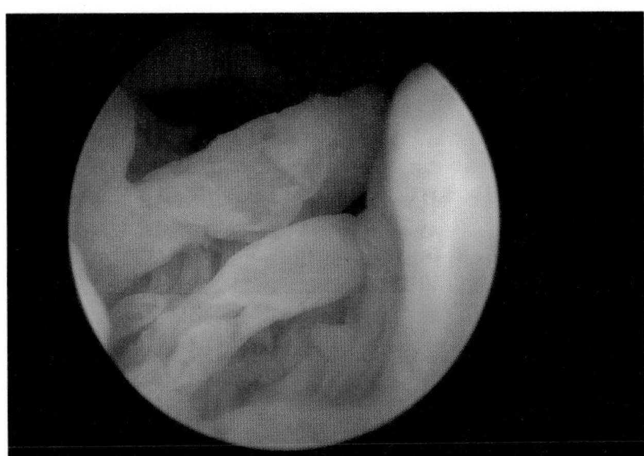

Fig. 5.3 Villous hypertrophy. Arthroscopic view of the synovial membrane in the knee of a patient with rheumatoid arthritis showing oedematous synovial villi.

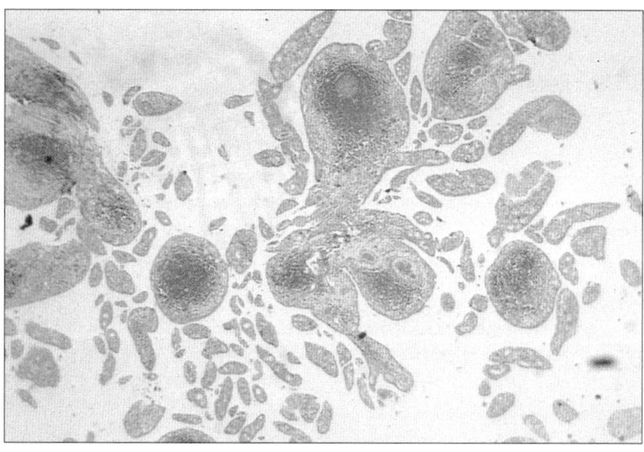

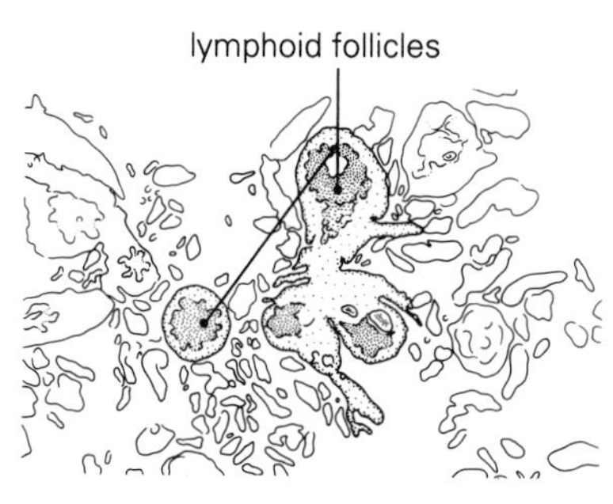

Fig. 5.4 Section of synovial membrane showing marked villous hypertrophy with cellular infiltration and aggregates organized into lymphoid follicles. H & E stain. Courtesy of Professor N. Woolf.

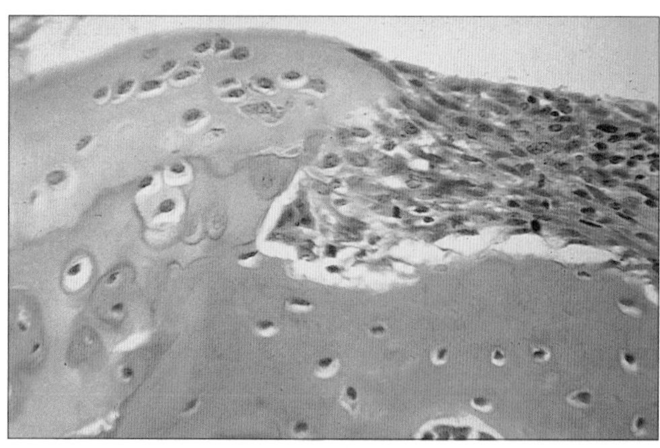

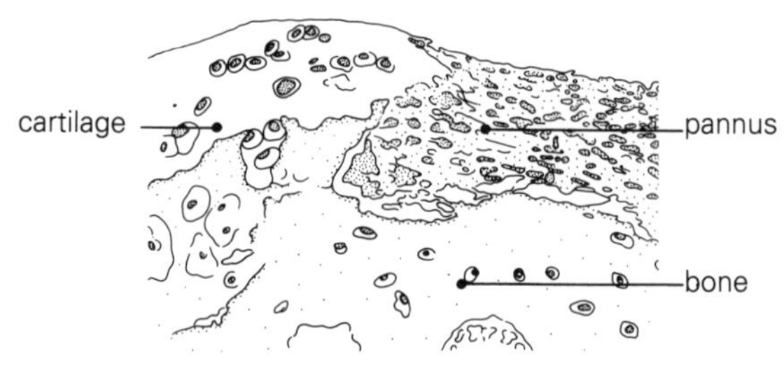

Fig. 5.5 Histology of pannus, seen as a layer of lymphocytes, macrophages and plasma cells overlying and eroding the cartilage. Note the tissue destruction at the pannus margin The layer below the cartilage is bone. H & E stain.

on microscopy shows proliferation of the lining layer with an inflammatory infiltrate. In some cases, invading lymphocytes become organized into lymphoid follicles, so called because their structure resembles that of lymph nodes (Fig. 5.4).

In terms of morbidity, the most important feature of rheumatoid arthritis is joint erosion which leads to deformity and, in some cases, severe disability. This destruction begins as a vasculitis associated with increased capillary permeability, oedema and inflammatory cell infiltrates in the affected joint. The synovial tissue becomes hypertrophied with finger-like processes and granulation tissue which extends into the cartilaginous areas as pannus (Fig. 5.5). It is thought that secretions by polymorphs and activated macrophages within the pannus cause erosion of cartilage and bone.

There is extensive expression of HLA-DR on T cells, B cells and synovial lining cells, indicating strong immunological activity. As a result of this, the synovial fluid contains immune complexes, cells and complement breakdown products. Immunofluorescence shows immune complexes in the dilated small vessels of the joint, suggesting a type III hypersensitivity, and cells producing rheumatoid factor in the synovium of the joint itself — a sign of ongoing inflammation.

These changes are first seen on X-rays as narrowing of the normal radiological space between the bones (due to loss of cartilage) and erosions (Fig. 5.6). Tendons and the joint capsule may also be involved, leading to disintegration of the whole structure of the joint and development of characteristic deformities associated with the disease (Fig. 5.7).

Extra-articular disease

About one-third of patients with RA attending hospital have systemic or extra-articular manifestations of the disease. These complications can be divided into three different pathological processes:

- fibrosing alveolitis, which presents as pulmonary interstitial inflammation and oedema, leading to fibrosis;
- vasculitis of the skin (infarcts/ulcers), nerves (neuropathy), and eyes (scleritis);
- granuloma formation, which appears as focal necrosis with surrounding macrophages and lymphocytes.

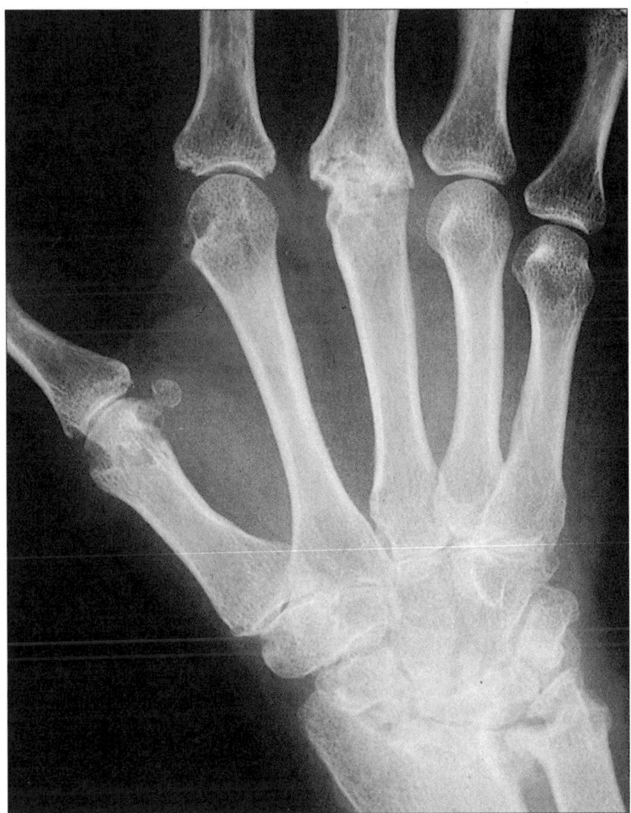

Fig. 5.6 X-ray of a hand from a patient with RA showing narrowing of the joint spaces with complete loss of joint space in the MCP joint of the middle finger. Erosions are seen as small 'bites' into the joint margins, which in this case are most obvious in the MCP joint of the thumb.

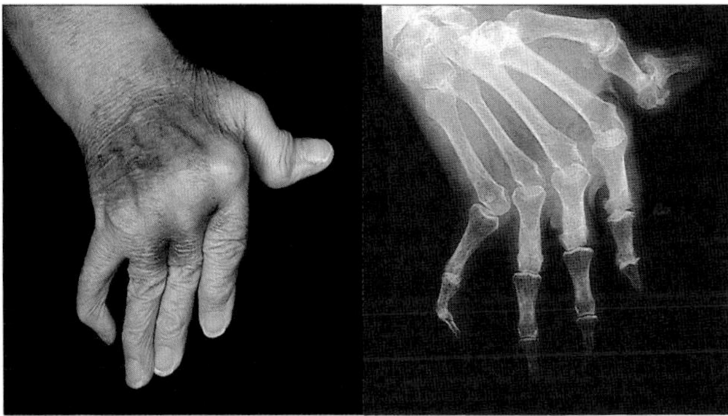

Fig. 5.7 Ulnar deviation in the hand of a patient with advanced RA, showing destruction of the ligaments around the joints which has resulted in dislocation of the MCP joints towards the ulnar side of the hand.

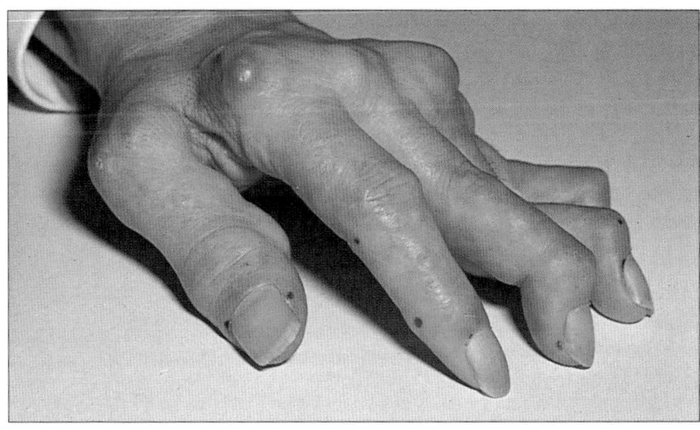

Fig. 5.8 Digital infarcts due to vasculitis in a patient with RA. Some infarcts are typically seen around the edge of the nails (peri-ungual infarcts). This patient has a second extra-articular manifestation, namely a nodule on the dorsal surface of the MCP joint of the index finger.

Extra-articular RA is almost always associated with a bad prognosis. Subcutaneous nodules, although of no more than nuisance value in themselves, are correlated with severe joint disease. Vasculitis also has serious prognostic implications. When detected as digital infarcts (Fig. 5.8), vasculitis is regarded as being part of a syndrome which has been called malignant rheumatoid arthritis. Felty's syndrome, in which vasculitis is a frequent feature, is defined as a combination of rheumatoid arthritis, lymphoid hyperplasia (lymphadenopathy or hepatosplenomegaly) and leucopenia. Fibrosing alveolitis (Fig. 5.9) is more common in men than women. It is not necessarily associated with severe joint disease but has a bad prognosis, with some estimates suggesting a five-year mortality of 50% from the time of diagnosis.

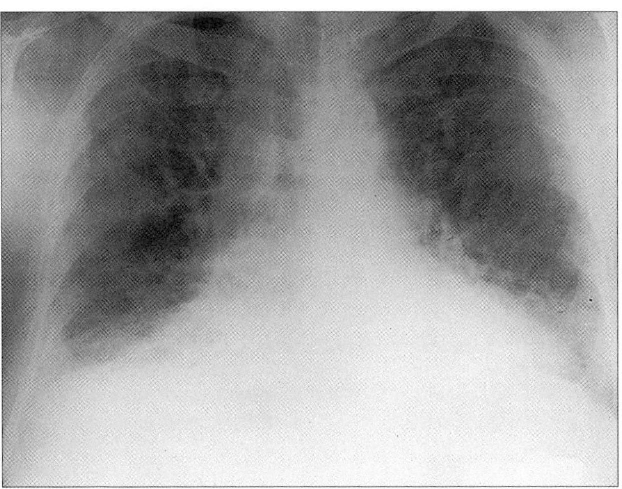

Fig. 5.9 X-ray of a patient with advanced fibrosing alveoltitis. There is increased shadowing (seen as pale, X-ray dense markings) in both lung fields, which would normally be nearly black. The shadowing indicates the presence of extensive inflammation and/or fibrosis.

AETIOLOGY OF RA

Like most autoimmune diseases, rheumatoid arthritis is thought to be caused by an interaction between constitutional and environmental factors. The autoantibodies form immune complexes, causing inflammation which, in the case of RA, is localized predominantly in the joint. The exaggerated inflammatory response includes the production of degradative enzymes which cause the destruction characteristic of the disease. The extra-articular features may be attributed to the same phenomenon occurring outside the joints.

Hormonal factors

The importance of hormones may be summarized as follows:

- RA is three times more common in women than men;
- the onset is usually after the menarche and before the menopause;
- the disease improves with pregnancy;
- there is a response to treatment with androgens.

Genetic factors

There is a tendency for RA to run in families. Many cases occur without a family history and these are known as 'sporadic RA'. Both forms of RA are associated with HLA-DR4 and, to a lesser extent, -DR1 (Fig. 5.10).

Class I (HLA-A and -B) and class III (complement allotype) antigens show less association with RA than class II. The frequency of B62 is increased, but this is probably because it is in linkage disequilibrium with DR4. There is also a complement gene, defined by a 30 kilobase DNA fragment (C4b 30), which is found in about 10% of cases of RA but very rarely in the general population.

Infectious agents

Many accept that autoimmunity in RA is triggered by a foreign antigen, usually microbial, in a genetically susceptible host. Studies performed over the last 40 years have suggested a variety of different agents, both viral and bacterial (Fig. 5.11).

Assumptions of causation are based either on claims that the organism has been isolated from a joint, or that patients with rheumatoid arthritis have been found to have an abnormal immune response to a particular agent. Data using either approach must be interpreted with caution. Many of the isolates can be attributed to the fact that the organism is part of the traffic through the joint rather than the cause of the inflammation. This may explain reports of diphtheroids and rubella in rheumatoid synovial membranes. Alternatively, as is probably the case with mycoplasma, contamination of cell lines grown *in vitro* may account for some claims in the literature.

Abnormal immune responses to several viruses and bacteria have been reported in RA. For example, titres of antibodies to Epstein-Barr virus (EBV) are elevated, although epidemiological studies have not supported an aetiological role. It is now thought that the high titres of antibodies to EBV antigens are due to defective T cell control of EBV infected B cells; in other words, the disease affects the immune response to the virus rather than vice versa. Similar mechanisms could account for abnormal serological findings relating to other infectious agents.

DR genes associated with RA

DR gene	Disease association	Disease subset
DR4	strong (RR ~6)	severe disease (Felty's syndrome) +ve rheumatoid factor
DR1	weak (RR ~2) (RR>2 in Jews, Indians & Spanish)	? fibrosing alveolitis seronegative RA
DR3	negative (?protective)	hypersensitivity to gold & penicillamine
DR2	negative (? protective)	mild disease

Fig. 5.10 DR4 occurs in over 90% of patients with Felty's syndrome, and could be regarded as a disease severity gene rather than a susceptibility gene. Both DR2 and DR3 appear to have modifying effects. RR = relative risk.

Microbial agents associated with RA

	High antibody titre	Organism in joint	Arthritogenic
Viruses			
rubella	+	+	++
EB virus	+	–	±
parvovirus	–	±*	++
Mycoplasma	–	+	+
Bacteria			
Proteus	–	–	+
mycobacteria	+	–**	–

* *a parvovirus-like agent has been identified*
** *cross-reactions between mycobacteria & proteoglycans have been described*

Fig. 5.11 Microbial agents associated with rheumatoid arthritis.

Animal models

Animal models may also give insight into aetiological or pathogenic mechanisms (Fig. 5.12), although no one model can be taken to reflect all stages in the pathogenesis of RA. The Glynn-Dumonde and collagen arthritis models demonstrate that localization of antigen to the joint is important in causing arthritis. In the former model antigen is injected into the joint and in the latter it is there already as one of the constituents of cartilage and other tissues. In the adjuvant model, joint inflammation may occur because of cross-reactivity between cartilage and mycobacterial antigens (recently demonstrated with T cell clones). The other models indicate that antigens could be ingested in the diet: in both the streptococcal cell wall and the Coombs' models the ingested antigens have been demonstrated within the synovium.

Spontaneously occurring diseases in animals are sometimes cited as models of RA. An example of this, an inbred mouse strain termed the MRL/lpr, develops an erosive arthritis associated with rheumatoid factors. However in colonies now being bred in this country, the arthritis appears to be mild and the most prominent features are those of systemic lupus erythematosus with disseminated vasculitis and nephritis associated with anti-nuclear antibodies.

Dogs also suffer from an erosive arthritis which is said to be associated with rheumatoid factors. However, the cause is unknown and no inbred strain suffering from RA-like disease has been developed. The usefulness of the dog is therefore limited as a potential model of RA.

The closest animal model of rheumatoid arthritis is the disease caused by the caprine arthritis-encephalitis virus; this is a lentivirus similar to the human immunodeficiency (AIDS) virus, which infects both macrophages and $CD4^+$ lymphocytes. It causes encephalitis and interstitial pneumonitis in both goats and sheep, and can also cause an erosive, destructive arthritis which is histologically similar to human RA.

Animal models of RA
Induced
Glynn-Dumonde Immunization with bovine immunoglobulin followed by injection into the joint.
Collagen type II Immunization with collagen type II in Freund's adjuvant.
Streptococcal cell wall Either in the diet or as intraperitoneal injections. Streptococcal antigens have been detected in the joint.
Milk diet in Old English rabbits 25% develop arthritis and antibodies to milk proteins (= Coombs' model).
Spontaneous
MRL/lpr mouse Also develops vasculitis, glomerulonephritis.
Lentivirus Caprine arthritis-encephalitis virus.

Fig. 5.12 Animal models of RA.

Diet and arthritis

The Coombs' model, and an earlier report that pigs fed on fish meal developed arthritis, suggests that diet alone can cause arthritis. In the case of the pigs, there is good evidence that synovitis is related to the presence of *Clostridia* in the intestine. It is possible that a similar alteration in bowel flora could cause arthritis in milk-fed rabbits. Arthritis also occasionally occurs in man after intestinal bypass operations when there is overgrowth of bacteria in loops of isolated intestine. In this case the disease process is not chronic or destructive like RA, but is more like a reactive arthritis.

There have been a number of studies on the effect of diet in the treatment of RA. These fall into two categories: those involving an increase in the polyunsaturated to saturated fat ratio, and those in which certain foods or food families are removed. The rationale behind the former is the production from eicosapentenoic acid of E3 prostaglandins and leukotrienes, which are significantly less inflammatory than those of the E2 series produced from the breakdown of arachidonic acid.

Although such diets have proved effective in inhibiting the development of adjuvant arthritis in rats and in delaying the onset of autoimmune nephritis in NZB x NZW F1 mice, no significant effect has yet been shown in man. A possible long-term adverse effect is increased neoplasia, which has been noted in rats fed a diet high in polyunsaturated fats.

Food allergy can cause arthritis, but this is normally associated with urticaria. Fasting has shown beneficial effects in RA, including:

- ↓ sympathomimetic activity
- ↓ acute phase proteins
- ↓ intestinal permeability
- ↓ mononuclear phagocyte function
- ↑ neutrophil bactericidal activity
- short-term objective and subjective improvement in joint disease

It has proved more difficult to identify particular foods which exacerbate the disease in individual patients, however recent double blind studies do suggest that this can occur.

Further controlled studies are necessary to evaluate the long-term effects of diet in RA and to assess the proportion of patients who are diet-responsive, together with a means of identification.

PATHOLOGY AND IMMUNOHISTOLOGY OF THE JOINT

The main areas of pathology within the joint can be divided into two parts: the synovial membrane and synovial fluid. For immunological studies the blood may be considered as a third (systemic) compartment (Fig. 5.13). One of the earliest changes within the joint is the proliferation of lining layer cells of the synovium, which becomes up to five cells thick rather than the 1–2 cell layers seen in normal joints. In the sub-membrane area there is proliferation of vascular endothelial cells with perivascular infiltrates of polymorphs and lymphocytes.

These aggregates may develop into the lymphoid follicles seen in some patients with more established disease. B cells are rarely seen in the synovium but when they do occur, it is usually near the centre, close to a blood vessel. Most of the cells within the aggregates are T cells, with dendritic cells tightly packed in between; outside the aggregates, the cell population is more mixed, with polymorphs, macrophages and plasma cells. The most important feature of this heterogeneous collection is that they represent all of the essential elements for a continuing immune response (see Fig. 5.17).

Synoviocytes and macrophages

Originally, two cell types in the lining layer were described and termed type A and B synoviocytes. With more advanced immunohistochemical techniques, three cell types are now recognized:

- a fibroblast-like cell of mesechymal origin, formerly called the type A synoviocyte;
- a monocyte-like cell, thought to be bone marrow derived, with cytoplasm rich in lysosomal enzymes and cell surface antigens which include class II, and both Fc and complement receptors;
- a non-phagocytic cell lacking most of the surface markers of monoctyes but strongly class II positive. These are thought to be from the same cell population as the dendritic cell of the sub-synovium or the veiled cell in the synovial fluid.

These last two correspond to the type B synoviocyte.

Cells of the monocyte-macrophage lineage have a central role in the pathogenesis of rheumatoid arthritis. Firstly, their presence as class II positive cells suggests that they

Cell types in blood & synovium in RA					
	T cells	B cells	CD4: CD8 ratio	DR +ve T cells	CD5 +ve B cells
blood	N	N	N	↑	↑
synovial fluid	↑	↓	↓	↑↑	?
membrane	↑	↓	↑	↑↑	?

5.6 **Fig. 5.13** Cell types in blood and synovium in RA.

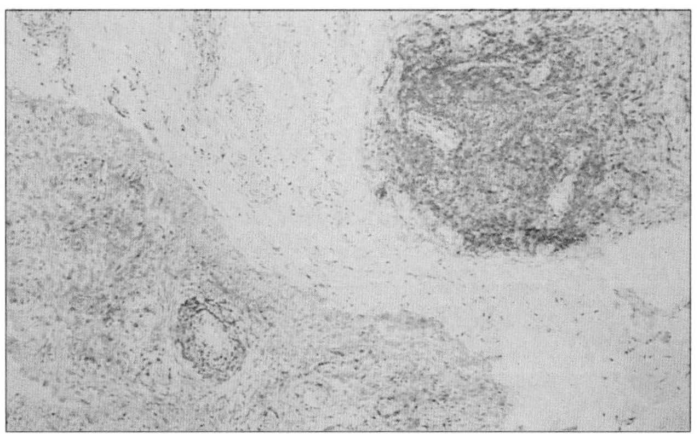

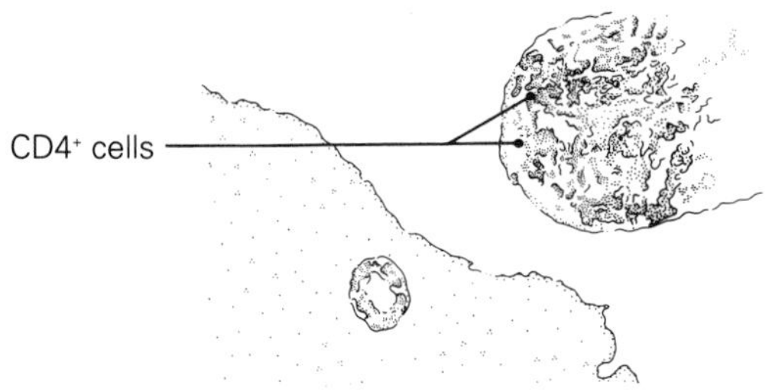

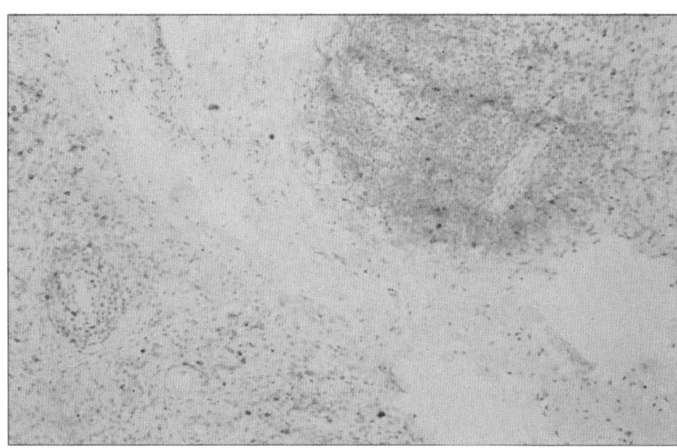

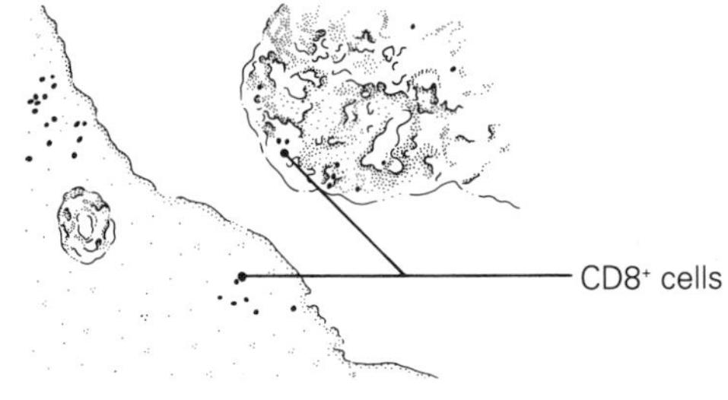

Fig. 5.14 Immunoperoxidase staining of RA synovial membrane. Upper: $CD4^+$ (helper) lymphocytes comprise the majority of cells within the aggregates. Lower: $CD8^+$ lymphocytes are scattered around the edge of the aggregates and within the inter-aggregate areas.

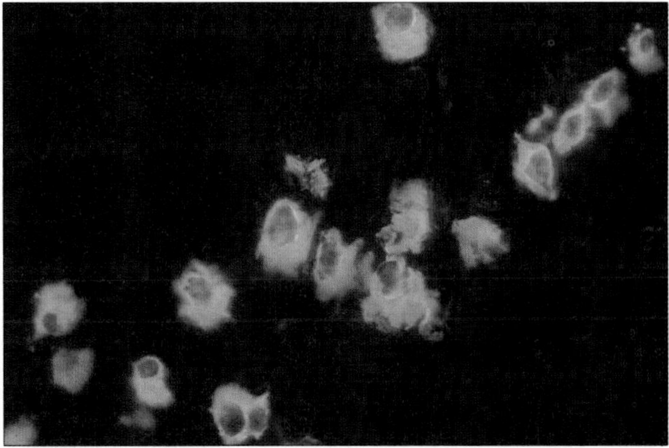

Fig. 5.15 Plasma cells in the synovium are visualized as cells with strong cytoplasmic immunofluorescence, detected by fluorescein conjugated anti-human IgM.

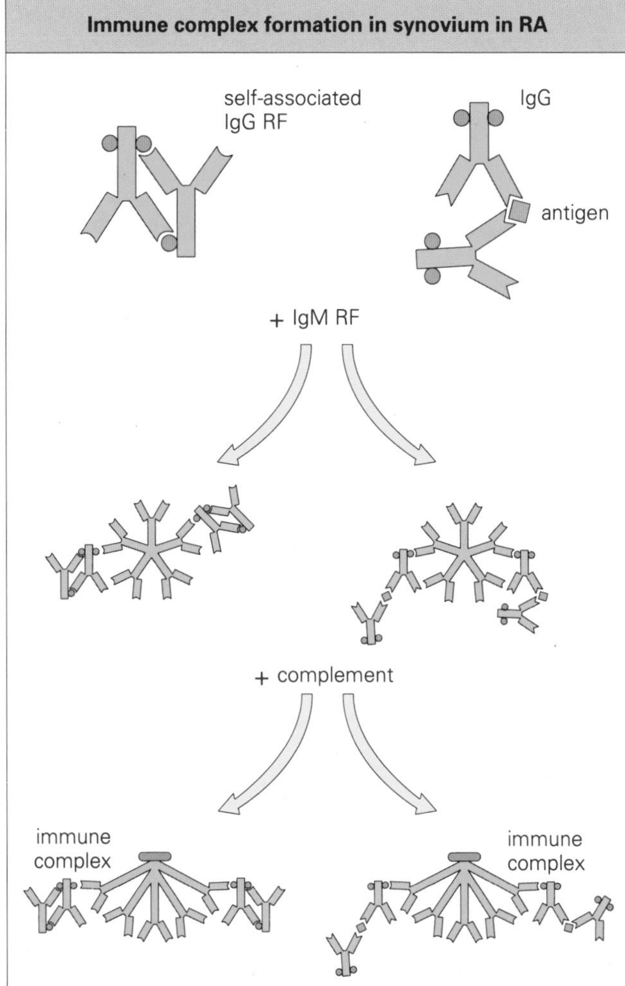

Fig. 5.16 The starting point for immune complex formation may be self-associated IgG — IgG rheumatoid factors (RF) — or IgG antibodies to an unknown antigen(s). In both cases the IgG then binds to IgM rheumatoid factor which fixes complement, thus producing an immune complex.

may be presenting the unknown antigen that initiates inflammation. Secondly, they are the predominant cell at the edge of the synovium where it is apparently eroding cartilage and bone (the cartilage–pannus junction). Most of the enzymes which cause this erosion appear to be macrophage-derived.

T cells

The majority of T cells in the synovium carry the CD4 (helper/inducer phenotype) and express class II antigens, indicating that they are activated. The CD4: CD8 ratio in the synovial membrane is increased, with estimates varying from 4:1 to 14:1. Within cellular aggregates almost every cell is $CD4^+$, and attached to or near dendritic cells (Fig. 5.14 upper). The $CD8^+$ (suppressor/cytotoxic) cells are thinly scattered and are usually found in small groups round the periphery of the aggregates (Fig. 5.14 lower).

By contrast, T cells in the synovial fluid are mostly $CD8^+$. The reason for this is unknown, but one explanation is that $CD8^+$ cells, being class II negative, are less 'sticky' than $CD4^+$ cells and migrate freely through the membrane into the synovial fluid, whereas $CD4^+$ cells are held up in the aggregates.

B cells

B cells are thinly scattered throughout the membrane, being found mainly in the centre of aggregates or around small blood vessels. They are normally class II positive but in the joint the density of expression is increased suggesting that, like T cells, they are also activated. Plasma cells, the terminal differentiation phase of B cells, are plentiful and are found dispersed through the synovium. This suggests that, having entered the joint via the blood vessels, B cells rapidly differentiate into plasma cells under the influence of the high concentration of B cell growth factors produced by the plentiful T cells within the joint.

The cytoplasm of plasma cells contains IgG, IgA and IgM (Fig. 5.15), much of which has rheumatoid factor activity. It has been suggested that IgG rheumatoid factors tend to react with themselves ('self-associate') and, either on their own or in combination with complement and IgM rheumatoid factors, form immune complexes (Fig. 5.16).

Polymorphs

Polymorphs are found within blood vessels, adhering to the vascular endothelium, in the perivascular infiltrate and in the synovial fluid, where they can account for over 50% of the cells present. Like B cells, they are infrequent in the synovial membrane, except in the vicinity of blood vessels and immediately under the surface. This suggests that they localize to the joint by sticking to endothelium and move rapidly through the membrane into the synovial fluid. Polymorphs have Fc and C3 receptors and, like macrophages, phagocytose immune complexes with the release of proteolytic enzymes. Neutrophils contribute further to inflammation by producing free oxygen radicals, which in turn are extremely cytotoxic and potent stimulators of the prostaglandin and leukotriene pathways.

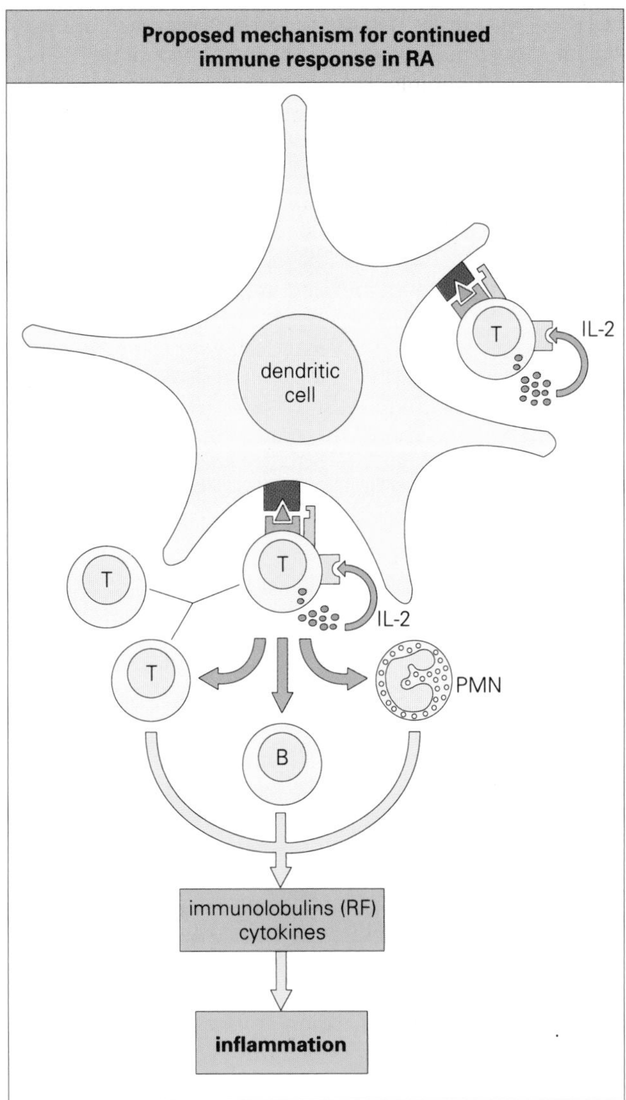

Fig. 5.17 Dendritic cells within aggregates present antigen to surrounding T cells (CD4+). The IL-2 produced by activated CD4+ cells promotes cell division as well as recruiting other inflammatory cells. This process occurs in the absence of control by CD8+ cells, which may be ineffective due to their relative distance away at the edge of the aggregates. This lack of control explains how the immune response in RA might self-perpetuate.

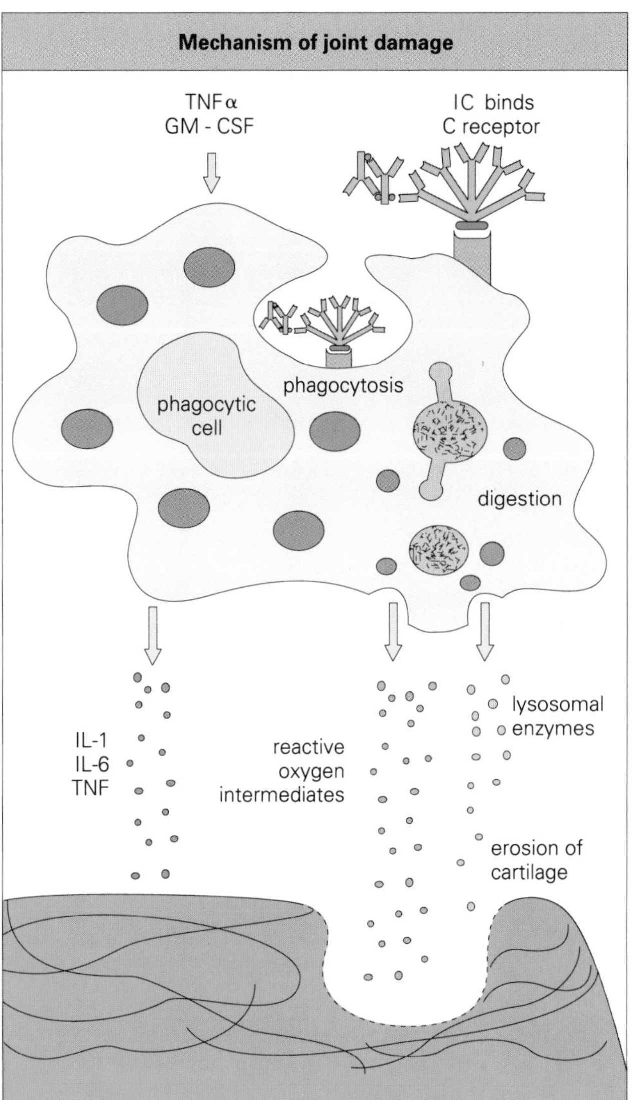

Fig. 5.18 Macrophages are activated by T cell-derived TNFα and GM-CSF and by the phagocytosis of immune complexes (ICs) containing rheumatoid factors and complement which bind to complement and Fc receptors. The cells release lysosomal enzymes, including collagenases, and reactive O_2 intermediates which cause erosion of cartilage and bone, a process further exacerbated by IL-1 and TNF mediated activation of chondrocytes and osteoclasts.

Cytokines

The activated T cells in the rheumatoid synovium secrete GM-CSF and high levels of TNFα, which stimulate the macrophages to produce further TNFα, IL-1 and IL-6. Earlier reports that IL-2 was deficient or absent are now being challenged and it is postulated that apparently low levels may be due to the masking effect of inhibitors or to excessive uptake by IL-2 receptors. Unexpectedlly, there is very little IFNα or TNFβ (lymphotoxin) despite abundant cellular mRNA; this is perhaps an inhibitory effect of transforming growth factor (TGF), another of the T cell lymphokines present in the joint.

Pathogenesis of joint damage

The immunopathology outlined above gives some idea of the mechanisms of joint damage. The antigen (still unknown) is presented by class II positive cells to $CD4^+$ lymphocytes (Fig. 5.17). These are activated and produce lymphokines which recruit more $CD4^+$ cells, B cells and polymorphs and stimulate macrophages. At the same time

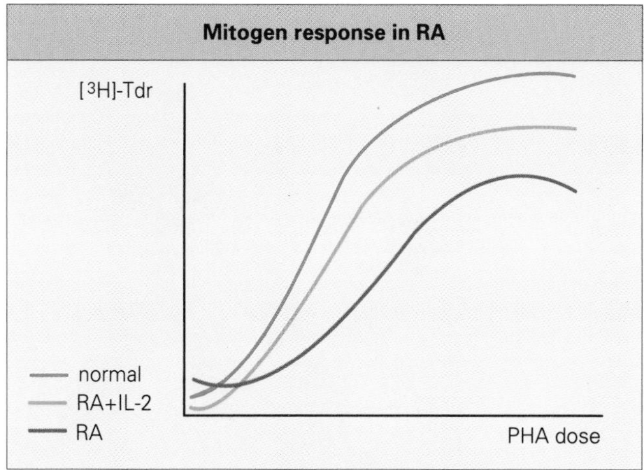

Fig. 5.19 After 3 days' culture in the presence of phytohaemagglutinin (PHA) peripheral blood mononuclear cells (PBMs) from both a patient with RA and a normal, healthy subject have responded in a dose-dependent manner. The RA patient has shown a lesser response, although this is partially restored by the addition of IL-2.

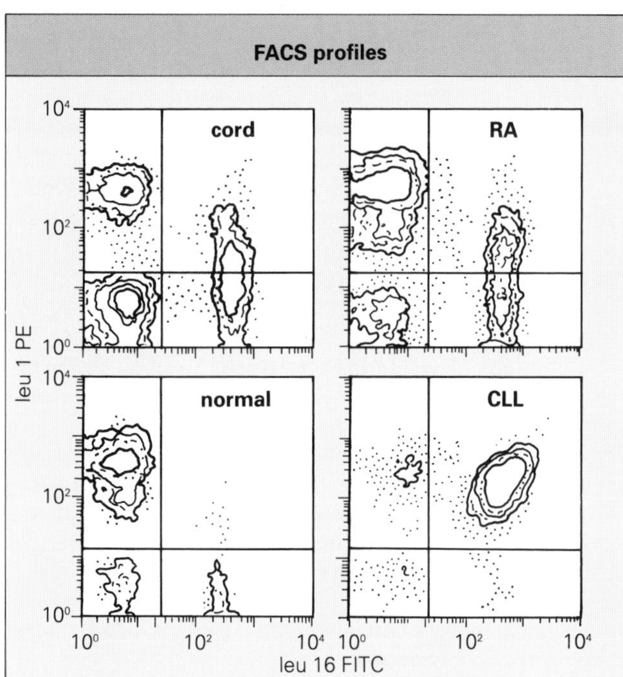

Fig. 5.20 Measurement of CD5+ B cells in lymphocytes from cord blood, from a patient with RA, from a healthy subject and from a patient with chronic lymphocytic leukaemia (CLL). The CD5 antigen is stained with Leu 1 antibody conjugated to phycoerythrin (PE); other B cells are stained with Leu 16 conjugated to fluorescein isothiocyanate (FITC). CD5+ B cells are seen in the top right hand panel of each profile. Almost all of the CLL B Cells are CD5+, and about 50% of the B cells from the cord blood and from the patient with RA are CD5 positive. Very few B cells from the normal control bear the CD5 marker. Courtesy of Dr Christine Plater-Zyberk, Kennedy Institute.

B cell growth factors cause the rapid maturation of B cells to plasma cells. These secrete rheumatoid factors which form immune complexes; these in turn are phagocytosed by macrophages and polymorphs, leading to further activation. The ensuing release of lysosomal enzymes and formation of reactive oxygen intermediates such as superoxide anion, hydroxyl radicals and hydrogen peroxide, produce erosion and destruction of cartilage and bone (Fig. 5.18). Release of IL-1 and TNF also causes direct damage to the joint by activating chondrocytes and osteoclasts as well as recruiting other inflammatory cells.

IMMUNOPATHOLOGY OF CELLS IN THE BLOOD

Although RA is primarily a disease of the joints, lymphoid cells in blood have been studied more than those in the synovial membrane. There are two reasons for this: firstly, the concept that RA is a systemic disease characterized by arthritis justifies the use of blood rather than joint cells; secondly, blood mononuclear cells are more easily obtained, separated and purified into their sub-populations.

T cells

The ratio of CD4+ to CD8+ cells in the blood of patients with RA is normal. Class II antigens, not usually expressed on circulating T cells, have been reported on 15% of T cells from RA patients. It is possible that these cells come from the joint, where the majority are class II positive or they may reflect stimulation in the blood as well as in the synovium. In contrast to the activation indicated by the high proportion of class II positive cells, peripheral blood mononuclear cells from RA patients respond poorly to mitogens in terms of thymidine uptake (Fig. 5.19). The response is increased by the addition of IL-2, indicating a functional deficiency in this cytokine. Another interpretation is that the T cells are already maximally stimulated as a result of the disease process and mitogens therefore have little additional effect.

B cells

Like the T cells and their subsets, B cell numbers are also normal in the peripheral blood from RA patients. However the B cell subset bearing the T cell antigen CD5 has been found to be increased (Fig. 5.20). This cell is of interest not only because it might indicate a specific B cell defect but also because a similar cell in autoimmune mice, the Ly-1 B cell, has been shown to secrete autoantibodies. CD5+ B cells are also found in fetal blood and in the blood of patients suffering from chronic lymphocytic leukaemia. This suggests that the cell is at an early stage of development and raises the intriguing possibility that there may be common mechanisms in the aetiopathogenesis of RA and certain lymphoid malignancies.

Also by analogy with T cells, B cells in RA show evidence of increased activation in culture. Unstimulated RA B cells spontaneously secrete immunoglobulin and rheumatoid factors, whereas cells from healthy donors

Autoantibodies in RA
anti-immunoglobulins anti-Fc (rheumatoid factors) anti-Fab anti-F(ab')$_2$ **antibodies to cellular antigens** anti-histones anti-single-stranded DNA antibodies to intermediate filaments antibodies to RA nuclear antigen **anti-collagen antibodies**

Fig. 5.21 Autoantibodies in rheumatoid arthritis.

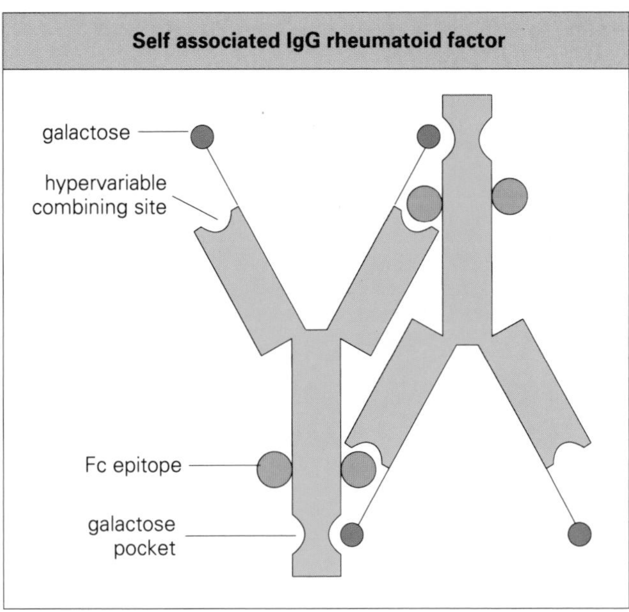

Fig. 5.22 IgG rheumatoid factor may self associate more avidly due to a galactose 'pocket' in the Fc region.

will only do so if stimulated with a B cell mitogen such as pokeweed mitogen or Epstein-Barr virus. Whether the immunoglobulin secreting cells in RA are from the $CD5^+$ B cell lineage remains unknown.

AUTOANTIBODIES AND IMMUNE COMPLEXES IN RA

Rheumatoid factors

The concept that RA is an autoimmune disease is supported by the variety of autoantibodies found in patients' serum (Fig. 5.21). The most important of these, now recognized for 50 years, are rheumatoid factors (RFs), which are antibodies that react with the patient's own immunoglobulin. The antigenic site most commonly recognized by RFs spans the C_H2 and C_H3 domains of the Fc fragment, although some react with Fab fragments or with pepsin digested immunoglobulins (pepsin agglutinators).

'Altered immunoglobulin'. RF binding to the Fc region binds more avidly if it can combine simultaneously with more than one Fc structure, as may happen if the target immunoglobulin is itself bound to antigen, or if it is aggregated or bound to any solid phase. RFs may be of IgM, IgA, IgG or IgE class, although IgM rheumatoid factors are the most frequently detected in RA. RFs are not disease specific: they occur in other connective tissue diseases such as SLE and Sjögren's syndrome and in some infections, such as rubella, leprosy and malaria.

As cells from healthy people will secrete IgM RFs after stimulation with polyclonal activators, it has been suggested that they are not necessarily pathogenic but may have a protective role in helping to clear immune complexes by binding more avidly to antigen-bound IgG, thereby helping to clear the antigen itself. It could be supposed that the high levels of RFs in RA are a response to the need for the clearance of high levels of antibody–antigen complexes. However, when such complexes are isolated and analysed by sensitive techniques such as immunoblotting, often only IgG and other immunoglobulins and complement components can be found; this suggests that immunoglobulins themselves are the antigen, with IgG RFs playing a unique role as both antigen and antibody.

Abnormal glycosylation. A recent and exciting discovery is that IgG in patients with RA is abnormally glycosylated with a galactose 'pocket' in the Fc region (Fig. 5.22). In normal subjects approximately 14% of the IgG Fc sugar groups lack the terminal galactose, compared with up to 60% in RA patients (Fig. 5.23). This glycosylation defect could lead to a conformational change in the Fc region which makes the molecules more autoantigenic, more likely to aggregate and to bind more avidly to RFs. Interestingly, abnormally glycosylated IgG is also found in patients with tuberculosis.

Antibodies to cellular antigens

Both tissue specific and tissue non-specific autoantibodies are found in RA (see Fig. 5.21). The mechanism for their generation is unknown, although antibodies directed at cytoskeletal antigens (Fig. 5.24) could be caused by polyclonal activation, as similar autoantibodies are found in infections with viruses known to be polyclonal activators, for example the Epstein-Barr virus in infectious mononucleosis. Cross-reactions with rheumatoid factors may be a second mechanism. Several investigators have found that rheumatoid factors isolated by affinity chromatography react not only with IgG, but also with DNA histones.

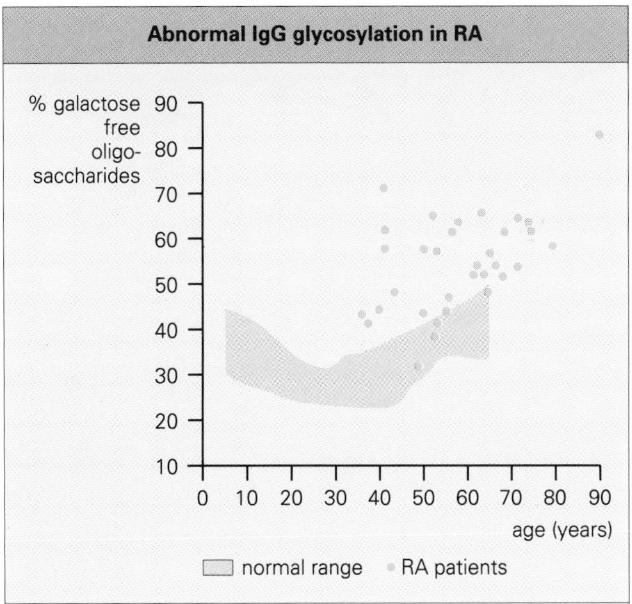

Fig. 5.23 Percentage of IgG sugars which lack terminal galactose showing the abnormal glycosylation of IgG in patients with RA. Modified from Pareth *et al.* (1987).

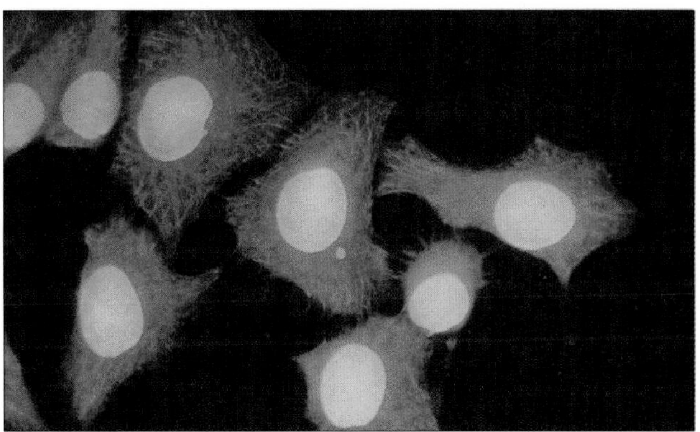

Fig. 5.24 Antibody to vimentin from a patient with RA detected by indirect immunofluorescence on HEP-2 cells, producing a green cytoplasmic filamentous staining pattern. The nucleus has been counterstained orange. Courtesy of Dr Martin Stocks, Kennedy Institute.

It is possible that cross-reactive RFs account for the antinuclear antibodies found in about 40% of RA sera. A third mechanism has been suggested to explain the generation of antibodies to structural tissues such as collagen. These are directed mainly against collagen type II, reacting preferentially with denatured collagen, and are thought to arise as a result of tissue damage rather than causing it.

Immune complexes

There is little doubt that immune complexes are of pathogenic importance in RA. In both the joint and in blood they consist mainly of IgG, IgM and complement components, suggesting that IgG itself may be the antigen, either as self associating IgG rheumatoid factors or as IgG altered by defective glycosylation. Alternatively, IgG may be bound to an autoantigen or even an extrinsic antigen. Complexed rheumatoid factors fix complement efficiently and deplete the level in the synovial fluid.

In patients with only articular disease, immune complexes are found mainly in the joints. In those with extra-articular disease, complexes are also detected in the blood. These circulating immune complexes cause vasculitis and other manifestations of systemic RA. In severe cases they can deplete blood complement levels, and the patient may develop clinical and serological features resembling systemic lupus erythematosus, although unlike SLE, immune complex glomerulonephritis is rare in RA.

DIAGNOSIS OF RHEUMATOID ARTHRITIS

Rheumatoid factors

The diagnosis of RA is based on clinical findings of a symmetrical polyarthritis and radiological erosions. The immunological test of greatest value is that for rheumatoid factors. These are normally detected by the agglutination of sheep red cells or latex particles coated with human or rabbit IgG (see chapter 30). More recently ELISAs have been developed, but these are not sufficiently standardized for routine laboratory use. Although not restricted to rheumatoid arthritis, rheumatoid factors, particularly in high titre, add weight to the diagnosis of RA and are associated with more destructive disease and a worse prognosis.

Other immunological tests

Most other commonly used tests are not specific for RA but are helpful in distinguishing an immunologically mediated arthritis from a degenerative or metabolic type such as osteoarthritis or gout.

The erythrocyte sedimentation rate (ESR) is the distance that the red cells fall in a tube of anti-coagulated blood in one hour. The test is crude but frequently performed because of its simplicity. Factors which cause an increase in ESR include the presence of acute phase reactants, anaemia and high levels of plasma immunoglobulins. Since all of these factors may be present in RA the ESR is often high.

Immunoglobulins and acute phase reactants such as C-reactive protein can also be measured individually. Although of limited diagnostic value, these tests can be helpful in assessing disease activity and are often used in monitoring response to treatment. Examination of joint fluid for complement levels is also occasionally used. Some centres perform biopsies of the synovium for diagnostic purposes, but like other tests they will not distinguish RA from other types of immune synovitis.

Some tests may be helpful in excluding RA by indicating an alternative diagnosis. For example antibodies to

Classification of juvenile chronic arthritis	
juvenile RA	similar to adult RA, seropositive & erosive nodules often present
pauciarticular	<5 joints involved associated with iridocyclitis anti-nuclear antibodies present
polyarticular	>5 joints involved rheumatoid factors negative
systemic JCA	severe systemic illness with fever & rash

Fig. 5.25 Classification of juvenile chronic arthritis.

DNA would indicate SLE, whereas anti-Ro (SS-A) or anti-La (SS-B) would suggest Sjögren's syndrome. Conversely the absence of such antibodies would favour a diagnosis of RA.

Immune complex assays have been examined extensively for their usefulness in diagnosing RA and other autoimmune diseases. In general they are technically difficult, subject to many artefacts and are not reproducible. Different assays may give completely different results on the same sera, probably because each tend to detect immune complexes with particular biological properties. Most assays give higher results in patients with extra-articular disease, reflecting the presence of circulating immune complexes. This extra serological information is outweighed by the considerable disadvantages of these tests and they are now rarely used.

DRUG TREATMENT

Although there is no cure for RA and little evidence that any of the currently available drugs affect the final outcome in terms of joint destruction and disability, several drugs give considerable relief of symptoms and improvement in functional capacity over the short term. The drugs are traditionally divided into first, second and third line, reflecting the order in which they would normally be used:

- first line (non-steroidal anti-inflammatory drugs — NSAIDS), for example aspirin and other prostaglandin synthetase inhibitors, such as indomethacin and ibuprofen;
- second line (anti-rheumatic drugs), for example gold salts (*Myocrisin*), *d*-penicillamine, sulphasalazine and hydrochloroquine;
- third line (steroids and cytotoxic drugs), for example prednisolone, azathioprine, cyclophosphamide and methotrexate.

Patients with RA who develop AIDS show complete remission of their arthritis. This indicates the importance of the $CD4^+$ cell in the pathogenesis of RA, and may provide a more specific target for immunosuppressive therapy in the future.

JUVENILE CHRONIC ARTHRITIS

In the past there was considerable confusion about the nomenclature and classification of arthritis in children. What is now known as juvenile chronic arthritis (JCA) was often called Still's disease or juvenile rheumatoid arthritis without recognition of the widely differing syndromes that it covered. The most widely recognized classification is that of Ansell, which divides JCA into four types (Fig. 5.25).

JUVENILE RA

Juvenile rheumatoid arthritis appears to be the same disease as adult rheumatoid, and its onset is almost always after the menarche. It is associated with DR4, most patients are RF-positive and tend to develop an erosive, destructive arthritis, the long-term effects of which tend to be more severe than in the adult disease. Treatment is as for adults except that steroids have the additional complication in children of inhibiting growth.

PAUCIARTICULAR AND POLYARTICULAR JCA

These forms of JCA occur in a much younger age group (2–5 years) and are associated with DR5 and DR8. The arthritis is less destructive and tends to result in fusion of joints rather than destruction. Pauci- and polyarticular JCA are regarded as different parts of the same disease spectrum. Rheumatoid factors are negative but some patients with pauciarticular JCA have anti-nuclear antibodies which are associated with iridocyclitis, a serious complication which can lead to blindness.

SYSTEMIC JCA

This form of JCA is the closest to the disease originally described by Still. The peak age of onset is around five years, but an adult form of Still's disease is now also recognized. The disease is characterized by fever, a rash (Fig. 5.26), arthritis and involvement of the monuclear–phagocyte system with enlargement of the liver and spleen. The diagnosis is made clinically, as there are no known serological or HLA markers. Systemic JCA is potentially fatal from septicaemia or liver failure, and is therefore often treated aggressively with a combination of steroids and cytotoxic drugs such as chlorambucil.

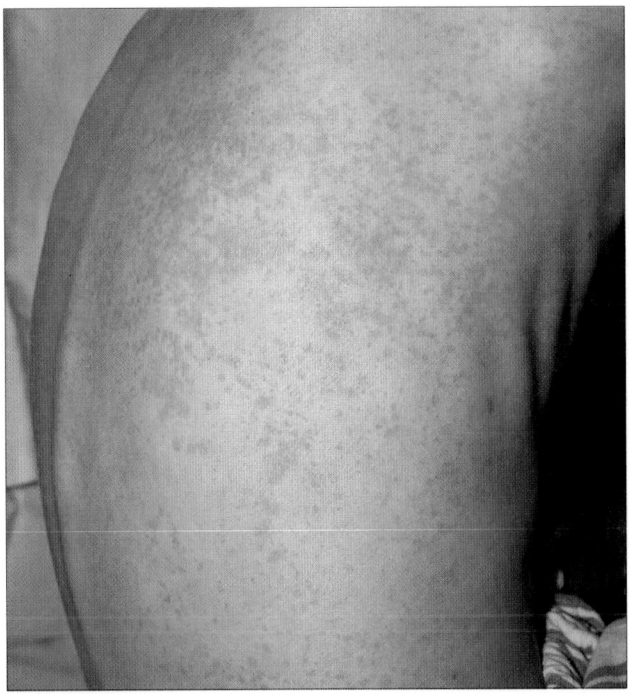

Fig. 5.26 Erythematous maculopapular rash on the back of a patient with systemic juvenile chronic arthritis.

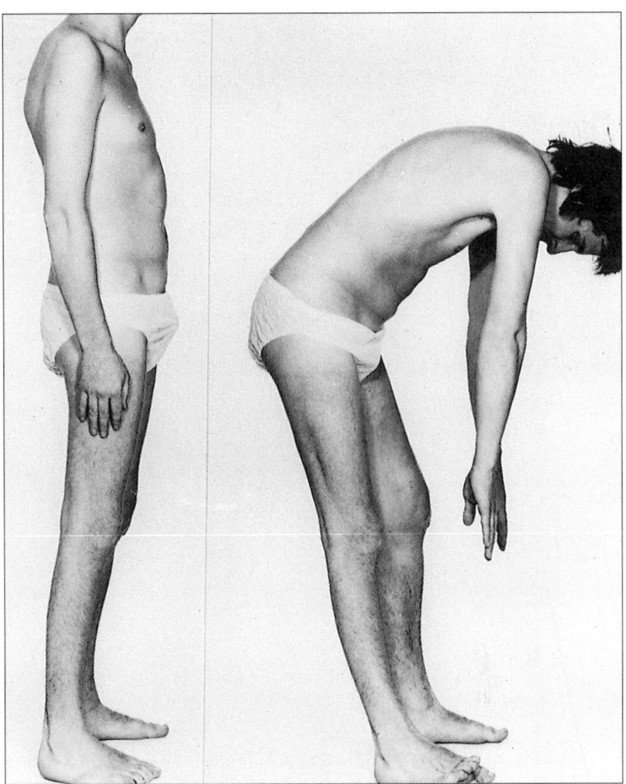

Fig. 5.27 Ankylosing spondylitis in a young man attempting to bend forward to touch his toes. The minimal flexion achieved is almost entirely due to movement at the hips, the spine being virtually rigid.

SERONEGATIVE SPONDYLOARTHROPATHIES

This group of disorders, so called because the sera are negative for rheumatoid factors and the arthritis usually involves the spine, may be divided into four groups:

- ankylosing spondylitis
- reactive arthritis
- arthritis associated with inflammatory bowel disease
- psoriatic arthritis.

Unlike other forms of arthritis, the spondyloarthropathies are more common in men; the onset is often in the late teens or early twenties, with an unexplained tendency to improve after the age of 40. The arthritis, but not necessarily the underlying disease, is strongly associated with HLA-B27. Patients with spondyloarthropathies may also develop uveitis.

ANKYLOSING SPONDYLITIS

Ankylosing spondylitis (AS) is the purest form of spondyloarthritis, with 95% of patients being HLA-B27 positive. It characteristically involves the spine (Fig. 5.27), where it causes ankylosis (fusion) of the apophyseal and sacroiliac joints, which on X-ray gives an appearance described as the 'bamboo spine' (Fig. 5.28). It may also affect the limbs, particularly the large joints such as the knees. Severe untreated cases may end up with a completely fused immobile spine.

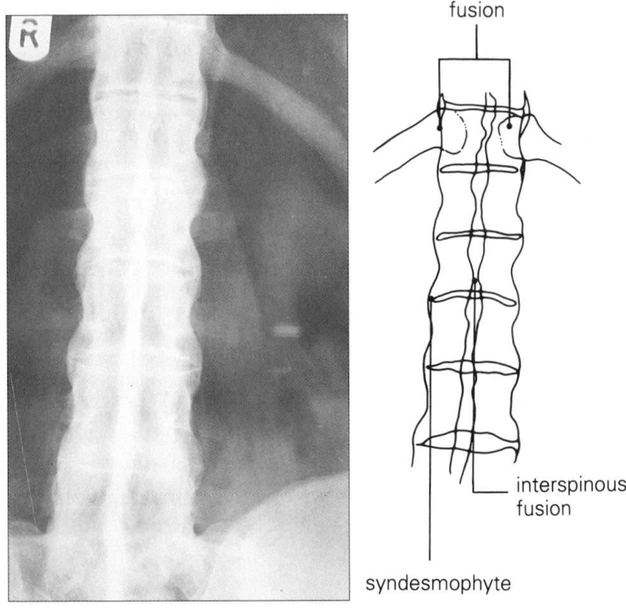

Fig. 5.28 X-ray of the lumbar spine in AS showing extensive ankylosis, producing the typical 'bamboo spine' pattern. There is also ossification of the dorsal interspinous ligament and fusion at the costovertebral joints. Courtesy of Professor P Dieppe.

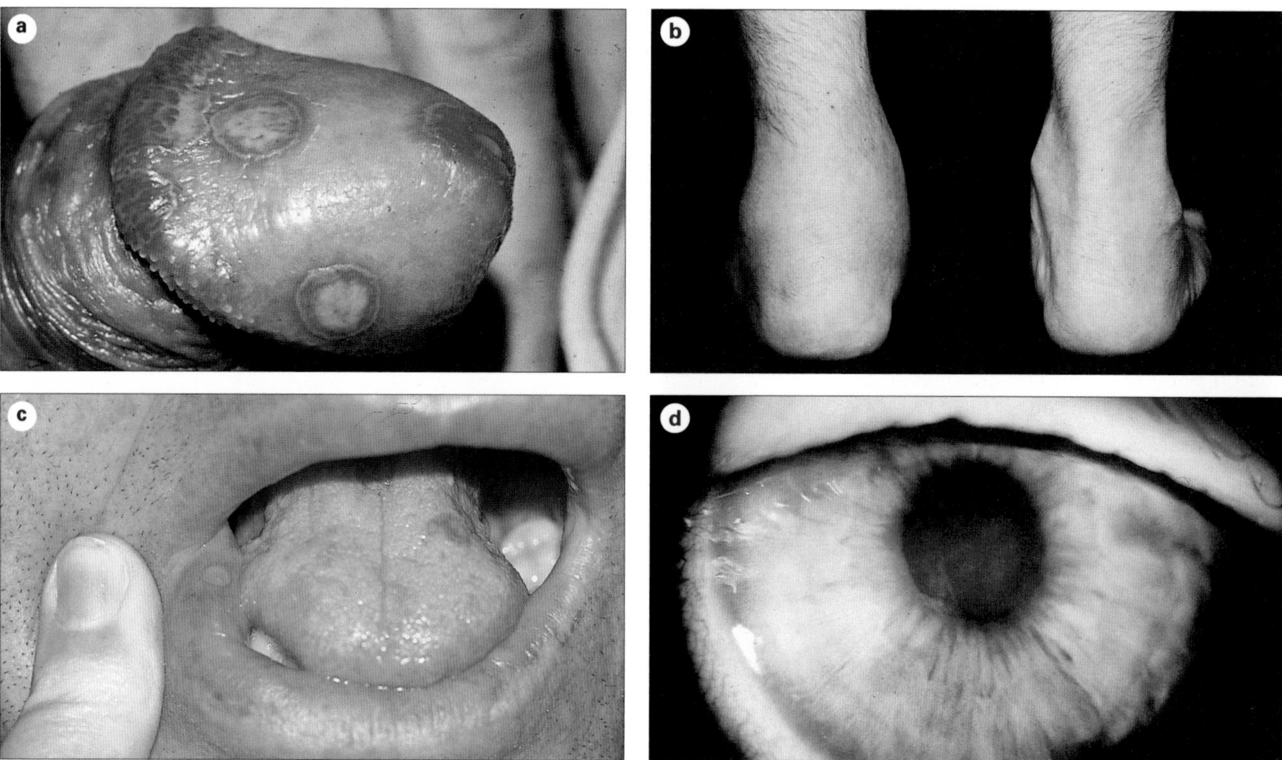

Fig. 5.29 Reiter's syndrome is characterized by (a) urethritis and balanitis of the penis, (b) thickening of the left Achilles tendon, (c) mouth ulcers, and (d) inflammation of the iris (iritis).

The recent finding of cross-reactivity between *Klebsiella* antigens and HLA-B27 sheds some light on the unknown aetiology of AS. These bacteria are found in higher numbers in the stools of patients with active AS than in controls and in subjects with quiescent disease. IgG and IgA antibodies are also much higher in patients than in controls, as is the level of total IgA. The cross-reaction between *Klebsiella* antigens and HLA-B27 is demonstrated by the fact that antibodies to the organism stain B27-positive cells and vice versa; this is a good example of molecular mimicry (see chapter 2).

Attempts to control the level of *Klebsiella* in the gut by antibiotics have failed, but putting patients on a low carbohydrate diet results in a substantial fall in anti-*Klebsiella* antibodies (and total IgA), a drop in acute phase proteins and in the sedimentation rate, and general clinical improvement.

Treatment is with NSAIDs and vigorous physiotherapy, primarily designed to prevent fusion of affected joints. Second line therapy with gold or salazopyrine is often successful in patients with active disease.

REACTIVE ARTHRITIS

This form of arthritis is so called because it appears to be due to an immunological reaction to an infectious organism. About 60% of patients are B27 positive. The infections are manifest either in the bowel as enteritis, or in the urinary tract, as urethritis or prostatitis. Organisms commonly associated with reactive arthritis include *Salmonella, Shigella* and *Yersinia* in the bowel, or *Chlamydia* as the cause of non-specific urethritis. The arthritis is similar to that of ankylosing spondylitis, although it tends to be less persistent and more likely to involve joints in the limbs than the spine. The triad of urethritis, arthritis and uveitis is termed Reiter's syndrome (Fig. 5.29). Patients with reactive arthritis may also develop genital ulcers.

Although the aetiology is known in many cases, the pathogenesis of reactive arthritis is obscure. The association with HLA-B27, a class I antigen, suggests that cytotoxic cells, which are class I restricted, may be involved. It is now known that whereas AIDS causes remission in RA, it has no effect in reactive arthritis or may actually make it worse. AIDS depletes $CD4^+$ cells but spares $CD8^+$, again suggesting that cytotoxic cells are of primary importance. Other observations which give clues to possible pathogenic mechanisms include claims of cross-reactivity between the B27 antigen and *Chlamydia* and *Yersinia,* and demonstrations of chlamydial antigens within affected joints.

Treatment of reactive arthritis is with antibiotics for the primary infection and NSAIDs for the arthritis. In some cases reactive arthritis can be persistent and active long after the primary infection has disappeared. In such cases second line anti-rheumatic drugs may be successful.

ARTHRITIS AND INFLAMMATORY BOWEL DISEASE

Inflammatory bowel disease (IBD) is a group of disorders in which chronic inflammation of the submucosa in the duodenum, ileum and colon leads to diarrhoea, protein loss (as mucus) and malabsorption syndromes. Coeliac disease (gluten-sensitive enteropathy), Crohn's disease and ulcerative colitis can all be associated with an arthropathy similar to reactive arthritis. It is thought that the arthritis may be secondary to bacterial infection of the bowel, the permeability of which is increased by chronic inflammation. Treatment of the bowel disease, for example by gluten withdrawal in coeliac disease or surgical resection of the colon in ulcerative colitis, results in improvement of the arthritis.

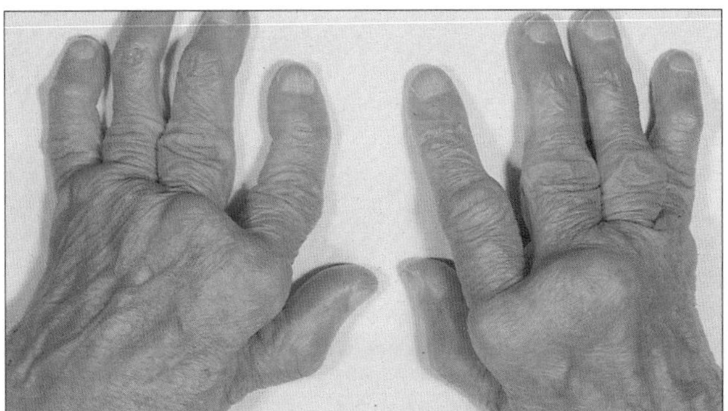

Fig. 5.30 Arthritis mutilans typically presents as subluxation of the MCP joints and foreshortening of the fingers due to bone erosion and resorption. All the fingers are involved in this case. Courtesy of Professor P Dieppe.

PSORIATIC ARTHRITIS

Psoriasis is a skin disease of unknown aetiology characterized by hyperactivity of keratinocytes leading to increased keratinization of the skin, giving it a scaly appearance. The arthritis associated with it may have a similar presentation to reactive arthritis (involving the spine or large joints), to rheumatoid arthritis, or may manifest as arthritis mutilans, a rare pattern of joint disease unique to psoriasis (Fig. 5.30). It is thought that some cases of so-called seronegative RA are psoriatic arthritis. The correct diagnosis may be missed, either because the psoriasis is so mild that it escapes notice, or because the arthritis precedes the skin disease. It is not known why psoriasis should lead to arthropathy, but treating the skin improves the arthritis.

FURTHER READING

Current Opinion in Rheumatology series. London: Current Science.

Currey HLF, ed. *Mason and Currey's clinical rheumatology (4E).* Edinburgh: Pitman Medical/Churchill-Livingstone, 1986.

Currey HLF. *Essentials of rheumatology (2E).* Edinburgh: Pitman Medical/Churchill-Livingstone, 1988.

Dieppe PA, Doherty M, MacFarlane DG, Maddison PJ. *Rheumatological medicine.* Edinburgh: Churchill-Livingstone, 1985.

Kelley WN, Harris ED, Ruddy S, Sledge CB, eds. *Textbook of rheumatology (3E).* Philadelphia: WB Saunders Company, 1989.

Lachmann PJ, Peters DK, Walport M, eds. *Clinical aspects of immunology (5E).* Oxford: Blackwell Scientific Publications, in press.

6

SLE & Other Connective Tissue Disorders

INTRODUCTION

These are non-organ-specific autoimmune diseases which form a spectrum, often with overlap between different diseases. Common pathological mechanisms could be type III hypersensitivity with immune complex deposition leading to vasculitis and other inflammatory processes.

SYSTEMIC LUPUS ERYTHEMATOSUS

CLINICAL FEATURES

The archetypal patient with SLE is a young (20–40 year old) woman with joint pains (but little overt arthritis), fever, and a facial rash involving particularly the 'blushing' area. Protein and red cells are found in the urine, and there is anaemia, a raised erythrocyte sedimentation rate (ESR), leucopenia, and elevated globulin levels (Fig. 6.1); mouth ulceration may also be present. There is a wide range of symptoms and signs (Figs 6.2–6.7), but the profile above will diagnose SLE with over 90% specificity.

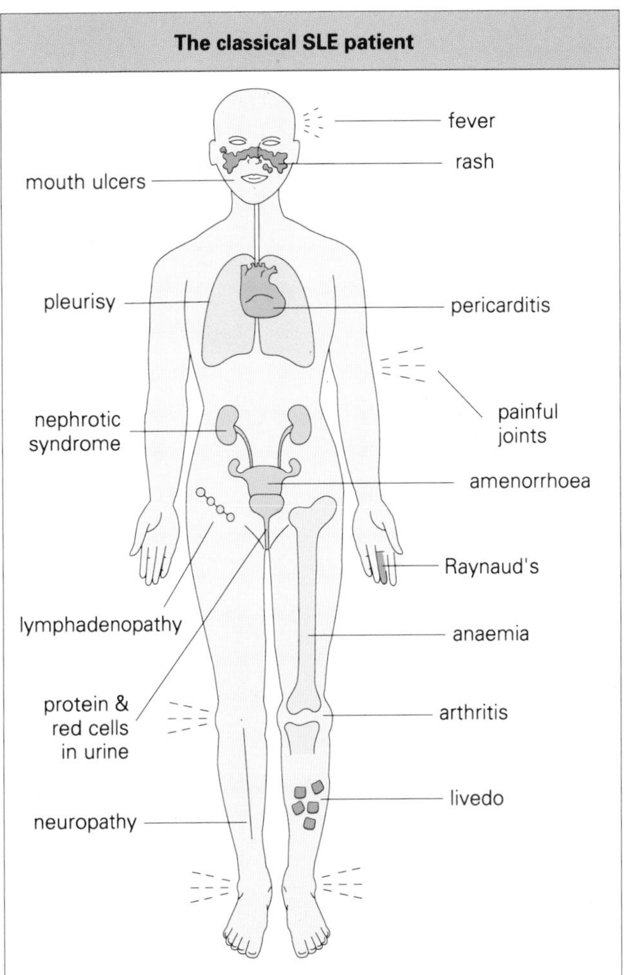

Fig. 6.1 The patient often loses hair rapidly during active disease, sometimes with frank alopecia. Headaches are common and may be migrainous.

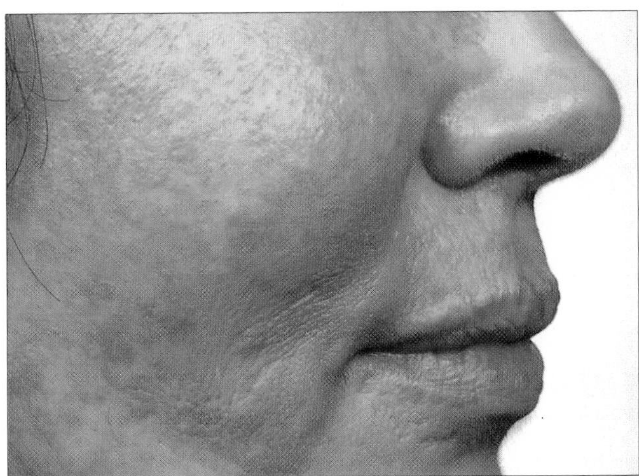

Fig. 6.2 Characteristic malar rash. Photosensitivity was thought to be due to the effect of UVA on thymine dimers with a presumed defect in DNA repair, but release of cytokines (such as IL-1) may be a more likely initiating process. Inflammation of sun-exposed areas may be rapid in onset, followed by blistering and subsequent atrophy.

Diagnostic accuracy

Testing for characteristic autoantibodies will increase the diagnostic accuracy even further. However, whilst classical lupus is quite easily suspected and diagnosed, there are patients with SLE-like disease who may be unlike the classical patient both in clinical presentation and prognosis. The relatively new information available, particularly on autoantibodies, helps to reveal these patients.

Patients with SLE can be classified using the criteria set out by the American Rheumatism Association (Fig. 6.8); these do not necessarily relate to disease severity.

Demography

Lupus is a disease of young women (90% female preponderance) thus, whilst rare in the population as a whole (prevalence 0.5–1.5/1000), it is a relatively common cause of chronic ill-health and death in young females. This is especially so for blacks: lupus is more common than rheumatoid arthritis in the Caribbean and also in North American blacks. The rank order of frequency is

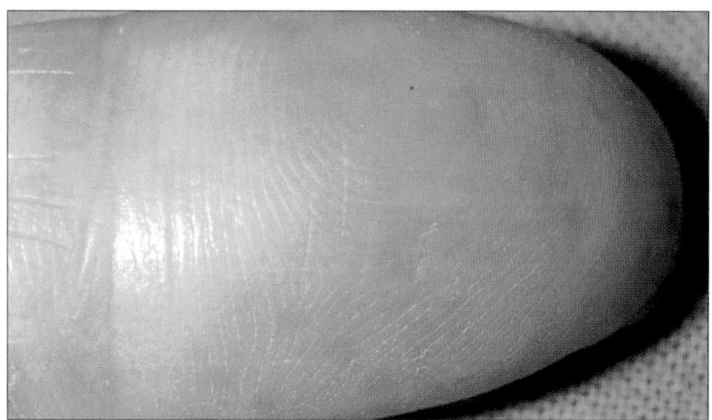

Fig. 6.3 Vasculitic lesions may affect both small and large vessels around the finger or toe nails and those of the pulps; the small vessel lesions may be painful but are not in themselves dangerous. The vasculitis of larger vessels may result in tissue necrosis, gangrene of digits or even limbs. Vasculitis is the pathology underlying such features as neuropathy and mesenteric arteritis.

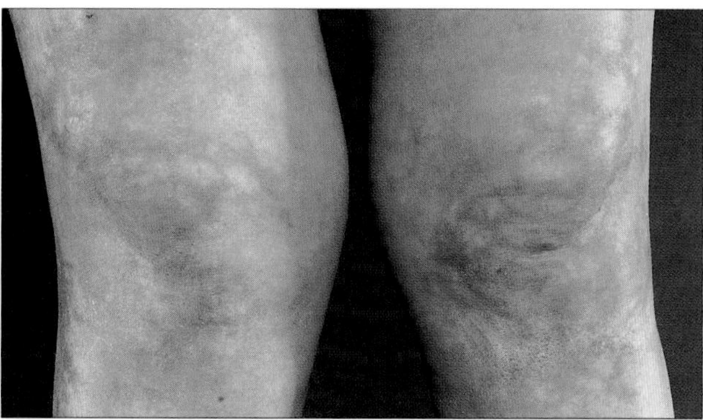

Fig. 6.4 Livedo reticularis can be seen in healthy people in the cold, but when widespread at room temperature it is a sign of pathological stasis of the arteriovenous network and may be associated with thromboembolism and lupus anti-coagulant syndrome.

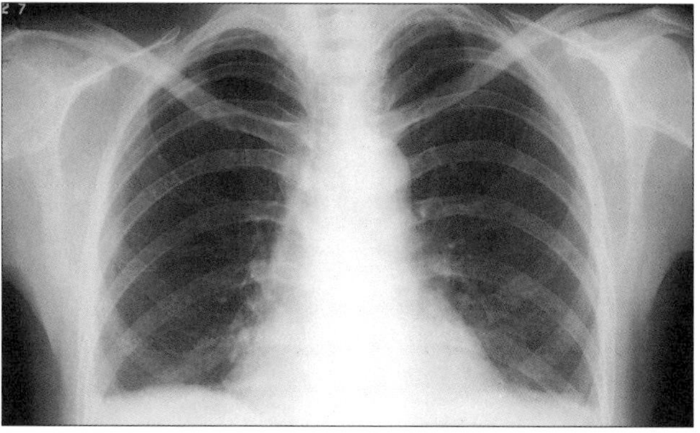

Fig. 6.5 Pleuritic pain, with or without sterile pleural effusion, and pericarditis are classical features and may be recurrent. Linear atelectasis of the lung may occur. The 'shrinking lungs' of lupus may become apparent over several months, resulting in chest constriction and abnormal lung function tests. This may stabilize over subsequent years.

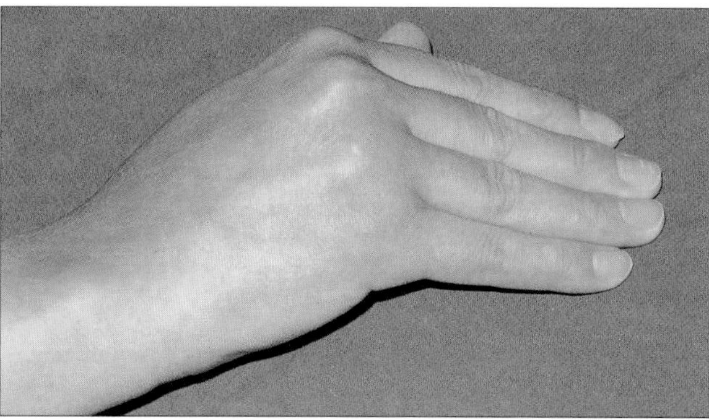

Fig. 6.6 Joints pains (arthralgia) are common, and the pain may be more severe and diffuse than in rheumatoid arthritis (RA). Swelling is not great compared with RA. Tendonitis is a prominent feature and contractures of tendons may lead to appearances superficially similar to the deformities of rheumatoid disease.

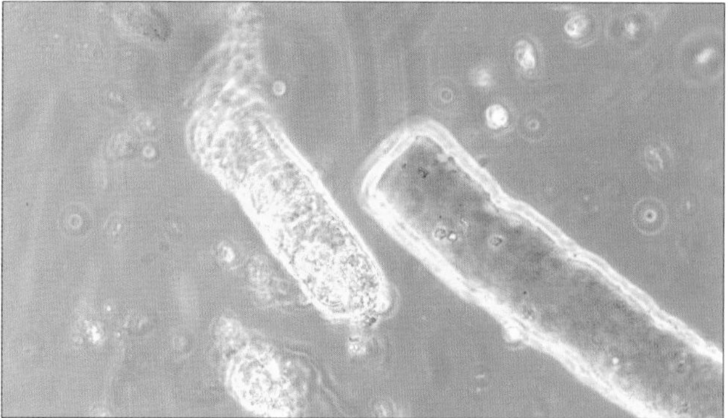

Fig. 6.7 Microscopy of fresh uncentrifuged urine is essential for detecting and monitoring nephritis where cellular casts of erythrocytes constitute an active urinary sediment. Renal involvement was formerly the most common fatal manifestation of the disease. Biopsy of patients with no clinical evidence of renal disease has revealed lesions in up to 70% of cases.

probably black > Chinese > Latin > Asian > white (Fig. 6.9), although population studies are not reliable enough to be sure about the frequency in coloured races worldwide.

IMMUNOLOGICAL RESPONSES

SLE is the most florid of the non-organ-specific autoimmune diseases. Clinical evidence for abnormally vigorous immune responses lies in splenomegaly and lymphadenopathy in the early stages of the disease. In contrast, patients with end-stage nephritis show the phenomenon of renal failure-induced 'immunosuppression' with amelioration of the non-renal aspects of the disease.

There is laboratory evidence of abnormal cellular and humoral immune responses with the presence of autoantibodies and polyclonal production of immunoglobulins.

Revised criteria for classification of SLE

mucocutaneous
malar rash discoid rash
photosensitivity
oral ulcers

arthritis
anti-nuclear antibody

serositis
pleuritis/pericarditis

renal disorder
persistent proteinuria/cellular casts

neurological disorder
seizures/psychosis

haematological disorder
haemolytic anemia/leucopenia/
lymphopenia/thrombocytopenia

immunological disorder
positive LE cell preparation/anti-DNA
anti-Sm/false positive serological test for syphilis

Fig. 6.8 Revised criteria (1982) for classification of SLE. The existence, whether simultaneously or successively, of four or more of these criteria constitutes a diagnosis of SLE.

However, the presence of autoreacting antibodies is quite compatible with a normal life, as seen in healthy subjects with circulating organ-specific and non-organ-specific autoantibodies.

Autoantibodies

Anti-nuclear antibody (ANA) is the major autoantibody in SLE (Fig. 6.10) and can be shown in a variety of ways. The fluorescent ANA test using a murine substrate has been superceded by cell lines such as HEP2 (Fig. 6.11 upper). Over 95 % of patients with SLE have ANA.

Antibodies to extractable nuclear antigens (ENA). These antibodies are designated in some instances by the initials of the patients in which they were first detected (for example Sm for Smith) or by description of the antigen (for example RNP for ribonucleoprotein). The frequencies of the antibodies vary with the populations of patients surveyed and the techniques used, for example Sm is found in 5% of whites with SLE and 25% of blacks and Chinese. In no instance does an antibody to a single ENA carry the same degree of specificity for disease as does that to DNA. In the case of the overlap syndrome, mixed connective tissue disease (MCTD), antibodies to RNP are regarded as necessary for diagnosis; however, this specificity is confined to those patients in whom there is no antibody to DNA. In contrast, in patients with SLE, antibodies to RNP are found quite frequently in association with anti-DNA.

Other autoantibodies have specificities for associated connective tissue diseases, for example anti-Ro/La for Sjögren's disease, anti-Jo-1 for respiratory involvement in polymyositis, anti-phospholipid antibody for the thrombocytopenia/thrombotic/livedo reticularis syndrome.

Antibodies to DNA. The most characteristic antibody in SLE is that to DNA. In its most specific form, it is directed against double-stranded DNA (dsDNA): antibodies to single-stranded DNA (ssDNA) are found in varying titre in a wide variety of infections, inflammatory and autoimmune diseases. The pivotal role of DNA as an immunogen is less certain because although anti-DNA–DNA complexes have been identified at sites of tissue damage in SLE (Fig. 6.12), attempts to identify the antigen in circulating immune complexes have failed.

In addition, experiments designed to reproduce SLE by immunizing animals (even lupus-prone strains) with DNA have also been unsuccessful. The avidity and specificity of anti-DNA antibodies may be important factors in their pathogenicity, but this may also be true of their

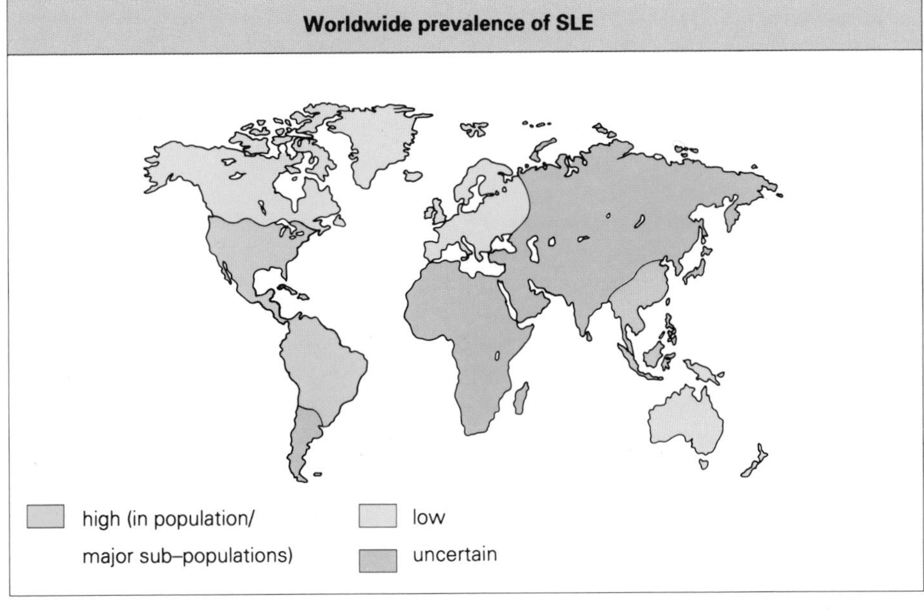

Fig. 6.9 Prevalence of SLE worldwide.

Autoantibodies in SLE	
Cell nuclei or components	
	whole nucleus
	DNA (ds, ss, z-type)
	RNA (ds, ss)
	nucleotides & polynucleotides
	histones (1–4)
Cytoplasmic components	
	La (SS–B)
	Ro (SS–A)
Specific cells	
	neurones
	lymphocytes
	erythrocytes
	platelets
Others	
	globulins (RFs)
	coagulant components & phospholipids
	thyroglobulin, microsomes

Fig. 6.10 Of those reacting with phospholipids, anti-cardiolipin antibodies are most often found.

cross-reactivity. The latter may explain the relationship between thrombocytopenia, renal disease and the lupus anticoagulant, as phospholipid molecules are common to all three.

Anti-double-stranded DNA antibodies correlate most clearly in renal, cerebral and cutaneous disease in SLE and are measured in complement fixation, immunoprecipitation and ELISA assays. The most specific way of identifying the anti-double-stranded native form of the antibody is to use *Crithidia lucilliae* as the substrate in a fluorescent assay.

Lupus 'band' test. The common involvement of the skin is reflected in the histological appearances, which show complement components and immunoglobulin deposited in a linear manner along the junction of the dermis and epidermis (Fig. 6.13). This constitutes the lupus 'band' test and is reasonably specific for lupus, provided the biopsy is taken from clinically uninvolved skin (immunoglobulin deposition is found in other non-lupus skin disorders). Interestingly, there may be a correlation between this and nephritis, providing further evidence of the ubiquitous nature of immune complex deposition.

Cross-reacting antibodies

An antibody which can react with a self antigen is not necessarily generated immunogenically by that antigen. Indeed, it is very difficult experimentally to induce antibodies to double-stranded DNA. Cross-reactivity between, for example, carbohydrate on the surface of bacteria and back-bone structures on nuclear proteins is a more likely explanation for the generation of anti-nuclear antibodies.

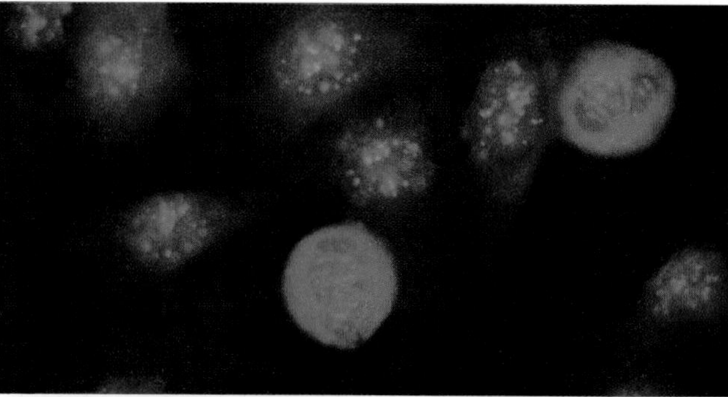

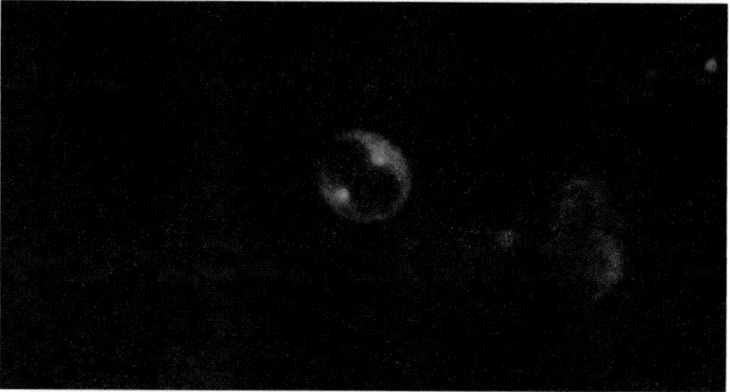

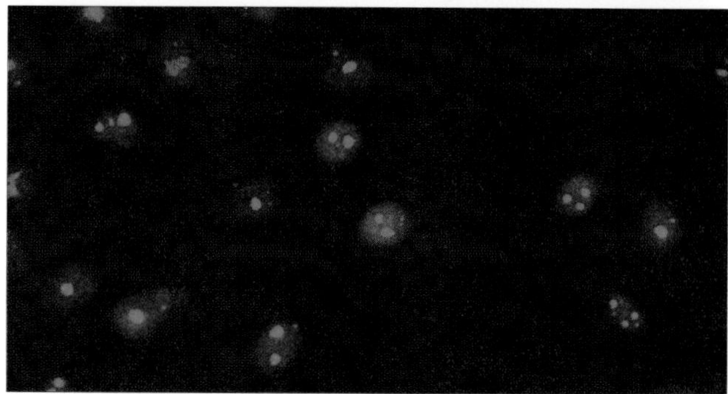

Fig .6.11 Anti-nuclear autoantibodies in SLE demonstrated using HEP2 cells. Upper: anti-nuclear antibodies. x500. Middle: anti-centromere antibodies. x800. Lower: anti-centriole antibodies. x500.

The idiotype network theory also provides for such cross-reactions.

Cellular immune function

Suppressor T cells. It has been suggested that the normal suppression of self-reaction, via Ts cells, is impaired in SLE. Ts cells are reduced in active SLE, as are natural killer cells, the autologous mixed lymphocyte reaction, IL-2 production and cell reactivity to interferon. Anti-lymphocyte antibodies are found, which may have a functional role, either in suppressing or stimulating normal reactions, and which may cross-react with neuronal tissue. Elevated levels of circulating interferon of an unusual, acid-labile type, as well as increased spontaneous polyclonal B cell activation is also found in active SLE. This could indicate 'block' of suppression or viral infection, which could be resultant or causal.

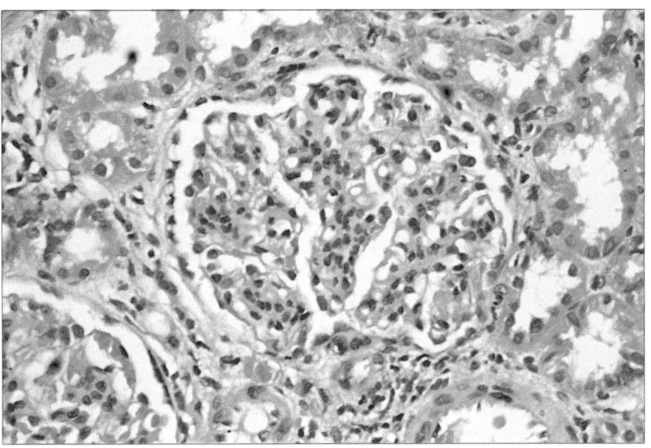

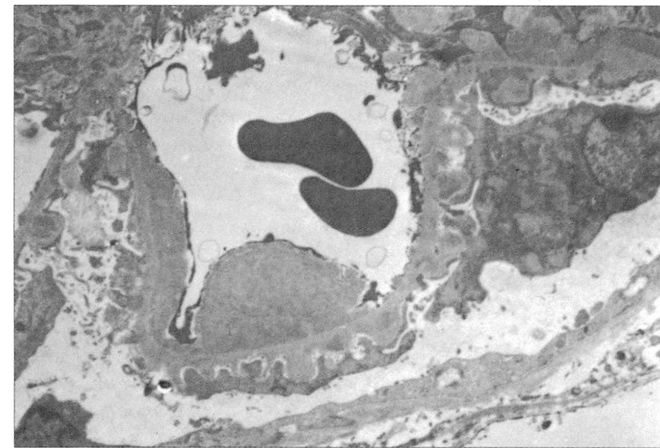

Fig. 6.12 Immune complexes in renal tissue. Left: light microscopy reveals thickening of the basement membrane. H & E stain. Right: electronmicroscopy shows immune complexes appearing as electron-dense sub-endothelial deposits.

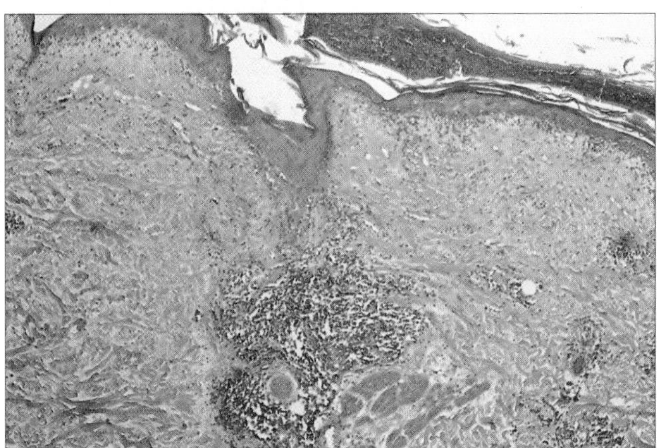

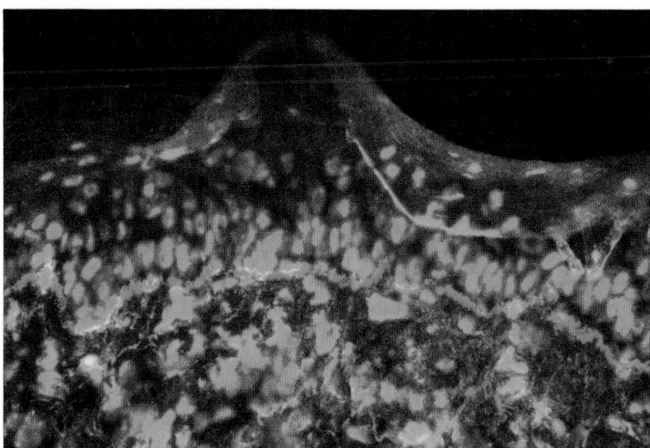

Fig. 6.13 Lupus 'band' test. Left: H & E stained section of skin showing slight thickening of the dermo-epidermal junction. Right: immunofluorescence reveals IgM and C3b at the same junction.

IMMUNOGENETICS

HLA associations

Autoimmune disorders in general are associated with the haplotype HLA-A1,-B8,-DR3. The association with HLA-B27 in spondyloarthropathies, and with DR4 in the synovitis of rheumatoid arthritis, is not seen in SLE. There are other associations, such as those between anti-Ro antibodies and DR3 and the supertypic antigen DRw52, and also between the syndrome known as subacute cutaneous LE and B8, DR3.

Complement

Complement consumption is a prominent feature of active SLE but there is also a link with inherited deficiencies of complement components. For example, about 6% of patients with SLE are heterozygous for C2 deficiency, compared with 1% of the normal population. These deficiencies tend to be of the early components, which react with immune complexes.

C3b receptors on erythrocytes (CR1) are reduced in SLE. This was initially thought to be a genetic deficiency, but closer study of active and inactive cases have revealed that it is secondary. There are probably other clinical subgroups with genetic associations yet to be described.

ANIMAL MODELS

The New Zealand Black (NZB) mouse develops autoimmune haemolytic anaemia. When crossed with the White strain (NZW), the F1 hybrid develops an autoimmune disease with many features of human 'anti-DNA'-type SLE. The existence of this murine analogue has permitted immunological manipulations which are not possible in patients.

Immunosuppression prolongs survival. The hormonal background of the mice can be altered by castration or treatment with androgens to demonstrate the importance of oestrogens on expression of disease. The potential

Murine lupus					
Strain	**Predominant manifestations**	**Influence of gender**	**Genes**	**Immunology**	**Survival (50%)**
NZB	haemolytic anaemia (glomerulonephritis) (reticulum sarcoma)	slight	polygenic	anti-RBC IgM hyperglobulinaemia immune complexes +	8 months
NZB/W F1	glomerulonephritis Sjögren's syndrome (haemolytic anaemia)	oestrogens accelerate, androgens retard	polygenic	anti-DNA (ds & ss) -RNA -gp70 -Sm antibodies immune complexes ++	8 months (F)
MRL lpr/lpr	glomerulonephritis lymphoproliferation periarthritis vasculitis Sjögren's syndrome	some androgen protection	lpr major accelerator	anti-DNA (ds & ss), -Sm, -thymocyte, -globulin (RFs) antibodies cryoglobulins T cell dysregulation hyperglobulinaemia	12–14 months
BxSB	severe proliferative glomerulonephritis	males worse	—	anti-DNA, -RBC -globulin, -thymocyte antibodies	6 months (M+F)

Fig. 6.14 Characteristics of the most studied types of murine lupus. Others include SWAN (Swiss anti- nuclear) and Palmerston North. All are genetically inbred strains. RFs = rheumatoid factors.

importance of the idiotype network is demonstrated by the use of anti-idiotypic monoclonal antibodies directed at anti-DNA antibodies to alter the natural history of the disease in NZB/W mice. The characteristics of the most studied types of murine SLE are given in Fig. 6.14. A lupus-like disease has been seen in dogs (beagles) with anti-DNA antibodies, but little further work has been reported using this model.

PATHOGENESIS

Immune complexes

SLE is often regarded as an immune complex disorder, however the levels of circulating complexes in patients with SLE varies widely and does not correlate well with either activity of the disease or clinical features.

Antigen. Circulating immune complexes (CICs), especially if complement-fixing, may contain pathogenetically relevant antigens. Free DNA can be found in the circulation after trauma, infection or treatment with corticosteroids, but efforts to find DNA (or other antigens) in complexes drawn from patients with anti-DNA antibodies have been unsuccessful.

Nephritis. Immune complexes are found in the basement membrane of patients' kidneys (see Fig. 6.12). This situation is difficult to reproduce in experimental non-autoimmune animals, where deposits tend to be in the mesangium. These findings support the suggestion that DNA (or other antigens) are deposited first, leach antibody from the circulation and subsequently set up inflammatory complement-induced lesions.

Saturation of the mononuclear-phagocyte system. A possible explanation for the vasculitis is that the mononuclear-phagocyte system (MPS) has become 'saturated' and is unable to clear the soluble complexes which are thought most likely to be pathogenic (Fig. 6.15). MPS function may be assessed by its ability to clear artificial complexes, such as radiolabelled heat-damaged or antibody-coated erythrocytes. Other, more toxic, materials such as carbon may be used only in experimental animals. Using such techniques, the clearance of complexes can be shown to be impaired in SLE and restored to some extent by plasma exchange (see chapter 29).

There are criticisms of this work: immune complexes are of widely varying sizes and red cells cannot be said to be representative of pathological complexes. Also, plasma exchange by itself does very little to improve SLE. Probably the largest potential clearance mechanism for circulating complexes is the complement receptor on erythrocytes themselves (CR1). Whether the reduction in CR1 which is seen in active SLE has any part to play in perpetuating the disease is not known.

Coagulation system

Recurrent thrombosis, sometimes over many years, is found in the sub-group of SLE patients with the lupus anticoagulant (LAC). This antibody is directed against the phospholipids of clotting Factors VIII and IX. Although LAC is detected by its effect in delaying the clotting time, it is actually associated clinically with a tendency to thrombosis, and pro-coagulant would better describe its effect. This is likely to occur through its interaction with endothelial surfaces. There is cross-reactivity of this antibody with phospholipid in cardiolipin (Fig. 6.16), producing false positive serum tests for syphilis. Immune

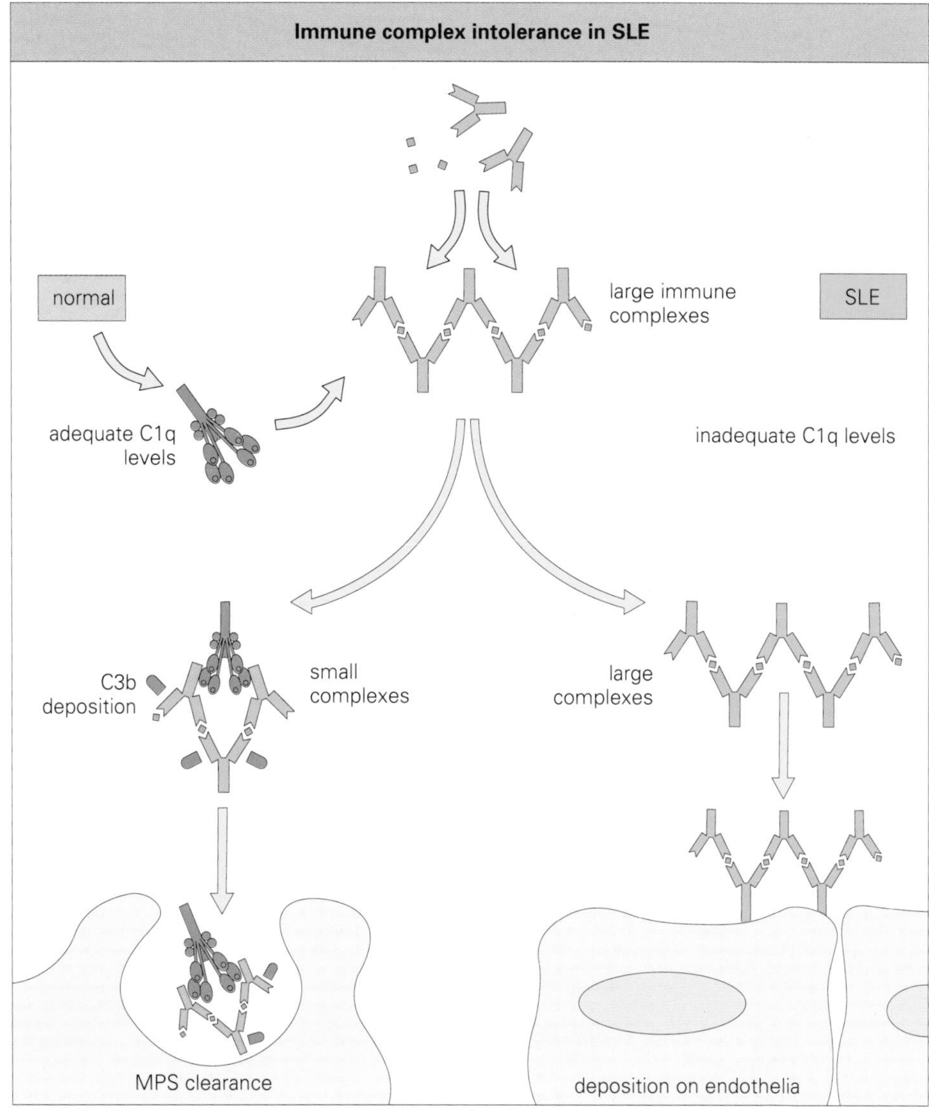

Fig. 6.15 In normal individuals, C1q activates the classical pathway, causing C3b binding which solubilizes immune complexes, facilitating MPS clearance. In SLE a low C1q level means that large immune complexes are not cleared and adhere to endothelial surfaces, causing inflammation.

thrombocytopenia is also found in some patients with anti-cardiolipin antibodies due to cross-reactivity with phospholipid on platelet membranes. LAC is also associated with recurrent spontaneous abortions in a small number of cases.

AETIOLOGY

The foregoing discussion indicates some of the ways or combinations of ways in which human lupus might arise:

- genetically-influenced immunoregulatory disturbances (for example failure of negative feedback suppression of antibody production);
- impaired ability to repair breaks in DNA;
- oestrogenic influences on self-recognition, and perhaps on antibody regulation;
- trigger factors, such as drugs and stress.

Patients may continue for months or years in normal health, yet with anti-nuclear antibodies, leucopenia, lymphopenia, a lupus anti-coagulant and elevated acute phase proteins. Then, suddenly, the disease becomes clinically active.

Role of infection

There is an impression that viral or bacterial infection may precede disease activation, but symptoms of viral infections (fever, malaise, chills, arthralgia) are thought to be produced by IFNγ, so that this mediator may actually be the herald of destabilization rather than a fresh or reactivated viral infection.

Immunization with influenza vaccine does not cause a flare of disease and does produce normal serum antibody levels, although in some patients there is a deficit of circulating lymphocytes capable of making an *in vitro* antibody response.

Electron-dense particles, identified as C-type viruses, have been seen in sections of SLE kidney, but this is not a regular finding. Various anti-viral antibody titres are

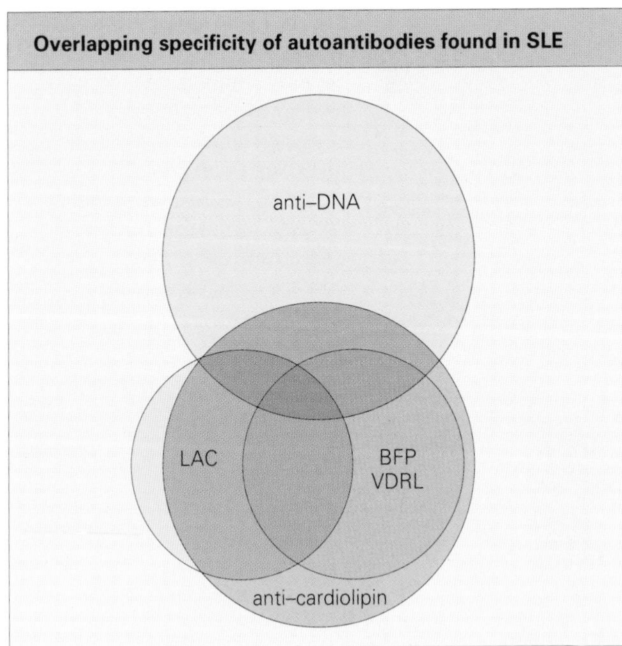

Fig. 6.16 Extent of cross-reaction between antibodies in SLE sera which bind dsDNA, cardiolipin and the lupus anticoagulant (LAC), and are falsely positive in the VDRL (Venereal Disease Reference Laboratory) test. Courtesy of Dr David Isenberg.

Therapy for SLE

non-steroidal anti-inflammatory drugs
— for symptomatic relief

anti-malarials
(chloroquine, hydroxychloroquine, mepacrine)
— for relief of rashes, arthralgia, serositis, fever, malaise

corticosteroids
(prednisone, prednisolone, methylprednisolone etc.)
— for severe flare & maintenance treatment

immunosuppressive drugs
(azathioprine, cyclophosphamide, chlorambucil etc.)
— in conjunction with steroids

adjunctive treatment
(splenectomy, plasma exchange, immunotherapy, bone marrow transplantation, hormone manipulation etc.)
— reserved for particular indications or experimental protocols

Fig. 6.17 The goal of SLE therapy is reduction of immune complex deposition. Splenectomy is unpredictable in SLE immune thrombocytopenia, for which iv gamma-globulin is a good temporary measure.

elevated, but probably reflect polyclonal activation. Retroviruses are contenders for involvement in autoimmune reactions, but there is no pathogenetic evidence for their presence in patients with SLE.

Drug-induced lupus

There is a clear link with extrinsic influences in the case of hydralazine- and procainamide-induced lupus. A patient who is DR4 positive, a slow-acetylator and hypertensive, and who is receiving hydralazine treatment has a very high chance of developing drug-induced lupus. This syndrome, which seldom involves the kidney or brain, will settle completely when the offending drug is withdrawn, but the ANA may remain positive for years. The relevant antibody system in procainamide-induced SLE is thought to be anti-H2a/b histone: in hydralazine-induced SLE the finding of inhibition of C4 binding by the drug may be relevant. Whether this is the case for the other drug-induced lupus syndromes is not known: a large number of drugs have been incriminated as rare causes, including antibiotics, anticonvulsants, anti-hypertensives and penicillamine.

THERAPY

Modes of therapy for SLE are shown in Fig. 6.17.

Drug reactions. Apart from drug-induced SLE, there is an increased frequency of reactions to sulphonamides and penicillins. This may yet prove to be concentrated in those patients who subsequently develop Sjögren's syndrome. Oestrogen contraception should be avoided in a patient with a history of thrombosis and in those with a lupus anticoagulant.

MONITORING

The care of patients with lupus is a continuous process of clinical observation and evaluating end-organ dysfunction. Certain 'process variables' such as acute phase responses are non-specific but valuable:

- ↑ ESR, ↓ white cell count, ↓ lymphocyte count, presence (but not level) of CICs. All indicate the potential for flare but do not correlate well with the need for treatment.
- ↓ Hb, ↓ platelet count, active urinary sediment, increasing proteinuria, & rising creatinine are all parameters of end-organ dysfunction which require action.

PROGNOSIS

Mortality in lupus has reduced greatly over the past two decades, to the extent that 95% of patients with lupus of all types can now expect to survive 10 years from diagnosis. Improved survival can be attributed to a mixture of more radical treatment with steroids and immunosuppression, combined with improved supportive measures such as antibiotics. Nevertheless, more sensitive diagnosis of

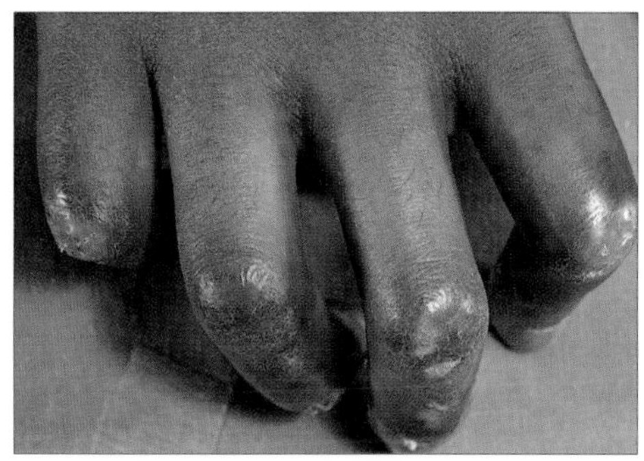

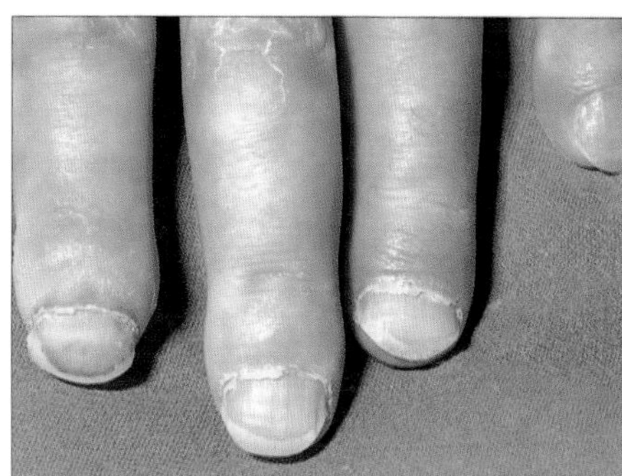

Fig. 6. 18 Scleroderma. Left: the skin on the hands is thickened and tethered. Right: Raynaud's phenomenon. This is an abnormal degree of vasospasm, incorporating a two or three phase colour response (white/ cyanotic then reactive hyperemia), usually in response to physical stimuli, but also to emotional stress.

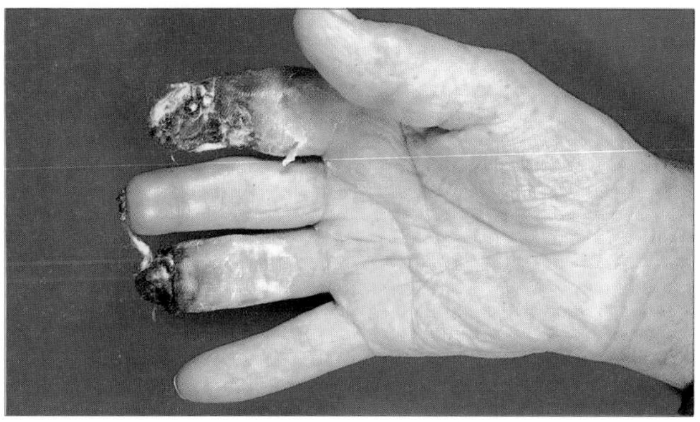

Fig. 6.19 Gangrene due to obliterative vasculopathy is one of the most common vascular manifestations of scleroderma.

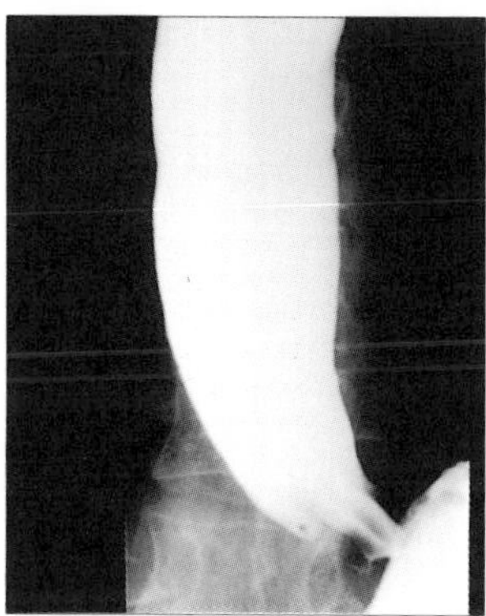

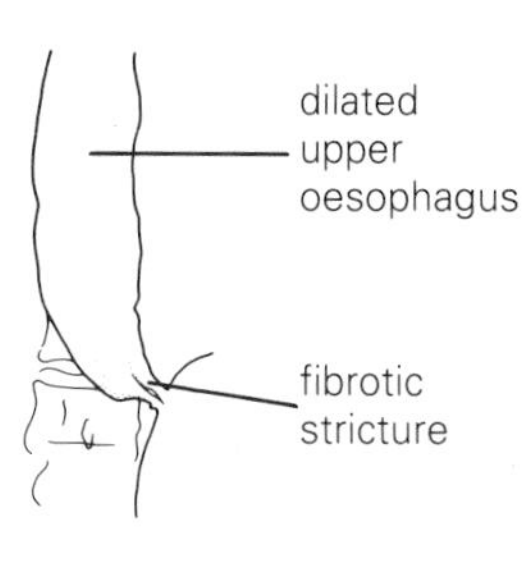

Fig. 6.20 Striated and smooth muscle atrophy with reflux oesophagitis is often a result of fibrosis and failure of the lower sphincter. In this case there is dilatation and immotility of the upper oesophagus, with fibrotic stricture of the lower portion. Courtesy of Dr Ian McNeil.

milder cases with lower intrinsic mortality have also contributed to the overall improvement in outlook.

Infection is the most common cause of death; this tends to occur in patients who have severe disease and who are being treated with some form of immunosuppression. The clinical factors which correlate with a high mortality rate are the development of renal failure, severe anaemia or pulmonary hypertension.

SCLERODERMA

Scleroderma is a term used to describe the physical feature of thickening of the skin and its tethering to subcutaneous tissues (Fig. 6.18); it also denotes the disease or syndrome (progressive systemic sclerosis), which is associated with smooth muscle atrophy and fibrosis of internal organs such as the intestinal tract, lungs and heart. Renal involvement with accelerated hypertension is the complication most likely to be fatal. As with all connective tissue diseases, females are more susceptible than males and most cases start in the fourth decade. The sub-types of the disease may be classified as follows:

- diffuse scleroderma and systemic sclerosis;
- sclerodactyly, CREST syndrome and related variants;
- overlap syndromes featuring scleroderma;
- limited forms such as morphoea (localized and diffuse) and linear scleroderma;
- scleroderma-like diseases, for example chronic GVHD and eosinophilic fasciitis;
- chemically-induced scleroderma variants due to vinyl chloride, bleomycin, trichloroethylene, pentazocine;
- scleroderma mimics such as porphyria cutanea tarda, carcinoid syndrome, amyloidosis, progeria, Werner's syndrome, lipoatrophy.

CLINICAL FEATURES

The main clinical features of scleroderma affect various systems as follows:

- skin — sclerosis, tethering, dyspigmentation, fingertip pits (pain and tenderness);
- vascular system — Raynaud's phenomenon (affects >90% of patients) and disease, nail fold lesions, obliterative vasculopathy, ulceration, gangrene (Fig. 6.19);
- gastrointestinal system — oesophageal hypomotility (Fig. 6.20), oesophageal reflux and stricture (dysphagia), intestinal stasis and dilatation (bloating, eructation, flatulence), malabsorption and diarrhoea;

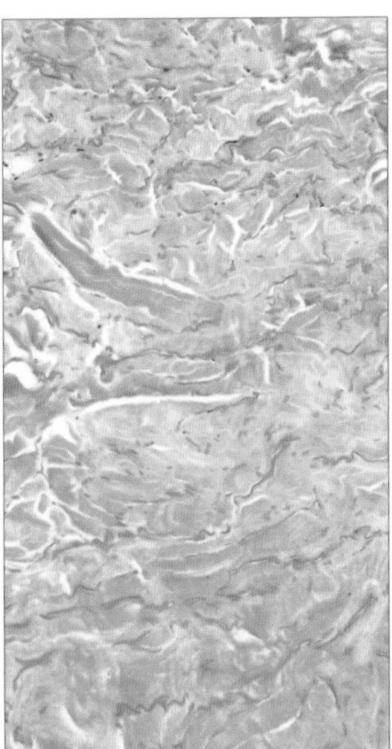
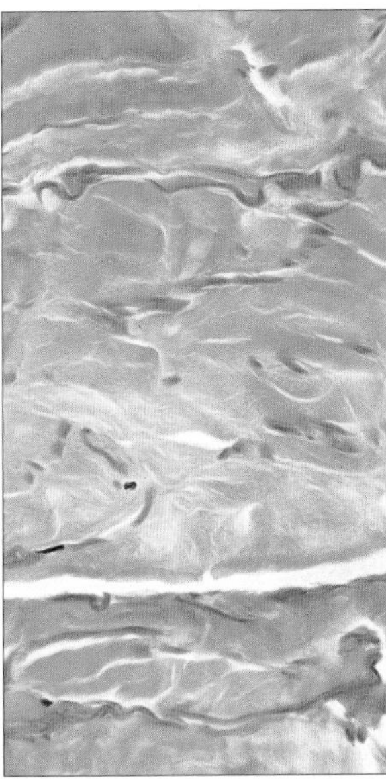

Fig. 6.21 Progressive systemic sclerosis: the dermal collagen fibres are swollen and eosinophilic. Courtesy of Dr P H McKee.

- musculoskeletal system — arthralgia, tendonitis, with rubs and contractures;
- cardiorespiratory system — bibasal interstitial fibrosis, pulmonary hypertension (cardiac fibrosis);
- neurological system — compressive neuropathies;
- renal system — proteinuria, azotaemia, hypertension;
- mucosae — sicca syndrome.

PATHOLOGICAL FEATURES

There is characteristically increased collagen deposition in skin (Fig. 6.21), subcutaneous tissues and internal organs, with associated oedema. There is also increased pro-collagen production by fibroblasts and subsequent cross-linking to form dense sheets. The thickened dermal collagen is of mature fibrous types I and III, with rather less mature tropo-collagen in the deeper layers. After this stage the inflammatory infiltrate (mostly activated T lymphocytes) lessens.

In graft-versus-host disease (GVHD) there is a cutaneous infiltrate of similar type, with similar clinical appearances and tethering of the epidermis which is atrophic. The sweat glands, hair follicles and rete pegs become sparse. There is little evidence of immune complex deposition although they may be found in the circulation.

In addition to the overt vascular manifestations of the disease, there are microscopic changes within and around small arterioles and capillaries, and perivascular inflammatory infiltrates leading to vascular obliteration or dilatation. These changes are found in the skin and internally, in the gut and kidney.

IMMUNOLOGICAL RESPONSES

Autoantibodies

Anti-nuclear antibodies (ANA) are found in over 90% of patients, the nucleolar pattern being most characteristic of scleroderma. There is a wide range of other reactive antigens, the titres of which are no guide to prognosis.

Soluble nuclear antigen. Antibody to a soluble nuclear antigen, Scl-70, is specific for scleroderma, but is found in only about 25% of patients with diffuse disease. Anti-centromere antibody (see Fig. 6.11) is associated with sclerodactyly in the variant termed CREST syndrome.

Precipitins. Other precipitins, Scl-4 and Scl-6, occur less frequently. Anti-RNP occurs in the overlap syndrome known as mixed connective tissue disease (MCTD). Many of the antigens which react with sera from patients with connective tissue diseases are located upon or associated with smaller nuclear ribonucleoprotein complexes and are known collectively as SnRNPs. Antibodies directed against these complexes are proving to be of importance in the further understanding of RNA recognition and splicing. Antibodies to the extractable antigens known as Ro/SS-A and La/SS-B are not usually found in classical diffuse scleroderma but are commonly seen in Sjögren's syndrome. Anti-Sm and anti-Jo-1 are not found in scleroderma.

The low incidence of anti-DNA antibody, with absence of immune complex deposition, yet the occurrence of nephropathy, highlights the heterogeneity of pathological processes in connective tissue diseases, especially in comparison with SLE.

Cell-mediated immunity

Lymphocytes. Circulating B lymphocyte numbers are normal but T cells may be reduced, possibly as a result of tissue sequestration. There is no consistent evidence of impairment in delayed-type hypersensitivity, but there may be some abnormalities in helper/suppressor function, principally augmentation of helper function.

Toxic peptide. There is clear evidence of abnormal cellular reactivity to various autoantigens, including collagens (especially types I and III) which predominate in the skin. A peptide which is toxic for endothelial cells, perhaps a lymphocyte product, has been identified in scleroderma sera.

Mitogen stimulated normal mononuclear cell cultures can produce a soluble factor which will stimulate skin fibroblasts to increase collagen production. Abnormalities in this factor may underlie increased collagen production.

ANALOGUES OF SCLERODERMA

Animal models

Mouse. There is no close animal model of the human disease. However, a mutant of the B10.D2 (58N)/Sn mouse demonstrates some features and is known as the tight skin or TSK mouse. The homozygote mutation is lethal; the heterozygote develops thickening and tethering of the skin which resembles scleroderma. There is over twice as much collagen in the skin as in non-mutant mice, both on an absolute basis and in terms of the collagen–DNA ratio. No involvement of internal organs is seen. The changes show that genetic mutation may cause increased connective tissue and collagen production, presumably as a result of fibroblast activity.

Chicken. There is also an inherited avian disease affecting a certain strain of White Leghorn chickens. Clinical features are oedema and loss of appendages, arthritis, vascular involvement of the skin and extremities and eventually considerable internal disease of the oesophagus and heart. Extensive collagen thickening is seen with a mononuclear cell infiltrate.

Rat. There is a greater similarity to human disease in the case of homologous disease in rats, in view of its scleroderma-like features and those seen in the human condition of GVHD (see below). The possibility of developing a realistic animal model of scleroderma exists.

Graft-versus-host disease (GVHD)

A delayed chronic GVHD develops in a varying proportion of recipients up to three months after an HLA-identical allogeneic bone marrow transplant. There are impressive similarities between this syndrome and scleroderma: GVHD also has features of Sjögren's syndrome, SLE and primary biliary cirrhosis, although clinically and pathologically there are some clear differences. For example, chronic GVHD has little oesophageal and virtually no renal involvement.

The wide variations in treatment regimens prior to transplantation make it difficult to interpret pathological findings. For example, cytotoxic drugs and radiotherapy produce basal layer skin damage and a degree of fibrosis, which might be the effect of relative survival of fibroblasts producing more collagen. The lichenoid dermatitis seen as part of acute GVHD, appearing shortly after transplantation, may persist and resemble the sclerotic skin of scleroderma.

IMMUNOGENETICS

There is some inconsistency in the reported frequencies of MHC association in scleroderma patients, probably due to different patient classification in the reported series as well as racial differences.

HLA associations

HLA-1, -B5 and -DR3 are probably increased in white patients with diffuse scleroderma, whereas HLA-DR6 is associated with localized disease in blacks. An association with the supertypic gene DRw52, which is in linkage disequilibrium with DR3, DR5 and DR6 has been reported, but since this is associated with the sicca syndrome, these sub-groups will need to be re-examined in order to define the clinical associations more clearly.

Complement genes. There is disagreement about the associations with complement genes, although there is probably a relationship with the C4AQo gene in diffuse disease. There is therefore good evidence of an association between scleroderma and several D locus antigens and complement genes, emphasizing the importance of immune responses to the development of the disease.

Clinical sub-groups. It is not clear if these HLA associations are with incompletely defined sub-groups, or a non-specific association between immune response genes and a liability to scleroderma which is then precipitated by non-immunological (environmental) factors. A hint that the former may be the case is in the association between the CREST variant and DR5, whereas the latter is exemplified by an association between DR5 and vinyl chloride disease, a clear example of an environmental precipitant. Individuals exposed to vinyl chloride were investigated and it was found that HLA-DR5 was raised in the group as a whole, with milder disease being associated with C4BQo and more severe disease with C4AQo.

DIAGNOSIS OF SCLERODERMA

This is a clinical diagnosis, supported by such findings as disturbed gut motility; skin biopsy and renal biopsy are rarely necessary. Nail-fold capillary microscopy (Fig. 6.22) is also a useful and simple clinical method of confirming the suspicion of vascular abnormalities.

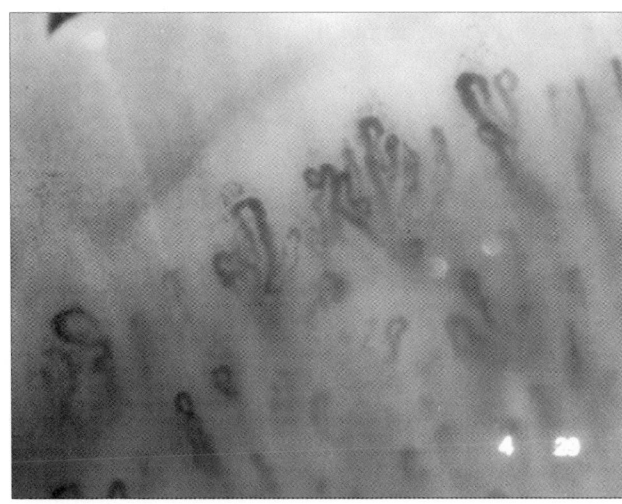

Fig. 6.22 Capillary microscopy gives dramatic evidence of vasculopathy in scleroderma.

PROGNOSIS

This is critically dependent on the sub-group:
- sclerodactyly (fingers only)
- hand and arm involvement
- diffuse, including trunk.

The worst prognosis for life is predicted by diffuse disease, renal and lung involvement, whereas relatively benign disease is found in patients with sclerodactyly alone and a positive anti-centromere antibody. A patient with Raynaud's phenomenon and a positive anti-nuclear antibody in high titre has a greater than 50% chance of developing a connective tissue disease in the future, scleroderma being more likely the more severe the Raynaud's.

TREATMENT

Controlled therapeutic trials have been few and inconclusive, largely because there is considerable variation in severity, the time course of the disease is long and spontaneous regression may occur. Widely available and commonly used treatments include:
- corticosteroids (low dose prednisolone)
- colchicine
- *d*-penicillamine — risk of toxicity demands close monitoring
- immunosuppression.

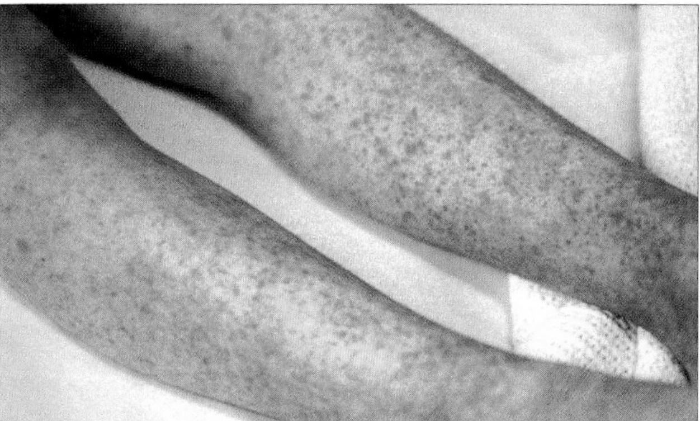

Fig. 6.23 Primary Sjögren's syndrome. The purpuric rash is characteristic and resembles that of Waldenström's macroglobulinaemia; it may be similarly mediated, in view of the frequent finding of hyperglobulinaemia.

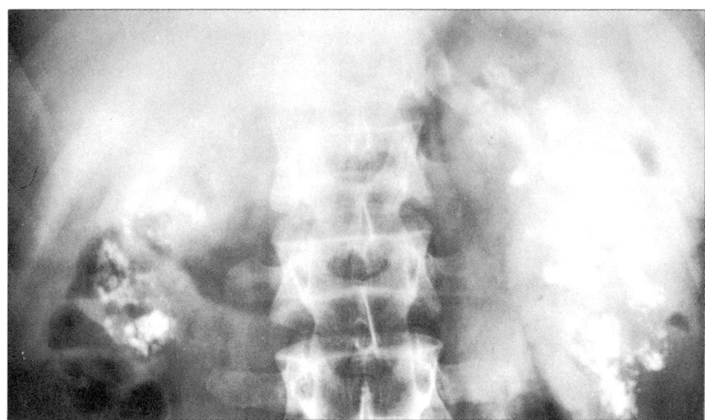

Fig. 6.24 Nephrocalcinosis in Sjögren's syndrome.

SJÖGREN'S SYNDROME

DEFINITIONS

The original description by Heinrich Sjögren, a Swedish ophthalmologist, was of patients with arthritis who suffered dryness of the eyes (xerophthalmia) and/or the mouth (xerostomia). The arthritis was subsequently shown to be usually rheumatoid in type. The term 'sicca syndrome' is used to indicate the components of mucosal dryness. The concept of Sjögren's syndrome has been extended and the following groups are recognized:
- primary Sjögren's syndrome (1° SjS) — sicca sydrome
- secondary Sjögren's syndrome (2°SjS) — sicca syndrome + SLE, scleroderma, polymyositis or primary biliary cirrhosis;
- Sjögren's syndrome with rheumatoid arthritis.

PRIMARY SJÖGREN'S SYNDROME

Local features

The most common causes of dryness of the mouth or eyes are physiological changes with ageing, the menopause and emotional disturbances. Strict criteria are needed to identify patients with immunologically mediated destruction of the salivary or lacrimal glands.

Exocrine glands. Whilst the emphasis is on the oral and ocular components, this is a disorder of exocrine glands in general, which led to the term 'autoimmune exocrinopathy'. Cutaneous and vaginal dryness can occur. Dry, inspissated respiratory mucus may present as bronchitis, and the pancreas or gastric mucosae are also often involved. Similarly, nasal dryness causes stuffiness and bleeding.

Systemic features

These patients do not often become systemically ill, although they may feel unduly fatigued, and have generalized aches and pains. Some may develop systemic features similar to SLE, for example Raynaud's phenomenon (see scleroderma) or vasculitis (Fig. 6.23).

Renal tubular acidosis (RTA) occurs in a small proportion of patients. It is identical to that found in the familial, non-autoimmune form and nephrocalcinosis may be the initial finding (Fig. 6.24). Perhaps all patients with autoimmune RTA represent part of the Sjögren's complex. The disease is papillary rather than cortical and biopsy may miss the lesion.

Immune responses and immunogenetics in Sjögren's syndrome			
Association	**Primary Sjögren's Syndrome**	**Secondary Sjögren's syndrome**	**RA/ Sjögren's syndrome**
synovitis	minor	minor	major
joint erosions	no	no	yes
vasculitis	yes	yes	less often
nodules	no	occasional	often
deformity	rare	sometimes	usual
lymphadenopathy	often	often	often (minor)
hyperglobulinaemia	usual	often	unusual
lymphopenia	sometimes	varies	rare
RF	usual	sometimes	usual
ANA	usual	usual	frequent (low titre)
anti-Ro (SS-A)	frequent	often	rare
anti-La (SS-B)	common	common	rare
DR3	usual	usual	infrequent
DR4	rare	rare	usual
B8/DQw1/2/C4A	often	often	rare

Fig. 6.25 Lymphopenia in secondary Sjögren's syndrome is commonly found, but only in active disease. Anti-Ro is usually associated with anti-La in primary Sjögren's syndrome, but may occur on its own in SLE, in which case the patients are usually DR2/3 and DQ1 positive.

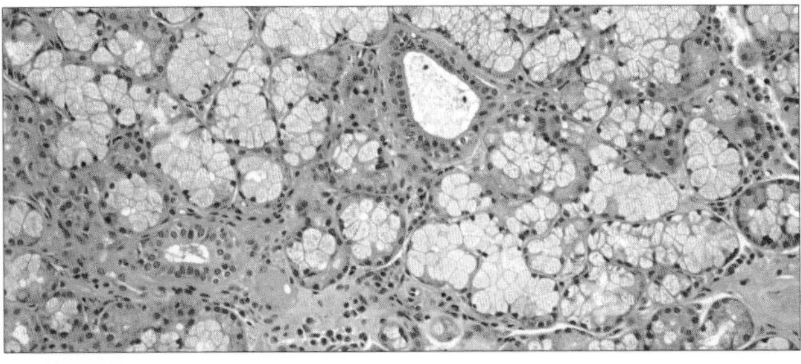

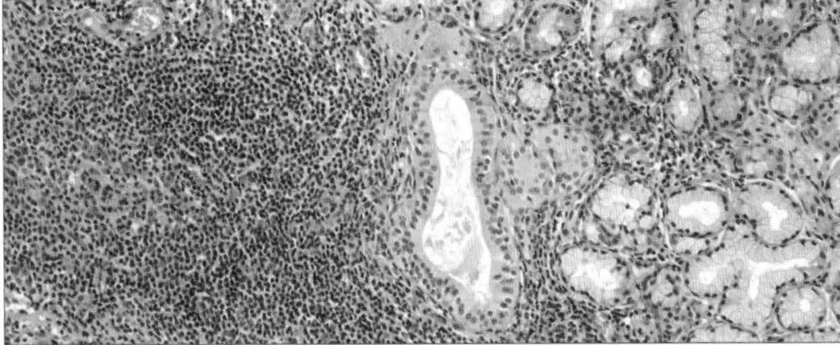

Fig. 6.26 Histology of salivary gland in Sjögren's syndrome. Upper: the normal gland has no lymphocytic infiltrate. Lower: in Sjögren's syndrome there is a dense mononuclear cell infiltrate around the salivary ducts.

The most common neurological finding is carpal tunnel syndrome with cranial nerves less frequently affected. A small minority of patients have diffuse, often subtle CNS involvement.

IMMUNOLOGICAL RESPONSES

Patients with Sjögren's syndrome lie on a continuum from benign to malignant lymphoproliferation. Hyperglobulinaemia is evidence of abnormal B lymphocyte hyperactivity. Lymphadenopathy is common and lymphocytic pneumonitis may develop, sometimes with massive pseudolymphoma.

Humoral immunity

Autoantibodies. The autoantibodies anti-Ro and anti-La were first described in patients with Sjögren's syndrome and termed anti-SjD and anti-SjT respectively. The same antibodies were subsequently but independently described as anti-SS-A and anti-SS-B by other authors, who noted a third antibody, termed anti-SS-C, in patients with RA but not in Sjögren's. This was further defined as having an affinity for Epstein-Barr nuclear antigen and called anti-RANA. This involvement with EB virus has been a matter of some debate (see below). Anti-nuclear antibodies are found in all types of SjS and do not indicate any particular disease severity.

Rheumatoid factors are almost universal in primary SjS and do not correlate with cartilage erosions as in patients with RA. Complement consumption is not a particular feature of SjS nor is there any obvious association with inherited disorders of complement.

Cell-mediated immunity

There is a relative deficiency of Ts cells in the circulation in most cases examined, which accords with the immunohistological picture (see below).

*Immunogenetics.*The supertypic genes DRw52 and -53 are associated with Sjögren's patients of all types, the former particularly with in SjS/RA. DR3 associates with anti-Ro/La in any clinical context. The haplotype HLA-B8, DR3, DW52 identifies at least 40% of patients with SjS but without RA, whereas DR4 is found almost exclusively in those patients with erosive arthritis.

The range of responses in the various types of Sjögren's syndrome is shown in Fig. 6.25.

PATHOLOGY

Salivary glands

The essential pathology of SjS lies in the exocrine glands, especially the salivary glands. The histology of the major parotid and submandibular glands is reflected in the minor labial glands in and around the mucosa of the lips. Biopsy of the latter is straightforward. The histology in SjS is fairly specific (Fig. 6.26): mononuclear cells form focal infiltrates around the salivary ducts. If plasma cells are present alone, they have less significance than if accompanied by foci of lymphocytes. $CD4^+$ cells predominate in the majority but $CD8^+$ T cells are also found. These findings, taken together with the expression of class II antigen and EBV DNA, indicates some form of autoreactive lymphocyte-mediated tissue damage, perhaps triggered by virus infection.

Association with malignancy

The frequency of B cell lymphoma is significantly increased in all patients with Sjögren's syndrome, as it is in patients with RA. It is not certain if this increase is accounted for by just those patients with Sjögren's syndrome. Pseudolymphoma is also a potentially malignant or a pre-malignant condition (Fig. 6.27). Pseudolymphoma, vasculitis or neurological involvement require corticosteroid treatment and the addition of cytotoxic drugs may further improve the response.

Drug reactions

There is a tendency in these patients to react adversely to antibiotics, particularly penicillin and suphonamides, and also to anti-rheumatoid medication such as gold salts and possibly penicillamine. DR2 is associated with drug toxicity of this type.

VARIANTS

CREST syndrome

The initials stand for calcinosis, Raynaud's, (o)esophagitis, sclerodactyly, telangiectasis. By definition, diffuse disease is not seen and the sclerodermatous skin is confined to the fingers, often with Raynaud's phenomenon. Vascular obliteration and oesophageal involvement may be severe, so this is not a benign disease, but renal involvement is not seen. About 60% of patients carry the anti-centromere antibody but do not have the anti-scl70.

Eosinophilic fasciitis (Shulman's syndrome)

This is characterized by rapid onset of skin oedema and thickening, often coming on after exertion and occurring most often in older men. It has a characteristic pathological picture in the skin provided the biopsy is taken deeply enough to include the sub-dermis. Treatment with corticosteroids seems to be very effective, however some patients may progress to true scleroderma.

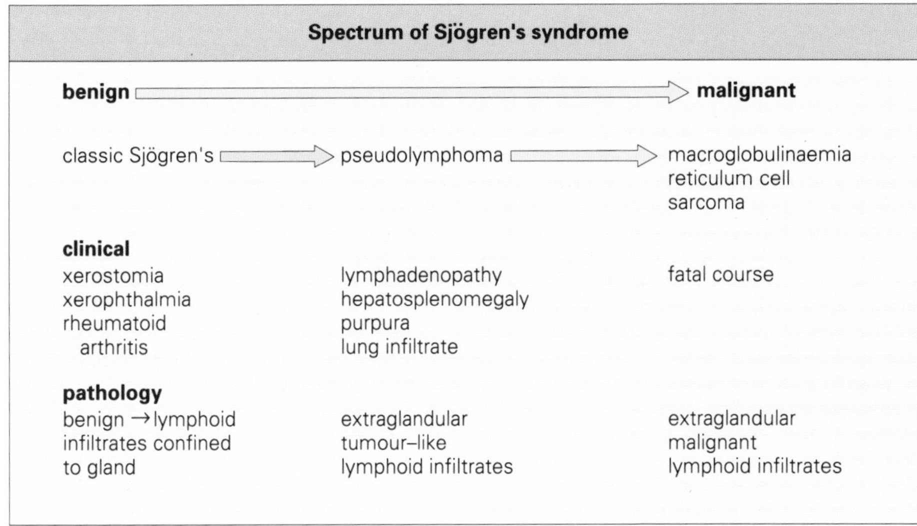

Fig. 6.27 Spectrum of Sjögren's syndrome (after Talal).

FURTHER READING

Dubois EL. *Systemic lupus erythematosus* (3E). Los Angeles: University of S. California Press,1987.

Pucetti A, *et al.* An immunoglobulin light chain from a lupus prone mouse induces autoantibodies in normal mice. *J Exp Med* 1990;**171**:1919–1930.

Kalunian K, *et al.* Characteristics of immunoglobulins associated with systemic lupus erythematosus: Studies of antibodies deposited in glomeruli of humans. *Arthritis & Rheum* 1990; **32**:513–522.

Worrall J, *et al.* SLE: A rheumatological view. Analysis of the clinical features, serology and immunogenetics of 100 SLE patients during long-term follow-up. *Q J Med* 1990;**NS74**:319–330.

7

Endocrine Disorders

ORGAN- VERSUS NON-ORGAN-SPECIFIC AUTOIMMUNE DISEASES

Autoimmune diseases in humans can be divided into organ-specific and non-organ-specific diseases on the basis of their immune response.

In non-organ-specific autoimmune disease, circulating autoantibodies (humoral immunity) and sensitized lymphocytes (cell-mediated immunity) are directed against antigenic determinants present in several tissues of the body. By contrast, organ-specific autoimmune disease is characterized by the presence of humoral and cell-mediated immunity directed mainly against cell constituents unique to the affected organ.

Immunologically based diseases of endocrine organs are almost always due to organ-specific autoimmunity (Fig. 7.1). Non-organ-specific autoimmune diseases are conditions which primarily involve the so-called rheumatological disorders (rheumatoid arthritis, systemic lupus erythematosus, dermatomyositis, scleroderma). The target organs most often affected are the joints, skin, kidney and muscles.

Organ- and non-organ-specific autoimmune diseases represent the opposite ends of a broad spectrum of different immune reactions which overlap considerably. Patients affected by an organ-specific disease, such as Hashimoto's thyroiditis, can also suffer from another organ-specific condition such as pernicious anaemia and vice versa, but it is rather unusual to find organ- and non-organ-specific diseases in the same subject.

Spectrum of classical endocrine autoimmune diseases
Thyroid disorders Hashimoto's thyroiditis primary myxoedema thyrotoxicosis (Graves' disease)
Gastric disorders fundal gastritis (type A) with or without pernicious anaemia autoimmune antritis (type B)
Other endocrine disorders insulin dependent diabetes mellitus (IDDM) autoimmune adrenalitis (Addison's disease) autoimmune hypogonadism & adrenalitis autoimmune hypophysitis autoimmune hypoparathyroidism vitiligo

Fig. 7.1 The majority of classical endocrine autoimmune diseases are organ-specific.

SPECTRUM OF ORGAN-SPECIFIC DISEASE

The concept of organ-specific autoimmunity was first introduced more than 30 years ago when anti-thyroglobulin antibodies were demonstrated by Roitt, Doniach and Campbell in the sera of patients affected by Hashimoto's thyroiditis, using a simple agar test (Fig. 7.2).

The concept of autoimmunity rapidly extended to include diseases of the stomach and adrenal glands following the discovery of antibodies to gastric parietal cells and to the adrenal cortex respectively. Subsequently, autoantibodies to the islet cells of the pancreas were detected in the serum of patients affected by insulin-dependent diabetes mellitus (IDDM), and autoantibodies to the endocrine cells of the adenohypophysis were documented in the serum of a proportion of patients with polyendocrine disease.

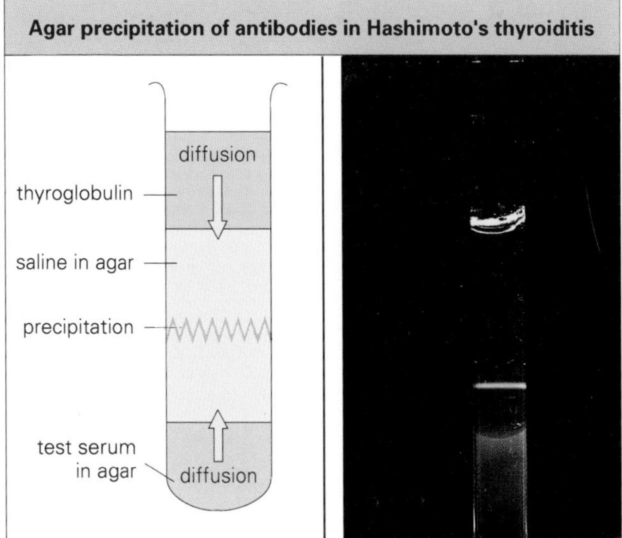

Fig. 7.2 Thyroglobulin antibodies in the serum of patient with Hashimoto's thyroiditis, demonstrated by precipitation in agar. Serum antibodies in the bottom layer of agar and thyroglobulin from the top layer diffuse towards the middle of the tube. If anti-thyroglobulin antibodies are present in the test serum, a zone of opaque precipitation will result.

Contribution of autoantibodies to diagnosis

The detection of serological markers of autoimmune disorders allows preclinical recognition of autoimmune endocrinopathies since autoantibodies can be present several years before the clinical condition develops. The frequency of such serological markers in the general population is quite low but rises with age. It is known that the larger the gland, the higher the titres of antibodies and the greater the likelihood that disease will develop in susceptible individuals.

It has been proposed that screening would be helpful in the following susceptible groups:

- patients with recognized autoimmunity to one endocrine organ, and their first degree relatives;
- patients with non-endocrine disorders that can be associated with endocrine autoimmunity (allergies, immune deficiencies) and their first degree relatives;
- middle-aged women with ill defined symptoms, such as fatigue and depression;
- patients with disorders of unknown aetiology. This may lead to the discovery of previously undescribed autoantibodies.

POLYGLANDULAR SYNDROMES

Since the beginning of the century it has been clear that more than one gland can be affected during the course of a patient's life; this process is characterized by a gradual destruction of the target epithelial cells and is associated with various degrees of lymphocytic infiltration. Claude and Gaugerot (1908) termed this syndrome 'polyglandular endocrine atrophy'. The concept of polyendocrinopathies has subsequently broadened to include patients affected by at least one endocrine disease who also possess a positive serological reactivity against other endocrine cell targets. It is now known that this is a much more common phenomenon than the full clinical expression.

The polyglandular failure diseases are linked by autoimmune phenomena, by similar immunogenetics and by the occurrence of multiple diseases in the same individual. The classical polyendocrinopathies are centred around the two most severe disorders — idiopathic hypoparathyroidism and autoimmune adrenalitis (Addison's disease).

Candida endocrinopathy (CE) & Schmidt's syndrome

Candida endocrinopathy, which occurs mostly in children of both sexes, revolves around hypoparathyroidism. It is so called because it associates with mucocutaneous candidiasis in 50% of paediatric cases (Fig. 7.3).

Schmidt's syndrome is a more common disorder which comprises the association between adrenalitis and thyroiditis. In later years Carpenter *et al.* found co-existing diabetes mellitus in 10 out of 15 patients and the concept was then extended to include this condition. The adrenalitis-thyroiditis-diabetes combination is more common and shows a female to male ratio of 3:1. Many cases start with thyrotoxicosis and Addison's disease occurring almost simultaneously; 40% of patients with the latter have at least one other overt disease. The frequency of vitiligo in patients with polyendocrine disease is 10–20%, much higher than that in the normal population.

Thyrogastric syndromes

It is not unusual to see thyroid and gastric autoimmunity in the same individual. Pernicious anaemia is at least five times more frequent in patients with thyroid disorders, and 10% of subjects with pernicious anaemia give a history of thyroid diseases. The serological overlap is even more common: parietal cell antibodies can be observed in 50% of patients with thyroid disorders. These findings suggested the existence of restricted forms of polyendocrine associations, which have been termed 'thyrogastric syndromes' (Fig. 7.4).

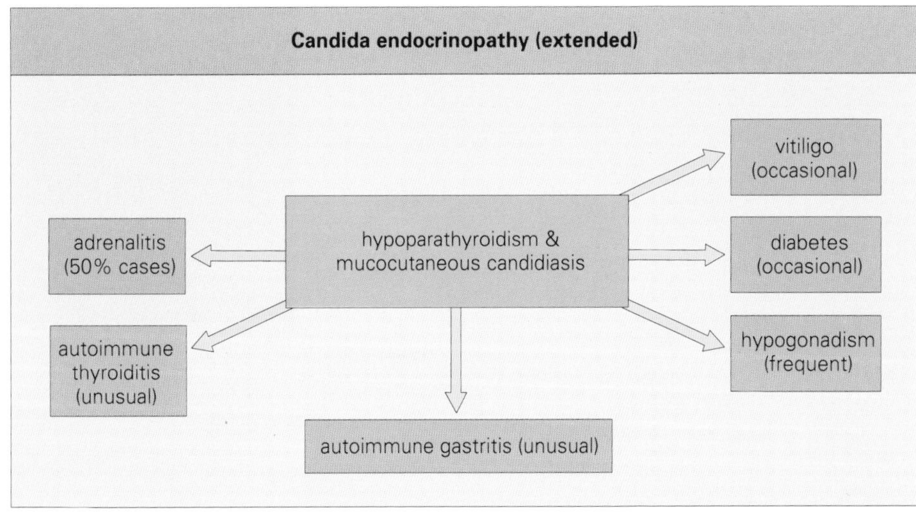

Fig. 7.3 Candida endocrinopathy is a rare disease with strong family connections. It is selectively concentrated in the population of Finland.

MECHANISMS OF ORGAN DAMAGE

Organ-specific autoimmunity is characterized by both humoral and cell-mediated immune phenomena, which in some cases can antedate the clinical outcome by many years. Humoral autoimmunity can affect target organs through:

- destructive mechanisms;
- stimulating mechanisms;
- blocking mechanisms.

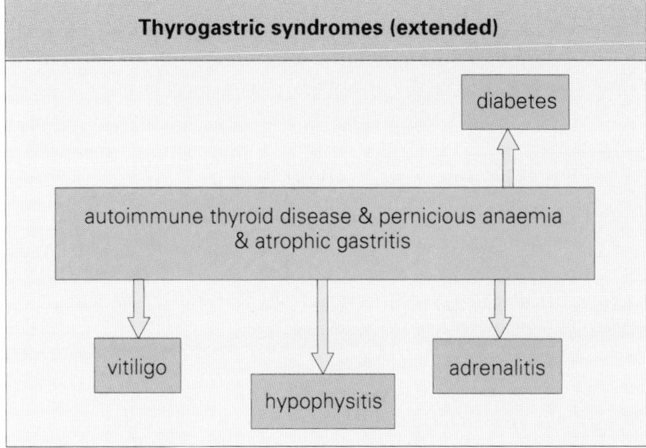

Fig. 7.4 Thyrogastric syndromes. It is common to see thyroid and gastric autoimmunity in the same patient, often with associated pernicious anaemia.

DESTRUCTIVE MECHANISMS

Cytoplasmic versus cell surface reactive autoantibodies

Cytoplasmic autoantibodies are invaluable tools for diagnostic and prognostic purposes. Their possible pathogenetic role lies in their ability to bind the corresponding autoantigens expressed on the cell surface. This is the prerequisite for activation of the complement cascade and binding by K cells. A precise definition of cell surface reactive autoantibodies requires the use of intact cells and the degree of practical difficulty is governed by the nature of each organ.

The data produced so far clearly indicate the existence of a heterogeneity within antigen-autoantibody systems between one endocrine gland and another and also between patients affected by apparently similar conditions (Fig. 7.5).

It is known that thyroid autoantibodies recognize cytoplasmic microsomal and cell surface microvillar autoantigens simultaneously in virtually 100% of cases, indicating an identity between the two thyroid autoantigens. Similarly, autoantibodies to gastric parietal cells recognize surface and cytoplasmic determinants in most cases, although 20% of patients with pernicious anaemia show only a cell surface reactivity. Conversely, in pancreatic islets conventional islet cell antibodies do not bind the cell surface in the majority of cases, and about 30% of diabetic sera which are negative for this specificity on tissue section show surface reactivity on live pancreatic cells. The extreme example of membrane restricted reactivity is shown by autoantibodies to melanocytes, which recognize cytoplasmic determinants in serum from patients with vitiligo in only a very small number of cases.

Circulating autoantibodies against organ-specific autoantigens

Tissue	Disease	Cytoplasmic Ab +ve surface Ab -ve	Cytoplasmic Ab -ve surface Ab +ve	Cytoplasmic Ab +ve surface Ab +ve
thyroid	thyroid autoimmune disease	—	—	100%
adrenal	adrenalitis/ Addison's disease	10%	—	90%
stomach	pernicious anaemia & chronic fundal gastritis	—	20%	80%
pancreatic islet cells	insulin dependent diabetes mellitus	50%	30%	20%
skin melanocytes	vitiligo	0.1% (9 cases)	~100%	1%

Fig. 7.5 Circulating autoantibodies against surface and cytoplasmic organ-specific autoantigens associated with destructive lesions. There appears to be heterogeneity among endocrine organs and among patients affected by similar clinical conditions.

Unique characterisitics of organ-specific autoantigen(s)		
Antibody specificity	**Autoantigens**	
	Biochemical characterization	**Molecular weight**
thyroid antibodies	thyroid peroxidase (TPO)	105–107 kDa
islet cell antibodies	glutamic acid dicarboxylase (GAD)	64 kDa (& other unidentified specificities)
melanocyte antibodies	?	75 kDa
gastric parietal cell antibodies	$Na^{+}K^{+}ATPase$	92 kDa

Fig. 7.6 Characteristics of autoantigens in destructive organ-specific disease. Autoantigen organ specificity is confirmed by absorption experiments. When sera containing both thyroid and gastric parietal cell antibodies are absorbed with thyroid extracts, the thyroid reactivity is lost but gastric antibodies are unaffected.

Characterization of autoantigens. It is remarkable that all organ- (and also non-organ) specific autoantigens so far isolated in different target tissues share certain biochemical properties, such as enzymatic activity, but clearly differ in others, such as molecular weights (Fig. 7.6).

STIMULATING AUTOANTIBODIES

Thyroid. It is now established that thyroid stimulating immunoglobulins (TSI) are present in up to 90% of cases of untreated Graves' disease. These antibodies, which are thought to be responsible for the clinical condition, are directed against the thyroid stimulating hormone receptor (TSH-R), and mimic the action of thyroid stimulating hormone (TSH) by promoting T3 and T4 production (Fig. 7.7).

There is evidence that TSH-R has more than one epitope, and this is reflected by the great variety of assays developed for measuring TSH-R antibodies. Some of these tests measure the ability of the antibody to bind to the receptor, whereas others measure stimulation of thyroid metabolic activities. It is now considered that binding and stimulation tests are complementary. The thyrotropin binding inhibiting immunoglobulin assay (TBII) measures the inhibition of binding radiolabelled TSH to intact thyroid cells, membranes and TSH-solubilized receptors. The thyroid stimulating immunoglobulin assay (TSI) measures the accumulation of cyclic AMP on an FRTL5 rat thyroid cell line.

Another type of antibody, possibly directed to the TSH-R, stimulates thyroid growth. This was intially demonstrated using a highly sensitive cytochemical bioassay and cytophotometry and the antibodies were found to be particularly associated with goitrous Graves' disease. Similar results were obtained by measuring tritium-labelled thymidine incorporation into reconstituted rat follicles or into an FRTL5 rat thyroid cell line.

Gastric. Stimulating antibodies have recently entered the field of gastric autoimmunity. Preliminary results show that among subjects with a duodenal ulcer who are also hypersecretors, approximately 40% possess immunoglobulins which can stimulate cyclic AMP production in parietal cell enriched suspensions prepared from the stomach of young male guinea pigs. These immunoglobulins could act either on the histamine receptors of gastric parietal cells, or on chief cells to stimulate pepsinogen secretion. In both cases, stimulation would lead to increased acidity of gastric secretions.

More work is required to confirm these data and those which demonstrate the existence of antibodies to adrenocorticotropic hormone receptor (ACTH-R) in the serum of patients with adrenocortical dysplasia.

BLOCKING AUTOANTIBODIES

The binding of autoantibodies to, or close to TSH receptors does not necessarily result in the functional stimulation of the receptor; it can, under certain cirucmstances, lead to receptor blocking (Fig. 7.8).

Thyroid. There is evidence that in primary myxoedema the clinical picture is influenced by TSH-R blocking antibodies which can stop the pathway of thyroid hormone synthesis either by inhibiting cAMP production, or by preventing regrowth of thyroid follicles despite increased pituitary output of TSH. Both types of blocking antibody may also be involved in transient neonatal hypothyroidism. Functional antibody blockers transmitted

Receptor stimulating autoantibodies in endocrine disease		
Disease	**Antigen**	**Effect**
Graves' disease	TSH-R	↑T3, T4
Graves' diease & non-toxic goitre & Hashimoto's thyroiditis	?	thyroid growth
duodenal ulcer	? histamine-R	↑gastric acid
Cushing's syndrome	? ACTH-R	↑steroids

Fig. 7.7 Receptor stimulating autoantibodies in endocrine disease.

Receptor blocking antibodies in endocrine disease		
Disease	**Antigen**	**Effect**
autoimmune thyroiditis	TSH-R (cAMP) ? TSH-R (growth)	blocks thyroid function blocks thyroid morphogenesis
fundal atrophic gastritis with pernicious anaemia	gastrin-R (on parietal cells)	inhibits gastric acid secretion
insulin resistant diabetes & acanthosis nigricans (type B)	insulin-R	↑ insulin dosage required
Addison's disease	ACTH-R	↓ steroid production
gonadal deficiency	gonadotropin-R (on ovarian cells)	infertility

Fig. 7.8 Antibodies blocking the ACTH-R in Addison's disease and antibodies blocking gonadotropin in gonadal deficiency are recent findings and still need confirmation.

through the placenta are thought to cause temporary hypothyroidism; these antibody blockers may affect the normal development of the thyroid in the fetus. It is postulated that they may be responsible for almost half the cases of athyreotic cretinism.

Stomach. Blocking antibodies have also been demonstrated in fundal gastritis. This condition, characterized by hypo- or achlorhydria, is associated with pernicious anaemia in extreme cases. Gastric parietal cell antibodies can be detected in the majority of patients. These have been shown to inhibit gastric acid secretion through a mechanism involving the inhibition of carbonic anhydrase activity on living gastric cells.

Pancreas. Like TSH-R antibodies, insulin receptor antibodies have been detected either by binding or by stimulation assay. Anti-insulin receptor antibodies were first observed in patients with severe insulin resistance and associated acanthosis nigricans; these patients' sera were able to inhibit the binding of ^{125}insulin to a lymphoblastoid cell line. Furthermore, antibodies to insulin receptors have been described in a group of untreated young diabetic patients, also with a binding assay but using rat adipocytes as substrate. The two antibodies appear to be directed against the same receptor, but have different immunological characteristics and produce two different clinical pictures. In one case, the binding of the insulin receptor leads to its blockage with consequent insulin resistance, whereas in the other, insulin requirement results. The insulin receptor antibodies associated with insulin resistance are IgG, and those seen in untreated young diabetics appear to be IgM.

CELL-MEDIATED IMMUNITY (CMI)

The role and significance of CMI in autoimmune endocrine disorders is much less clear than that of humoral immunity. This is mainly due to the technical difficulties involved in studying complex cellular functions in terms of both the activities of individual cells and their role within the intricate networks which consititute the immune system.

T cell function

The most popular, and arguably the most controversial test has been the leucocyte migration inhibition test (LMT) which, in expert hands, has given positive results with specific antigens or organ extracts in most endocrine diseases (Fig. 7.9). In individual cases, however, CMI correlates poorly with the presence of circulating antibodies to these organs. Confirmation by more reliable assays for lymphokine release from antigen-stimulated T cells is

Leucocyte migration inhibition tests (LMT) in endocrine autoimmune disease					
Antigen	thyroid microsomes	intrinsic factor & gastric homogenates	adrenal extracts	pancreatic extracts/ insulin	parathyroid extracts
Disease positivity	Graves' disease Hashimoto's thyroiditis	pernicious anaemia	Addison's disease	insulin dependent diabetes mellitus	idiopathic hypopara-thyroidism

Fig. 7.9 The LMT is positive in 30–50% of newly diagnosed diabetes patients and then tends to become negative after insulin treatment. In Graves' disease, the LMT is positive regardless of the derivation of the symptoms; circulating antibodies vary inversely with thyroid function, treatment and disease intensity.

Hypothyroidism & thyrotoxicosis : contrasting clinical features				
	Symptoms	**Signs**	**Tests**	**Treatment**
Hypo-thyroidism	fatigue, cold, constipation, weight gain, muscle cramps, menstrual irregularity, inability to concentrate, depression	dry skin, puffy face & hands, anaemia, hoarse voice, slow reflexes, bradycardia, cardiac enlargement	↓ total serum T4 ↓ free T4 ↓ serum free T3 ↑ TSH	thyroxine replacement
Thyro-toxicosis	palpitations, fatigue, sweating, weight loss, excitability	goitre, nystagmus, tremors, hot clammy skin, muscle wasting, dyspnoea, tachycardia, exophthalmos (atrophic variant) & pretibial myxoedema	↑ T3 & T4 ↓ TSH thyroid auto-antibodies TSI	anti-thyroid drugs; 131 iodine or surgery in case of relapse

Fig. 7.10 The clinical spectrum of thyroid diseases runs from hypothyroidism at one extreme to thyrotoxicosis at the other.

required to establish these ideas more firmly. Antigen purification is the greatest problem in the LMT since the presence of a mitochondrial fraction could contaminate the microsomal preparations.

Recently, a migration inhibition factor (MIF) assay has been used to examine suppressor activity: the results suggest that the production of MIF by autoreactive T cells in insulin dependent diabetes mellitus and Graves' disease is due to a deficiency of antigen-specific suppressor T cells.

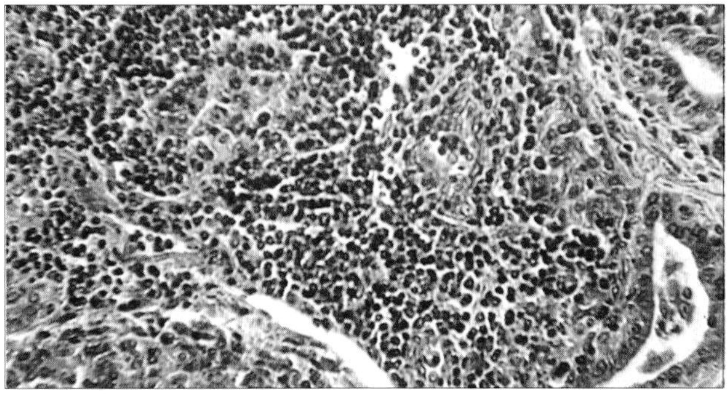

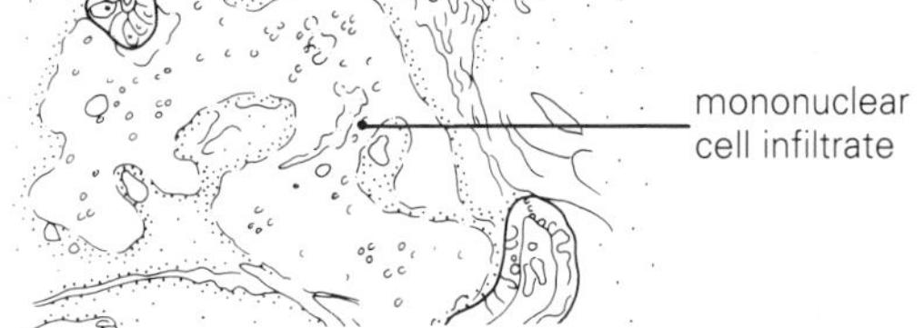

Fig. 7.11 Autoimmune thyroiditis. There is intense, diffuse infiltration of the gland by mononuclear lymphoid cells, which invade and destroy the thyroid follicles. Courtesy of S D Deodhar & R M Nakamura.

ORGAN–BASED DISEASE

THYROID

Clinical spectrum of thyroid autoimmune disease

Since 1956, when thyroid changes and lymphocytic infiltration were reproduced in experimental animal models and circulating thyroglobulin precipitating antibodies were found in patients with Hashimoto's thyroiditis, immense progress has been made in the understanding of autoimmune thyroid disease. This condition has continued to be a useful model of autoimmunity. It is now known that many clinical variants of thyroiditis share a common morphological picture and have to be regarded under this common denominatior.

Thyroid autoimmune disease constitutes a spectrum of conditions, with primary myxoedema at one end, running through the different variants of Hashimoto's thyroiditis, to Graves' disease at the other end. The clinical picture is summarized in Fig. 7.10. Clinical experience shows that thyroid autoimmune diseases seldom present in a 'pure' form, and they may also progress from one form to another in the same patient. The typical thyroiditis lesion, seen to different extents in all forms, is illustrated in Fig. 7.11.

Primary myxoedema (atrophic variant of thyroiditis). This is the most common form of spontaneous hypothyroidism in adults. It represents the last stage of a chronic inflammatory process similar to chronic lymphocytic thyroiditis, occurring in about 25% of treated patients with goitres and in a small proportion of those with thyrotoxicosis treated with anti-thyroid drugs. Women are affected at least five times more frequently than men, and more than

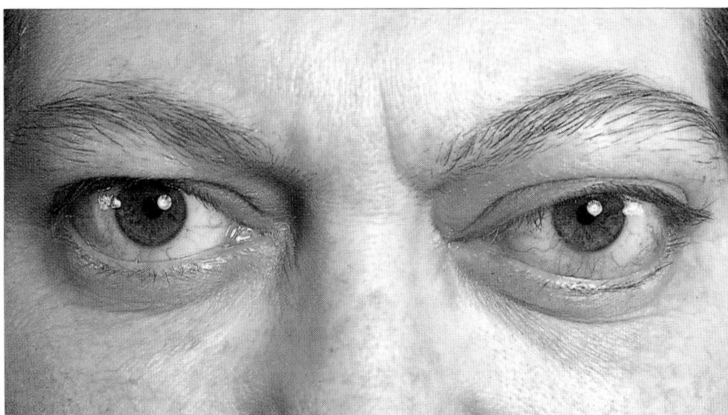

Fig. 7.12 The typical clinical appearance of Graves' disease includes exophthalmos and lid retraction, as seen in this case.

70% of cases are diagnosed after the age of 50. The onset in adults causes a generalized slowing down of the metabolism, with deposition of glycosaminoglycans in intracellular spaces (mainly skin and muscle). The role of TSH is important in the early stages of decompensation, since cases with a markedly raised serum TSH level are usually the quickest to respond to thyroxine treatment.

Hashimoto's thyroiditis. This is a common cause of hypothyroidism associated with goitre, but the patient may be unaware of the condition until the goitre becomes very large. It is the result of lymphocytic infiltration of the thyroid. At least three forms have been described: the juvenile thyroiditis variant, the oxyphil variant, and the rare fibrous variant which occurs mainly in elderly women. All variants exhibit high levels of thyroid autoantibodies in most cases.

In Hashimoto's thyroiditis different clinical stages can be observed. The initial stage is characterized by the presence of goitre, with normal TSH levels and thyroid function. This stage can progress to clinically compensated hypothyroidism with goitre, normal thyroid function, but increased levels of TSH. Subsequently, the goitre can be found in association with uncompensated or clinical hypothyroidism, in which TSH levels are raised, T4 is low, and T3 is normal or low.

Of the women with goitre and elevated TSH, 5% per year develop hypothyroidism. Occasionally patients with thyroiditis can develop transient hyperthyroidism due to episodic release of thyroid hormone from damaged cells. This clinical entity has been observed in pairs of identical twins and in members of the same family. T4 replacement leads to disappearance of the goitre in 30% of patients after 5–10 years; only 10–20% fail to show any reduction in size after years of treatment with T4.

Graves' disease. This is the most common cause of thyrotoxicosis. The female to male ratio is 5:1. The condition can occur at any age, but the peak incidence is around 20–40 years. Graves' disease can occur with or without exophthalmos (Fig. 7.12) or goitre. The course of the disease is characterized by remissions and exacerbations.

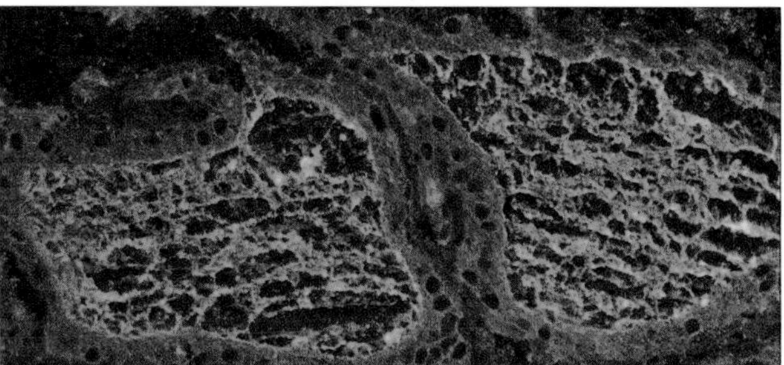

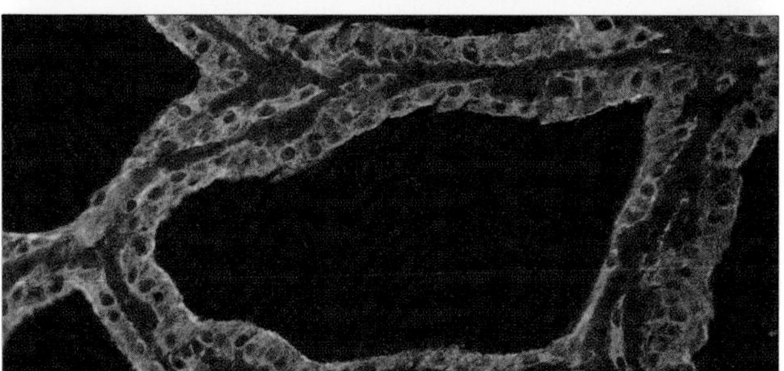

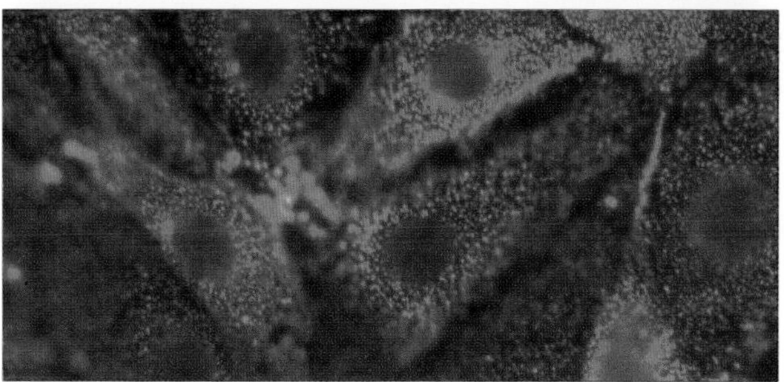

Fig. 7.13 Immunofluorescent staining of thyroid antigen. Upper: thyroglobulin. Cryostat section of human thyroid fixed in methanol at 56°C for 10 minutes and incubated with serum from Hashimoto's patient. The reaction is detected by applying fluorescein isothiocyanate (FITC)-rabbit anti-human Ig. A floccular appearance is evident within the thyroid follicles.x250. Middle: TPO antigen. Unfixed cryostat section of human thyroid stained with serum from Hashimoto's patient. Fluorescence is detected as above and is restricted to the cytoplasm of the thyroid epithelial cells lining the follicles.x250. Lower: TPO. Two day monolayer of thyroid cells incubated with serum from a patient with Hashimoto's disease and stained with rhodamine isothiocyanate (TRITC)-rabbit anti-human Ig.

Radioactive iodine treatment or surgery can be performed after the patient has been prepared with anti-thyroid drugs.

Spectrum of thyroid antibodies

The cornerstone of immunological diagnosis of human thyroiditis is the demonstration of autoantibodies to a specific thyroid antigen. These autoantibodies can be directed against thyroid cytoplasmic structures, cell surface components and thyrocyte receptors. Cytoplasmic autoantibodies are directed against the thyroglobulin and thyroid peroxidase (TPO) autoantigens (Fig. 7.13). Anti-thyroglobulin antibody is found in 50–70% of patients with various forms of chronic thyroiditis and in a third of patients with hyperthyroidism. Approximately 70% of patients with autoimmune thyroiditis possess antibodies, which recognize TPO. The percentage increases up to 95% in patients with Hashimoto's thyroiditis.

The thyroglobulin and TPO antibodies vary independently of each other in the serum, thus it is essential to titrate both in every goitrous patient and in all cases of suspected thyroid deficiency. TPO antibodies tend to occur early, while thyroglobulin antibodies can occur later when cellular destruction may release high quantities of thyroglobulin. It is known that TPO antibodies correlate better with clinical thyroid disease. However, a few cases of advanced myxoedema react only with thyroglobulin, having lost their TPO antibodies with the progressive destruction of the thyroid gland. Thyroid autoantibodies increase with age in the normal population (5% in children versus 40% in the elderly).

A third cytoplasmic antibody is also occasionally found. The reaction is attributed to a 'second' colloid antigen (Fig. 7.14), but it cannot be absorbed with thyroglobulin; the antigen appears to be a non-iodinated form of colloid protein.

Native thyroglobulin, although secreted, is not expressed on the surface of the thyroid follicular cells, in contrast to asialo-agalactothyroglobulin (Fig. 7.15), the thyroglobulin precursor; this may indicate that the precursor molecule is the possible relevant immunogen for the induction of thyroglobulin autoreactive sera. Microsomal and thyroglobulin antibodies occur in up to 80% of cases of thyrotoxicosis but are of less diagnostic importance, as the disease is caused by thyroid stimulating immunoglobulin (TSI) reacting with TSH receptors.

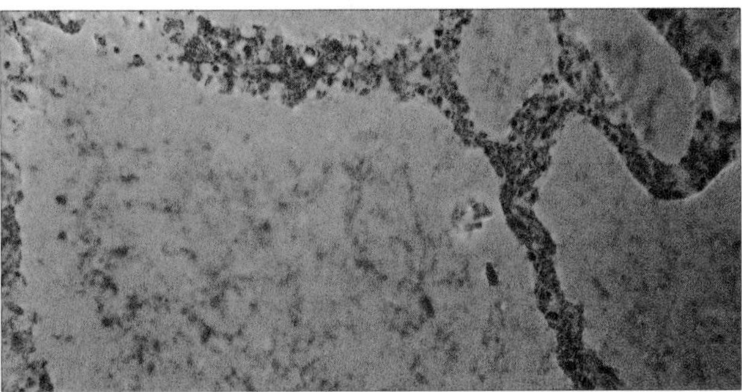

Fig. 7.14 Immunofluorescent staining of second colloid antigen. Cryostat section of human thyroid stained as in Fig. 7.13 lower. A homogeneous pattern of fluorescence is seen in the thyroid follicles.

STOMACH

According to the Strickland and McKay (1973) classification, two forms of gastritis exist (Fig. 7.16):
- type A — chronic fundal gastritis
- type B — antral gastritis

Type A is considered to be the precursor of pernicious anaemia (PA), in which the mucosal atrophy is more marked. As cited above, hypochlorhydria, high levels of serum gastrin and parietal cell antibodies (PCA) can be present in this type of chronic gastritis (Fig. 7.17), but there are no anti-chief or anti-mucus cell antibodies, despite the specific destruction of corresponding cells. In addition, intrinsic factor antibodies (IFAb) can be detected in the serum and gastric juice of patients with PA. The serum IFAb are IgG and do not affect B_{12} absorption, whereas the IFAb secreted directly into the gastric juice are IgA and appear to contribute to PA by inactivating the remaining traces of IF produced by atrophic mucosa. Conversely, PCA do not affect B_{12} absorption but appear to affect gastric acid secretion.

More recently, antibodies to gastrin-producing cells have been demonstrated in a proportion of patients with type B antral gastritis. This variant of gastritis is commonly associated with gastric ulcers, or follows partial gastrectomy. Alcohol and nicotine are also thought to be precipitating factors.

PANCREAS: DIABETES MELLITUS

Clinical features

This syndrome is characterized by altered metabolism and hyperglycaemia, due to either a failure of insulin secretion or a decrease in biological function, or both. Diabetes has been classified according to whether patients treated successfully are dependent (type I; IDDM) or non-dependent (type II; NIDDM) on insulin.

Type I most commonly occurs in young subjects. It is

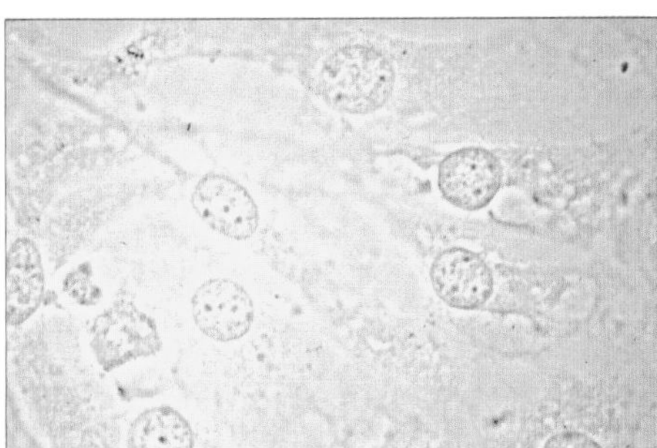

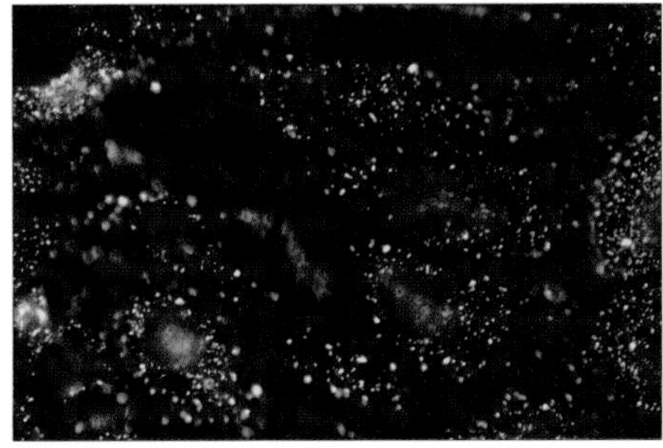

Fig. 7.15 Asialo-agalacto-thyroglobulin on thyroid cells in culture. Left: a two day monolayer of human thyroid cells (phase contrast). Right: after incubation with asialo-agalactothyroglobulin, rabbit anti-thyroglobulin Ig is added, followed by FITC-goat anti-rabbit Ig. Courtesy of Professor R Pujol-Borell.

Comparison of type A & B chronic gastritis		
	Type A	Type B
sex ratio F : M	3:1	2:1
age	~50 years	~50 years
fundal atrophy	80%	27.5%
antral atrophy	13.3%	92.5%
gastrin levels	↑	↓
association with polyendocrine disease	60%	12.5%
PCA	60% (female) 20% (male)	20%
S-PCA	100%	n.d.
gastrin-R blocking Ab	common	rare
IFAb	30%	20%
gastrin cell Ab	rare	10%

Fig. 7.16 In type A gastritis associated with pernicious anaemia, the prevalence of parietal cell antibody (PCA) increases in up to 90% of cases and that of intrinsic factor (IFAb) to 56% of adults and to 100% in children. Surface-reacting PCA (S-PCA) correlates with PCA in 80% of cases. Modified from Doniach, D *et al.* (1982).

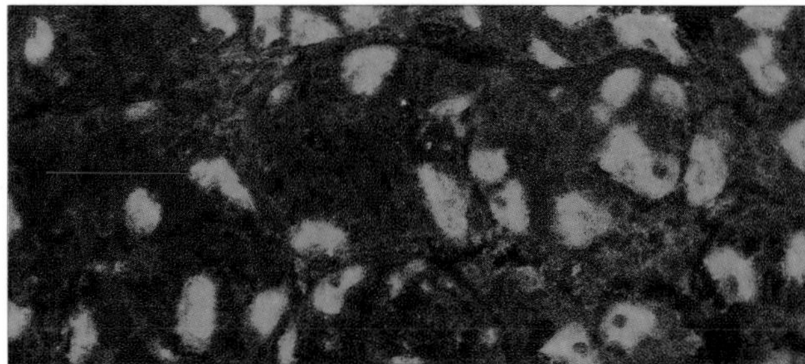

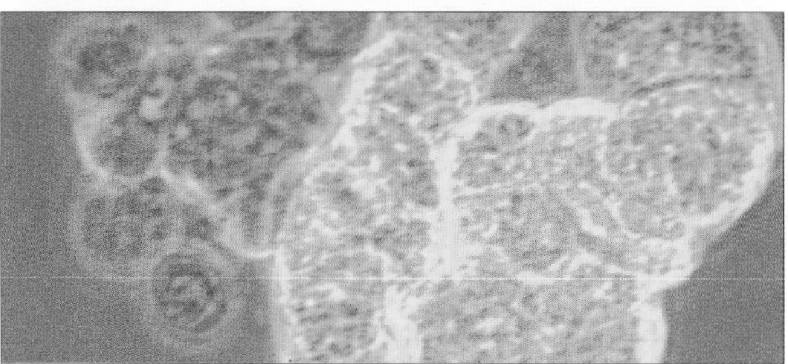

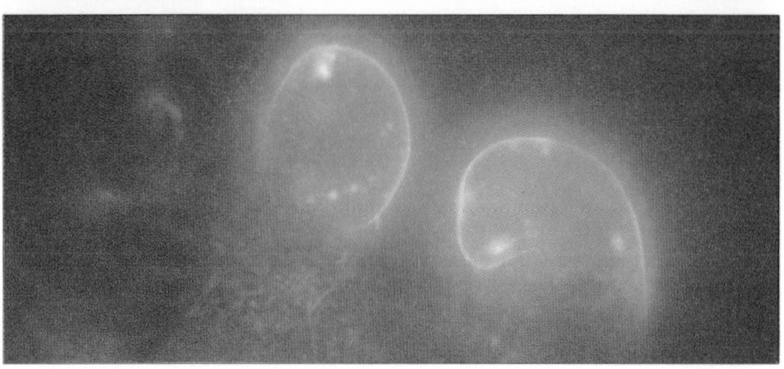

Fig. 7.17 Immunofluorescent staining of human parietal cells in stomach. Upper: cytoplasmic parietal cell antibody (PCA). Cryostat section of human stomach incubated with PA serum and FITC-rabbit anti-human Ig. The reaction is localized to the parietal cells. Middle: surface reacting PCA. Phase contrast of viable suspension of human stomach cells. Lower: the same preparation is then stained for indirect imunofluorescence with PA serum. Surface staining is restricted to the parietal cells.

characterized by polyuria, polydypsia, weight loss, normal/increased appetite, fatigue and visual disturbances. Insulin deficiency leads to excessive accumulation of glucose and fatty acids, with consequent hyperosmolality and hyperketonuria.

Type II comprises a group of milder forms, occurring predominantly in adults, of whom 85% are obese. The remaining 15% have an absent or delayed early phase of insulin release in response to glucose. The condition usually presents insidiously, with initial signs of chronic skin infections or generalized pruritus and vaginitis. A family history of mild diabetes is usually reported.

Immunological features

It is now clear that IDDM, in spite of the acute onset of clinical symptoms, is the result of a long, latent, but progressively damaging process to pancreatic β cells. Clinically, this latency period is characterized by the loss of the first phase of insulin response to intravenous glucose and by the presence of islet cell antibodies (ICA) which can be detected months or even years before the clinical onset.

It is now universally accepted that type I and not type II diabetes is the result of an autoimmune mechanism selectively directed against pancreatic β cells. The hypothesis of an immune basis for type I diabetes was suggested in the mid-1960s with the elegant description of insulitis, a process characterized by lymphocytic infiltration around the islet cells (Fig. 7.18); this was found in approximately 68% of pancreases obtained from patients with juvenile diabetes who died soon after the clinical onset of the disease. In the following decade, the detection of circulating antibodies reacting with the cytoplasm of all islet cells (ICA) in the majority of patients with newly diagnosed type I but not type II diabetes has subsequently confirmed the suggestion that only type I is of immunological origin.

The first account of ICA was followed by the description of several other species of islet cell antibodies in the sera of diabetes patients; these are complement fixing islet cell cytoplasmic antibodies (CFICA), surface reactive islet cell antibodies (ICSA) and cytotoxic islet cell antibodies.

There is also a compelling amount of evidence indicating that genes in the HLA-D region of the short arm of chromosome 6 confer susceptibility to IDDM (see chapter 2). It is known that at least 90–95% of Caucasian IDDM patients have HLA-DR3 or DR4 or both genes, compared

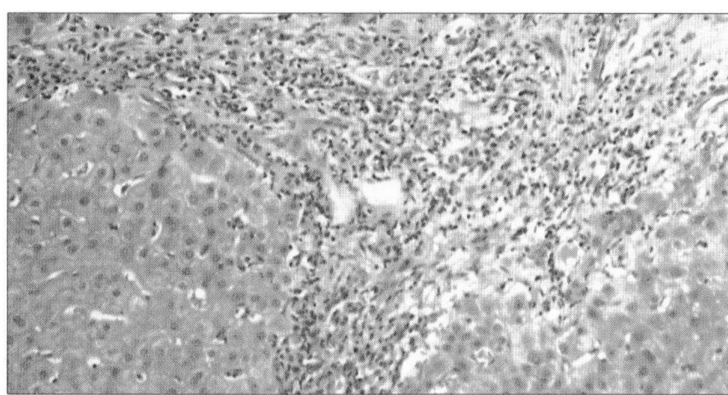

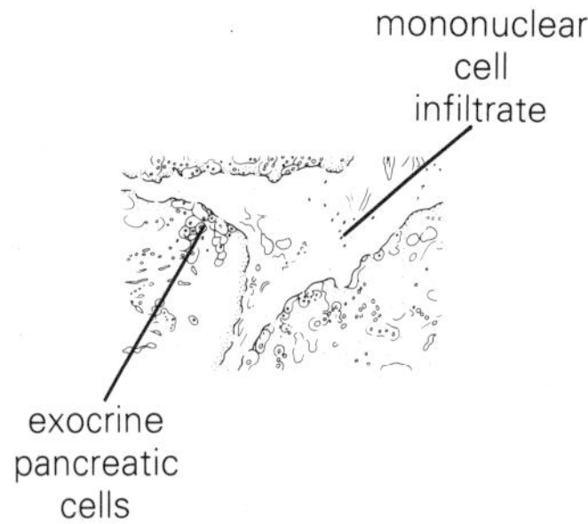

Fig. 7.18 Insulitis. There is mononuclear cell infiltration of a pancreatic islet, with relative sparing of exocrine pancreatic cells. H & E stain.

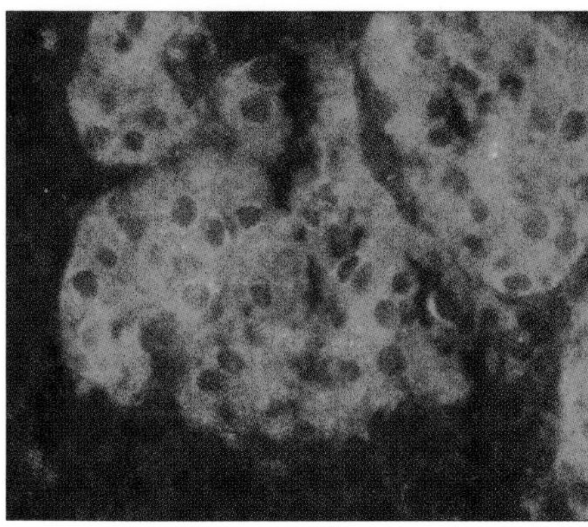

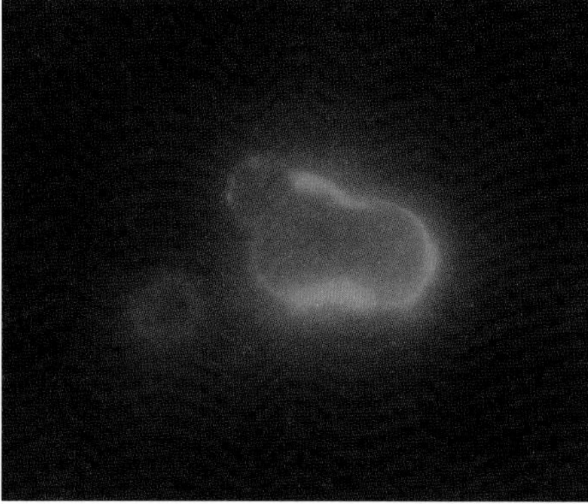

Fig. 7.19 Immunofluorescent staining of islet cells. Left: cytoplasmic reactivity. Cryostat section of human (blood group O) pancreas stained with diabetic serum. The antibody reaction is confined to the islet cells. Right: surface cell reactivity. Viable fetal pancreatic β cells (blood group O) stained with diabetic serum, showing cell surface reactive antibody. Courtesy of Professor R Pujol-Borell.

with 50–60% in the general population. More recently it has emerged that IDDM susceptibility is even more closely related to the DQ rather than the DR locus.

Relevance of autoantibodies in IDDM. ICA is an organ-specific antibody, which is present in 70–80% of patients at diagnosis but tends to disappear thereafter; in the general population ICA is detected in 0.4% of subjects. It does not retain a pathogenetic role, but is considered an invaluable tool for diagnostic and prognostic purposes as only a few individuals lacking this specificity develop IDDM. In approximately 50% of cases it is able to fix complement. This property appears to reflect high titres of antibody and may select individuals at highest risk. It represents a polyclonal autoimmune response exclusively of IgG, in contrast to the wider class distribution of antibodies in thyroid and gastric autoimmune diseases. The antibody reacts with the cytoplasmic structures of glucagon, somatostatin and insulin cells, suggesting that the endocrine cells in the islets share a common autoantigen (Fig. 7.19 left).

ICA is also a useful marker for defining heterogeneity within diabetic patients: 10% of patients with NIDDM who have persistent ICA and a low C-peptide response to arginine infusion tend to progress to overt IDDM. Similarly, genetically predisposed individuals and subjects with a milder form of diabetes who have ICA are more prone to becoming diabetics.

Surface reactive islet cell antibodies (ICSA) would appear to have greater pathogenetic significance than ICA since they might represent the initial attack against the plasma membrane of viable β cells (Fig. 7.19 right). They have complement fixing ability and show ADCC activity. ICA, however, retains its usefulness for routine screening since there is an unexpectedly high incidence of ICSA (20–25% against a predicted 6–10%) in first degree relatives and because of the high variability in ICSA determination among different groups. Measurement of ICSA still requires better standardization procedures.

Anti-insulin antibodies (IAA). The full insulin autoimmune syndrome was first described in Japan in patients with spontaneous hypoglycaemia and thyrotoxicosis. The attacks of hypoglycaemia may persist for months but then tend to remit spontaneously. Based on this observation it was anticipated that anti-insulin antibodies could be found in newly diagnosed IDDM patients prior to insulin treatment. IgG IAA have recently been demonstrated in 16–32% of newly diagnosed diabetic patients and in a proportion of subjects 'at risk' of IDDM (twins or first degree relatives of IDDM subjects).

Despite assay differences, IAA are now considered an important humoral marker in IDDM. However, the present state of the art indicates that a high titre of ICA and/or CFICA with or without the detection of IAA has to be considered the best predictive marker of autoimmune aggression.

ADRENAL

Following the advent of antibiotic treatment, most cases of Addison's disease (53–60%) are now caused by autoimmune destruction of the adrenal cortex. This process results in deficient adrenal production of glucocorticoids and mineralocorticoids, leading to adrenal failure. It is an unusual form of autoimmunity and occurs mainly in women.

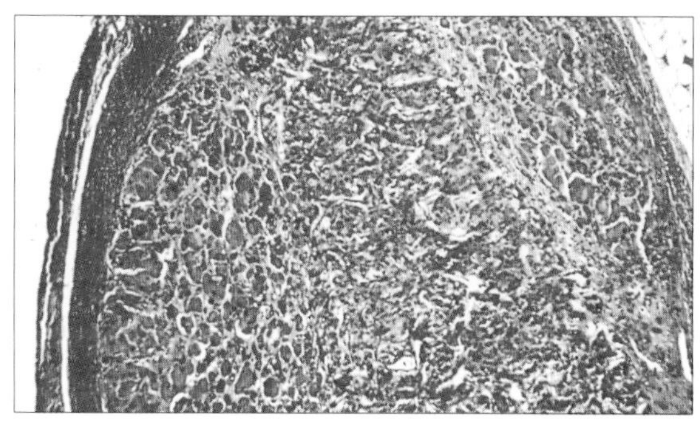

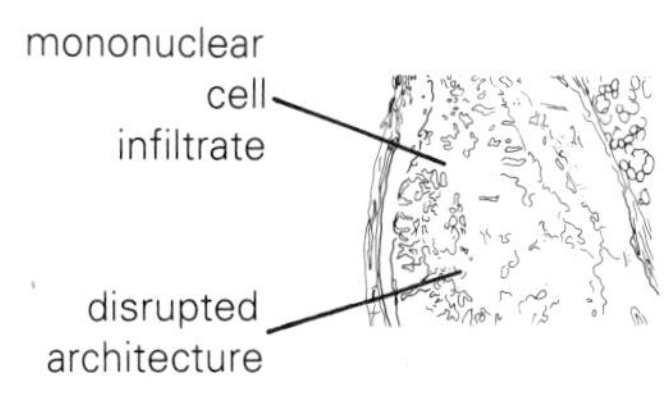

Fig. 7.20 Adrenalitis. Focal mononuclear cell infiltration is visible within the adrenal gland, causing disruption of the normal architecture. Courtesy of S D Deodhar & R M Nakamura.

Clinical and laboratory features

One of the earliest features is hyperpigmentation, appearing initially in the nail beds, areolas, palmar creases and paravaginal area; this then extends to the rest of the skin and mucous membranes. Other symptoms include weakness, fatigue, amnesia, weight loss, hypotension, gastrointestinal symptoms and hypoglycaemia; all are caused by adrenocorticoid failure. Mineralocorticoid deficiency results in renal sodium loss and potassium retention, inducing hyponatraemia, hyperkalaemia and acidosis.

Immunological features

The autoimmune process has been documented by the morphological picture of adrenalitis (Fig. 7.20), and by the presence of autoantibodies (Fig. 7.21) which can react with all three layers of adrenocortical cells (or less frequently with either the glomerulosa cells or the fasciculata and reticularis cells). The clinical significance of the different patterns is unknown, but could indicate the presence of heterogeneity within this condition. The autoantibodies are IgG and are usually present in low titres (less than 1/60). In 50% of cases the adrenal antibodies are able to fix complement; this feature is considered a predictive marker for developing disease.

Autoantibodies are found mainly in patients with isolated Addison's disease (38–79%). They occur to a lesser extent in patients with polyendocrine disease (7%) in which adrenal failure does not necessarily follow, and are found very occasionally in patients with thyrotoxicosis, or pernicious anaemia, or diabetes (1–3%). The prevalence in the general population is very low (0.7%). It has been shown that 90% of positive cases also have an antibody directed against specific adrenal surface antigens.

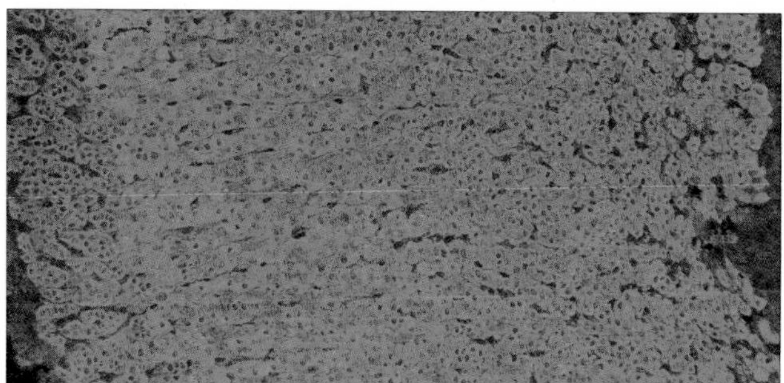

Fig. 7.21 Immunofluorescent staining of the adrenal cortex. The cytoplasm of the granulosa and fasciculata cells reacts with serum from a patient with Addison's disease.

Immunofluorescent staining of steroid cells by St-Abs-containing sera

Organ	Reactive cells	Remarks
adrenal cortex	all 3 layers (less often 1–2)	all St-Abs can be absorbed out with adrenal homogenates
human testis	Leydig cells	common origin & equivalent function
human ovary	interstitial & hilum cells	
Graafian follicle	theca cells	common antigen
corpus luteum	paraluteum cells	
	lutein cells (3 patterns)	3 separate antigens
human placenta	trophoblast	doubtful specificity

Fig. 7.22 Immunofluorescent staining of steroid-producing cells by sera containing steroid cell antibodies (St-Abs). Courtesy of D Doniach, G F Bottazzo & H Drexhage.

GONAD AND PLACENTA

Steroid-producing cell antibodies (St-Abs) are a group of antibody systems which cross-react with steroid-producing cells in the ovary, testis, and placenta and have so far been detected only in sera that also react with human adrenal cortex. 50% of sera from Addison's patients who have other associated polyendocrine diseases and 22% of isolated Addison's disease cases have St-Abs. These specificities can be absorbed out with adrenal homogenates.

Steroid cell antibodies have various patterns in corpus luteum and other ovarian structures and nearly all stain the Leydig cells in the testis (Fig. 7.22). Whether patients with St-Abs have an increased tendency to premature menopause and ovarian failure or infertility is still a controversial issue.

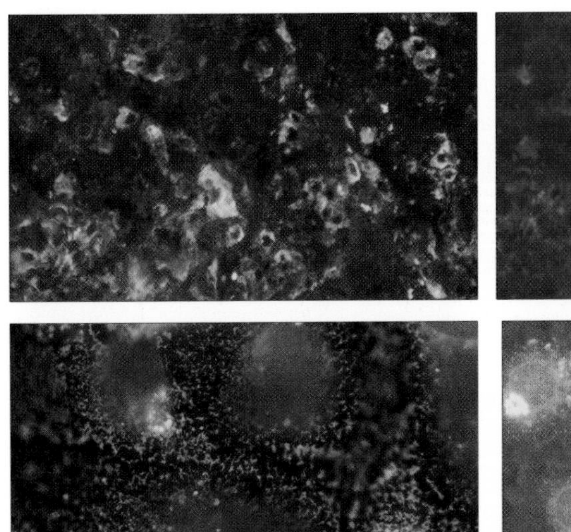

Fig. 7.23 Immunofluorescence in prolactin (PRL) cells of pituitary. Left: cryostat section of human pituitary stained with serum from a patient with polyendocrine disease (fluorescein). Right: the same preparation is then counterstained with a monoclonal antibody to PRL (rhodamine).

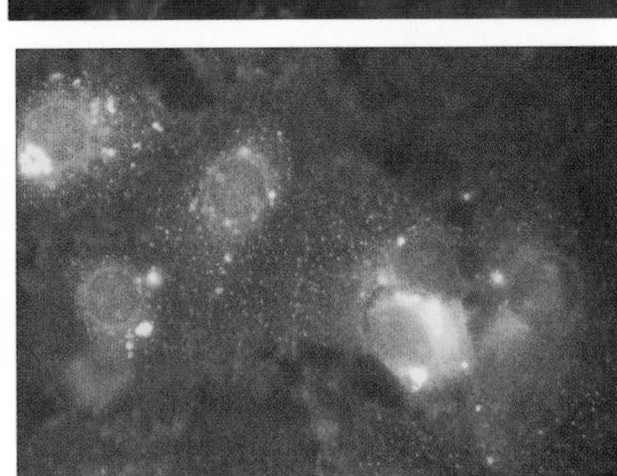

Fig. 7.24 Parathyroid surface reacting antibodies. Left: two day culture of human parathyroid cells from parathyroid adenoma stained by indirect immunofluorescence with serum from a hypoparathyroid patient showing speckled surface staining. Right: the cell surface reaction is not seen after incubation with $F(ab')_2$ fragments of IgG from the same patient.

PITUITARY

Clinical features

The first case of lymphocytic hypophysitis was described in 1962 by Goudie and Pinkerton in a woman with Hashimoto's thyroiditis. Compared to other endocrine organs, autoimmune diseases of the pituitary are quite rare, the existence of lymphocytic hypophysitis reflecting a possible underlying autoimmune mechanism of endocrine cell destruction. This has been a relatively recent finding, with almost ten years elapsing before autoantibodies to pituitary endocrine cells were reported.

A survey of 16 cases of documented hypophysitis showed a prevalence in females (only one male case), with a higher occurrence during pregnancy and the puerperium. Subjects aged 22–74 presented with symptoms of hypopituitarism requiring hormone replacement, together with a variety of autoimmune disorders and/or circulating organ-specific antibodies.

Immunological features

Currently, there is no standardization procedure for the detection of pituitary cell antibodies. The choice of substrate is still controversial. The shortage of human surgical specimens has led several groups to make use of rodent pituitary, which is known to produce heterophile reactions. There is now evidence that primate pituitary may be a more suitable substrate for pituitary autoantibody screening. It is not clear why pituitary prolactin cell antibodies (Fig. 7.23) are the most common type of pituitary autoantibody to be detected. These specificities were first observed in 10% of patients affected by polyendocrine disease. They have not been found in severe panhypopituitarism, but can occur in patients with various partial pituitary defects. Antibodies to growth hormone cells have been identified in only three patients with growth hormone defects, after an extensive search in a selected group of 220 children. Adrenocorticotropic hormone (ACTH) cells present a special difficulty because they appear to have Fc receptors, and so virtually all immunoglobulins react with them. To prove that these antibodies exist, it is necessary to digest the patient's immunoglobulins with pepsin to obtain $F(ab')_2$ fragments.

No human serum has yet been found to react with all pituitary cells, implying that the gland does not possess a 'common' antigen comparable with those of the thyroid, adrenal and pancreas.

PARATHYROID

Immunological features

Only one group has reported the existence of circulating cytoplasmic antibodies to parathyroid chief cells; these were found in the sera of a sub-group of patients with primary hypoparathyroidism. Conversely, positive results were obtained by leucocyte migration inhibition in 7 out of 10 cases of hypoparathyroidism. Recently, autoantibodies were demonstrated binding to the cell surface of dispersed cell cultures of human parathyroid derived from adenomatous glands in 8 out of 23 patients with idiopathic hypoparathyroidism. These results are, however, controversial as parathyroid cells from adenomas appear to express *'de novo'* surface antigens which are not present in normal or hyperplastic parathyroid tissues (Fig. 7.24). The reaction disappears after incubation of adenomatous parathyroid cells with the $F(ab')_2$ fragments derived from the patient's immunoglobulin, indicating that this phenomenon is not the result of an antigen–antibody reaction.

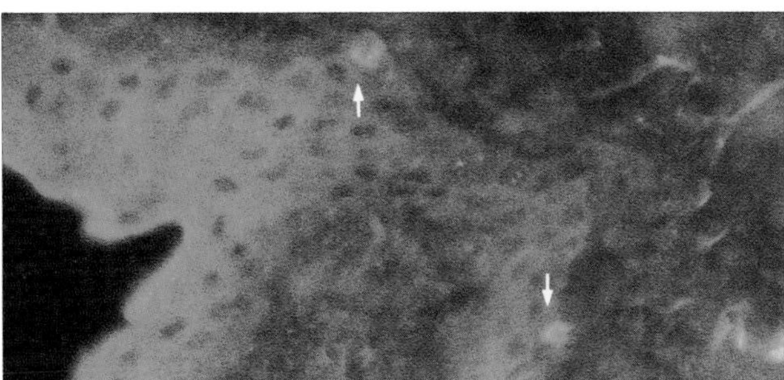

Fig. 7.25 Immunofluorescent staining of melanocytes (arrows). Cryostat section of human skin stained with a serum positive for melanocyte antibodies.

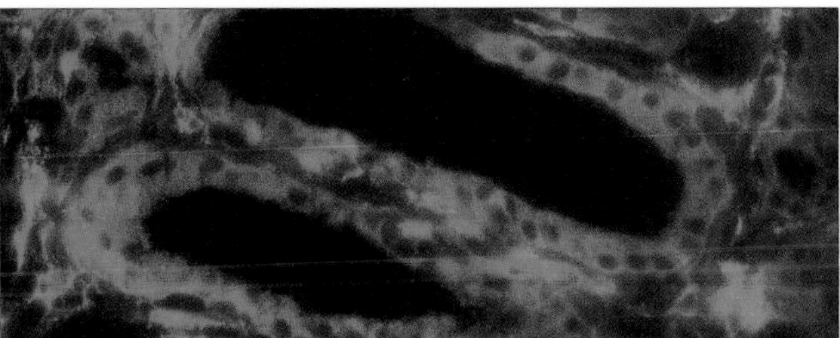

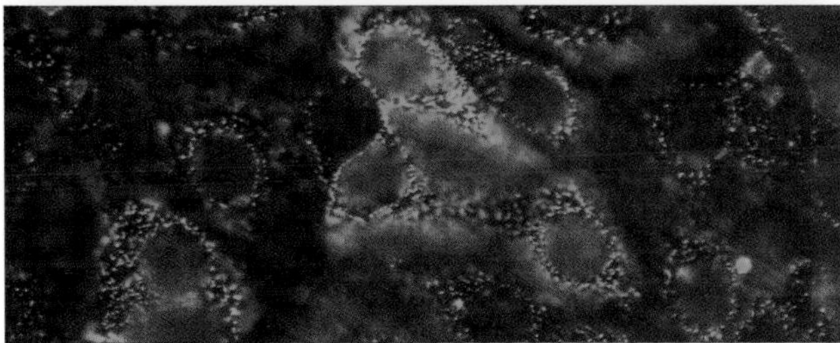

Fig. 7.26 Inappropriate DR expression in thyrocytes from patient with Graves' disease. Upper: cryostat section of human thyroid stained by immunofluorescence with anti-DR monoclonal antibodies (non-polymorphic region). DR-positive cells are visible in the lamina propria and the cytoplasm of the epithelial follicular cells is also stained. Courtesy of Dr B Dean. Lower: two day monolayer of human thyroid cells stained by immunofluorescence with anti-DR monoclonal antibodies (non-polymorphic region). The surface of the thyrocytes is stained.

SKIN

Cytoplasmic reacting autoantibodies to melanocytes are a rare finding: only nine cases have been reported so far, these occurring in patients with vitiligo associated with polyendocrine disease. Vitiligo is a disorder caused by a defect in melanocytes which leads to failure of melanin formation. The lesion can be localized or generalized. A complement fixing test has to be employed to enhance the detection ability as persistent negative results are obtained with classical immunofluorescent labelling. However, when using an immunoprecipitation technique, virtually all sera from patients with vitiligo appear to react with the melanocyte surface antigen (Fig. 7.25), indicating the existence of antigenic heterogeneity in the antigen–antibody system.

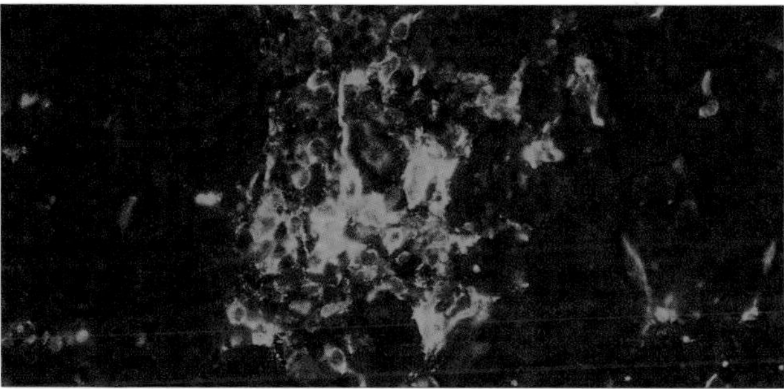

Fig. 7.27 Inappropriate DR expression in islets from a patient who died of newly diagnosed diabetes. Cryostat section of 'diabetic' pancreas stained by immunofluorescence with an anti-DR monoclonal antibody (non-polymorphic region). The cytoplasm of the endocrine cells (β cells) is stained. The section was counterstained with anti-insulin to confirm the specificity of the reaction. Courtesy of Dr B Dean.

HLA AND AUTOIMMUNE DISEASE

Population and family studies have indicated various genetic associations within autoimmune endocrinopathies. The strongest and most clear cut of these are with the HLA complex. The HLA system is located on the short arm of chromosome 6 and contains genes which control the ability of the individual to respond immunologically when exposed to various 'foreign' antigens (see chapter 2).

INAPPROPRIATE EXPRESSION OF HLA IN AUTOIMMUNITY

Thyrocytes from patients with Hashimoto's thyroiditis, from most patients with Graves' disease and from a proportion of subjects with non-toxic goitre exhibit *'de novo'* expression of HLA-DR molecules. The intensity of immunostaining follows the pattern DR > DP > DQ; a correlation was observed between HLA-DR expression and high titres of microsomal antibodies (Fig. 7.26), and between DQ and high titres of thyroglobulin antibodies. Similarly a *'de novo'* class II expression was detected in pancreatic islets taken from patients who had died of diabetes. The immunostaining was restricted to insulin containing islets and double immunofluorescent labelling showed that class II expression was confined to β cells (Fig. 7.27). Islets which had lost their β cells did not show this reaction, and inappropriate expression could not be seen in islets from cystic fibrosis or chronic pancreatitis specimens. Class I molecule staining was shown to be enhanced in affected glands.

Role of class I and II gene products in pathogenesis

It has been postulated that the transition from a non-specific inflammatory reaction in which lymphokines are locally released to an autoimmune response would occur as a consequence of the inappropriate expression of class II molecules on endocrine cells. The cause of the initial inflammation is unknown but it is possible that latent viruses or cytokines that they induce (?IFN) play a role in this initiation.

Failure of down regulation of HLA-DR expression, for example due to a deficit in antigen specific suppressor cells or a breakdown of the idiotype/anti-idiotype system, will finally trigger an autoimmune attack and influence its severity and direction. The assumption that autoreactive T cells are also present in normal individuals constitutes the basis of this hypothesis. The most relevant organ-specific immunological events would be the presentation of endocrine autoantigens to T helper cells and the consequent response, directed against the same organ which initiated the reaction.

FURTHER READING

Doniach D, Bottazzo GF, eds. Endocrine and other organ orientated autoimmune disorders. In *Clinical immunology and allergy.* Volume I.London: Baillière-Tindall, 1987.

Ludgate M, Vassart G. The molecular genetics of three thyroid autoantigens: thyroglobulin, thyroid peroxidase and the thyrotropin receptors. *Autoimmunity.* 1990; **7**:201–211.

Rose NR, Mackay I, eds. *The autoimmune diseases.* London: Academic Press, 1985.

Volpé R, ed. *Autoimmunity and endocrine disease.* New York, Basle: Marcel Dekker, 1985.

8

Renal Disorders

CLASSIFICATION OF RENAL DISEASES

Some of the most important diseases that affect the kidney are summarized in Fig. 8.1. The term glomerulonephritis (GN) applies only to immunologically triggered inflammation that is largely restricted to the glomerular tuft. Sometimes the larger vessels in the kidney are affected by the vasculitic process, leaving the glomeruli relatively unharmed. These systemic vasculitides are also regarded as having an immunological basis, since they are caused by the trapping or deposition of immune complexes in vessel walls.

In acute tubulo-interstitial nephritis (ATIN), the tubules bear the brunt of the damage. Lesions may be produced by non-immunological mechanisms which include toxins, ischaemia, infection and drugs, but allergic reactions to a wide variety of drugs may produce similar lesions, so-called allergic ATIN.

KIDNEY SUSCEPTIBILITY TO IMMUNE-MEDIATED DAMAGE

The kidney is damaged as an innocent bystander in many conditions. It has a rich blood supply (25% of cardiac output) and a unique fenestrated capillary bed (of hemiarterioles) which forms the glomerular tuft (Fig. 8.2). The high glomerular capillary pressure, ultrafiltration and the density of negatively charged glycoproteins on the glomerular filtration barrier all increase the kidney's susceptibility to circulating substances of potential toxicity.

A number of macromolecules, for example DNA, may stick preferentially in the glomerular tuft. Positively charged molecules are trapped, particularly under the epithelial cells of the glomerular filtration barrier and, if antigenic, may lead to the formation of immune complexes *in situ* in the glomerular tuft. Preformed complexes may be deposited in the mesangium and in the sub-endothelial zone for largely haemodynamic reasons. Glomerular cells bear Fc and complement receptors which may also enhance the deposition of immune reactants.

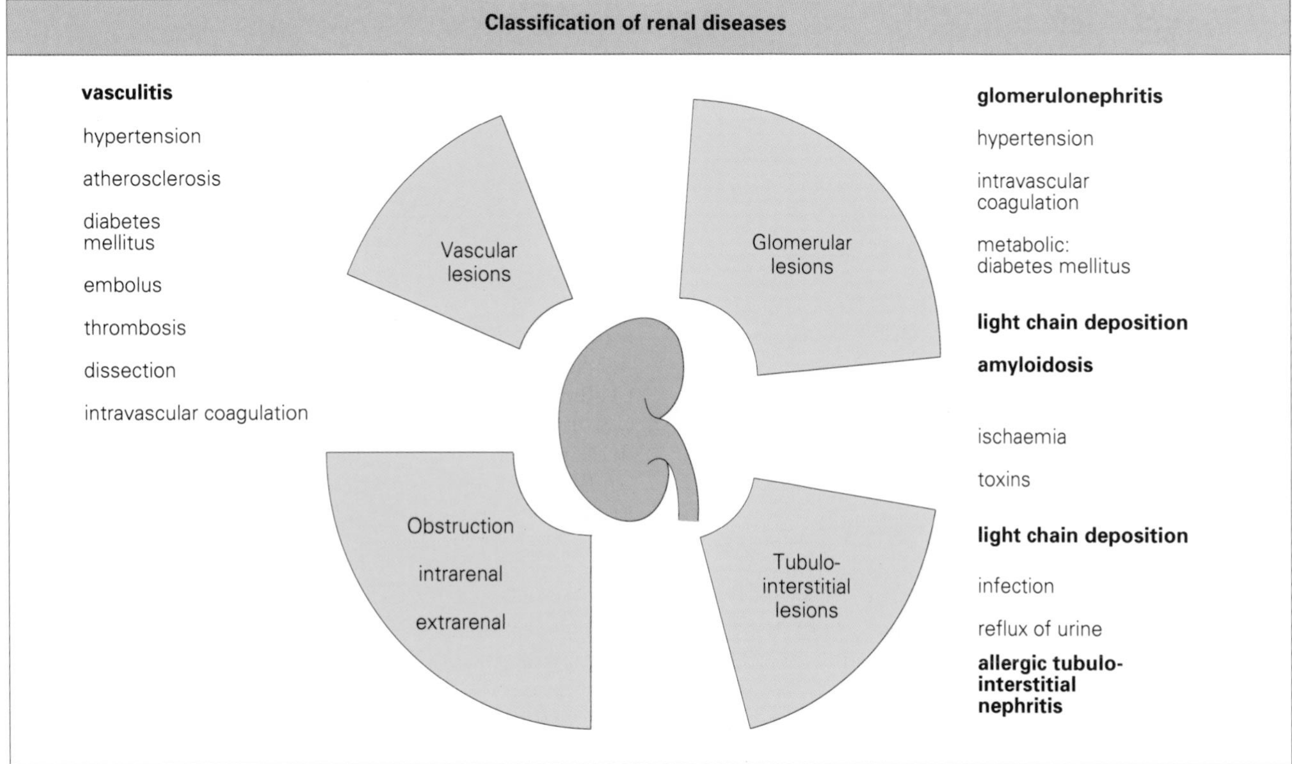

Fig. 8.1 Disorders with an immunological basis are shown in bold type.

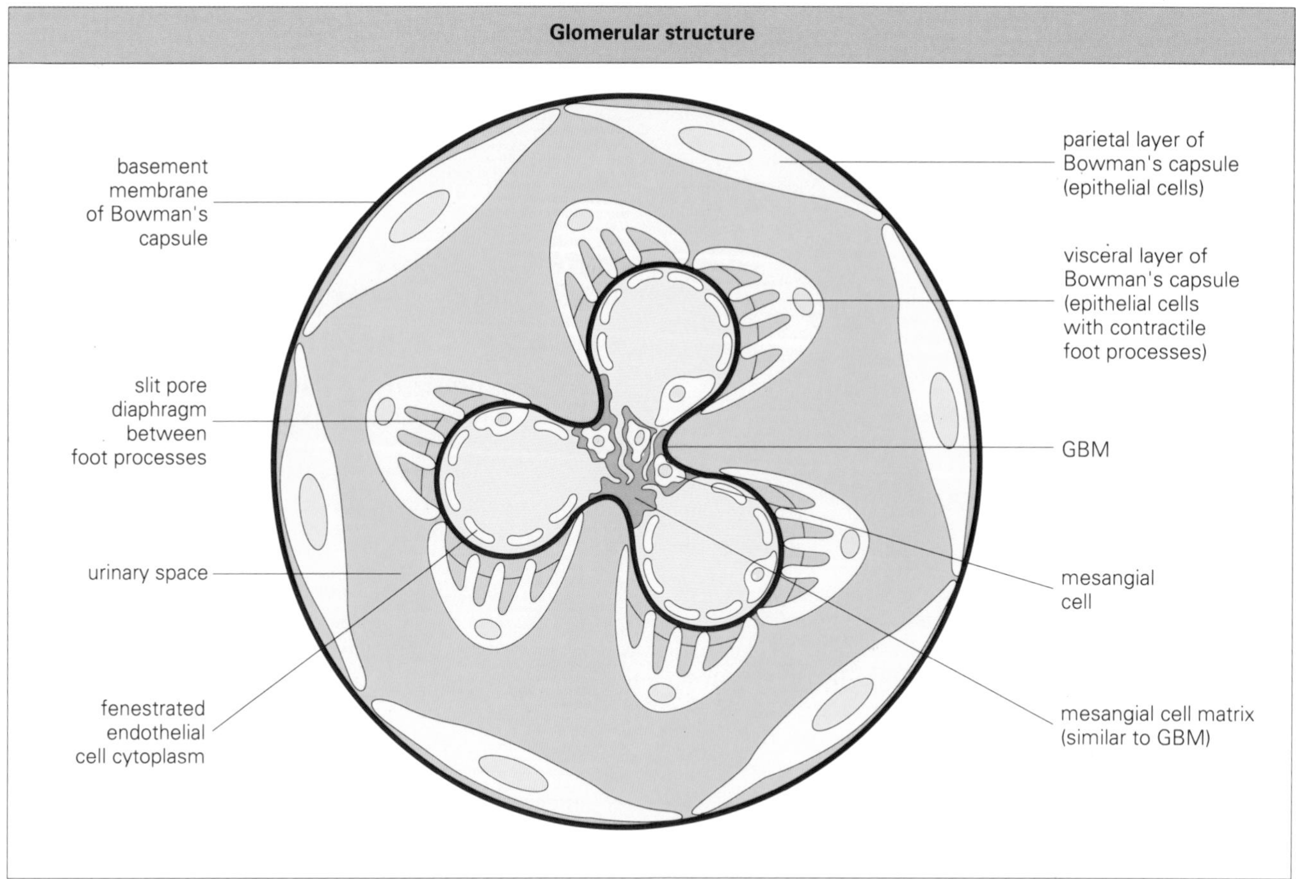

Fig. 8.2 The glomerulus is a vascular network which invaginates the blind-ended tube of epithelial cells that forms the nephron. The capillary loops can be considered as hemiarterioles, as the mesangial cells at the neck of the capillary loops are contractile and share properties with smooth muscle cells. The barrier for ultrafiltration consists of a fenestrated layer of endothelial cell cytoplasm, glomerular basement membrane (GBM) and the epithelial cell slit pores. The filtration barrier is highly permeable to small molecular weight substances and is covered with negatively charged glomerular sialoprotein which impedes the passage of anionic molecules.

GLOMERULONEPHRITIS

ANIMAL MODELS

The development of animal experiments has laid a firm basis for the immunopathology of human GN. Some of the pertinent models are discussed below.

One-shot (acute) serum sickness

A large single intravenous dose of foreign protein, usually bovine serum albumin (BSA), is given to an animal, most frequently a rabbit. The disappearance of labelled BSA from the circulation is shown in Fig. 8.3. Studies have shown that the vasculitis is complement- and PMN-dependent, but the GN is largely monocyte-macrophage dependent. Steroids reduce glomerular inflammation but do not prevent the glomerular localization of immune complexes. This model is analogous to the acute self-limiting post-infectious GN in humans.

Chronic serum sickness

In this model, a daily intravenous injection of antigen is given for several months, after which the injected rabbits fall into one of four groups (Fig. 8.4). The chronic BSA model has provided evidence that a degree of immune deficiency (low affinity or low titre antibody), with failure to eliminate rapidly circulating antigen, may predispose to GN. It also indicates that the larger immune complexes (ICs) localize to the mesangial or sub-endothelial areas, while smaller complexes may well be incapable of tissue localization. Sub-epithelial deposits are probably formed *in situ* rather than being deposited already formed from the circulation.

Heyman nephritis

Rat glomerular and tubular epithelial cells share an antigen variously known as Fx1A, brush border antigen or GP330. Intravenous immunization with this antigen or its antibody results in typical membranous changes with sub-epithelial deposits of Ig, complement and tubular antigen.

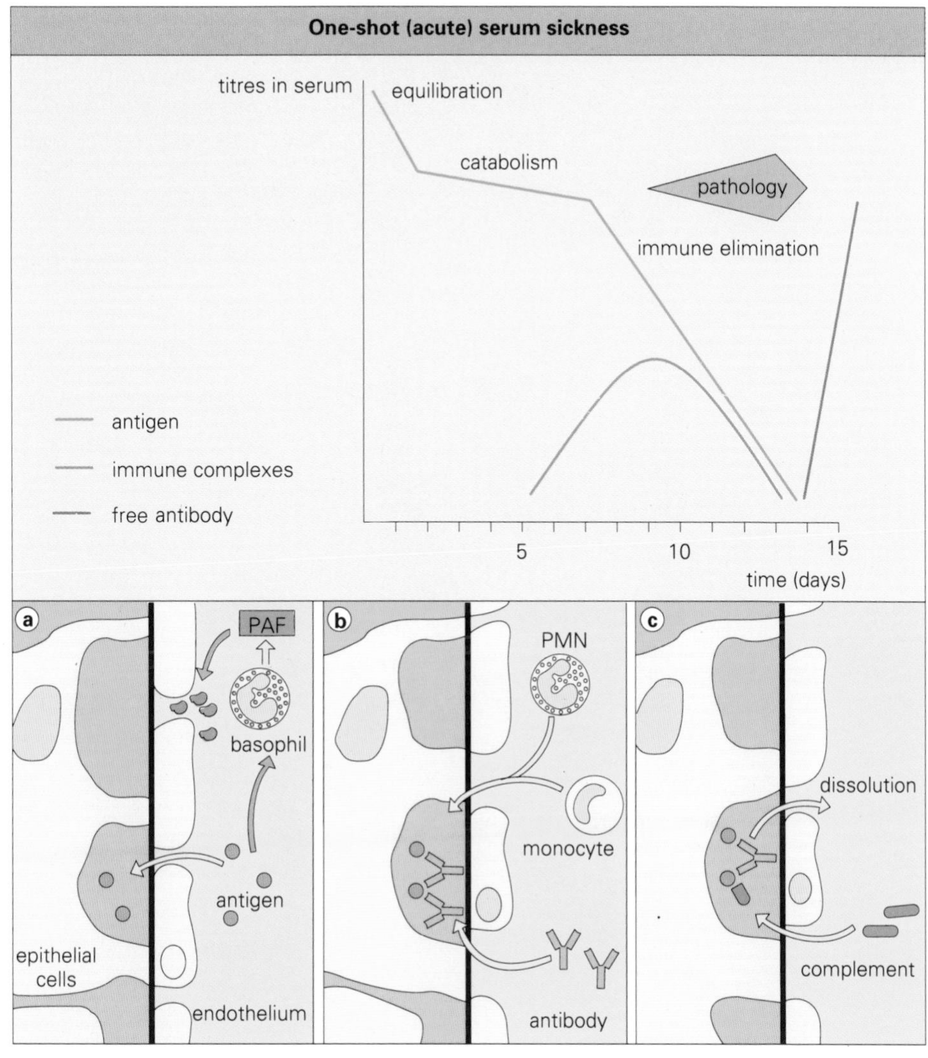

Fig. 8.3 Upper: following antigen (BSA) injection there is a period in which antigen equilibrates in extracellular fluids; it is then slowly catabolized, and declines rapidly after antibody synthesis begins at day 5. Immune complexes are present at days 5–13, coinciding with the incidence of vasculitis and glomerulonephritis. Lower: kidney pathology. a) in the early stages antigen may deposit in sub-epithelial spaces, and in some cases can activate basophils to release PAF. b) antibody binds to antigen; neutrophils and monocytes are attracted to these sites and cause pathological damage. c) in the late phase, complement deposition occurs, which may contribute to complex dissolution.

Antibody reacts with the antigen which caps and is shed from the glomerular epithelial cells, appearing as discrete sub-epithelial deposits (Fig. 8.5).

Although no equivalent antigen has been convincingly demonstrated in man, this model shows that antibody can react with antigens on the far side of the GBM and it is likely that the terminal complement components (membrane attack complex — MAC) are largely responsible for the glomerular damage seen in human membranous GN.

Masugi nephritis (nephrotoxic serum nephritis)

Antibody to GBM can be raised by the repeated immunization of sheep with glomeruli. The sheep eventually develop progressive GN and die from renal failure (Steblay model). Sera from such sheep have been used to produce acute GN in rats, guinea pigs and rabbits (Masugi model/nephrotoxic serum nephritis, NTS) (Fig. 8.6). Damage to the glomerulus occurs rapidly after the injection of heterologous anti-GBM antibody (heterologous phase) and is made more severe by autologous antibody to the foreign immunoglobulins (autologous phase). The model can be 'telescoped' by pre-immunizing with gamma-globulin from the same species that provides the nephrotoxic serum, in which case the heterologous and autologous phases occur simultaneously.

Subcutaneous staphylococcal abscesses or bacterial lipopolysaccharide will exacerbate glomerular injury, presumably by stimulating the acute phase proteins and priming other non-specific inflammatory mediator pathways. The Steblay and NTS models are the equivalent of Goodpasture's syndrome in humans (anti-GBM antibody-mediated GN).

Cationic antigens. In the chronic BSA model, a striking difference in immune complex deposition can be achieved by altering the isoelectric point of the BSA antigen used (Fig. 8.7). Naturally-occurring cationic antibodies may behave similarly, fixing sub-epithelially and reacting with specific antigen later. As with Heyman nephritis, the cationic BSA model, with its deposits on the far side of the GBM, is dependent on MAC for proteinuria. In congenitally C6-deficient rabbits, cationic BSA produces sub-epithelial deposits but minimal proteinuria.

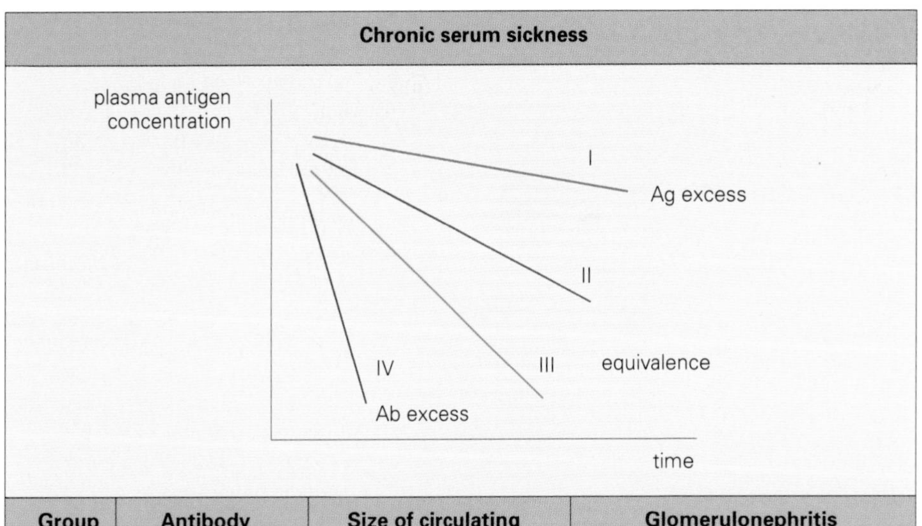

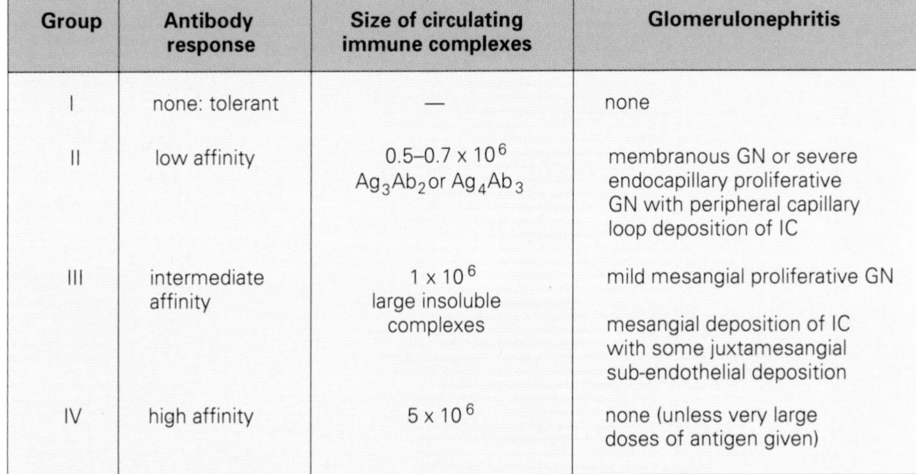

Group	Antibody response	Size of circulating immune complexes	Glomerulonephritis
I	none: tolerant	—	none
II	low affinity	0.5–0.7 x 10^6 Ag_3Ab_2 or Ag_4Ab_3	membranous GN or severe endocapillary proliferative GN with peripheral capillary loop deposition of IC
III	intermediate affinity	1 x 10^6 large insoluble complexes	mild mesangial proliferative GN mesangial deposition of IC with some juxtamesangial sub-endothelial deposition
IV	high affinity	5 x 10^6	none (unless very large doses of antigen given)

Fig. 8.4 Group I animals become tolerant to the antigen, make no antibody and develop no lesions. The other groups (II, III and IV) make antibody of various affinities and the development of both renal and extra-renal lesions is influenced by the relative concentration of antigen to antibody, i.e. the size of the immune complex (IC) formed.

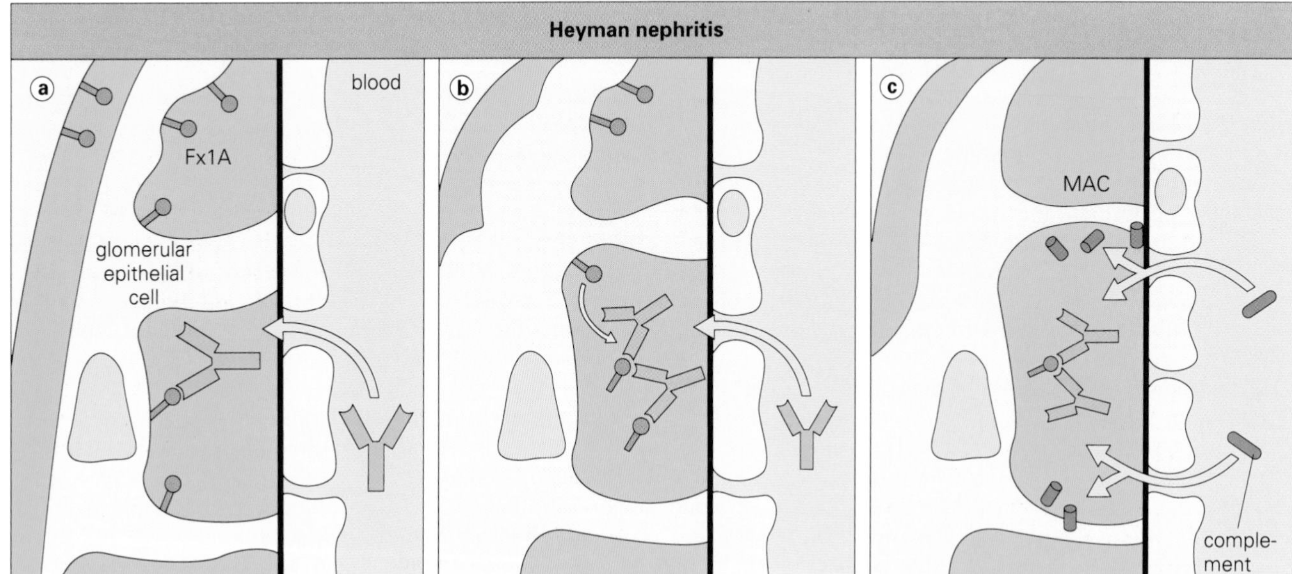

Fig. 8.5 a) serum antibody traverses the glomerular basement membrane and binds to Fx1A. b) the antigen is shed from the epithelial cells forming deposits of sub-epithelial complexes. c) complement activation and formation of the C5b–9 membrane attack complex (MAC) is largely responsible for the pathology, since cobra-venom-treated or C6-deficient animals do not develop proteinuria. Polymorph depletion does not protect the glomerulus from damage.

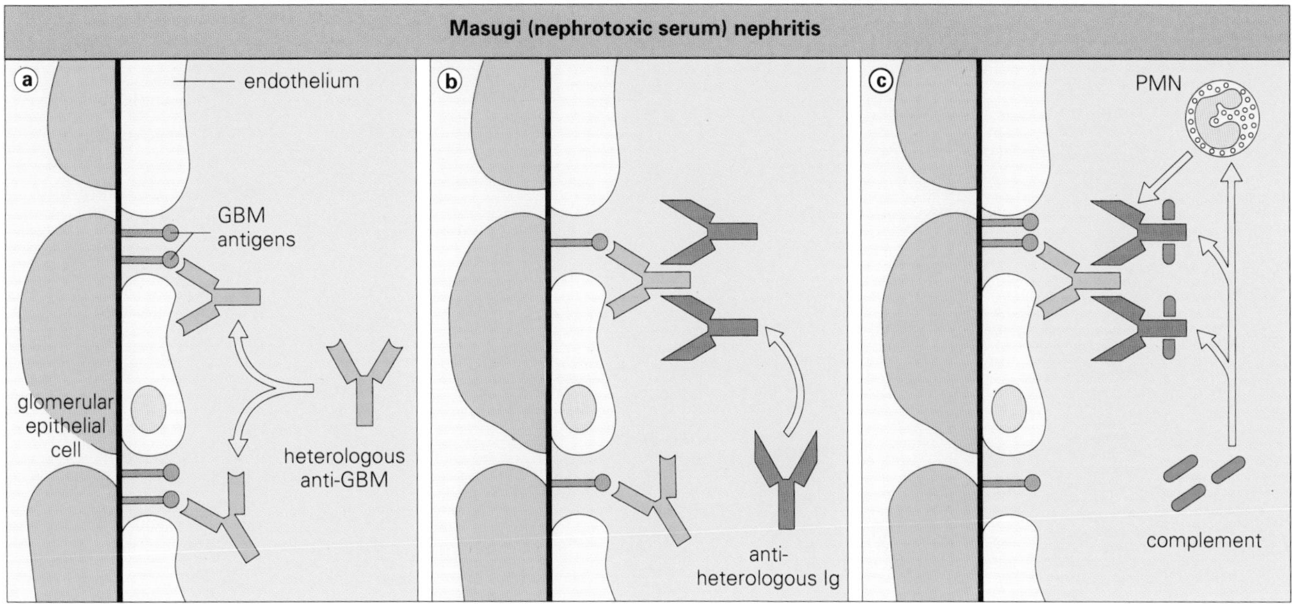

Fig. 8.6 Animals are injected with heterologous antibodies to basement membrane antigen. a) in the initial phase these antibodies bind to the GBM. b) complexes are then built up with autologous (anti-heterologous) antibody to the foreign Ig. c) complement adds to the complexes and polymorphs accumulate by complement-dependent and -independent mechanisms, and produce immunopathological damage. Proteinuria increases and renal failure rapidly develops with crescentic GN.

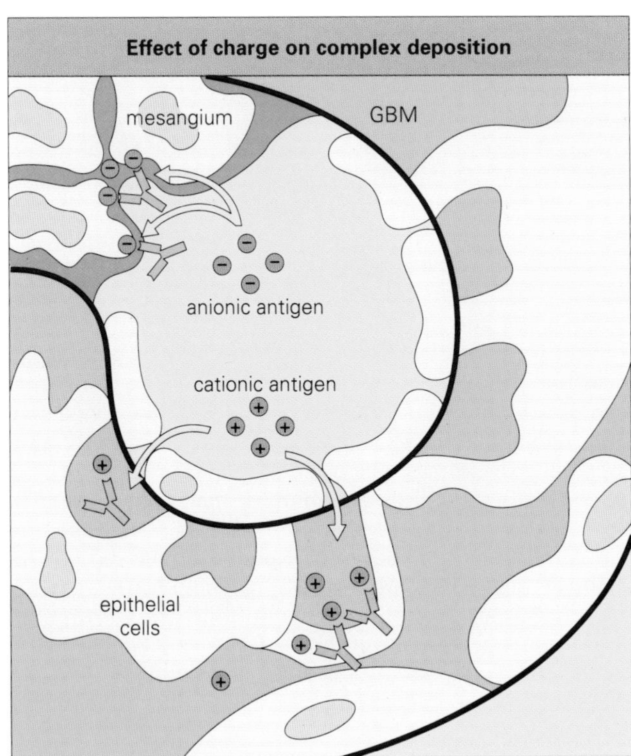

Fig. 8.7 Cationic BSA antigen (pI ≥ 9.5) can readily traverse the GBM, producing sub-epithelial deposits, while anionic BSA (pI = 4.5) tends to localize in the mesangium.

Injection of preformed immune complexes. Almost all such experiments have failed to produce either significant glomerular lesions or sub-epithelial deposits. It is possible that complexes made *in vitro* dissociate after injection. When localization of exogenous complexes does occur, it is usually mesangial, even when complexes made from brush border antigen and its antibody are used.

GN with large insoluble complexes

Large complexes form with polyvalent antigens at equivalence or in antibody excess. If ferritin or BSA is injected into the renal arteries of previously immunized animals, a severe GN with mesangial and sub-endothelial deposits can be produced. Although it was previously thought that large complexes would be preferentially removed by the mononuclear-phagocyte system (MPS), it seems likely that they can be trapped in the glomerulus, particularly if the MPS is deficient or saturated. The net charge on the IC may also be important, with cationic IC being deposited sub-endothelially, while anionic IC can only localize to the mesangium.

Conclusions from animal studies

GN has an undoubted immunological basis. Sub-epithelial complexes are probably formed *in situ*, where antigen (or antibody) may preferentially localize, either because of charge (cationic) or non-immunological binding. Once there, antibody, antigen and complement can penetrate the GBM.

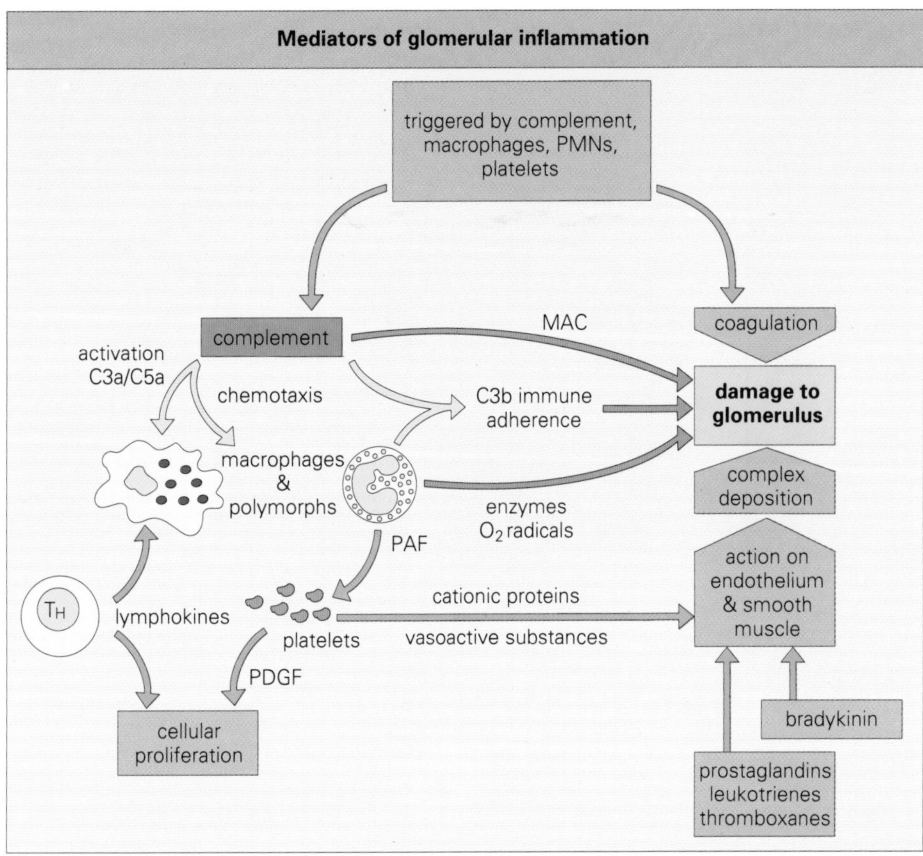

Fig. 8.8 Glomeruli are damaged by a combination of inflammatory mediators which include complement, the coagulation cascade, arachidonic acid metabolites and cells. Much of so-called glomerular proliferation represents invasion by monocytes. Polymorphs are occasionally seen applied to denuded areas of basement membrane in certain forms of glomerulonephritis. The complement cascade is one of the most important mediators of the inflammatory response. PDGF=platelet-derived growth factor; MAC=membrane attack complex.

Large, insoluble complexes are trapped in the mesangium. If present in sufficient quantities (or cationic) deposits also develop in the sub-endothelial space. Here, they meet PMNs and activate the other mediators of glomerular injury.

Genetic factors influence both the quality of the immune response (for example antibody affinity) and probably also, as yet poorly defined, variations in the non-specific inflammatory mediators. Environmental factors are also likely to be important, and include general nutrition as well as exposure to various infectious agents, which may be the source of the antigen in the immune precipitate.

MEDIATORS OF INFLAMMATION

The mediators of inflammation which appear to be important in producing glomerular damage after antibody or immune complexes have been deposited in the glomerular tuft are summarized in Fig. 8.8. An understanding of these mediators may suggest points at which treatment can be directed.

Monocytes and macrophages

Some of the 'proliferative' lesions in the glomerular tuft represent invasion and infiltration by monocytes. Crescents are partly composed of macrophages, and stud-
8.6 ies on human biopsies confirm the presence of these cells in many glomerular lesions (acute post-streptococcal GN, SLE, cryoglobulinaemia and crescentic GN).

Complement

Complement activation occurs early after antibody or complexes fix in the glomerular tuft, and attracts and activates PMNs, monocytes and platelets. C3a and C5a are potent anaphylatoxins and the terminal components of complement produce the MAC (C5b, 6, 7, 8 and 9) which may be the major cause of glomerular damage in membranous GN and several other conditions.

Complement also has a beneficial role in helping to dissolve complexes and promote antigen and immune complex elimination by opsonization. Certain congenital complement deficiencies are associated with GN and lupus-like syndromes.

Red cells as well as polymorphs, macrophages and B cells bear a receptor for C3b, termed CR1. Once bound, the immune complexes are transported on the red cell to the liver, where they are released, taken up by the hepatic macrophages and cleared, reducing the amount of immune complexes available for tissue deposition. Reduced CR1 activity on the red cell could lead to tissue deposition of immune complexes.

Platelets and coagulation

Platelets. Platelet consumption is increased in several forms of human GN, and platelet antigens can be demonstrated in the glomerular tuft. Platelets have a wide range of biological activities, including the release of mitogens such as platelet-derived growth factor, cationic protein, enzymes and vasoactive substances. Platelet depletion and anti-platelet agents can ameliorate some types of GN both in animal studies (Masugi and acute serum sickness) and in human GN (mesangiocapillary).

Platelet activating factor (PAF), released from a variety of cells, plays an important role in the inflammatory response. In terms of glomerular inflammation, PAF may cause platelet aggregation with the release of cationic proteins (neutralization of glomerular polyanions) and other platelet-derived mediators. It attracts polymorphs and monocytes which then release enzymes and superoxides. Glomerular capillary permeability would be increased and glomerular blood flow altered by PAF-induced mesangial cell contraction. Such changes could augment immune complex deposition and cause glomerular damage via polymorphs and macrophages.

Coagulation. The coagulation system can be activated via exposed collagen and basement membrane, both of which activate Factor XII (Hageman factor), which in turn can activate the kinin system. Activated platelets, PMNs and macrophages release a variety of enzymes including prothrombinases, which also initiate coagulation.

In animal studies, heparin therapy or defibrination reduces crescent formation in the nephrotoxic serum nephritis model, although anticoagulants or defibrination have a minimal protective effect on the IC models of GN. In human studies, fibrin is present in glomerular crescents, and other coagulation proteins can be demonstrated in the glomerular tuft in some cases(SLE, Henoch-Schönlein purpura and MCGN). Treatment directed at interrupting the platelet and coagulation pathways has been disappointing when used alone, but may have a role as an addition to standard immunosuppressive treatment.

Non-specific factors: acute phase response. Many of the mediators of inflammation act as acute phase reactants. Intercurrent infection may 'prime' these inflammatory pathways so that, if a specific trigger is activated, the resulting tissue damage is particularly severe. The importance of this non-specific effect can be seen in anti-GBM disease where intercurrent infections precipitate worsening renal function and lung haemorrhage in patients with Goodpasture's disease.

HLA and GN

The formation of CICs is a normal part of the immune response. The glomerular localization of complexes, whether from the circulation or assembled *in situ*, can be viewed as unwanted and probably as abnormal if outside the mesangium. Observations from the chronic serum sickness model in rabbits suggest that a poor antibody response is more likely to be associated with GN. Studies with different strains of mice have shown that strains producing lower affinity antibody and strains with less efficient mononuclear-phagocyte systems are those that develop spontaneous GN. In humans, it has been claimed that patients with membranous GN tend to produce low affinity antibody and this suggests that a degree of immune system incompetence may be at the root of GN. The quality of the immune response may well be controlled by genes close to the HLA genes on chromosome 6. Many studies have related HLA types to particular forms of GN, and further studies have suggested that, within individual types of GN, certain HLA types may be associated with a particularly poor prognosis.

CELL-MEDIATED IMMUNITY AND GN

It seems certain that GN is not an entirely humoral affair. T cells modulate the humoral response and are likely to indirectly affect the production of GN. The nude mouse (T deficient) develops a much less severe GN in the chronic serum sickness model. B cell hyperactivity *in vitro* has been demonstrated in several types of GN (IgA nephropathy, SLE, Henoch-Schönlein purpura) and may be due to impaired T-suppressor cell regulation. Impaired Ts cell generation after ConA stimulation has been found in patients with membranous GN.

The presence of T cells in the kidney in GN has been demonstrated using monoclonal antibodies, particularly in patients with proliferative lesions and those with the multisystem vasculitides. Occasional T cells are seen in close proximity to macrophages and may well modulate their activity.

It has been suggested, but never adequately confirmed, that T cells might produce a potent permeability factor or other lymphokine that could account for the proteinuria in nephrotic syndrome associated with the minimal change lesion (see below).

HUMAN GN

The interrelations between the initiating factors in GN, the mediators of inflammation and tissue damage, and the host's response, are very complicated. It has to be remembered that the kidney and its glomeruli have a limited repertoire of responses to a wide variety of insults. The same insult in different individuals may produce different lesions and, conversely, the same lesions in different individuals may be the end result of different insults.

Assessment of GN has to be made at three separate levels and then the patient fully assessed. The cause, histology and the clinical syndrome all need to be carefully defined. It is worth noting that the histology is really the reaction to the cause and should not necessarily be taken as a specific disease entity in itself. Some histological appearances probably do represent specific disease entities, but many do not.

Cause

In most cases no cause can be identified. Antibodies to GBM can be found in the circulation of patients with anti-GBM disease by a sensitive radioimmunoassay.

Antigen–antibody systems in human glomerulonephritis		
group	**examples**	**lesion**
virus	hepatitis B EBV, CMV	membranous GN
bacteria	streptococci	diffuse endocapillary proliferative GN
	staphylococci	diffuse endocapillary proliferative GN
protozoa	*Plasmodium falciparum*	proliferative GN
	Plasmodium malariae	membranous or mesangiocapillary GN
worms	*Schistosoma (mansoni & japonicum)*	variable — mesangiocapillary GN
drugs	gold	membranous
	penicillamine	membranous
vaccines	DPT	diffuse proliferative GN
	pertussis	diffuse proliferative GN
tumours	lymphomas	minimal change
	solid tumours (bronchus, colon)	membranous GN
endogenous antigens	thyroglobulin	membranous GN
	DNA (SLE)	variable

Fig. 8.9 Many cases (>90%) of GN are associated with evidence of immune complex deposition in the glomerulus. A minority (approximately 5%) is caused by an anti-GBM antibody. In some cases, no immune reactants can be demonstrated (minimal change lesion and some examples of focal segmental glomerulosclerosis and crescentic GN). Although still conventionally grouped with GN, the pathogenesis of such cases is not understood.

Circulating plasma immune complexes correlate poorly with the presence or absence of GN and the activity of the underlying disease. In biopsy material, immunofluorescence or immunoperoxidase techniques demonstrate the presence of glomerular immunoglobulin and complement. A linear pattern of staining along the GBM showing deposition of immunoglobulin is typical of anti-GBM antibody-mediated disease. Granular, discontinuous or a 'lumpy-bumpy' staining for immunoglobulin implies immune complex disease and electron microscopy defines the precise localization of the complexes. Even if immune complexes have been demonstrated in the glomerular tuft, it is often not possible to define the antigen, despite the growing list of those known to be associated with human GN (Fig. 8.9).

GN can be subdivided into cases forming part of a more generalized disease such as one of the multisystem vasculitides, cases where a clear cause can be identified (for example drug-induced or post-infectious), and cases where the cause remains unknown (primary or idiopathic GN).

Histology

The histological features of the major types of GN are summarized in Fig. 8.10.

In minimal change GN, the glomerulus is normal to light microscopy, but electron microscopy shows foot process fusion (Fig. 8.11). Membranous glomerulonephritis is typified by thickening of the basement membrane without an increase in glomerular cells (Figs 8.12 & 8.13), and electron-dense deposits are visible in the sub-endothelial spaces (Fig. 8.14).

The various forms of proliferative glomerulonephritis show an over-cellular glomerulus caused by cellular proliferation of endothelial, epithelial and mesangial cells together with invasion of the glomerular tuft by monocytes. In type I membranoproliferative (mesangiocapillary) glomerulonephritis, the mesangial area expands and extends around the capillary loop between basement membrane endothelial cells. A second layer of basement membrane is then deposited, giving double contours. In type II membranoproliferative GN, the basement membrane is partly replaced by linear electron-dense deposits (Fig. 8.15).

In focal segmental glomerulosclerosis the glomeruli show areas of hyalinosis and sclerosis. Focal necrotizing glomerulonephritis is typified by areas of necrosis and disruption of basement membrane. This may be a forerunner of full-blown crescentic GN.

A crescent forms when fibrin enters Bowman's space and stimulates proliferation of cells outside the capillary loop (Fig. 8.16). These cells are now thought to be largely invading monocytes, although histologically they appear to be formed by proliferation of the parietal area of Bowman's capsule. In 20–30% of cases, immunofluorescence shows the classical linear deposition of immunoglobulins along the basement membrane typical of anti-GBM antibody-mediated disease (Fig. 8.17). Granular deposits are seen in 30–50% of cases and no deposits on immunofluorescence can be detected in the remaining 20–50% of cases.

Clinical syndromes

There is no simple relationship between histological appearances and clinical features. Generally, proteinuria is associated with loss of glomerular polyanions and foot process fusion.

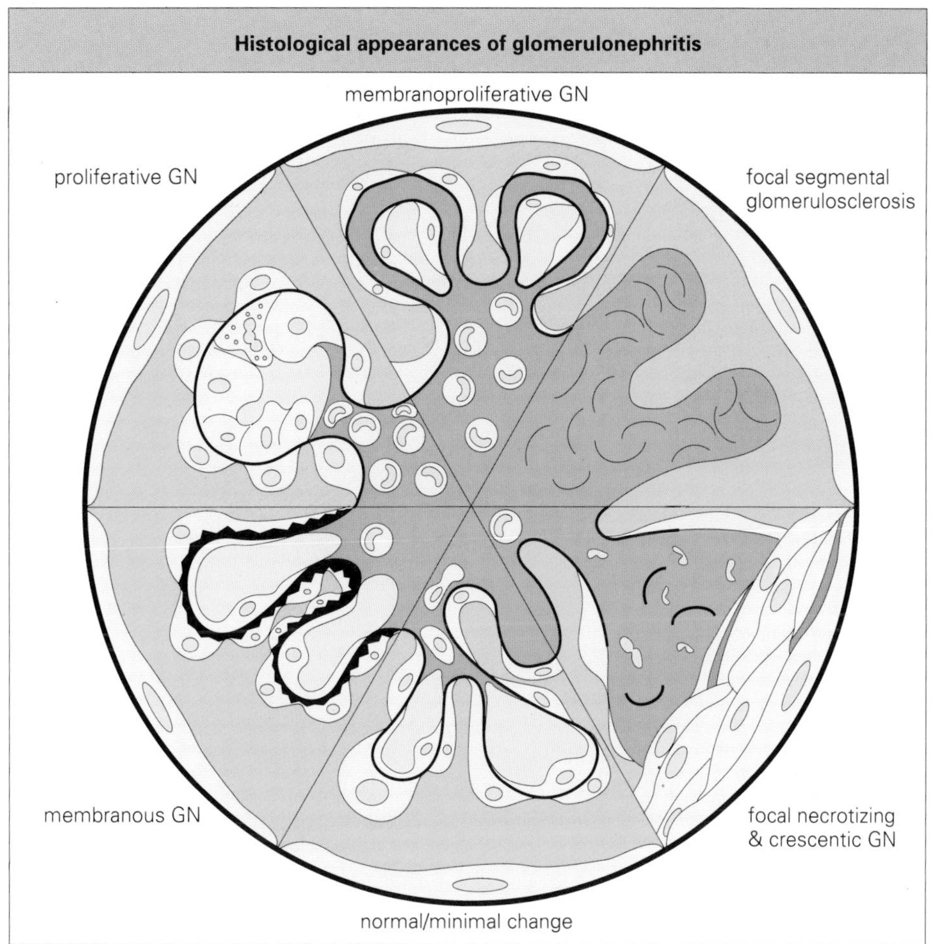

Fig. 8.10 Comparison of the histological appearances of different types of glomerulonephritis.

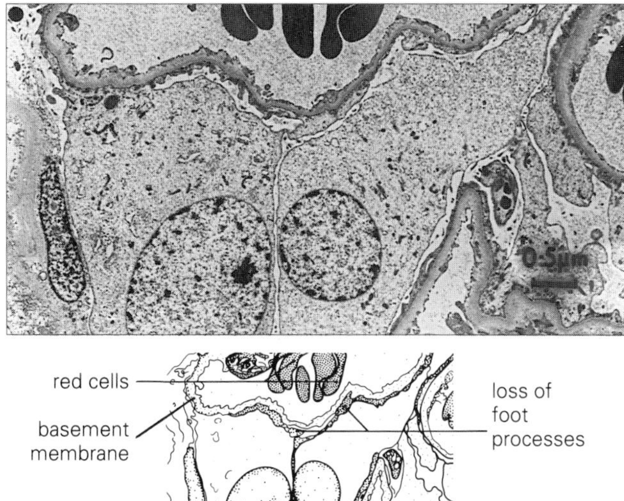

Fig. 8.11 EM of minimal change lesion showing foot process fusion. The upper part shows a capillary loop containing red cells. The basement membrane is normal. Two large epithelial cells are applied to the basement membrane with loss of the epithelial cell foot processes. This is associated with loss of the glomerular polyanion and results in a marked increase in membrane permeability to negatively charged molecules.

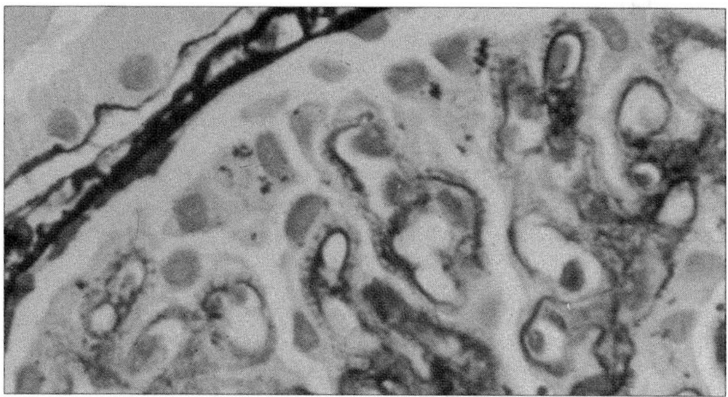

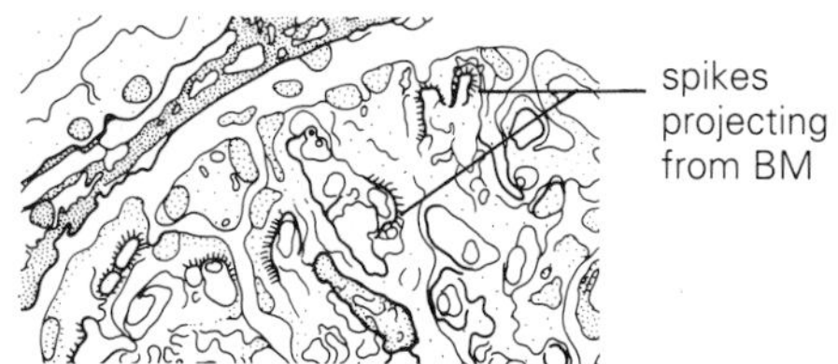

Fig. 8.12 Basement membrane thickening in membranous glomerulonephritis. Spikes are visible projecting from the basement membrane into the sub-epithelial zone. These are formed as new basement membrane is laid down around immune complexes. Electron microscopy (see Fig. 8.14) demonstrates these immune complexes. Silver stain.

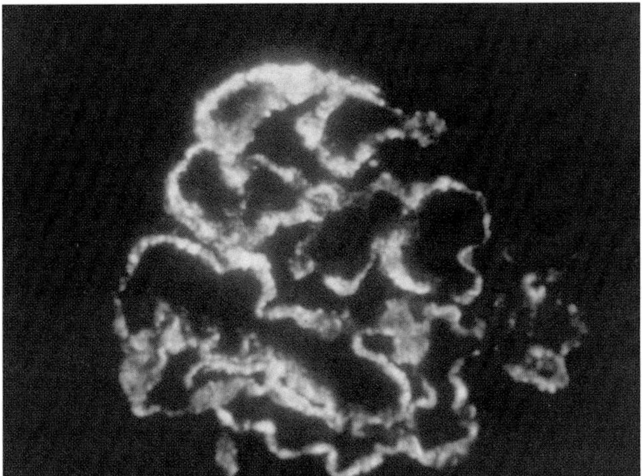

Fig. 8.13 Granular peripheral capillary loop deposits of immune reactants in membranous glomerulonephritis. The basement membrane is outlined by a 'lumpy-bumpy' granular and discontinuous deposition of immunoglobulins and complement. These can be demonstrated using a fluorescein-conjugated antibody to human immunoglobulins and complement. This pattern is typical of immune complex glomerulonephritis.

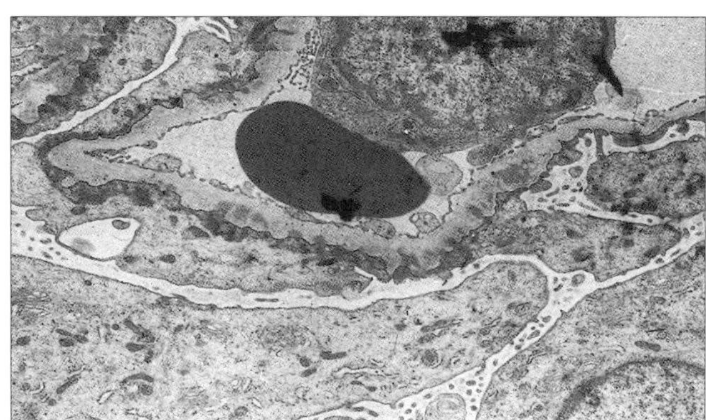

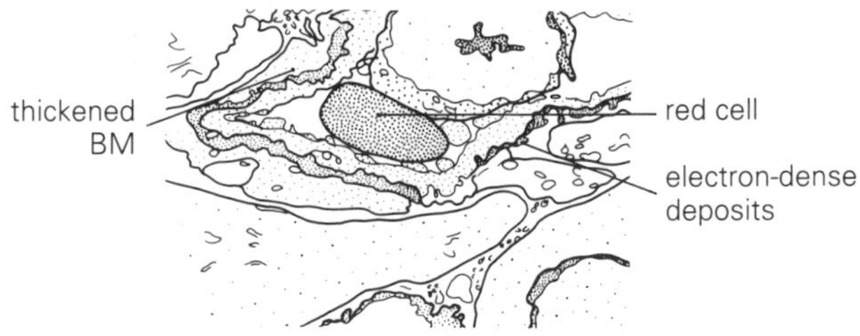

Fig. 8.14 Membranous glomerulonephritis. A single red cell is seen within a capillary loop. The basement membrane appears thickened and electron-dense deposits are clearly identifiable along the sub-epithelial surface of the basement membrane. Some deposits have become incorporated into basement membrane as more is laid down around the complexes.

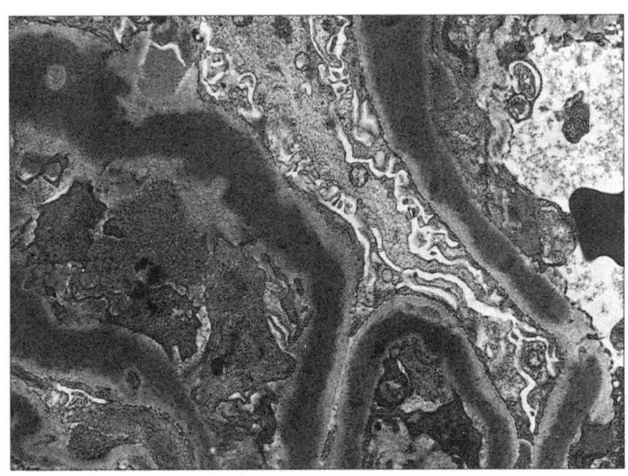

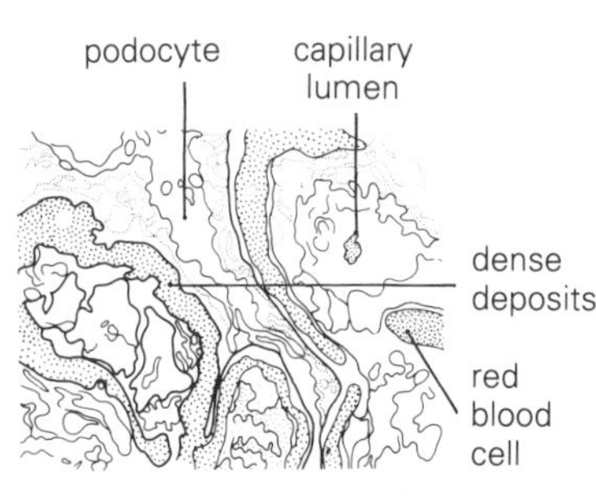

Fig. 8.15 Type II mesangiocapillary glomerulonephritis. The basement membrane has been replaced by a ribbon-like dense thickening. This variation of mesangiocapillary glomerulonephritis is often called dense deposit disease. Courtesy of Professors A W Asscher & D B Moffat & Dr E Saunders.

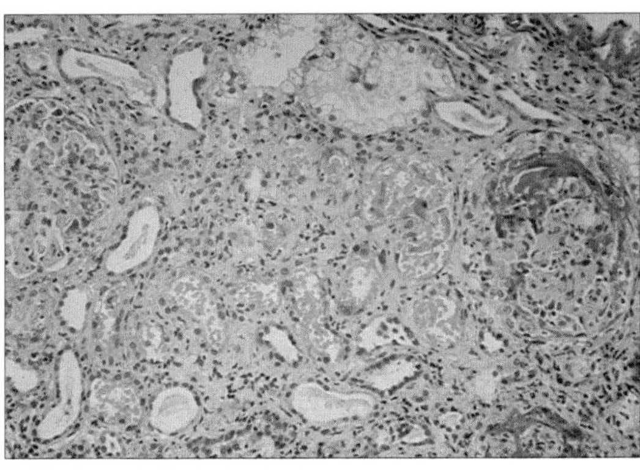

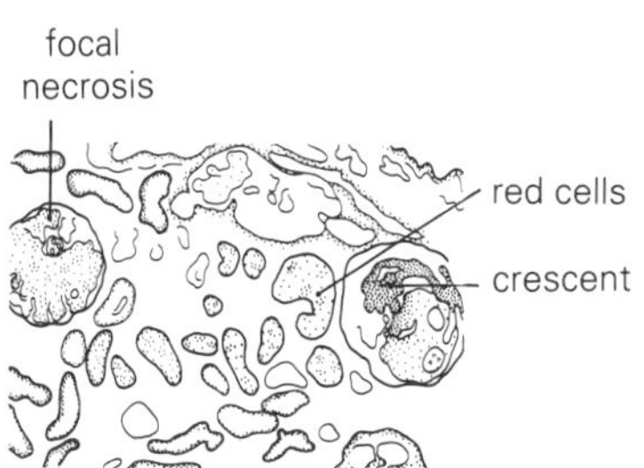

Fig. 8.16 Crescentic glomerulonephritis. Two glomeruli are shown. The glomerulus on the right is surrounded by a large crescent. The glomerulus to the left shows an area of focal necrosis involving the upper third of the glomerular tuft. Red cells, which stain yellow in this preparation, are seen within the tubules.

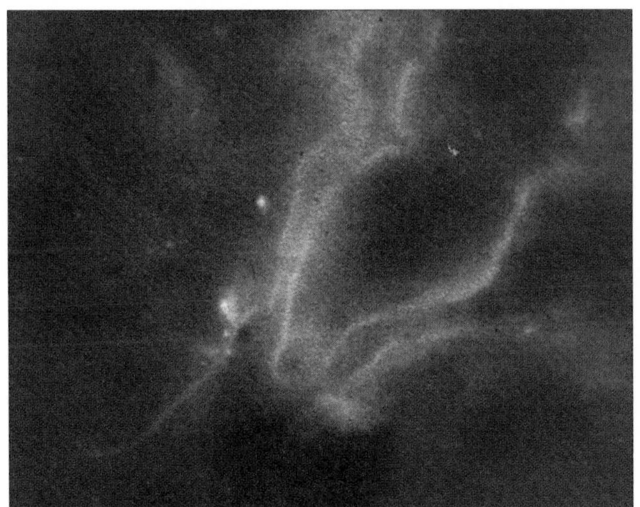

Fig. 8.17 Linear basement membrane fluorescence in anti-GBM antibody-mediated disease. This is a high power view of glomerular basement membrane stained with a fluorescein-labelled anti-human immunoglobulin. The entire basement membrane is uniformly stained, producing linear fluorescence. This pattern is typical of the fixation of autoantibody to glomerular basement membrane.

Haematuria tends to be found in patients with proliferative lesions. Once glomerular damage has advanced to the point of impairment of glomerular filtration rate, hypertension is common. The major clinicopathological correlations are summarized in Fig. 8.18. Treatment is based on histology as well as the clinical picture, which includes the context in which the GN has developed (for example post-infection or part of a multisystem vasculitis).

Treatment

Supportive treatment. This is required in most patients. Infection is treated with antibiotics, and hypertension must be obsessionally controlled with anti-hypertensives. Persistent hypotension and oliguria in patients with the nephrotic syndrome may be improved by albumin infusions. Control of hyperlipidaemia may be helpful in chronic nephritis not responding to immunosuppression. Patients with moderate or severe renal failure (a low GFR) require a low protein diet (0.5g/kg/day), which reduces glomerular hyperperfusion and may protect the surviving glomeruli.

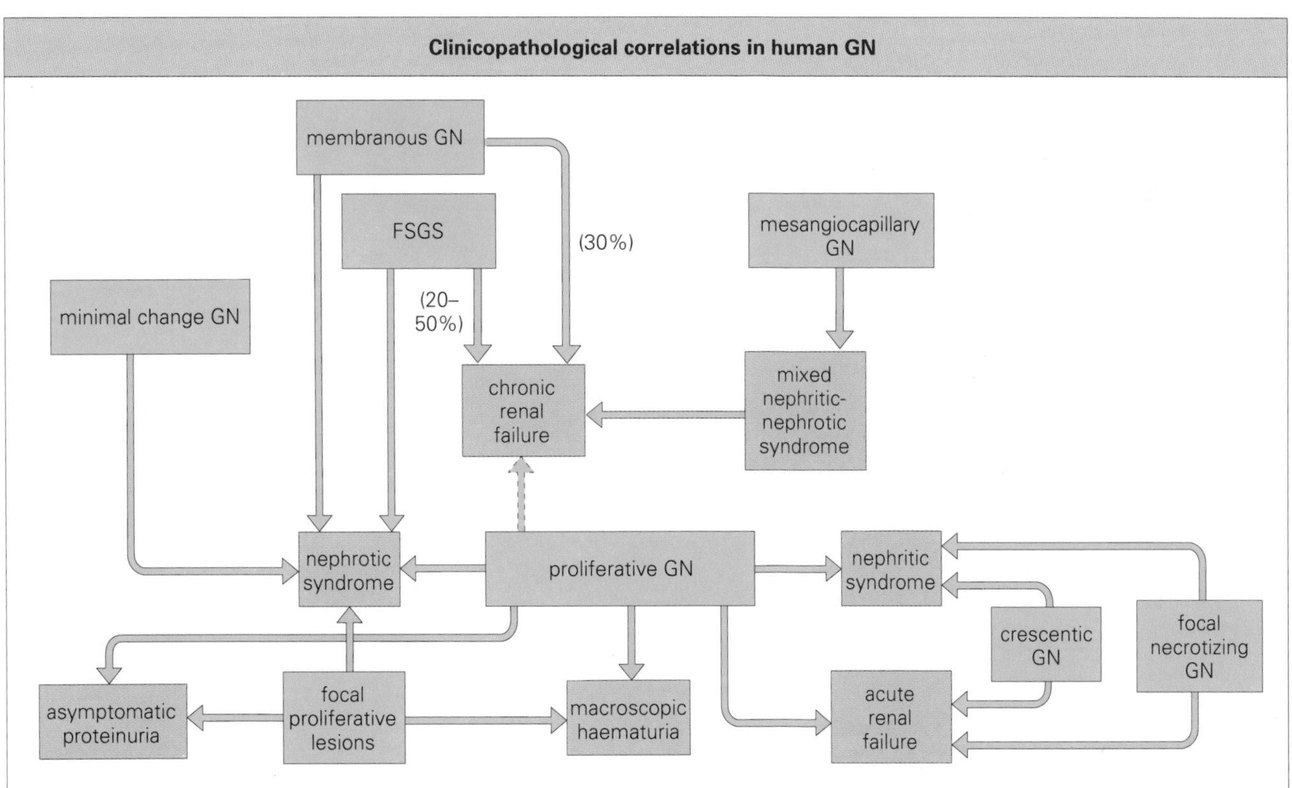

Fig. 8.18 Although there is considerable overlap in the clinical syndromes produced by the individual histological variants of GN, some general trends can be defined, as shown here. Proliferative GN has a very variable clinical picture and prognosis. Within the broad category of a proliferative glomerulonephritis there are probably still several disease entities to be defined. FSGS = focal segmental glomerulosclerosis.

Immunosuppression. The need for such treatment and the drugs used depend upon histological disease and clinical course (Fig. 8.19). Cyclosporin A will induce remissions in minimal change GN, possibly by inhibition of lymphokine production, but is not useful in other types, and can be harmful, being nephrotoxic at high doses. It can also cause angioedema in SLE due to inhibition of C1 esterase inhibitor function.

Plasma exchange (see chapter 29) removes soluble mediators of inflammation as well as antibodies and circulating immune complexes. The clinical effects occur within days, faster than drugs, which take seven to ten days to show much effect. Plasma exchange is combined with steroids and cytotoxic drugs to prevent rebound after a course of treatment (Fig. 8.20). For immune complex or vasculitic diseases, five to ten treatments are usually sufficient. In anti-GBM antibody-mediated GN, a more prolonged course of plasma exchange may be necessary to remove antibody from the circulation.

Adequate controlled trials to define the precise place of plasma exchange are not available. Anti-GBM antibody-mediated GN has such a bad prognosis when treated by drugs alone that most authorities consider plasma exchange the treatment of choice. Impending acute renal failure, despite steroids and cyclophosphamide, may be another indication.

ANTI-GBM ANTIBODY-MEDIATED GN

Anti-GBM antibody-mediated GN is a severe and often fulminating disease caused by deposition of an autoantibody to basement membrane antigens in the glomeruli and sometimes, but not always, in the lungs (Goodpasture's syndrome).

It is not known why the autoantibody appears. Production may be triggered by a virus infection or by exposure to hydrocarbon fumes in susceptible individuals (HLA-DR2).

Pathogenesis

IgG antibodies (IgG1 or IgG4) of a restricted allotype (Gm2) fix to antigens expressed on various basement membranes. The antigen involved is a non-collagen glycoprotein found on the inner aspect of the GBM, the alveolar septal basement membrane, the choroid plexus and some tubular basement membranes. Fixation to just the GBM is seen in 50–60% of cases. Lung involvement seems clearly related to smoking.

Treatment of GN based on histological types

Lesion	Treatment
minimal change GN	tapering course of high dose oral prednisolone 6 – 8 week course of cyclophosphamide (x1) for multiple relapsers cyclosporin A (? inhibits lymphokine production)
membranous GN (severe nephrotic syndrome, impaired GFR)	removal of cause (e.g. gold, *d*- penicillamine, tumour) limited course of high-dose, alternate day prednisolone
mesangiocapillary GN	anticoagulants and anti-platelet agents
proliferative GN	supportive treatment only unless: nephrotics — ? trial of steroids impending ARF — immunosuppression ± plasmapheresis
focal segmental glomerulosclerosis	steroids combination steroids & cytotoxic drugs
focal necrotizing GN crescentic GN	immunosuppression ± plasma exchange

Fig. 8.19 Focal necrotizing GN may produce renal failure in days. Immunosuppression and plasma exchange should be used only if the renal biopsy does not show extensive scarring. ARF=acute renal failure; GFR=glomerular filtration rate.

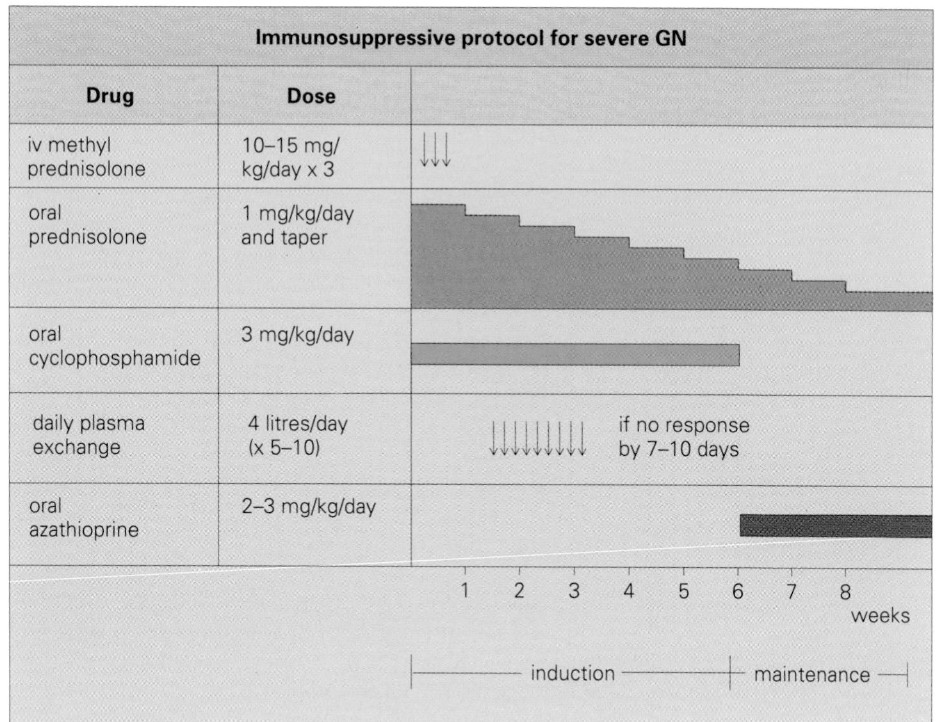

Immunosuppressive protocol for severe GN
Drug
Dose
iv methyl prednisolone
10–15 mg/ kg/day x 3
oral prednisolone
1 mg/kg/day and taper
oral cyclophosphamide
3 mg/kg/day
daily plasma exchange
4 litres/day (x 5–10)
if no response by 7–10 days
oral azathioprine
2–3 mg/kg/day
1 2 3 4 5 6 7 8
weeks
induction
maintenance

Fig. 8.20 Steroids and immunosuppression form the mainstay of treatment of aggressive glomerulonephritis in which renal function is deteriorating. Failure to respond to steroids and cytotoxic drugs is usually an indication to introduce plasma exchange. Intravenous methylprednisolone is sometimes used to attempt to gain control of very active inflammation while oral cytotoxic drugs have time to work.

Clinical presentation

The disease is rare, with a peak incidence in spring and early summer. Slightly more males than females are affected, with a mean age at presentation of 45–50 years. A bimodal age distribution with a peak in young adult life and another peak in the 60s has been noted.

Initial renal presentation may be a nephritic or nephrotic illness. Rapidly developing renal failure then occurs, with about half the patients requiring dialysis at or near the time of presentation. Hypertension is usually absent in the early stage of presentation.

Lung haemorrhage is present in just under half the cases, particularly in younger males. It can vary from the occult to the massive which is rapidly fatal. In most patients, systemic symptoms such as joint pains, rashes, fevers and other clinical features typical of the multisystem vasculitides, are remarkable by their absence.

Investigation

All patients have detectable anti-GBM antibody in their blood. Renal biopsy reveals a focal proliferative or focal necrotizing GN, usually with extensive crescent formation. On immunofluorescence, linear GBM deposition of IgG is almost invariable (see Fig. 8.17), with about half the cases having demonstrable C3 in addition. Other immunoglobulins are occasionally found (IgA 19%, IgM 8%).

Lung haemorrhage is suggested by the finding of an anaemia which is out of proportion to the duration and severity of the renal impairment. The most sensitive test is a rise in the diffusing capacity for carbon monoxide (K_{CO}) caused by the trapping of inhaled carbon monoxide by fresh interstitial lung haemorrhage. The chest X-ray may show any of several changes, from minimal interstitial shadowing to a complete 'white-out'.

Treatment

Once the diagnosis has been made, treatment is started immediately (Fig. 8.21). Second courses of plasma exchange may be needed in the few patients in whom antibody titres rebound. In most patients, the antibody has cleared by eight weeks. Intercurrent infections which may exacerbate both lung bleeding and nephritis should be promptly treated. Smoking is forbidden. Fluid overload should not be allowed to develop as it too can precipitate an acute lung haemorrhage. Ventilation and dialysis support may be needed, particularly if treatment is started late or is inadequate.

Prognosis

Renal function can usually be preserved in patients with a serum creatinine under 600mmol/litre at presentation and who are not yet dialysis dependent. Oligoanuric patients who are dialysis dependent do not usually recover any useful kidney function.

Lung haemorrhage is an important cause of death (5–10%), which is prevented by prompt treatment with plasma exchange. Patients who present without lung haemorrhage but with advanced dialysis dependent renal failure should probably not be treated aggressively but maintained on dialysis until antibody levels disappear and transplantation becomes possible.

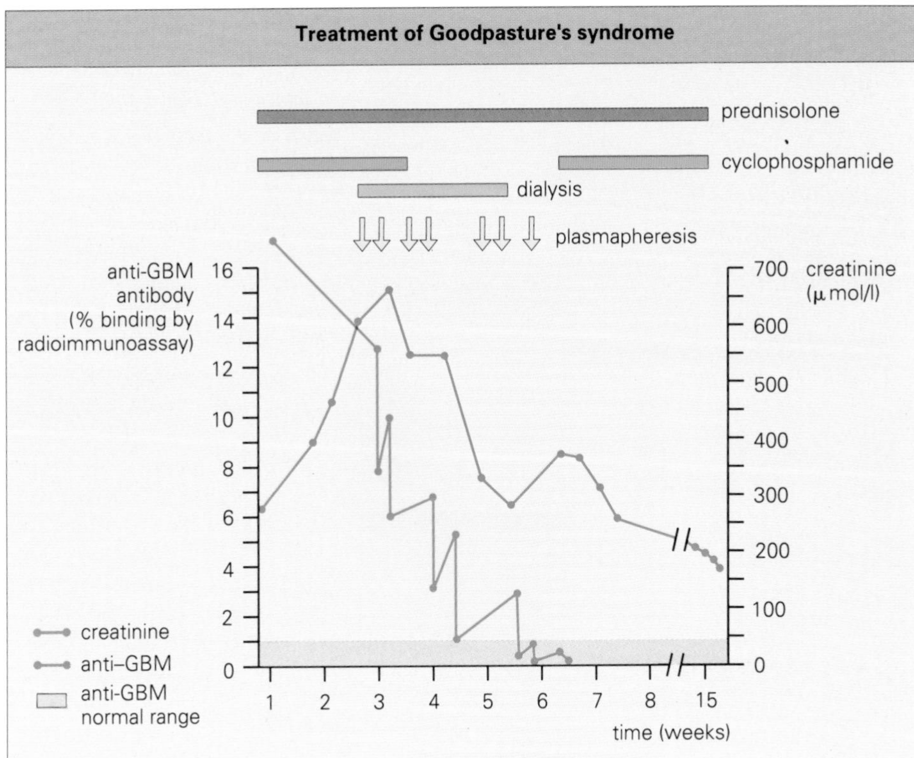

Fig. 8.21 Plasmapheresis combined with prednisolone and cyclophosphamide therapy is responsible for the rapid removal of anti-GBM antibody from the circulation. Renal function, as indicated by the plasma creatinine level, improves after a period of dialysis with this treatment. Modified from Lockwood, C.M. *et al* (1975).

Renal transplantation

The current practice is to defer transplantation for at least 12 months after the last detectable raised anti-GBM antibody titre in the blood. If this is done, recurrence in the new graft is very rare. There is no evidence to support bilateral native kidney nephrectomy prior to transplantation.

THE MULTISYSTEM VASCULITIDES

These diseases form an important group, as renal involvement is not only common but is readily amenable to treatment (Fig. 8.22).

Systemic lupus erythematosus (SLE)

Renal involvement correlates with the presence of a low plasma C3 and plasma C4, suggesting classical pathway activation. Some workers have suggested that the mesangial and sub-endothelial glomerular deposits found in renal lupus are associated with high titres of precipitating or high affinity antibody to DNA. Membranous GN with deposition of immune complexes at a sub-epithelial site is considered to be a relatively inactive renal lesion in lupus, and is associated with lower titres of low affinity antibody. Free DNA is capable of fixing to the GBM of mice and can then react with antibody. The GN in SLE could develop in this manner (see chapter 6).

Multisystem vasculitides commonly associated with GN

disease	treatment
systemic lupus erythematosus (SLE)	steroids ± cytotoxic drugs plasma exchange if necessary
polyarteritis	steroids + cyclophosphamide plasma exchange if necessary
Churg–Strauss syndrome	steroids: renal involvement usually mild occasionally may require cyclophosphamide
Wegener's granulomatosis	cyclophosphamide + steroids plasma exchange if necessary
Henoch-Schönlein purpura (HSP)	expectant & supportive treatment usually sufficient rarely needs aggressive treatment
subacute bacterial endocarditis (SBE)	antibacterial chemotherapy expectant: rarely needs immunosuppression
cryoglobulinaemia	plasma exchange + cyclophosphamide

Fig. 8.22 Multisystem vasculitides commonly associated with glomerulonephritis and their relevant treatment.

Polyarteritis
Unlike SLE, this disease tends to affect slightly older males. The microscopic variety produces a focal necrotizing GN, which may progress to a full-blown crescentic GN. The prognosis is worse than in SLE and treatment is usually more aggressive. Late relapses, even several years after acute attacks, are not uncommon.

A raised PMN count and a high C-reactive protein suggest active disease. A variant of the neutrophil cytoplasmic antibody described for Wegener's granulomatosis is helpful, both diagnostically and for assessing disease activity.

The macroscopic variety of polyarteritis, so-called polyarteritis nodosa (PAN) affects larger blood vessels and is associated with severe hypertension (see chapter 11). It produces aneurysm and thrombosis in the affected vessels. The renal lesions are usually infarcts and ischaemic lesions.

Wegener's granulomatosis
Diagnosis can be difficult despite the classical triad of midline and respiratory tract granulomas, GN and evidence of a widespread vasculitis (see chapter 12). Biopsies often fail to demonstrate a granulomatous reaction, revealing only non-specific inflammation and necrosis. Recently, however, an antibody to cytoplasmic antigens in ethanol-fixed PMNs, which appears specific for Wegener's granulomatosis, has been described. The renal lesions of Wegener's granulomatosis are similar to those seen with microscopic polyarteritis.

Bacterial endocarditis
Patients presenting with fever, heart murmurs and glomerulonephritis, should be assumed to have bacterial endocarditis until proved otherwise (see chapter 11). In acute endocarditis, there is a considerable antigen load provided by a relatively heavy load of virulent micro-organisms. Patients may be considered to be in antigen excess. The resulting GN is usually a diffuse proliferative GN with sub-epithelial immune complex deposition.

In subacute bacterial endocarditis, the number of micro-organisms present is much lower and a strong antibody response is usually evident. Such patients are in antibody excess. The resulting immune complexes are thought to produce a mild and more focal proliferative GN.

The presence of rheumatoid factor in high titres and a low C3 and C4 correlate with the presence of GN in endocarditis. With effective antibiotic treatment the GN usually resolves fully. Occasional patients develop acute renal failure with a crescentic GN and may need immunosuppression in addition to anti-microbial therapy.

A number of cases of endocarditis associated with GN have been reported in which complement activation occurs due to the presence of a complement activating factor, presumably produced by the offending micro-organism. A minority of cases of GN and endocarditis are notable for the complete absence of glomerular immunoglobulin deposits. The pathogenesis of the GN in these cases is unknown. The direct and non-immunological fixation of bacterial products in the glomerulus is possible.

Renal involvement in hepatitis B
Three main renal lesions occur as a consequence of hepatitis B infection, the result depending on the relative proportion of antibody to antigen:

- chronic hepatitis B carriers usually have a chronic membranoproliferative GN. If e antigen (molecular weight 200kDa) predominates, the complexes can penetrate the GBM and produce a membranous lesion. The surface antigen (molecular weight 2000 kDa) forms complexes restricted to the mesangial and sub-endothelial area, and leads to a membranoproliferative appearance.
- patients with hepatitis B may present with a disease indistinguishable from idiopathic polyarteritis nodosa. This large vessel vasculitis is thought to occur when the patient is in a state of (surface) antigen excess.
- other patients may present with the clinical syndrome of cryoglobulinaemia but are thought to be in antibody excess, producing large amounts of antibody to surface antigen. Unless tested for hepatitis B specifically, such patients may be misdiagnosed as suffering from essential mixed cryoglobulinaemia. Occasionally, an acute serum sickness-like illness may be associated with acute hepatitis B.

Until recently, there has been no effective treatment for hepatitis B-associated glomerular lesions. Indeed, immunosuppression potentiates viral replication and may worsen liver disease. However, the advent of interferon offers the possibility that some of these diseases will clear if the virus can be eradicated.

ACUTE ALLERGIC TUBULO-INTERSTITIAL NEPHRITIS

A hypersensitivity reaction occurs, focused on the tubules. The usual cause is a drug (Fig. 8.23). It is certain that this condition is underdiagnosed, and with the expanding use of the non-steroidal anti-inflammatory drugs (NSAIDs), it is also probably increasing.

Pathogenesis
Drugs or their metabolites may be bound to, or present on, the surface of tubular cells or tubular cell basement membranes. When so exposed, the drug acts as a hapten and triggers an immune response. In some instances, the reaction is associated with antibodies to tubular basement membrane, but in many cases the reaction is thought to be largely T cell mediated.

Histology
A diffuse mononuclear cell infiltrate consisting of variable proportions of both T and B cells is seen around the tubules (Fig. 8.24). Tubular damage can be quite marked, with rupture of the tubular basement membrane and

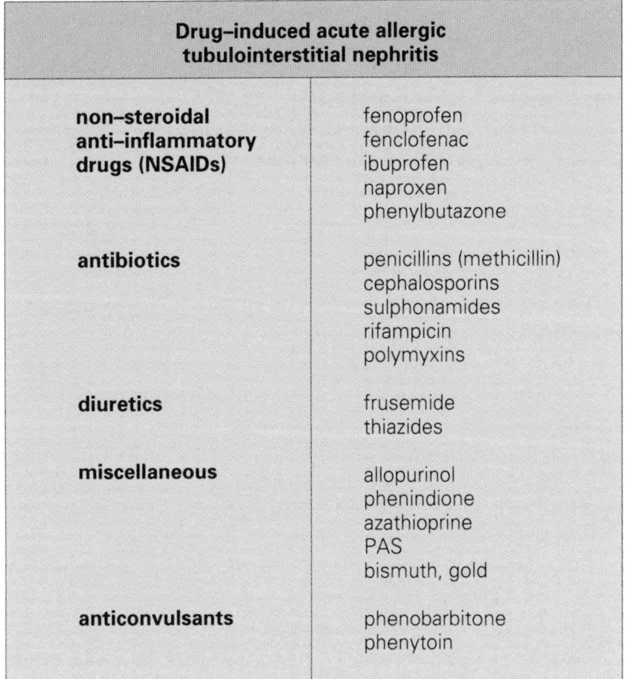

Drug-induced acute allergic tubulointerstitial nephritis	
non-steroidal anti-inflammatory drugs (NSAIDs)	fenoprofen fenclofenac ibuprofen naproxen phenylbutazone
antibiotics	penicillins (methicillin) cephalosporins sulphonamides rifampicin polymyxins
diuretics	frusemide thiazides
miscellaneous	allopurinol phenindione azathioprine PAS bismuth, gold
anticonvulsants	phenobarbitone phenytoin

Fig. 8.23 Most of these drugs are used in patients with a wide variety of renal diseases. Under these circumstances, diagnosis of a superimposed allergic tubulo-interstitial nephritis is particularly difficult but, nevertheless, very important.

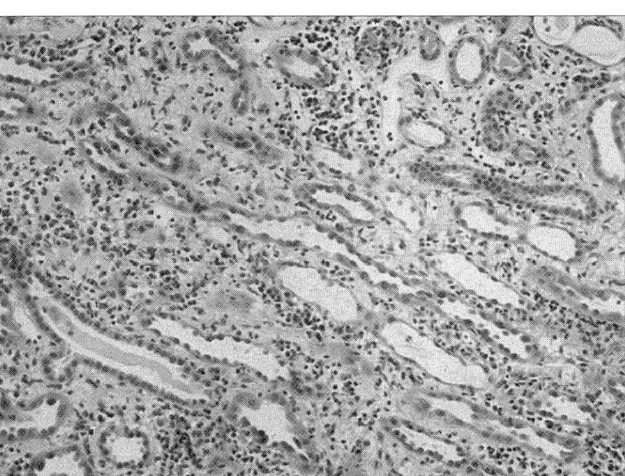

Fig. 8.24 Acute allergic tubulo-interstitial nephritis. There is a dense mononuclear cell infiltrate in and around the tubules. Eosinophils are present and are typical of this condition.

sloughing of the tubular cells. In some instances there may be numerous eosinophils amongst the inflammatory cells. Minor glomerular lesions may be seen, particularly in cases associated with the non-steroidal anti-inflammatory drugs, which produce quite heavy proteinuria and foot process fusion. Immunoglobulin deposits are usually absent.

Clinical features

Acute allergic tubulointerstitial nephritis may present silently, sometimes with heavy proteinuria (particularly in the cases associated with NSAIDs). In some patients, features that suggest an allergic reaction are present with fevers, rashes and joint pains.

Investigation

Eosinophilia may be present. Acute or acute-on-chronic renal failure may occur. The urine deposit contains numerous tubular epithelial cell casts and red cells. In some cases, numerous eosinophils are present and can be demonstrated with specific stains. Proteinuria can be heavy, producing the nephrotic syndrome. A renal biopsy is usually diagnostic, but acute tubular necrosis from toxic or ischaemic insults looks similar, as it can be associated with quite a marked mononuclear cell infiltrate. Drug withdrawal is essential. Steroids may hasten recovery.

IMMUNE COMPLEX-ASSOCIATED TUBULO-INTERSTITIAL NEPHRITIS

The granular deposition of immunoglobulins and complement along the tubular basement membrane may be seen in patients with SLE. In some, the tubulo-interstitial changes can be more marked than the glomerular changes. Whether the deposits represent the deposition of immune complexes from the capillary circulation or assembly *in situ* is not known.

ANTI-TUBULAR BM ANTIBODY-ASSOCIATED TUBULO-INTERSTITIAL NEPHRITIS

Linear staining of the tubular basement membrane for IgG and complement is occasionally found. Some cases occur with anti-GBM antibody-mediated acute GN. Other cases appear to be drug induced (methicillin and phenytoin).

DENSE DEPOSIT DISEASE (TYPE II MCGN)

The electron-dense deposits present in type II MCGN that replace the GBM may also be seen in the tubular basement membrane. Alternative pathway components of the complement cascade and IgM have been reported along the tubular basement membrane and also in the basement membrane of Bowman's capsule.

AMYLOIDOSIS

Amyloidosis is the tissue deposition, usually widespread, of a proteinaceous material derived from the polymerization of partially degraded proteins or polypeptides. The basic structure of amyloid is that of a β-pleated sheet, and accounts for its unique staining properties.

Classification

Parent proteins or polypeptides that may give rise to amyloid have been identified from shared amino-acid sequences. It seems probable that there are many different sorts of amyloid. Systems of classification are now based on the different parent protein or polypeptide (Fig. 8.25). Excessive production or accumulation of these precursor molecules occurs, and they then undergo partial protein degradation in an attempt at clearance. Polymerization of the resulting fragments produces amyloid fibrils.

Clinical features

Amyloid classically presents as hepatosplenomegaly and proteinuria. Despite marked hepatomegaly, there is usually little evidence of parenchymal liver dysfunction. The proteinuria is heavy (nephrotic syndrome) and is associated with a progressive decline in renal function, producing end-stage chronic renal failure. Gut deposition can be extensive and troublesome, leading to malabsorption, bleeding and diarrhoea. Skin deposits also occur causing macules, plaques and purpura. Peripheral nerve involvement is particularly common in the familial forms. The cardiac manifestations of amyloid are as important as the renal consequences (see chapter 11).

Diagnosis

Tissue biopsy is necessary to confirm the diagnosis of amyloidosis. There is a risk of haemorrhage, so that the less invasive biopsies are preferred to renal and liver biopsy whenever possible. Bleeding occurs because arteriole infiltration with amyloid prevents constriction. There may also be a bleeding diathesis, as factor X can be bound by amyloid fibrils. Thick (6mm) tissue sections stained with Congo red are the best material with which to demonstrate amyloid. When thus stained, amyloid fibrils exhibit apple-green birefringence under polarized light (Fig. 8.26). This phenomenon is abolished by potassium permanganate treatment of tissue sections if the amyloid is AA, but not if it is AL.

Classification of amyloid	
Parent protein	**Amyloid type**
light chains (AL)	primary amyloid
protein A (AA)	secondary amyloid
calcitonin	amyloid associated with medullary carcinoma of the thyroid
β_2-microglobulin	amyloid of chronic renal failure (dialysis)
pre-albumin	senile amyloid

Fig. 8.25 AL amyloid is derived from the variable region of the light chains, usually lambda. AA amyloid is derived from an acute phase protein (protein A), produced by the liver in response to infection or inflammation.

Management

Treatment is unsatisfactory. An identifiable underlying cause should be treated. Steroids may be used to control the chronic inflammatory conditions, but their use in animal models increases the deposition of amyloid. Regression can occur if the underlying cause is eradicated, but well documented cases of regression are rare. Colchicine can prevent deposition of amyloid if started early in familial Mediterranean fever. Its use in other forms of amyloidosis is not usually helpful. The alkylating agents (chlorambucil or cyclophosphamide) have been used in the treatment of B cell-associated AL amyloid (multiple myeloma), as well as of amyloid associated with chronic inflammatory disease (Still's disease in children). Some success has been reported, but there must be reservations about the use of these potent and toxic drugs.

Once the nephrotic syndrome of renal failure develops, patients with amyloidosis should be offered full renal support. Dialysis and transplantation are not contraindicated. Long-term survival is limited by an increased incidence of serious sepsis and by the consequences of cardiac involvement.

Prognosis

Prognosis depends on the presence of serious underlying disease. Patients with amyloid due to multiple myeloma may survive for only 6–12 months. A much better prognosis is possible with secondary amyloid if the underlying disease can be well controlled.

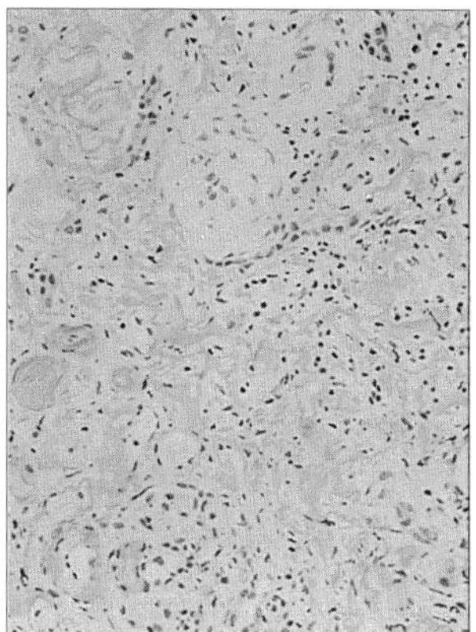

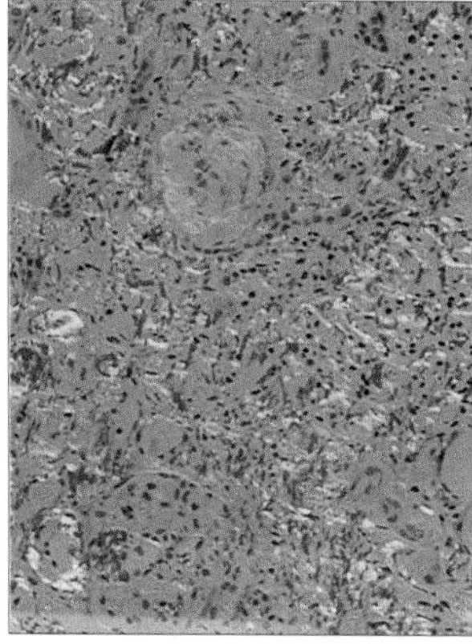

Fig. 8.26 Renal biopsy in amyloidosis. Amyloid deposits demonstrated by Congo red stain (left) show the birefringence typical of amyloid fibrils under polarized light (right).

FURTHER READING

Cameron JS, Healy MJR, Adu D. The Medical Research Council trial of short term high dose alternate day prednisolone in idiopathic membranous nephropathy with nephrotic syndrome in adults. *Quart J Med* 1990; **74(274)**: 133–156.

Cameron JS. The natural history of glomerulonephritis. *Contrib Nephrol* 1989;**75**:68–75.

Couser WG, Abrass CK. Pathogenesis of membranous nephropathy. *Ann Rev Med* 1988;**39**:517–530.

Couser WG. Mediation of immune glomerular injury. *J Am Soc Nephrol* 1990;**1(1)**:13–29.

Jennette JC, Falk RJ. Antineutrophil cytoplasmic autoantibodies and associated disease. *Am J Kidney Dis* 1990;**15(6)**:517–529.

Johnson RJ, Couser WG. Hepatitis B infection and renal disease: Clinical immunopathogenetic and therapeutic considerations. *Kidney Int* 1990;**37**:663–676.

Kelly CJ. T cell regulation of autoimmune nephritis. *J Am Soc Nephrol* 1990;**1(2)**:140–149.

Kyle RA. Monoclonal gammopathies and the kidney. *Ann Review Med* 1989;**40**:53–60.

Meyrier A. Treatment of glomerular disease with cyclosporin A. *Nephrol Dial Transplantation* 1989;**4(11)**:923–931.

Pierucci A *et al.* The role of eicosanoids in human glomerular disease. *Adv Exp Med Biol* 1989;**259**:389–421.

Rees AJ, Andres GA, Peters DK, eds. Symposium on pathogenetic mechanisms in nephritis. *Kidney Int* 1989;**35(4)**:921–1033.

Sweny P, Farrington K, Moorhead JF. *The kidney and its disorders.* Oxford: Blackwell Scientific, 1989.

9

Neurological Disorders

INTRODUCTION

Similarities between the nervous and immune systems

The nervous and immune systems are both concerned with recognition, possess memory and communicate by soluble substances. In fact lymphocytes possess receptors for neurotransmitters such as acetylcholine, dopamine, encephalins and endorphins and there are many examples of antigenic cross-reactivity between the two systems, typified by Thy 1 which is present on T cells and brain synaptosome membranes.

INTERACTION BETWEEN CNS AND IMMUNE SYSTEM

Normally the brain is shielded from the immune system and this can be attributed to:

- low levels of lymphocyte traffic through the brain;
- lack of conventional lymphatic drainage from the brain;
- low level of MHC expression on neurons and glia;
- absence of dendritic cells, or other cells capable of activating resting T cells;
- the blood-brain barrier, which restricts the movement of immunologically important molecules into the brain parenchyma.

Nevertheless, when immune reactions do develop in the CNS there are profound changes which may include extensive lymphocyte infiltration, particularly around the venules, the induction of MHC molecules, and localized disruption of the blood-brain barrier.

Movement of cells and antibody into the CNS

The endothelium in the brain differs from that in other tissues in having continuous tight junctions and specialized transport molecules. The endothelium and its associated astrocyte foot processes form a barrier which restricts the passage of large molecules into the brain. Consequently, the levels of immunoglobulin in the CSF are less than 1% of the plasma level, and this is also true of most complement components; even in severe encephalitis immunoglobulin levels do not exceed 5% of the serum level.

Lymphocyte traffic. The endothelium also controls the level of lymphocyte traffic through the brain which is low in comparison to other tissues. This may be related to its structural specialization, or a low level of endothelial adhesion molecules to signal to passing lymphocytes. The level of adhesion molecules is increased by cytokines such as interferon (IFN) and tumour necrosis factor (TNF). Activated lymphoctyes adhere more effectively to brain endothelium than resting lymphocytes, which suggests that immunological events could alter the rate of lymphocyte migration into brain. This may occur in multiple sclerosis (Fig. 9.1).

The migratory route of lymphocytes through the brain is debated, as there is no lymphatic drainage from the parenchyma. However, antigens from the brain can reach cervical lymph nodes to sensitize lymphocytes in the periphery.

Antigen presentation in the CNS

The level of MHC expression on cells in the normal brain is very low, although neurons, oligodendrocytes, endothelium and astrocytes express low to moderate levels of class I, but no class II. Microglia, which belong to the mononuclear phagocyte lineage, may express low levels

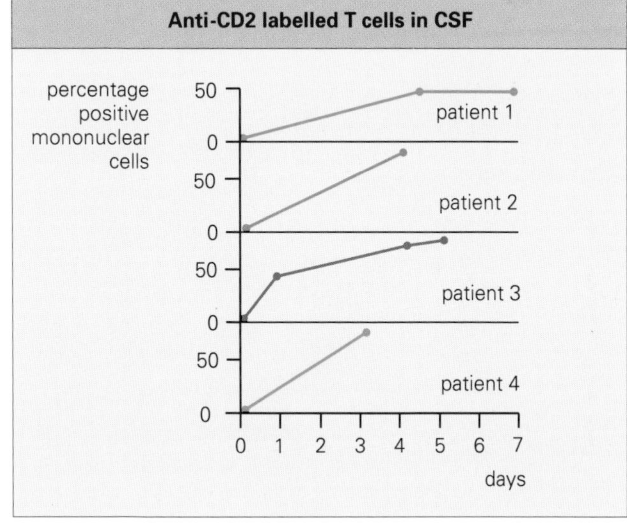

Fig. 9.1 To show cell migration, 4 MS subjects were infused with anti-CD2 and the number of labelled T cells examined in the CSF. Between 1 and 8 days later a significant proportion of the CSF T cells were labelled, showing migration of cells from the circulation into the CSF. Free antibody did not cross the blood–brain barrier. Modified from Hafler & Weiner (1987).

of class II, as well as class I in the resting state. Cytokine (for example IFN) activation of CNS cells induces selective increases in MHC expression depending on the cell type (Fig. 9.2).

It is not clear which cells in the brain could present antigen to incoming T cells, and it seems likely that the initial sensitization to antigen originating from the brain must occur in the periphery, possibly in cervical lymph nodes. Several cell types are potentially capable of presenting antigen, once sensitized lymphocytes have entered the brain, with the microglial cell being the most probable candidate. While astrocytes and brain endothelium can present antigen to $CD4^+$ cells *in vitro*, it is doubtful whether they express sufficient class II molecules to interact with incoming T cells *in vivo* in low grade immune reactions such as multiple sclerosis. Class II interactions are probably confined to the resident microglial cells, except in severe immune reactions. On the other hand, any cell may theoretically present antigen to class I restricted T cells and other infiltrating cells such as macrophages and B cells, which enter the brain, can present antigen to activated T cells.

Effector phase of the immune response

Antibody and complement. The type of immune reaction which develops in the CNS depends on the initiating stimulus. Oligoclonal antibody bands seen in the CSF in multiple sclerosis indicate local production of antibody, although these clones can sometimes also be detected in serum. The specificity of this locally produced antibody is inconsistent, and has not shed light on the aetiology of the disease. Conversely in viral encephalitis, virus specific antibody may be produced in brain parenchyma. In diseases such as sub-acute sclerosing pan-encephalitis (SSPE), which is thought to be caused by defective measles virus, there is a high titre of anti-measles antibody both in serum and CSF.

The role of complement mediated damage is debatable in view of the low levels of complement components normally found in the CSF. However, macrophages can synthesize some components locally at sites of immune reactivity and there is evidence that low levels of complement mediated damage can occur to oligodendrocytes, without causing actual cell death.

Cell-mediated immunity. Cell-mediated immune reactions can be subdivided broadly according to whether they are produced by cytotoxic T cells, by cytokine release from helper T cells, or by macrophage or myeloid cell mediated cytotoxicity.

Microglia, which belong to the mononuclear phagocyte lineage and TNFα, are important producers of IL-1 in the CNS, although astroyctes stimulated by viral infection can also generate IL-1. IL-1 can enhance lymphocyte proliferation, macrophage activation, and in man appears to alter the expression of endothelial cell adhesion molecules. Endothelium itself can generate some colony stimulating factors, as well as IL-1 and IL-2, but the major source of cytokines during immune reactions in the brain is thought to be the infiltrating $CD4^+$ T cells.

Summary

In the induction of immune reactions of the CNS, antigen from the brain enters the peripheral lymphoid tissue to sensitize T cells. The level of cell traffic through the brain is enhanced by activation of lymphocytes or the brain endothelium, and if a sensitized T cell enters the CNS and encounters antigen on a microglial cell, it is stimulated to release cytokines which increase cell migration. The incoming T cells, B cells and macrophages then mediate the effector stages of the immune response, while local disruption of the blood–brain barrier leads to an increase in the levels of immunologically important molecules, which further contribute to these reactions.

Induction of MHC molecules on CNS cells				
Cell type	Normal cells		Cytokine activated cell	
	MHC class I	MHC class II	MHC class I	MHC class II
neuron	(+)	–	+	–
oligodendrocyte	(+)	–	+	–
microglia	+	(+)	++	++
astrocyte	+	–	++	+
brain endothelium	+	–	++	++

9.2 **Fig. 9.2** *In vitro* induction of MHC molecules on cells from the CNS.

MULTIPLE SCLEROSIS

CLINICAL FEATURES

Multiple sclerosis is the most common crippling neurological disorder of young adults in predominantly Caucasian populations and it is characterized by a tendency for small multifocal patches of demyelination (plaques) to occur throughout the CNS at irregular intervals over several decades. The clinical features are a faithful expression of this pathology and include weakness or paralysis, sensory disturbance, gait disorders, tremor, dementia, bladder and bowel disturbance, pain and fatigue.

Severe demyelination prevents the conduction of nerve impulses through myelinated axons; partial myelin injury results in delayed conduction, inability to transmit fast trains of impulses, spontaneous discharge often provoked by mechanical displacement, and the substitution of continuous for saltatory conduction.

Several new lesions develop annually in the minority of patients, each evolving over weeks, but of these only a minority are symptomatic. Symptoms are rapidly produced

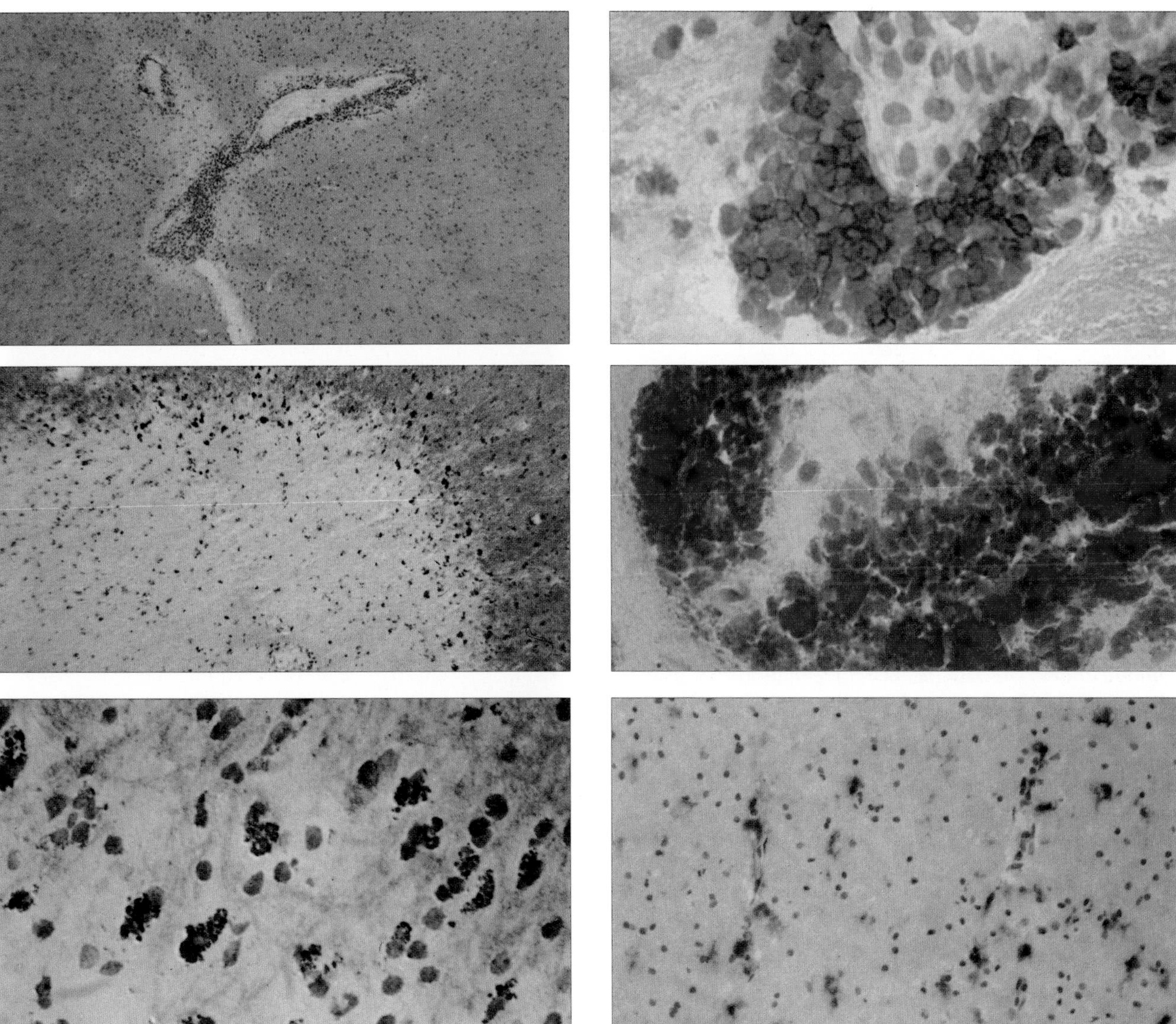

Fig. 9.3 Multiple sclerosis. Upper: an early plaque showing perivascular cuffing and some loss of myelin. Middle: plaque stained for myelin basic protein showing loss of myelin and a hypercellular border. Lower: macrophages with intracellular myelin at the plaque border. Courtesy of Dr N Woodroofe & Dr G M Hayes.

Fig. 9.4 Pathology of MS plaque. Upper: perivascular cuffing with dark-rimmed $CD8^+$ cells in the area of cell accumulation. Middle: the perivascular area stained with Oil Red-O showing intracellular neutral lipid — a breakdown product of myelin in macrophages. Lower: increased MHC class II expression in microglia in unaffected MS brain. Courtesy of Dr N Woodroofe & Dr G M Hayes.

when certain parts of the CNS such as the optic nerves, brain stem and cervical portion of the spinal cord are affected, whereas lesions in other areas, including the periventricular white matter, are rarely detectable.

Pathological features of the plaque

Plaques are usually confined to the CNS (Fig. 9.3) although infrequently they occur in the peripheral nerves. In the earliest stage of plaque development, T lymphocytes and macrophages attach to the lining of cerebral vessels and migrate across the brain's endothelial barrier. Notably, the infiltrate appearing on the abluminal surface contains many cells bearing activation markers such as the IL-2 receptor. As the plaque develops, $CD8^+$ lymphocytes concentrate at the lesion edge (Fig. 9.4 upper) while $CD4^+$ cells are found within the core; B lymphocytes and antibody can also be detected. Consequently, there is an accumulation of inflammatory cells within the brain parenchyma. Eventually macrophages attach to the myelin lamellae and systematically strip the sheaths from short segments of myelinated axons (Fig. 9.4 middle). These fat-laden macrophages are described as foamy or glitter cells. In the acute plaque oligodendrocytes are also damaged and show ultrastructural features consistent with

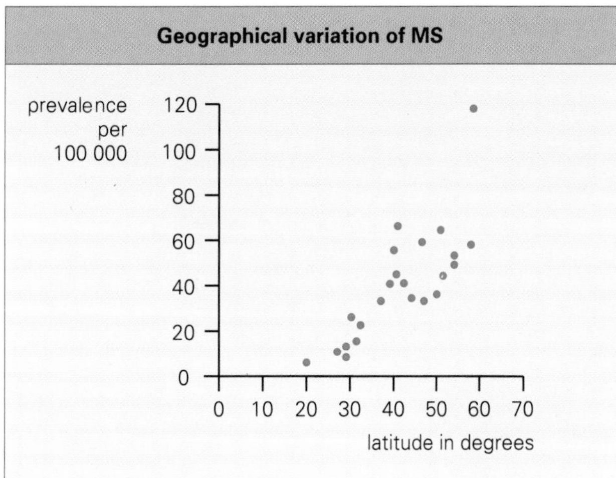

Fig. 9.5 The prevalence of MS is strongly affected by geographical location. It is much commoner in temperate climates, as is shown by the relationship with latitude. Migration studies show that geographical location exerts an effect within the first 15 years of life.

Relative risk of multiple sclerosis associated with known susceptibility genes

Gene locus	Chromosome	Relative risk
HLA class II		
DPw4	6	5.4*
DQw1	6	10.5
DR2,4, or 6	6	3.4
T cell receptor		
alpha T	14	11.0
beta T	7	3.0
Immunoglobulin		
Gm 3:γ3	14	3.5
Regulation of inflammation		
Pi (M3)	14	3.0
sibling		20.0
identical twin		500

* not found in all series of patients
T defined region idiotopes

Fig. 9.6 Relative risk of MS associated with some of the known 'susceptibility genes'.

osmotic shock, but significant remyelination can also be demonstrated. In the chronic lesion, when perivenular lymphocytic infiltration and myelin laden macrophages are no longer present, the plaque consists of naked axons, some of which later degenerate, and there is astrocytic overgrowth and oligodendrocyte depletion. There is also increased MHC class II expression on microglia (Fig. 9.4 lower), even in unaffected brain.

IMMUNOGENETICS

Multiple sclerosis (MS) primarily affects whites, whereas blacks, Orientals and to some extent Indians and Hispanics are relatively resistant. However, these racial trends are modified by geographic location (Fig. 9.5), so that the risk for whites raised in Australia is less than half that for those in Northern Europe. Similarly the disease is present in the black population of North America and the United Kingdom.

About 15% of patients with MS have an affected relative, usually a sibling, and concordance may be as high as 70% in identical twins. Pedigree analysis does not suggest a Mendelian pattern of single gene inheritance and it is likely that several genes interact in conferring disease susceptibility.

HLA-D locus. An association between the development of MS and the presence of HLA-DR2 or the closely linked allele DQw1 has been shown, especially in Northern Europe. Different specific associations are seen in many non-European populations of MS patients, for example DR4 in Italians and Jordanian Arabs. In multiply affected families the disease does not always segregate in association with an HLA haplotype. Genotyping confirms the association with polymorphisms of DR and DQβ chains but unlike diabetes, there is no disease specific sequence peculiar to the form of DR2 or DQ1 found in patients with MS. These observations indicate that, at best, the class II HLA association can only account for a fraction of the genetic susceptibility implicated by classical genetic methods.

T cell receptor. Analysis of restricted lengths of the T cell receptor show that particular re-arrangements of the T cell α and β variable region genes carry an increased risk approximately comparable to that conferred by the presence of the class II HLA gene. These non-linked genes may have complementary effects which account for a major component of disease suceptibility, if they occur together in an individual. The relative risk of MS associated with various susceptibility factors is shown in Fig. 9.6.

AETIOLOGY

Viruses

Heritability has been estimated at under 60% in MS, while genetic factors that increase susceptibility are also present in a significant proportion of the unaffected population. This suggests that environmental triggers are also involved. Prevalence rates are influenced by geography before the age of 15, but attempts to identify the

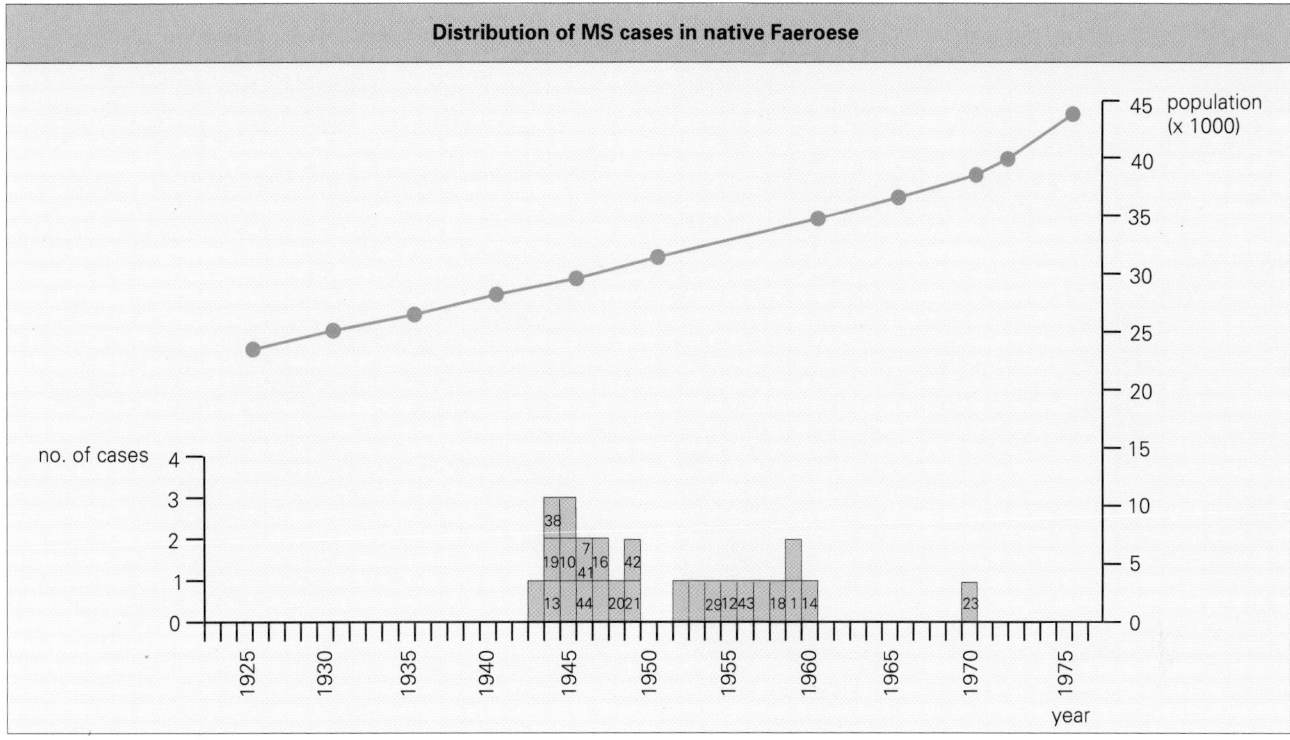

Fig. 9.7 The distribution of MS cases in the Faeroes as defined by year of clinical onset. British troops landed there on 13 April 1940 after the fall of Denmark and stayed for 5 years. This would seem to be a 'point-source' epidemic associated with the arrival of the troops. Modified from Kurtzke & Hyllested (1979).

Animal models for MS

Experimental autoimmune encephalomyelitis (EAE)

CNS viral infections
immune response to viral neoantigens

CNS viral infections
with consequent autoimmunity

Fig. 9.8 EAE is the most relevant model to MS research. Viral infections can lead to two types of CNS damage: an immune response to viral neoantigens causing CNS inflammation e.g. Theiler's viral encephalitis and visna in sheep; an infection with consequent T cell-mediated (and transferrable) autoimmunity, e.g. immune hepatitis virus and measles virus in rats.

environmental and presumably infective factor that underlies these epidemiological patterns have been unsuccessful. Despite this, it seems reasonable that a viral factor is responsible; epidemiological evidence shows that 40% of new clinical events are associated with a presumed viral infection and 10% of all infections occurring in patients with MS are followed by a new relapse. MS seems to follow common viral infections, but does not involve persistent infection with one particular virus. During adolescence there is a 'window of vulnerability' when this is most likely to occur, so the relative risk of contracting MS increases with age of infection with measles, mumps, rubella and EBV to a maximum between 12 and 15. This could explain the association with temperate climates and higher socioeconomic groups in which viral infections tend to be postponed to later ages. The interesting epidemic of MS in the Faeroes in the 1940s may have been associated with a virus 'transmitted' by the Second World War garrison stationed there (Fig. 9.7).

Animal models

Restricted access to affected tissue at times when the lesions are evolving has meant that research into the mechanisms of myelin injury has depended on animal models. Researchers have investigated three types of model, as shown in Fig. 9.8.

Experimental autoimmune encephalomyelitis (EAE). The immunization of small animals with homogenized brain or spinal cord, encephalitogenic extracts or myelin basic protein in adjuvant, produces an encephalitis which has been likened to MS. T cells from these immunized animals can adoptively transfer the clinical and pathological effects of the disease, which suggests that EAE, and by analogy MS, is mediated by T cells sensitized to myelin

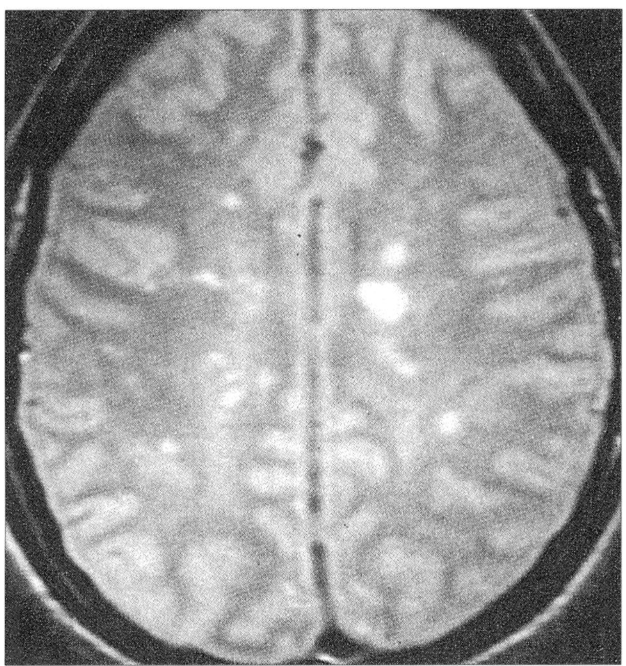

Fig. 9.9 Magnetic resonance imaging (MRI) is a very sensitive indicator of the presence of MS, showing typical lesions in over 90% of definite cases; this case shows multiple bilateral lesions. Courtesy of Dr W Kucharczyck.

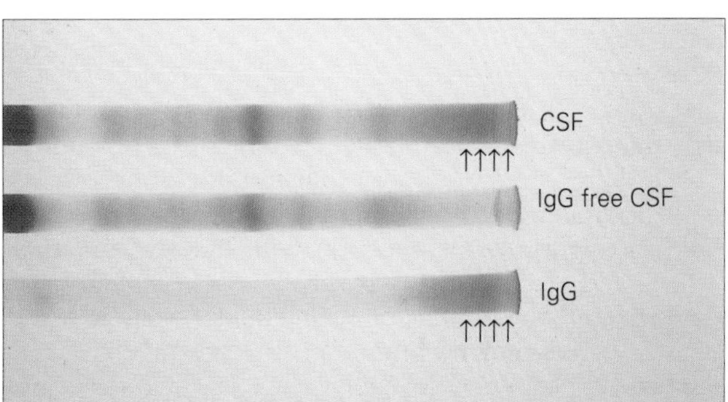

Fig. 9.10 Electrophoresis of CSF in MS. Oligoclonal bands (arrows) in CSF which are absent when IgG is removed by immune adsorption. The eluted IgG, when re-examined, contains the oligoclonal bands. Courtesy of Dr D Perkin.

Treatment of MS

non-specific immunosuppression
TLI, drugs, plasma exchange, anti-CD4

anti-viral agents
IFNs, methisoprinol

anti-inflammatory agents
ACTH, steroids, Ca^{++}chelators

non-specific immunomodulation
levamisole, thymic hormones, IFN-inducers, α-fetoprotein, tolerance induction (oral myelin, co-polymer 1)

specific immunomodulation
monoclonal antibodies, immunopotentiation

drugs
affecting spasticity, weakness & tremor

Fig. 9.11 The various treatments tried in MS. TLI = total lymphoid irradiation.

basic protein. However, this conclusion is unsatisfactory at a clinical level because EAE is a monophasic disease whereas the course of MS is multiphasic. Further research has shown that it is possible to produce a relapsing variant of EAE by altering the protocol for immunization with myelin basic protein and using young animals.

Another problem with this conclusion is the observation that immunization with minor constituents of the myelin membrane or even antigens in the cerebral endothelium can also lead to EAE. To complicate matters even further, EAE cannot be induced by T cells when the animal is depleted of complement and macrophages. This shows that experimental demyelination requires both cellular and humoral factors.

INVESTIGATION OF MS

The most discriminating test for MS is magnetic resonance imaging which demonstrates widespread lesions in over 90% of patients (Fig. 9.9), including a high proportion of those with clinically isolated demyelination. However, the abnormal signals are not specific for MS and can also be seen in other inflammatory diseases or with advancing age.

An inflammatory response is seen in the CSF, with an increase in cell count and total protein, and evidence for intrathecal immunoglobulin synthesis which can be detected quantitatively or by the electrophoretic demonstration of oligoclonal bands (Fig. 9.10). No other marker of biological activity has been identified despite intensive investigations of the phenotype and function of the peripheral blood lymphocytes. There is a deficiency in non-specific T suppressor activity in the peripheral blood and the CD8 suppressor T cell population shows increased β-adrenergic receptors, as in sympathectomized animals. Other blood cells are also activated: monocytes and granulocytes show increased prostaglandin and leukotriene secretion, release of free oxygen radicals and lysosomal enzyme activity; platelets are more adherent.

The detection of myelin basic protein in urine has been proposed as a measure of disease activity but this requires

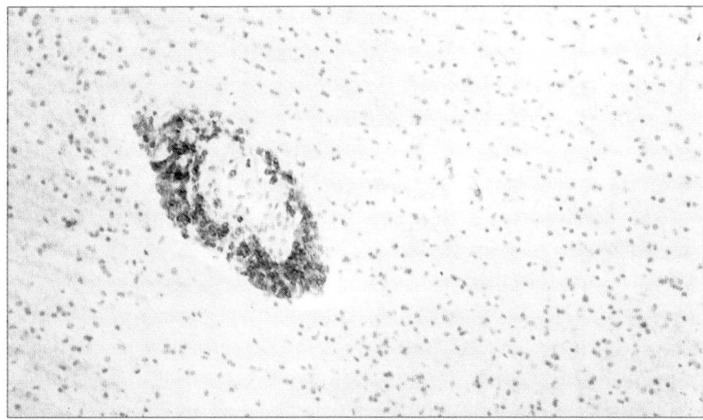

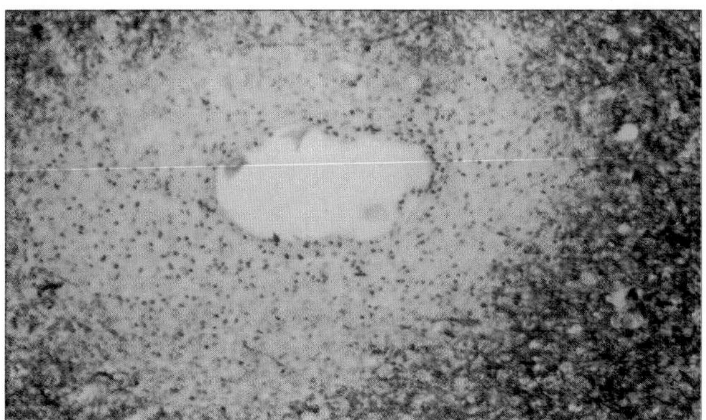

Fig. 9.12 The perivenous exudates (upper) are associated with demyelination (lower). The demyelination is believed to be effected by the action of monocytes emeging from the vessel. Courtesy of Dr N Woodroofe & Dr H Okazaki.

a very sensitive assay and has not yet achieved widespread use.

TREATMENT

Therapeutic approaches are outlined in Fig. 9.11.Patients who remain minimally disabled over several decades are not treated. Those experiencing new symptoms or exacerbations of existing complaints often improve with corticosteroids, usually administered intravenously as a pulsed high dose of methyl prednisolone and this regimen may also help those with chronic progressive disease. However, the main challenge is still to influence the long term course of the disease, especially in patients with minimal handicap but who are starting to deteriorate.

Several attempts have been made to stimulate the immune response in the belief that this would enhance the putative defect in suppressor function or purge the nervous system of latent virus but these are either neutral in their effect or, as in the case of IFNγ, increase disease activity. Conversely, there is preliminary evidence that IFNβ, which has many properties that are antagonistic to IFNγ, may stabilize the disease in patients with chronic progressive MS.

Immunosuppression has been used more extensively, but the results are disappointing. It is possible to stabilize the chronic progressive disease and reduce the relapse rate by immunosuppression, but in most trials toxic doses have been required to achieve slight effects. However, short pulses of intravenous cyclophosphamide may achieve fairly prolonged stabilization and keep adverse effects to a minimum. Specific immunosuppression may become an effective treatment once the antigen(s) initiating MS are determined.

POST-INFECTIOUS NEUROLOGICAL DISORDERS

PARAINFECTIOUS ENCEPHALOMYELITIS

Clinical and pathological features

Acute disseminated encephalomyelitis occurs 10–14 days after smallpox vaccination or a few days or weeks following an exanthem or a non-specific upper respiratory tract infection. Pathologically the characteristic lesions are perivenous exudates (Fig. 9.12 upper) which are usually concentrated in the white rather than in the grey matter. They consist of a fibrin deposition and an infiltration of mononuclear lymphocytes (CD5/8 positive T cells) and macrophages around swollen endothelial cells. Demyelination also occurs (Fig. 9.12 lower). There is a more severe form in which haemorrhagic changes and polymorphonuclear leucocytes are more prominent.

Pathogenesis

Few patients presenting with this condition have been investigated, although histologically the disease is similar to EAE, and is transferable by T cells.

A delayed hypersensitivity (type IV) reaction is likely and lymphocytes sensitized to myelin basic protein have been reported in a few patients with perivenous encephalitis or after rabies immunization. In the haemorrhagic form a type III (Arthus) reaction may occur, but immune complexes containing myelin basic protein have not been found in the few cases studied and this form is still only transferable with cells.

In man the disease is monophasic and this is also true of EAE, where T suppressor cells are thought to be involved in protection against further episodes.

Aetiology

It is not known how the viral infection initiates the damaging immune reaction, but one possibility is that the viral antigen alters host cell membrane antigens so that they are no longer recognized as self and become the subject of an autoimmune reaction. Usually the virus is not detectable in the brain when the immune reaction becomes apparent. In some natural animal infections, for example coronavirus infection in rats, demyelination and inflammation occur; lymph node cells can transfer the disease, with its histological resemblance to EAE, to normal recipients. An alternative is that viral infection of the immune system alters immune regulation and allows self reactivity to occur.

The major organsims associated with parainfectious encephalomyelitis are shown in Fig. 9.13.

TREATMENT

Treatment of acute disseminated parainfectious encephalomyelitis with corticosteroids is controversial, with some studies showing benefit and some not. A short course seems reasonable if there is no evidence of ongoing infection, especially if cerebral oedema is prominent.

GUILLAIN-BARRÉ SYDROME (GBS)

In 1916 Guillain and Barré gave their name to a rapidly progressive predominantly motor neuropathy associated with a high CSF protein but no pleocytosis. 75% of patients with GBS give a history of preceding respiratory or gastrointestinal infection and serological studies confirm recent infection with a variety of agents, of which herpes viruses (CMV and EBV) and *Campylobacter jejuni* are the most common. Acute motor neuropathy, which may involve bulbar function, reaches its maximum within four weeks and, in about 75% of cases, resolves within the next few months. Approximately 5% of cases succumb in the acute stage, usually from the consequences of an associated autonomic neuropathy.

The aetiology is unknown, but it is suggested that an infection triggers an immune mediated attack on peripheral nerve myelin. Peripheral nerves show perivascular lymphocytic infiltrates, and electron microscopy reveals macrophages appearing to separate myelin lamellae. The most plausible aetiological hypothesis so far postulates that infective agents have similar epitopes to the myelin constituents. Plasma exchange (see chapter 29) has been shown by controlled trials to improve weakness and shorten recovery time. Steroids have not been shown to be beneficial.

REYE'S SYNDROME

Reye's syndrome was first described in 1963, and follows a prodromal illness such as influenza, varicella or other febrile event. Two to five days later there is an

Parainfectious encephalitis			
Organism	**Incidence**	**Timing**	**Comment**
vaccinia (smallpox vaccination)	219/10 ^{6} † 25 – 50%	3 days – 2 weeks	local response to vaccination & ↑L.N. in axilla also seen may occur with use of recombinant vaccinia as a vector for viral genes
measles	1/1000 † 14%	EEG slowed from 1 day pre-rash	not related to immune dysfunction or to severity of measles attack live attenuated viral vaccine is 1000 x less likely to cause encephalitis
varicella-zoster (chickenpox)	420/10 ^{6} † 11.25% (associated with ↓CMI)		often predominantly cerebellar rapid diagnosis by precipitation assay for viral Ag treat with immune globulin, transfer factor, IFN, cytosine arabinoside, acyclovir
rubella	1/6000 † 20%	2–4 days from onset of rash	adult > child diagnosis by rubella-specific IgM in serum
in mumps, infectious mononucleosis & influenza the host immune response is probably important in causing CNS disease			

Fig. 9.13 Similar changes can also occur following mumps, infectious mononucleosis and influenza. In these the host immune response is also probably important in causing CNS disease.

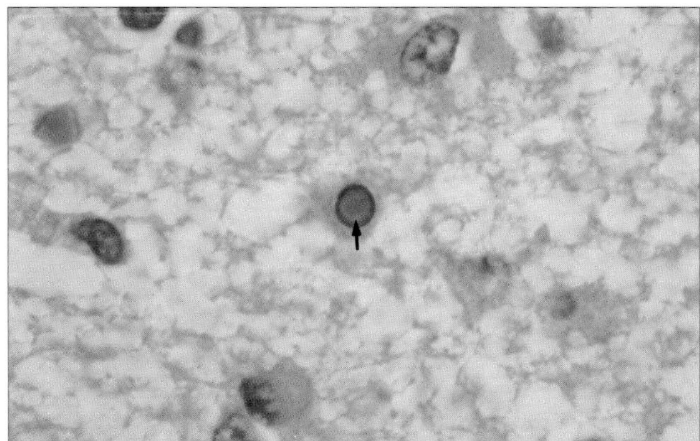

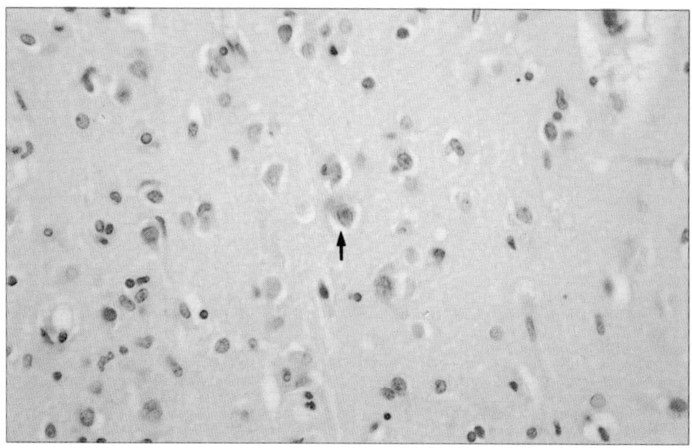

Fig. 9.14 Viral inclusion body in SSPE. Left: the chromatin ring of the nucleus surrounds the viral inclusion body (arrow). Right: the inclusion (arrow) is stained by anti-measles antibody thus confirming this as the aetiological agent. Courtesy of Professor L W Duchen & Dr F Scaravelli.

encephalopathy with massively raised liver enzyme levels, but no jaundice. There is cerebal oedema and fatty change in the viscera, especially the liver, heart and kidney. Hypoglycaemia and coma may ensue. In contrast to EAE, there is remarkably little inflammation in the CNS. Electron microscopy reveals mitochondrial abnormalities in both the liver and brain, and mitochondrial enzymes are reduced. A toxin, possibly interacting with salicylates, is thought to be responsible.

Treatment is based on the reduction of cerebral oedema and maintenance of blood sugar. This is done with intravenous mannitol and glucose.

SUB-ACUTE AND CHRONIC ENCEPHALOMYELITIS

SUB-ACUTE SCLEROSING PAN-ENCEPHALITIS (SSPE)

Clinical and pathological features

This is a rare, late manifestation of measles infection. The syndrome usually starts with involuntary movements and progresses over a period of months with deteriorating intellectual function, dementia and eventually death. Similar syndromes occur more rarely after rubella, mumps and Russian spring–summer encephalitis. All these are single stranded RNA viruses with envelopes in part derived from host cell membranes.

The macroscopic features are white matter gliosis and atrophy; microscopically there is inflammation with lymphocytes, macrophages and plasma cells occurring in perivascular cuffs and the parenchyma. The plasma cells produce IgG which is present as oligoclonal bands in the CSF and is mostly directed against measles virus antigens. In the nuclei of neurons and oligondendrocytes, there are tubular inclusion bodies (Fig. 9.14 left) which resemble those of measles virus, and measles antigen is demonstrable in the brain by immunocytochemistry (Fig. 9.14 right)

It has proved difficult to culture viruses from the SSPE brain, except occasionally by co-culture; this probably reflects the fact that the virus is incomplete.

Pathogenesis

The majority of children with SSPE have had classical measles, and 50% of them were infected under 2 years of age. Consequently it is possible that the measles virus survives in the CNS in a non-lytic state. Notably several studies have failed to confirm the suggestion that SSPE children are immunodeficient. However, recent research has found that some patients lack an immunological response to measles M protein, although they do respond to other measles virus proteins. Cultured SSPE brain cells do not make M protein, which is responsible for viral assembly. It is probable that this deficiency results in a failure of assembly and therefore there is no lytic release of virus and extracellular immune mechanisms cannot function. Instead there is slow direct transfer of virus from cell to cell by cell fusion, which is followed by cell death.

Treatment

Isoprinosine, an anti-viral agent, probably slows the progression of neurological disability. Immunization against measles virus should decrease the incidence of SSPE since the condition is much rarer in immunized patients.

CHRONIC ENCEPHALITIS WITH UNCONVENTIONAL AGENTS

Clinical and pathological features

Creutzfeldt–Jacob disease is a rare progressive fatal degenerative disease of the CNS. It is transmissible, but has a long incubation period of 18 months to many years. Other similar diseases are known, for example Kuru in New Guinea, scrapie in sheep, bovine spongiform encephalopathy (BSE) in cattle and transmissible mink encephalopathy. These are all thought to be caused by 'slow viruses', which are now renamed prions.

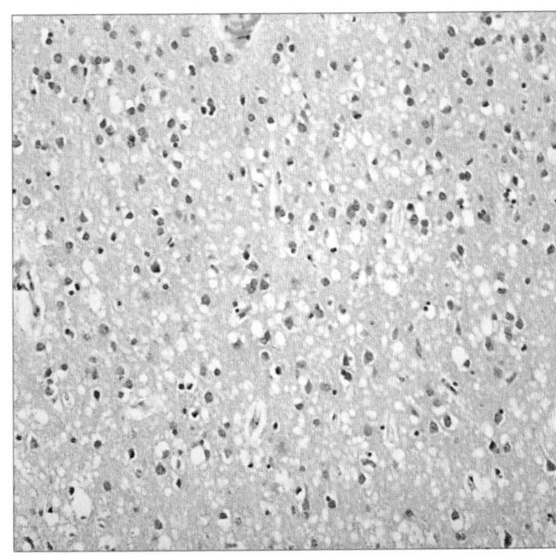
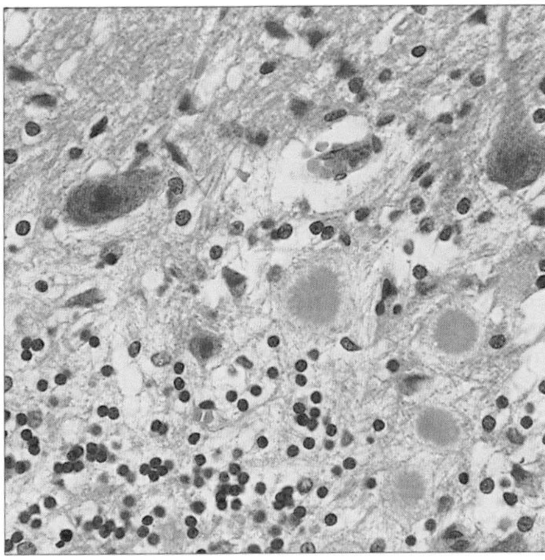

Fig. 9.15 Creutzfeld-Jacob disease. Left: spongiform encephalopathy in a patient who was treated with human growth hormone preparation 20 years previously. Right: typical amyloid plaques in the cerebellum of the same patient. These are identical to those seen in Kuru. This is one of the few cases clearly shown to be due to transmission from one human to another. Courtesy of Professor L W Duchen & Dr F Scaravelli.

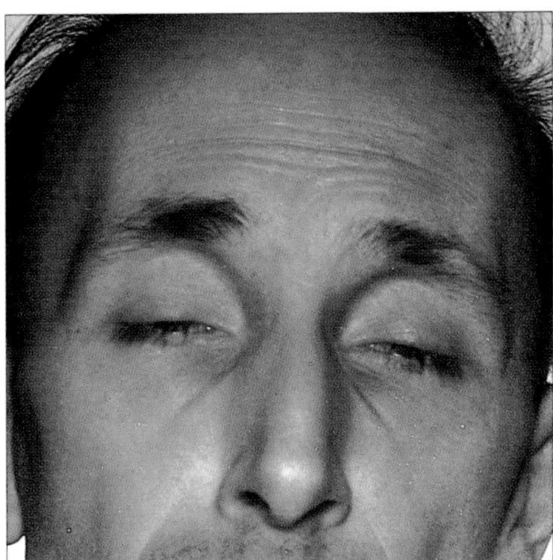
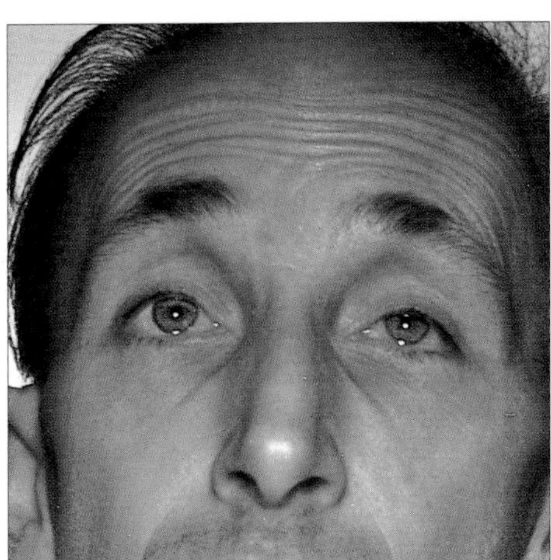

Fig. 9.16 Myasthenia gravis. Left: ptosis before the injection of anticholinesterase (edrophonium). Right: following a diagnostic single test dose there is a transient improvement in muscle power. Courtesy of Dr D Perkin.

Pathologically there are multifocal areas in the grey matter where neurons are lost, with gliosis and a spongy change in the parenchyma (Fig. 9.15). There may also be microscopic plaques of amyloid-like material, but there is no inflammation.

Pathogenesis

The transmissible agents responsible are resistant to heat, formalin, alkylating agents, ultraviolet radiation and to most lipid solvents, proteases and nucleases. However, they are inactivated by prolonged autoclaving, oxidizing agents, extremes of pH and biphenol. The likely structure is a small nucleic acid with a polypeptide. In 1984 Merz *et al.* reported particulate structures consisting of 2–4 twisted filaments each of which was 4–6 nm in diameter.

Transmission of Kuru probably occurred by cannibalism and the disease is now dying out. Creutzfeldt–Jacob disease has occasionally been iatrogenically transferred by corneal transplant, intracranial electrodes or pituitary extract. There is also a 15% familial inheritance in an autosomal dominant fashion. Scrapie behaves as a recessively inherited disease.

Immune response

Until recently no immune response had been demonstrated to these agents. However, Bendheim and colleagues injected rabbits with the membrane-rich portion of Scrapie brain, resulting in an antibody against Scrapie prion protein. There is no known treatment for these conditions.

AUTOIMMUNE NEUROLOGICAL DISORDERS

MYASTHENIA GRAVIS (MG)

Clinical features

Myasthenia gravis is a disorder of neuromuscular transmission characterized by abnormal fatigability of skeletal muscle that can range from transient double vision or ptosis (Fig. 9.16) to life-threatening bulbar and respiratory muscle paralysis. It occurs from infancy to extreme old age. The prevalence is 5–9 per 100,000 and the incidence 2–4 per million. All races can be affected. Other autoimmune diseases occur at increased frequency in MG.

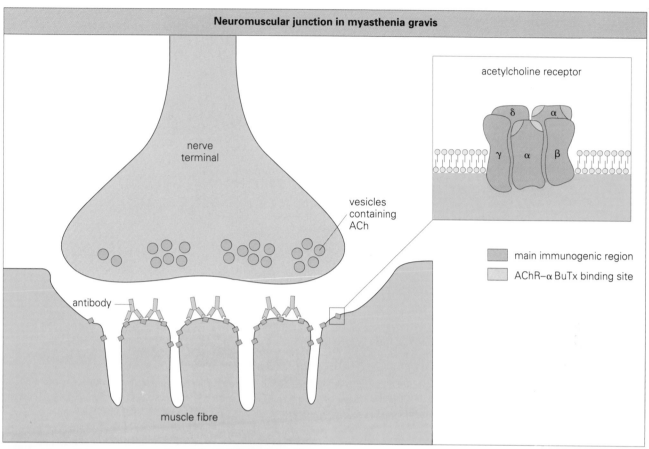

Neuromuscular junction in myasthenia gravis

nerve terminal
vesicles containing ACh
antibody
muscle fibre
acetylcholine receptor
δ α γ α β
main immunogenic region
AChR–α BuTx binding site

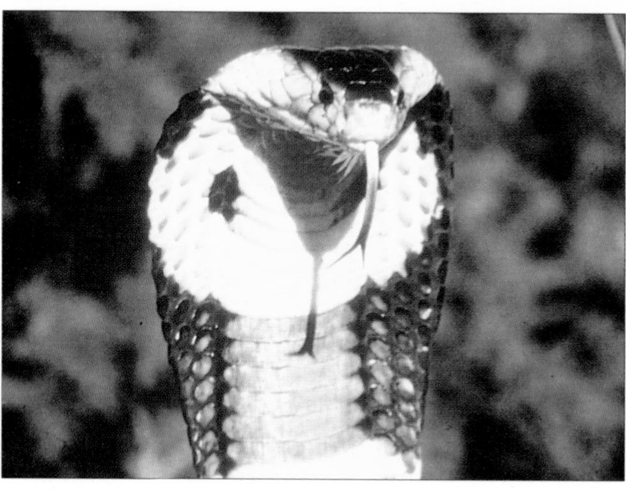

Fig. 9. 17 In MG, antibodies bind to the α subunit of the acetylcholine receptor (AChR). Left: the toxin from the Thai cobra is a specific ligand for the α subunit of the acetylcholine receptor.

Neonatal myasthenia is present in about 12% of babies born to MG mothers, and is due to placental transfer of maternal autoantibodies.

Immunopathology

The primary abnormality in MG is a decrease in the number of functional acetylcholine receptors (AChRs) at the post-synaptic muscle membrane (Fig. 9.17). This has been shown by using the snake toxin, α-bungarotoxin (BuTx), a specific ligand for the α-subunit of the acetylcholine receptor. As a result of receptor loss, the muscle endplate potential (generated by the release of acetylcholine from the nerve terminal) is reduced in amplitude, and is often insufficient to trigger a muscle action potential and contraction. Clinical electromyography shows an abnormal decrement in the muscle action potential and increased jitter in the firing relationships of pairs of muscle fibres innervated by the same motor unit.

Research has shown that receptor loss is brought about by IgG anti-AChR antibodies:

- IgG anti-AChR antibodies are detectable in the serum of 85–90% of MG patients with generalized disease,

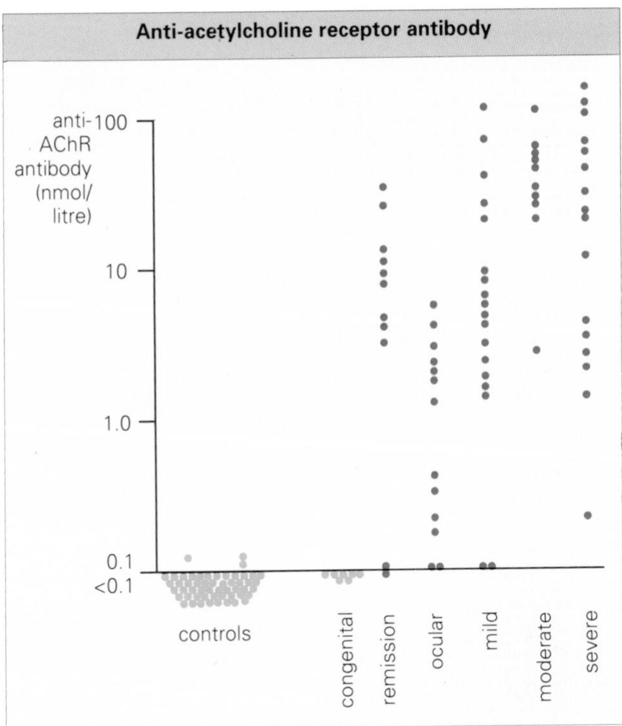

Fig. 9.18 Levels of anti-acetylcholine receptor antibody in myasthenia gravis with varying disease severity. Data courtesy of Dr A Vincent.

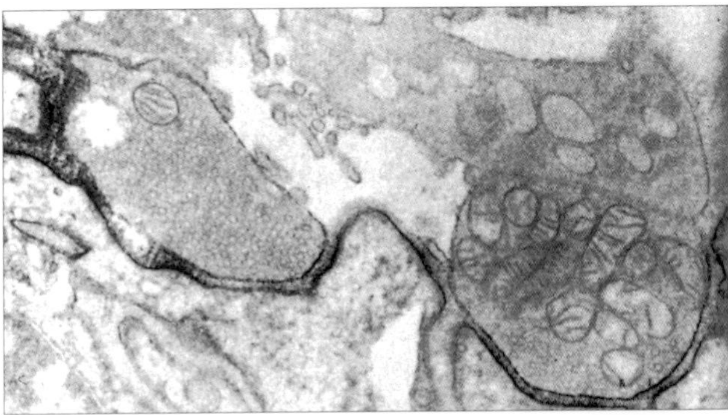

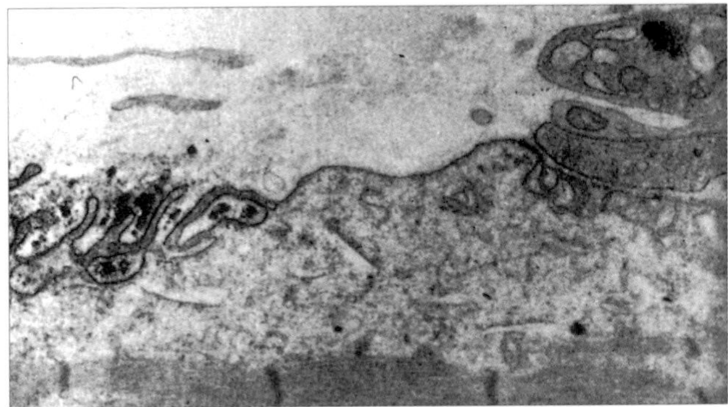

Fig. 9.19 Electron micrographs showing IgG autoantibody (upper; ×1300) and complement C9 (lower ×9000) localized at the motor endplate in MG. Courtesy of Dr A G Engel.

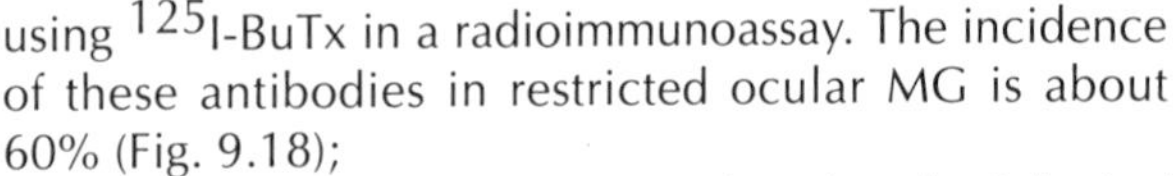

using ^{125}I-BuTx in a radioimmunoassay. The incidence of these antibodies in restricted ocular MG is about 60% (Fig. 9.18);

- MG IgG injected into mice transfers the physiological changes of the disease;
- animals immunized with xenogenic or allogeneic AChR develop IgG anti-AChR antibodies, and clinical and electrophysiological changes of MG;
- immunocytochemistry has demonstrated IgG at the post synapatic membrane of MG muscle (Fig. 9.19)
- plasmapheresis transiently reduces serum antibodies and other serum factors, and is usually accompanied by clinical improvement;
- many patients also respond to immunosuppressive drug treatment.

At least three mechanisms of AChR loss are recognized (Fig. 9.20).

Anti-AChR antibodies

The antibodies in MG are of the IgG class. All subclasses can be represented, but IgG1 and IgG3 usually predominate. Many of these antibodies bind to the α-subunit of the AChR in the main immunogenic region, but other subunits (for example γ) are certainly implicated. Heterogeneity of the fine specificity of these antibodies can be shown by competition studies using monoclonal antibodies that bind to different regions of the AChR molecule. Anti-AChR idiotypes also appear to be diverse; substantial idiotype sharing has not been demonstrated.

Immunogenetics

HLA association. Association of MG with particular immune response genes is influenced by race. In Caucasians, MHC (HLA) associations, taken together with thymic pathology and age at onset, have enabled three main patient subgroups to be identified

- A) young onset, non-thymoma;
- B) old onset, non-thymoma;
- C) thymoma.

In group A there is a strong association with the HLA haplotype A1, B8 and DR3 while in group B there is a weaker association with B7 and DR2; no strong association is seen in group C. In Chinese and Japanese patients, young onset cases with restricted ocular myasthenia are frequent, and in these an association with the Bw46, DR9 haplotype is seen.

IgG heavy chain markers. Associations with immune response genes are not limited to the MHC, or to other genes at neighbouring loci (for example, class III) on chromosome 6. Strong association with immunoglobulin heavy chain markers (Gm) have been seen in Japanese subjects, but the associations are weak in Caucasians; however, RFLP typing using a probe for the Cμ switch region

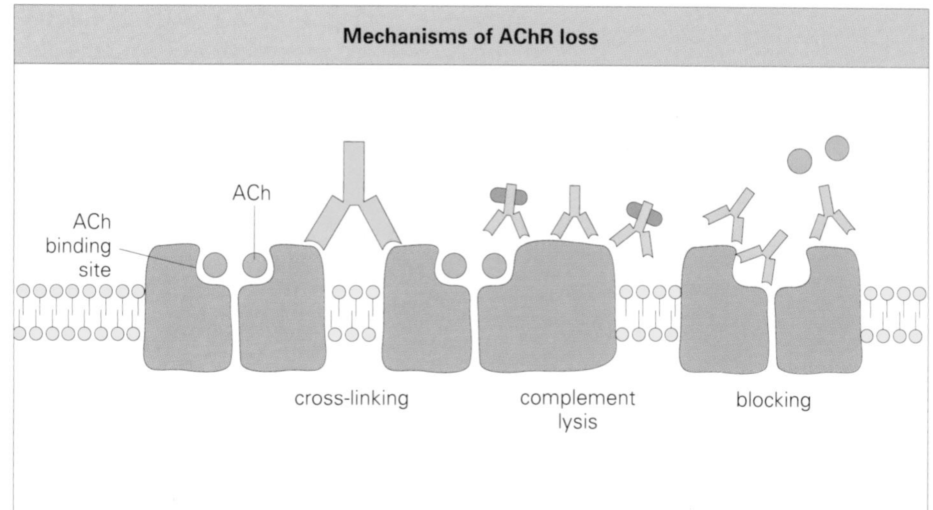

Fig. 9.20 Cross-linking of adjacent AChRs by the divalent antibody leads to accelerated internalization and degradation, with consequent synaptic loss of AChRs. C3 and C9 have been identified at the post-synaptic membrane of MG muscle, and also coating degraded products in the synaptic cleft. In severe MG, the prominent post-synaptic folding of the normal muscle membrane is reduced, leading to a simplified appearance. Some MG sera appear to block agonist activity at the endplate.

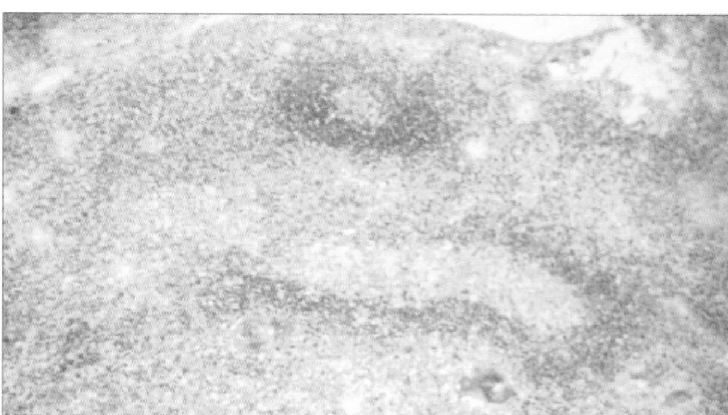

Fig. 9.21 Thymus from a patient with myasthenia gravis showing lymphoid follicles with surrounding T cell areas. Courtesy of Dr M Schluep.

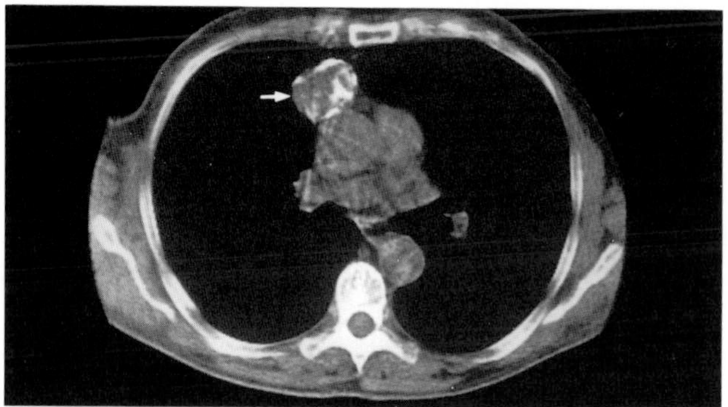

Fig. 9.22 Myasthenia gravis. CT scan of the mediastinum showing a thymoma. Courtesy of Dr D Perkin.

shows a strong association in old-onset Caucasian MG patients.

The HLA association may not reflect the limited number of class II molecules (for example DR3) capable of presenting AChR peptides, since T cell cloning studies using recombinant human α-subunit polypeptides indicates that the other class II isotypes are also implicated.

Thymus

Group A (young onset). In group A, the medulla contains lymphoid follicles with T cell areas surrounding germinal centres (Fig. 9.21), and, in well developed cases, fenestration of the laminin layer normally separating the cortex from the medulla. The germinal centres contain immune complexes, lymphoblasts, follicular dendritic cells and $CD4^+$ T cells, and are surrounded by a mantle of IgD^+ B cells; these appearances suggest local antibody production. In confirmation of this, thymic cell cultures from MG patients (but not from controls) spontaneously synthesize anti-AChR antibodies. Other sites of synthesis include peripheral blood cells, bone marrow and lymph node. The rate of anti-AChR synthesis by thymic cells córrelates strongly with the serum antibody titres, and fine specificities (defined by competition studies) closely match those in the patient's serum. The thymus is also enriched with AChR reactive T cells. These findings imply the presence of antigen in the thymus. This has been shown directly using monoclonal anti-human AChR antibodies, which strongly stain myoid (muscle-like) cells. These are found principally in the medullary epithelial bands, and also in the septal regions. The myoid cells appear to express HLA class II. Myoid cells are present at similar frequency in MG patients and controls, the frequency declining with age.

Group B (late onset). In group B cases, the thymus usually shows an atrophic appearance, and anti-AChR antibody synthesis in culture occurs only in a small proportion of cases, with the amounts produced being small.

Group C (thymoma). These tumours probably arise from a rare cortical epithelial stem cell that is positive for both cortical and medullary epithelial cell markers (Fig. 9.22). There is sometimes medullary hyperplasia in the attached non-tumour thymus. Some anti-AChR specific monoclonal

Clinical subgroups in myasthenia gravis				
	Young onset (55%)	**Thymoma (10%)**	**Old onset (20%)**	**Ab negative (15%)**
thymus	hyperplasia	thymoma	atrophy	↑T cell areas?
age of onset	<40 years	any	>40 years	any
sex incidence	F>>M	M=F	M>F	M>F
anti-AChR titre	high	intermediate	low	absent
weakness	generalized	generalized	generalized/ocular	gereralized/ocular
HLA (Caucasians)	B8, DR3	–	B7;DR2	–
Su (2.6/2.6kb)	+/–	–	++	–

Fig. 9.23 A summary of the clinical heterogeneity of patients with myasthenia gravis.

antibodies stain thymoma tissue, indicating the possible presence of antigenic determinants that can cross-react with AChR.

A summary of the clinical heterogeneity in MG is shown in Fig. 9.23.

T cell reactivity

Peripheral blood T cells from MG patients proliferate in the presence of AChR, and T cells lines and clones can be raised to this antigen. The response appears to be principally to the α-subunit. T cells from control subjects can also respond, although the proportion of responders appears smaller when the antigen used is the recombinant human AChR α-subunit. With the latter approach, several different regions of the α-subunit have been shown to contain T cell epitopes, for which the restricting class II isotypes appear to include HLA-DP and DQ, as well as DR. T cell epitopes specific for MG have yet to be defined.

Treatment

Most young onset cases improve or become asymptomatic within 1–2 years of thymectomy. In thymoma cases, thymectomy is undertaken to prevent local invasion but usually this does not improve myasthenic weakness. In late onset cases, there is little firm evidence to promote thymectomy. In those failing to respond to thymectomy, or in whom the operation is not possible, treatment with prednisolone (usually given on alternate days), and in severe cases combined with azathioprine (2.5 mg/kg body weight), appears to be the most effective regime. The response to treatment is slow, typically requiring many months for the full response. Plasmapheresis may induce a short term remission, and in severe cases is a useful adjunct to immunosuppressive drug treatment (see chapter 29). Anti-cholinesterase medication provides symptomatic treatment.

LAMBERT–EATON MYASTHENIC SYNDROME

Clinical features

The Lambert–Eaton myasthenic syndrome (LEMS) is much rarer than myasthenia gravis. LEMS is characterized by proximal muscle weakness, depressed tendon reflexes, and autonomic changes including dry mouth, constipation, and sexual impotence in males. It is associated with small cell lung cancer (SCLC) in 60% of cases, and in this form is thus a paraneoplastic disorder (see below); in the remaining cases, no cancer can be detected despite prolonged follow-up. LEMS usually develops after the age of 30 years but occasional cases have been described in children or adolescents.

Immunopathology

The primary physiological abnormality in LEMS is a reduction in the number of packages (quanta) of acetylcholine released by the nerve terminal in response to a nerve impulse, although the size of each package is normal. The release of transmitter depends upon opening voltage-gated calcium channels (VGCCs), the resulting influx of Ca^{2+} leads to vesicle exocytosis. Clinical electromyography shows a greatly reduced resting compound muscle action potential amplitude, that enhances following maximum voluntary contraction of the muscle (owing to pre-synaptic facilitation).

Impaired transmitter release in LEMS appears to be due to a reduced number of VGCCs brought about by IgG anti-VGCC antibodies (Fig. 9.24). Evidence for this includes:

- freeze-fracture electron microscopy shows reduced active zones and active zone particles (that represent VGCCs) at the nerve terminals of LEMS patients;
- injection of LEMS IgG transfers the physiological and morphological changes of LEMS to mice;
- LEMS IgG blocks $^{45}Ca^{2+}$ flux into cultured human SCLC line cells (see below);
- IgG anti-VGCC antibodies can be detected in a proportion of LEMS cases;
- IgG has been demonstrated at the nerve terminal in the region of active zones in LEMS injected mice;
- plasmapheresis can induce a short-term improvement in the neurological syndrome, and immunosuppressive drug treatment can result in sustained improvement in LEMS cases who do not have cancer.

Down-regulation of active zone particles (VGCCs) appears to be brought about by cross-linking of adjacent

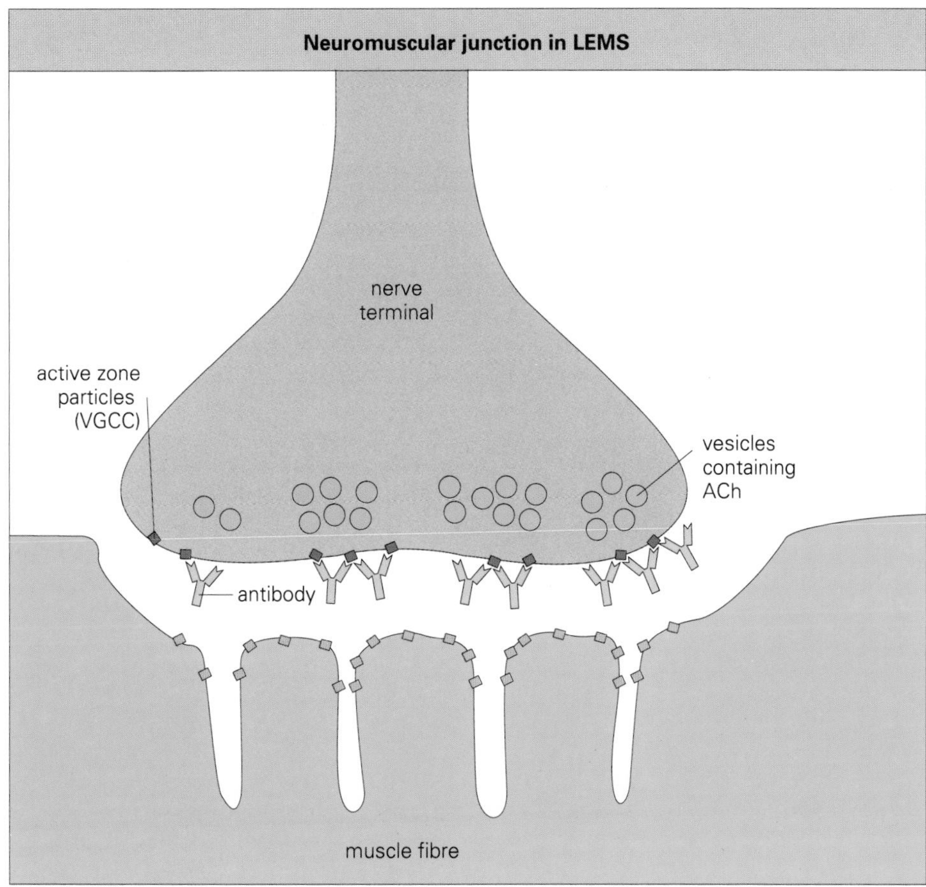

Fig. 9.24 Antibodies directed against the voltage-gated calcium channels (VGCCs) leads to reduced transmitter release. This is in contradistinction to the antibodies directed against the distal part of the neuromuscular junction (as in MG) which are more frequent.

particles by divalent antibody. There is no morphological evidence favouring complement mediated lysis, and C5 deficient mice are as susceptible to LEMS IgG injection as those with normal complement.

Anti-VGCC antibodies. These IgG antibodies can be detected at raised titre in a proportion of patients, using ^{125}I-omega-Conotoxin labelled VGCCs. Titres appear to be higher in those without SCLC than in those in whom a tumour is present.

Immunogenetics. The frequency of the HLA-B8-DR3 haplotype is increased both in SCLC-LEMS and in those in whom no cancer is detected. As in MG, there is also a significant association with IgG heavy chain genes as shown by restriction fragment length polymorphism (RFLP) typing using a Cμ switch region probe (Su).

Role of small cell cancer

LEMS appears to associate specifically with SCLC; association with other tumours may be a chance occurrence. SCLC is thought to be of neuroectodermal origin and therefore may share antigenic determinants with the CNS. SCLC has been shown to express VGCCs e.g. depolarization of an SCLC cell line (by high external K^+ concentration) increases radiolabelled Ca^{2+} influx. This stimulated $^{45}Ca^{2+}$ influx can be blocked by LEMS IgG but not by control IgG, suggesting that in SCLC cases LEMS may be triggered by VGCC determinants in the tumour. In support of this is the clinical observation that resection of the primary tumour or its treatment by radiotherapy or chemotherapy is typically followed over the next 6–12 months by clinical improvement, or remission of the neurological disorder. In addition, inhibition of Ca^{2+} flux by the patient's serum correlates with the severity of the electromyographic defect.

Treatment

Symptomatic treatment with 3,4-diaminopyridine, a preparation that increases nerve evoked transmitter release from motor nerve terminals, is often helpful. In cases in whom no cancer is suspected (e.g. non-smokers, with a history of more than 4 years), treatment with prednisolone and azathioprine, as in myasthenia gravis, usually results in clinical improvement, and remission can occur in some cases. In SCLC associated LEMS, treatment of the primary tumour will often be followed by neurological improvement. Prednisolone is also probably beneficial in this group of patients.

FURTHER READING

Mossman S, Vincent A, Newsom-Davis J. Myasthenia gravis without acetylcholine receptor antibody: A distinct disease entity. *Lancet.* 1986; **i**: 116–118.

Newsom-Davis J. Myasthenia gravis. *Med Int.* 1987; **48**: 1988–1991.

Newsom-Davis J. Autoimmunity in neuromuscular disease. *Ann NY Acad Sci.* 1988; **540**: 25–38.

O'Neill JH, Murray NMF, Newsom-Davis J. The Lambert-Eaton myasthenic syndrome: A review of 50 cases. *Brain.* 1988; **111**: 577–596.

Sommer N, Willcox N, Harcourt GC, Newsom-Davis J. Myasthenic thymus and thymoma are selectively enriched in acetylcholine receptor-reactive T cells. *Ann Neurol.* 1990; **28**: 312–319.

Vincent A, Lang B, Newsom-Davis J. Autoimmunity to the voltage-gated calcium channel underlies the Lambert-Eaton myasthenic syndrome, a panneoplastic disorder. *TINS.* 1989; **12**: 496–502.

Willcox N, Vincent A. Myasthia gravis as an example of organ-specific autoimmune disease. In: Bird G, Calvert JE. *B lymphocytes in human disease.* Oxford: Oxford University Press, 1988: 469–506.

10

Gastrointestinal & Liver Disorders

GASTROINTESTINAL DISORDERS

The mucosal immune system

The gastrointestinal tract is exposed to a vast antigenic load in the form of dietary and bacterial antigens. The intestinal mucosa plays a major role in preventing activation of harmful immunological mechanisms by either excluding antigens or processing the antigens which are absorbed. In the human fetus, lymphocytes appear in the developing intestinal mucosa at about 12 weeks and increase to term. However, following delivery, there is a marked increase in the lamina propria and intra-epithelial cells in response to feeding.

The intra-epithelial lymphocytes are all T cells and the majority (around 90%) have the suppressor-cytotoxic phenotype. Recently, 12–15% of these cells have been found to bear γδ T cell receptor (TCR) in contrast to the usual αβTCR. Intra-epithelial lymphocytes do not bear surface immunoglobulin. They are frequently seen in close association with macrophages, which lie in the lamina propria adjacent to the basement membrane of the epithelium (Fig. 10.1). The lamina propria contains both T and B cells, and the majority of the T cells are of the helper phenotype ($CD4^+$).

Secreted immunoglobulin. The plasma cells of the lamina propria secrete predominantly IgA, with only a small proportion (<20%) synthesizing IgG or IgM. IgA is synthesized as a dimer with two IgA molecules linked by the J chain. The dimer then combines with the secretory component, which acts as a receptor on the serosal surface of the epithelial cell, to form secretory IgA. This complex is thought to traverse the epithelial cell to be secreted into the gut lumen. These mechanisms also apply to secretory IgM.

Peyer's patches. These are specialized areas of lymphoid tissue in the gastrointestinal tract, occurring in the ileum. In experimental animals, Peyer's patches are a major site of entry of antigen into the mucosal immune system. Uptake of antigen occurs through M cells, which are antigen processing cells within the epithelium covering the dome of the Peyer's patch. The processes of the M cells are closely applied to the underlying T_H cells, thus within the Peyer's patch there is both T and B cell sensitization.

Furthermore, there is a sub-population of T cells, known as switch cells, which control the isotype differentiation of B cells. This ensures that the B cells which leave the Peyer's patch are pre-committed to differentiate into IgA-producing plasma cells when they home back into the intestinal lamina propria after reaching the systemic circulation. In this way, the lamina propria becomes populated with both T and B cells which are sensitized to gut antigens. The mechanism involved in selective homing depends on the interaction between complementary molecules on the lymphocyte and the local endothelial cell.

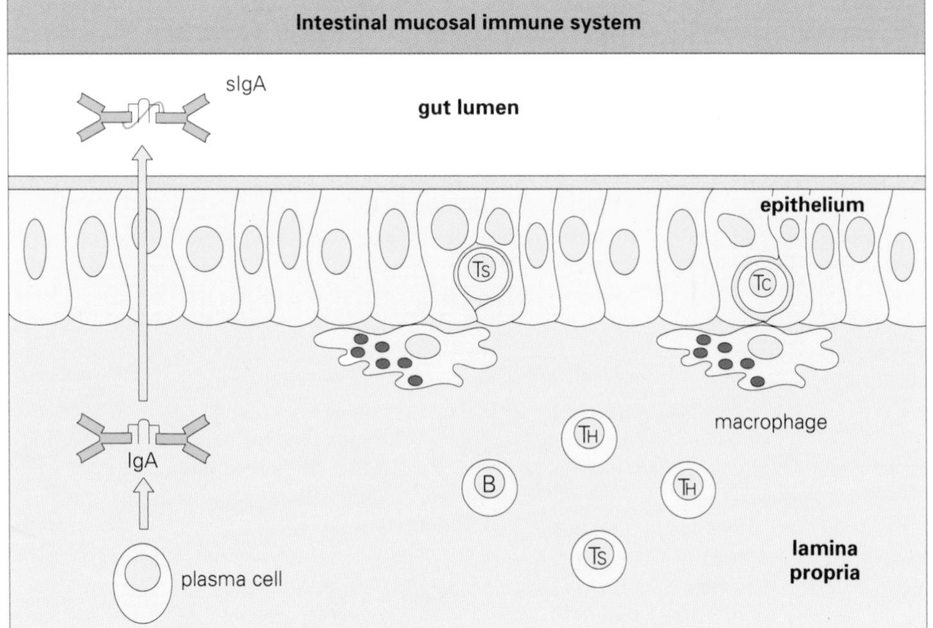

Fig. 10.1 The epithelium contains T_S and T_C cells, often in close approximation to macrophages in the lamina propria. These cells exhibit large quantities of HLA class II molecules on their surface. B and T (mostly T_H) cells are also present in the lamina propria, as are IgA-secreting plasma cells. Secretory IgA (sIgA) picks up its secretory component as it passes through the epithelium.

Classification of gastritis		
Type	**A**	**B**
distribution		
antral inflammation	±	+++
parietal cell canalicular antibody	+++	±
intrinsic factor antibody	+	-
G cell mass	↑	normal or ↓
serum gastrin	↑	normal

Fig. 10.2 Classification of gastritis, showing the features differentiating the lesion of pernicious anaemia (type A) from gastritis associated with non-immunological conditions (type B).

GASTRITIS

Gastritis may be classified as immune (type A, pernicious anaemia) or non-immune (Type B) (Fig. 10.2). Histologically, both types show a chronic atrophic gastritis, but in patients with type A gastritis the antrum is relatively spared, whereas type B is predominantly an antral gastritis and is associated with the presence of *Helicobacter pylori.* The gastric atrophy seen in the body of the stomach in patients with pernicious anaemia leads to achlorhydria and failure to secrete intrinsic factor, resulting in vitamin B_{12} malabsorption. The mucosal lesion is probably immunologically mediated, since patients with this disease show antibody and lymphocyte proliferative responses to mucosal antigens, predominantly the secretory canaliculus of the parietal cell and intrinsic factor, but antibodies to gastric epithelial cells and gastrin-producing cells occur in a few patients. Pernicious anaemia (PA) is a familial disorder and is frequently associated with other autoimmune diseases. However, it is only weakly associated with HLA antigens (predominantly HLA-A3 and -B7, although there is a stronger association with HLA-DR2 and -DR4).

Antibody to the parietal cell canaliculus

This antibody is best detected by immunofluorescence (Fig. 10.3); it reacts with an antigen concerned in acid secretion (H^+ K^+ ATPase) in the microvilli of the secretory canaliculus of the parietal cell. It is present in the serum of

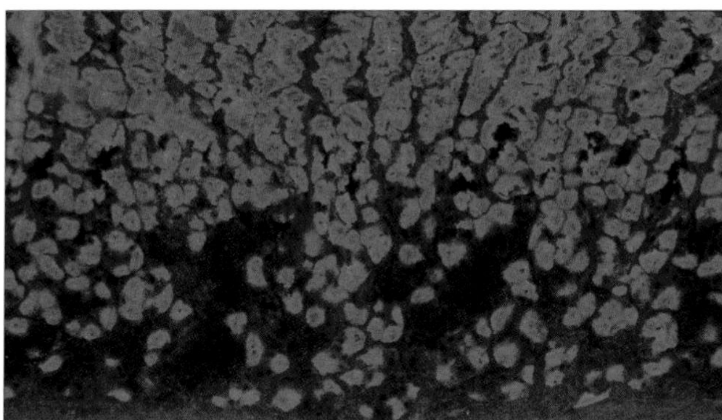

Fig. 10.3 Antibody to the parietal cell canaliculus. This antibody, present in the sera of patients with pernicious anaemia, has been demonstrated by immunofluorescence using a section of monkey stomach. x160.

Incidence of antibodies to parietal cell canaliculus	
Condition	**%positive**
pernicious anaemia (PA)	95
relatives of PA patients	30
iron deficiency	30
autoimmune thyroid disease	30
Addison's disease	30
juvenile diabetes mellitus	30
normal subjects <60 years	16

Fig. 10.4 Antibody titres are generally higher in PA patients.

95% of patients with PA, and is normally IgG. The antibody is synthesized, at least in part, within the lamina propria of the stomach and can be found in gastric juices. It is also present in the serum of other groups of patients, as shown in Fig. 10.4. Whether circulating antibody has any effect on human parietal cell function is not known. However, IgG has been shown to inhibit acid secretion in an *in vivo* preparation of bullfrog gastric mucosa, and repeated injections of the antibody into rats has produced a fall in acid secretion, but not any histological changes.

Antibodies to intrinsic factor

Intrinsic factor (IF) is a glycoprotein synthesized in most species by the gastric parietal cells. It is essential for vitamin B_{12} absorption in the ileum, as the ileal receptors will bind only the IF-B_{12} complex and not B_{12} alone. Failure to provide intrinsic factor is the cause of B_{12} malabsorption in patients with pernicious anaemia. As parietal cells are destroyed, IF secretion is diminished and the biological activity of secreted material is inhibited by antibodies. These patients may have two different antibodies to IF:

- Blocking antibody. This is directed towards the binding site for vitamin B_{12} on the intrinsic factor molecule. It is found in about 70% of patients with pernicious anaemia and in a few patients with thyroid disease;

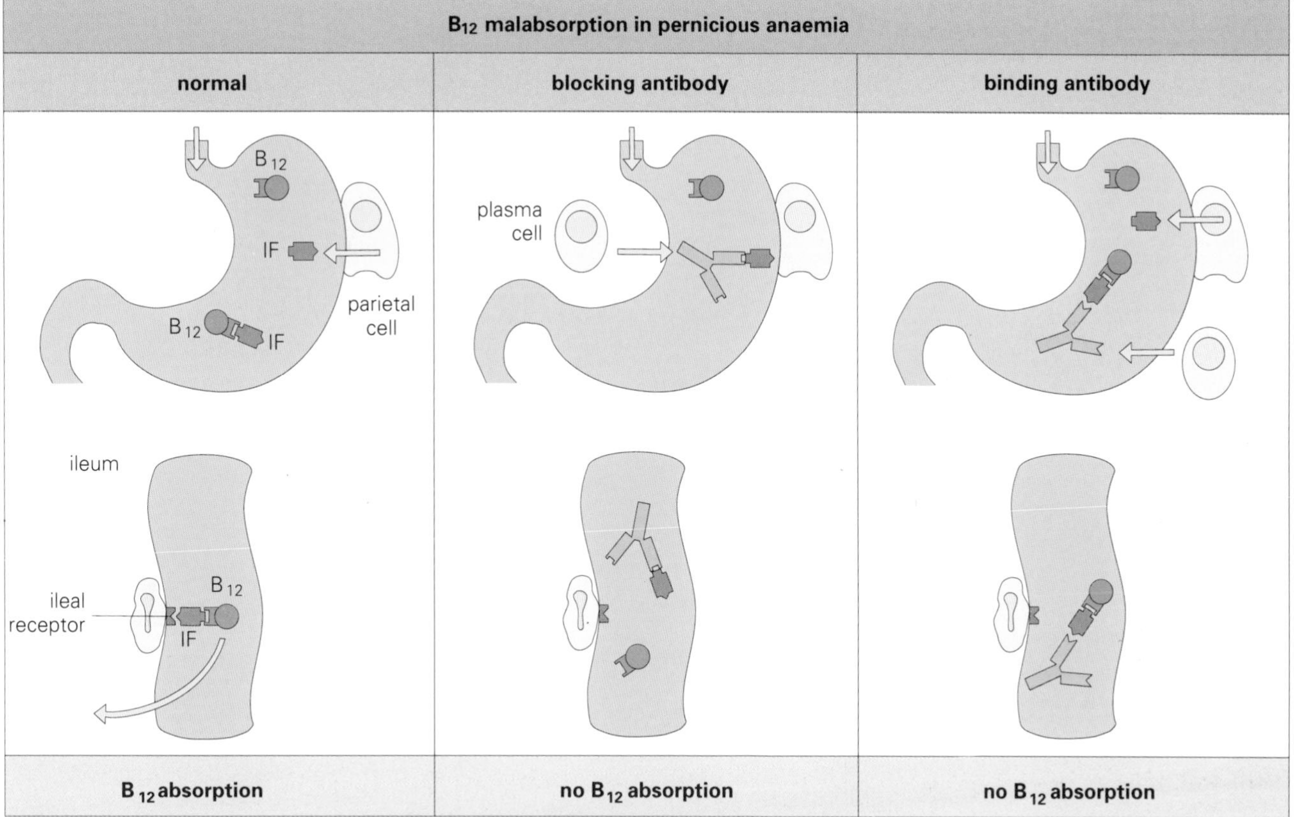

Fig. 10.5 The two antigenic determinants on the intrinsic factor (IF) molecule provide binding sites for blocking (type I) and binding (type II) antibodies, both of which are found in the gastric juice of patients with PA. Blocking antibody prevents B_{12}-IF complex formation: binding antibody prevents the complex from binding to ileal receptors.

Effect of IF antibodies on B_{12} absorption

Antibodies present in		B_{12} absorption
serum	gastric juice	
+	-	↓
-	+	↓↓
+	+	↓↓↓

Fig. 10.6 The effect of antibody to IF on B_{12} absorption in patients with pernicious anaemia.

- Binding antibody. This is directed towards another determinant remote from the B_{12} binding site. It occurs in 35–40% of patients with pernicious anaemia, and is found only in the presence of blocking antibody (Fig.10.5).

Due to local production both antibodies occur more commonly in the gastric juice than in the serum of patients with pernicious anaemia. They are normally of the IgG class in serum, but may be IgG or IgA in gastric juice. That their presence in gastric juice may compromise B_{12} absorption even further by combining with the small amounts of IF that may be secreted, has been confirmed by measuring B_{12} absorption in PA patients who have been given an additional source of IF and correlating the results with antibody status. Patients with IF antibodies in serum and gastric juice absorb very little B_{12} compared with those who have antibody in the serum only (Fig. 10.6).

Effects of corticosteroids in pernicious anaemia

Although the absorption of vitamin B_{12} may increase following corticosteroid therapy, the mechanisms involved are not understood. It has been shown in some studies that steroid therapy allows parietal cells to regenerate with some increase in IF secretion. However, there is poor correlation between the changes observed in B_{12} absorption and those in IF production or in the titre of IF antibodies. It is possible that steroids affect B_{12} absorption by non-immunological means, for example cell turnover or changes in the ileal receptor. Fig. 10.7 shows data based on one patient in whom steroids increased B_{12} absorption with a concomitant increase in IF secretion and a fall in IF antibody titre.

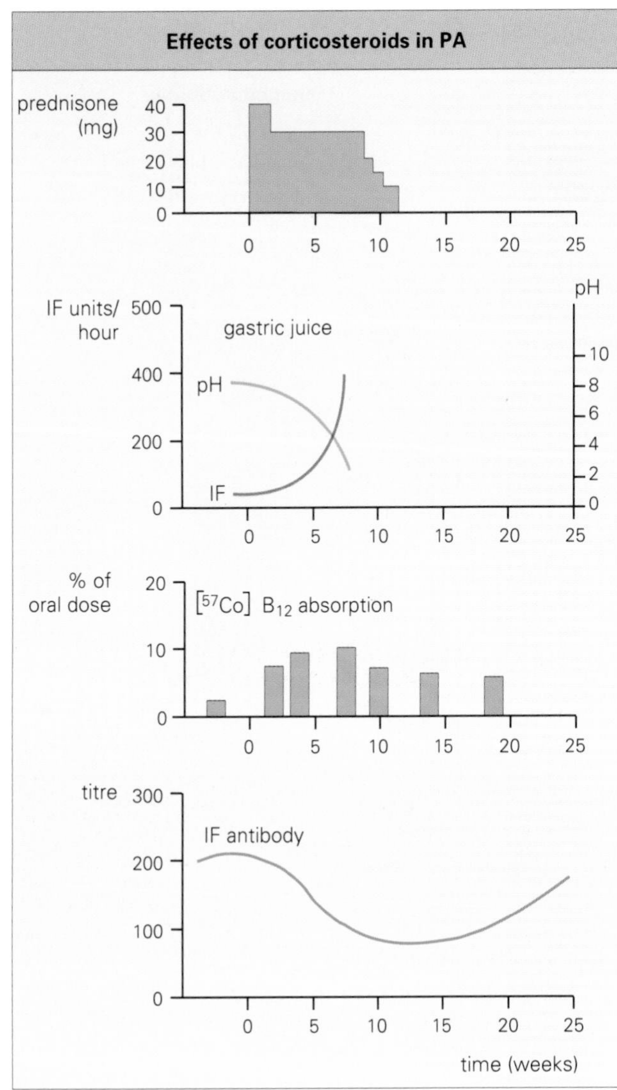

Fig. 10.7 The effects of corticosteroids in a patient with pernicious anaemia.

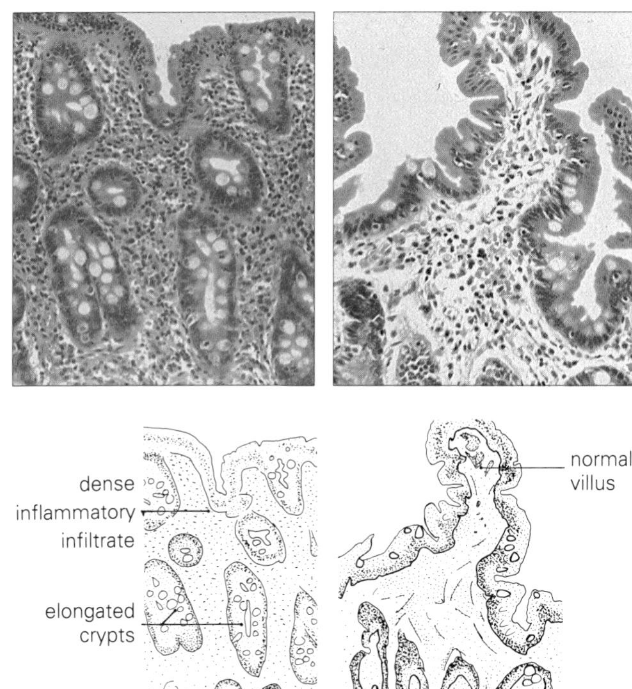

Fig. 10.8 Coeliac disease. Left: histological appearance of a jejunal biopsy from a patient with coeliac disease showing flattened villi, elongated crypts and a dense inflammatory cell infiltrate. Right: biopsy taken from the same patient after three months on a gluten-free diet showing more normal villi.

COELIAC DISEASE

Coeliac disease is due to an adverse reaction to dietary gluten resulting in small intestinal mucosal damage and subsequent malabsorption. The three hypotheses proposed for the pathogenesis of the disease, which are not mutually exclusive, are:

- an enzyme deficiency resulting in the accumulation of toxic peptides;
- an immunological response to a gluten component;
- gluten acts as a toxic lectin.

The mucosal lesion is characterized by flattening of the villi, elongation of the crypts, and an inflammatory infiltrate of lymphocytes, plasma cells and eosinophils (Fig. 10.8 left). These changes affect mainly the proximal small intestine and are largely reversed once the patient is treated with a gluten-free diet (Fig. 10.8 right).

Humoral and cellular immune responses to gluten fractions have been described in patients with coeliac disease, but they are not specific for this condition and may, therefore, represent secondary immune responses to increased antigen absorption through an abnormal mucosa. Gut permeability is increased, at least to small molecules, as shown by [^{51}Cr]-EDTA absorption (Fig. 10.9). However, these patients often have high titres of circulating antibody to gluten fractions which then fall following treatment with a gluten-free diet (Fig. 10.10).

Cellular reactions. Cellular hypersensitivity to gluten has been shown using inhibition of leucocyte migration. Recently, an amino acid sequence of α-gliadin (a protein fraction derived from gluten) has been identified which has considerable homology with an early protein (Elb) of adenovirus 12. Cellular immune responses to both the gliadin and viral peptide sequences have been shown in patients with coeliac disease but not in controls. The hypothesis that follows from this suggests that an immune response to adenovirus 12 in a genetically susceptible individual might break oral tolerance to gluten peptides and thus initiate mucosal inflammation.

Whether both humoral and cellular mechanisms are important in inducing tissue injury is unknown. However, in experimental situations, such as graft-versus-host reactions, T cell activation can cause villous atrophy.

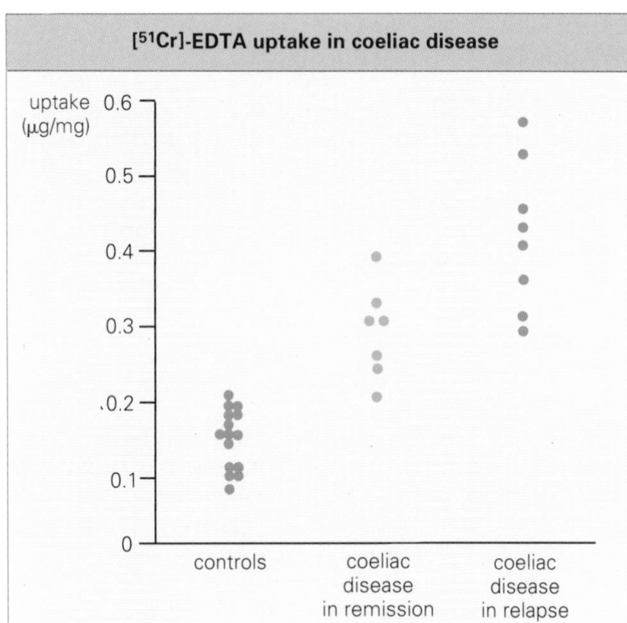

Fig. 10.9 Altered gut permeability in coeliac disease is indicated by increased uptake of [^{51}Cr]-EDTA. In this experiment the most marked abnormality was seen in patients in relapse, but this persisted in patients in remission, suggesting that the defect might be a primary factor in coeliac disease. The increased permeability may allow passage of toxic fragments of gluten into the lamina propria. Modified from Bjarnason and Peters.

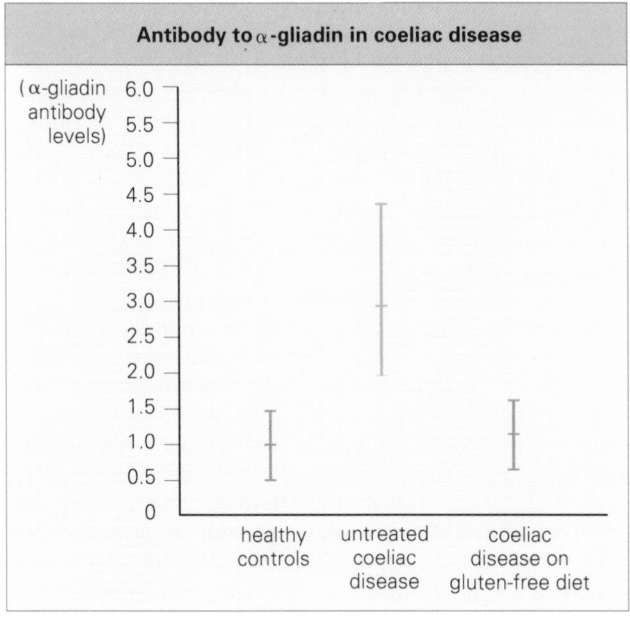

Fig. 10.10 Antibody levels to α-gliadin are significantly higher in untreated coeliac patients than in those on a gluten-free diet, who show levels comparable to healthy controls. The mean ± standard deviation is shown for each group. Modified from O'Farrelly *et al.*

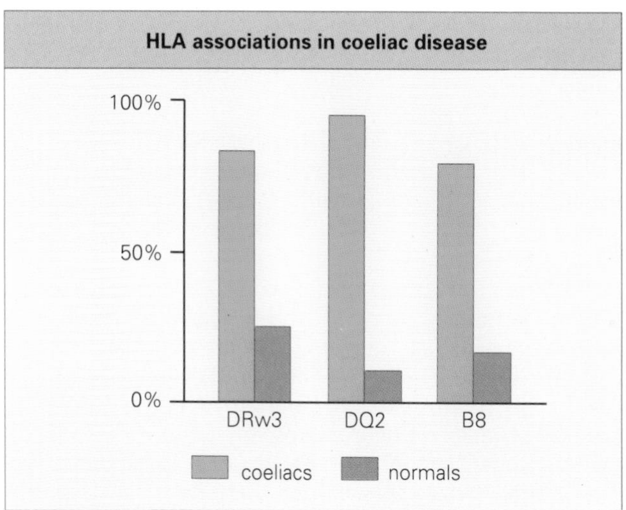

Fig. 10.11 Immunological markers of coeliac disease, showing HLA associations.

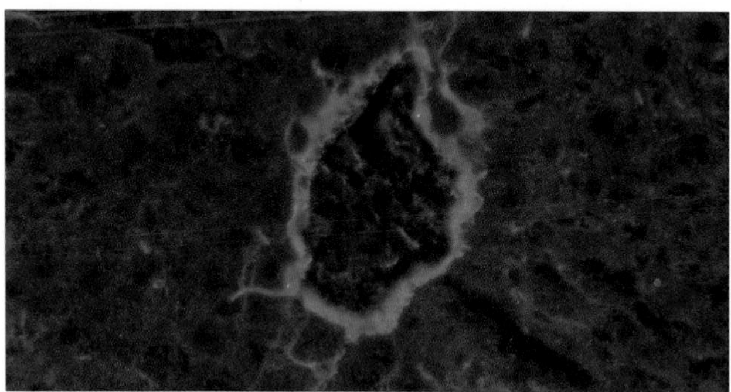

Fig. 10.12 The reticulin antibody (RI pattern). Serum from a patient with untreated coeliac disease has been layered onto a section of liver and stained with a fluorescein-conjugated antibody to human immunoglobulin. x250.

Immunological markers of coeliac disease

Coeliac disease is strongly asociated with HLA-DRw3 and -DQ2 and secondarily associated with HLA-B8 (Fig. 10.11) in Northern Europeans. There is a familial incidence, but discordance in identical twins has been reported.

Serum immunoglobulin concentrations may be normal, but a low IgM and a raised IgA are commonly seen in untreated patients; these return to normal following treatment with a gluten-free diet. Isolated IgA deficiency occurs in about 2% of patients with coeliac disease. This is not corrected by treatment, but there is otherwise no difference between these patients and those without IgA deficiency.

Serum IgG and IgA antibody to reticulin may be useful in the diagnosis (Fig. 10.12). IgG has been reported in 90% of untreated children and in 36% of adults, whereas IgA antibody is found in approximately 80% of coeliacs and in only 13% of controls. About 20% of patients with Crohn's disease and other gastrointestinal disorders may also have this antibody. The titre falls following treatment with a gluten-free diet in both children and adults. The significance of the reticulin antibody is unclear, but there may be antigenic cross-reactivity between gluten and reticulin.

Immune response following gluten challenge
Once dietary treatment has commenced, the mucosa returns almost to normal within a few months. If patients are then challenged with gluten, mucosal damage occurs. Within a few hours of such a challenge, alterations in electron microscopic appearances occur — mainly damage to the microvillous brush border. In addition, the activity of brush border enzymes falls and there is an increase in the number of intra-epithelial lymphocytes present in relation to the number of epithelial cells. Marked changes on light microscopy can be seen during the subsequent few days in the majority of patients. Fig. 10.13 summarizes the various immune responses that have been reported following such a challenge. There is a rapid but transient fall in CH_{50} (complement activity as expressed by 50% haemolysis), and a gradual rise in antibody titres to reticulin and fraction III (a peptic-tryptic digest) of gluten.

Coeliac disease and dermatitis herpetiformis
More than 95% of patients with dermatitis herpetiformis have an abnormal jejunal mucosa. The lesion is patchy and responds to a gluten-free diet. These patients have a high frequency of HLA-DRw3 and HLA-B8 haplotypes; the remaining 5% do not show these HLA associations. The immunological phenomena found in patients with coeliac disease also occur in dermatitis herpetiformis associated with a coeliac mucosal lesion. Hence, antibodies to gluten and reticulin, circulating complexes, and cellular hypersensitivity to gluten fractions have been described in such patients. The skin lesions and deposits of IgA and C3 within the skin are described in chapter 14.

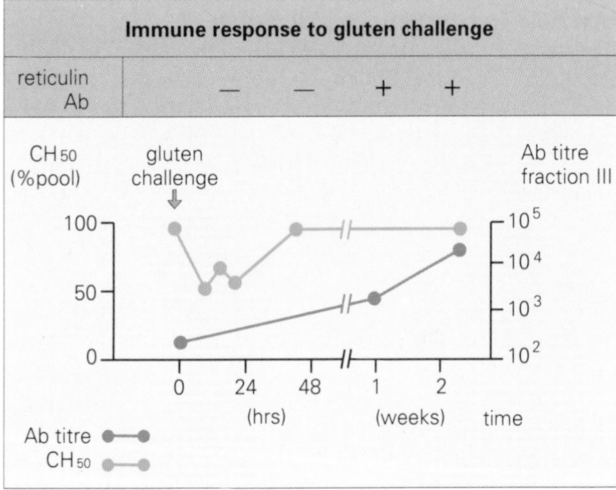

Fig. 10.13 A patient who had been in remission on a gluten-free diet was challenged with gluten, causing a rapid but transient fall in CH_{50}, followed by a more gradual increase in titre of gluten and reticulin antibodies.

OTHER FOOD-SENSITIVE SMALL INTESTINAL ENTEROPATHIES

In children a number of other foods, such as cows' milk and soya, have been found to cause alterations in the small intestinal mucosa that are similar to those of coeliac disease. These changes are often transient and improve more quickly than coeliac disease when the food is avoided. The mechanism of damage is not known.

ULCERATIVE COLITIS AND CROHN'S DISEASE

Ulcerative colitis is a disease of the colon, beginning in the rectum and extending proximally to a variable extent. It frequently affects the entire colon but never causes significant involvement of the small intestine. Crohn's disease may affect any part of the gastrointestinal tract, although an ileocolitis is the most common distribution. Occasionally, Crohn's disease may be confined to the colon, and when the entire length is involved it may be difficult to distinguish between the two diseases.

Histologically, ulcerative colitis affects primarily the colonic mucosa, which becomes infiltrated with neutrophils, plasma cells and eosinophils. As the inflammation becomes more severe there is ulceration of the surface epithelium, loss of goblet cells, and formation of crypt abscesses (Fig. 10.14 left). In contrast, Crohn's disease causes a transmural inflammation involving lymphocytes, plasma cells and eosinophils (Fig. 10.14 right); the gland architecture and goblet cells are usually well preserved. The hallmark of Crohn's disease is granuloma formation, which is seen in about 70% of patients.

Immunopathology
The aetiology of both diseases is unknown. No clear evidence for an infective agent has been found although recently *Mycobacterium paratuberculosis* has been isolated from a few patients with Crohn's disease. There is a familial incidence of about 10% but no strong HLA association, except in patients who also have ankylosing spondylitis (who have a high incidence of HLA-B27).

Many humoral and immune phenomena have been described, and it seems likely that immunological effector mechanisms may be responsible for causing chronic disease. Serum concentrations of immunoglobulins are normal, as are lymphocyte counts, although some workers have reported reduced T cell counts in Crohn's disease. However, T cell numbers and the ratio of helper to suppressor cells remain within the normal range in both diseases. In terms of function, there may be reduced suppressor cell activity during active disease, but this returns to normal once the disease goes into remission.

Immune complexes and complement metabolism. Immune complexes have been demonstrated in the sera of patients with ulcerative colitis and Crohn's disease using a wide variety of techniques. They are small (less than 19S) and contain IgG. However, until a specific antigen can be

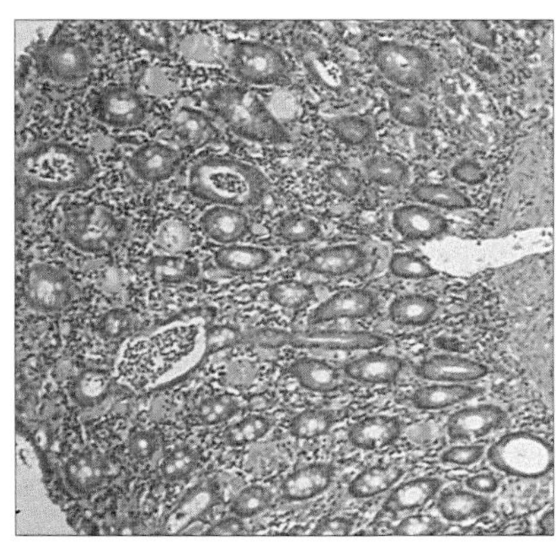

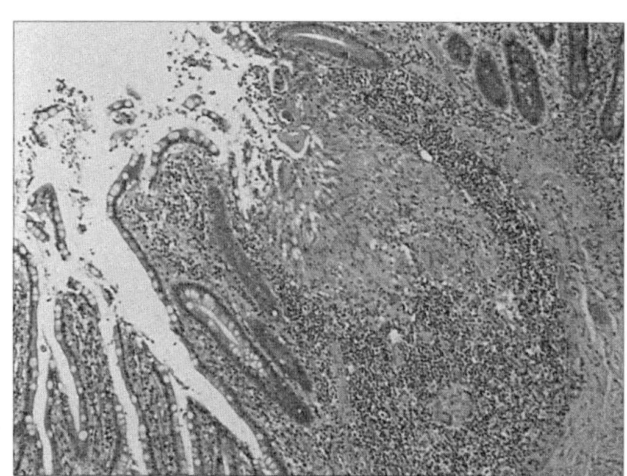

Fig. 10.14 Inflammatory bowel disease. Left: histological appearance of ulcerative colitis, showing a dense inflammatory cell infiltrate, crypt abscess formation and loss of goblet cells. Right: Crohn's disease, showing a dense lymphocytic infiltrate, focal ulceration and granuloma formation.

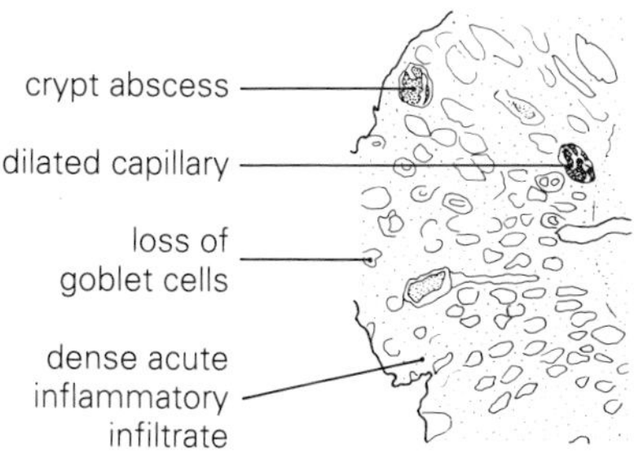

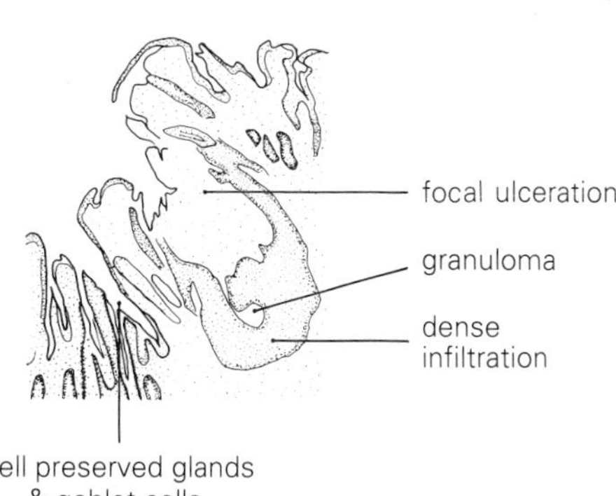

identified, it is not possible to determine whether they are true antigen-antibody complexes or whether they represent aggregated IgG. They are found most frequently in patients with active disease and in those with associated acute arthropathy, uveitis or erythema nodosum. In patients with Crohn's disease, circulating complexes are associated with colonic disease and are less commonly found in patients with ileal disease. Serum concentrations of C3, Factor B, C1 inhibitor and C3b inactivator tend to be high in active disease, and fall towards normal when the patient goes into remission. Concentrations of C1q, C4 and Factor H are normal. Increased catabolism of complement can nevertheless be shown for C1q and C3 by the use of metabolic turnover studies. Further evidence for continuing complement activation is shown by a positive correlation between the length of history and the titre of immunoconglutinins (antibodies to activated C3).

Immunological reactions to bacteria. Patients with Crohn's disease and ulcerative colitis have higher antibody titres to bacterial antigens (*E. coli* and *Bacteroides*) than normal subjects. This antibody, part of which is formed locally within the inflamed mucosa, cross-reacts with a lipopolysaccharide contained in the colonic goblet cells. The colonic autoantibodies found in these diseases (15–20%) probably arise as a result of an immune response to the bacterial flora. Cell-mediated hypersensitivity to *E. coli* antigens has been shown using the techniques of lymphocyte transformation and leucocyte migration inhibition, although not all workers have been able to confirm this.

Lymphocyte cytotoxicity. Peripheral blood lymphocytes from all patients with ulcerative colitis and Crohn's disease are able to kill colonic epithelial cells *in vitro*. This is not seen in healthy subjects and is rarely found in patients with other intestinal diseases. The reaction is independent of complement and is mediated by a cell bearing an Fc receptor but without T or B cell markers. It is specific for colonic epithelial cells and is lost only when the colon is resected. Cytotoxicity can be inhibited by prior incubation of the patients' lymphocytes with either lipopolysaccharide extracts of *E. coli* or the sera of other patients with inflammatory bowel disease. The situation is further complicated by the finding that normal lymphocytes will become cytotoxic to colonic epithelium when incubated with either *E. coli* extracts or with sera from patients with inflammatory bowel disease (Fig. 10.15). Recently, lymphocytes isolated from the colonic mucosa of patients with ulcerative colitis or Crohn's disease have also been shown to be cytotoxic to colonic epithelial cells. The precise immunological mechanisms involved in the cytotoxic reaction and the significance of these *in vitro* findings to the pathogenesis of mucosal inflammation are unknown.

Mucosal immune responses

The normal colonic epithelium does not express HLA-DR molecules but these antigens are strongly expressed when inflammation occurs (Fig. 10.16). This is not specific for inflammatory bowel disease but also occurs in infectious colitis, in graft-versus-host disease, and in the colonic mucosa adjacent to carcinomas. There is some evidence that colonic epithelial cells expressing these molecules may be able to present antigen to T cells. Hence, it is possible that this is one mechanism involved in the pathogenesis of chronic inflammation.

Evidence for an alteration in immunoregulatory control within the mucosal immune system is not convincing. Studies using cells isolated from colonic mucosa to measure T suppressor activity or helper activity for immunoglobulin synthesis have produced highly variable results. Mucosal lymphocytes from patients with either ulcerative colitis or Crohn's disease appear to release interleukin-2 (IL-2) less readily than mucosal cells from healthy individuals, and their ability to express surface receptors to IL-2 may be diminished. Whether these minor *in vitro* changes in immunoregulatory molecules are also significant *in vivo* is unclear.

Recent attention has focused on the mucosal macrophages which are a highly heterogeneous population with respect to phenotype. In inflammatory bowel disease there is an increase in dendritic or 'veiled' cells, which are antigen-presenting cells, and there is also a selective increase in macrophages bearing Fcγ receptors ($3G8^+$) and epithelioid cells ($RFD9^+$). This pattern is unique to ulcerative colitis and Crohn's disease. The functional significance of these observations is unknown.

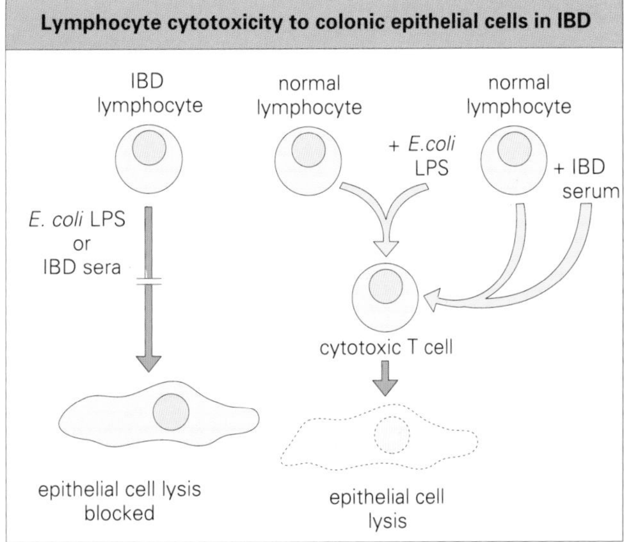

Fig. 10.15 Lymphocytes from patients with inflammatory bowel disease (IBD) can kill colonic epithelial cells. This is blocked by addition of *E. coli* lipopolysaccharides (LPS) or sera from patients with IBD. Normal lymphocytes also become cytotoxic to epithelial cells when incubated with either *E. coli* or IBD sera.

LIVER DISORDERS

The normal liver contains a few lymphocytes and plasma cells which are mainly distributed in the portal tracts within the liver sinusoids. There are also macrophage-like cells called Kupffer cells which are phagocytic and line the walls of the sinusoids.

In many forms of liver disease there is a marked increase in inflammatory cells, especially lymphocytes and immunoglobulin-producing cells. In primary biliary cirrhosis there is histiocytic infiltration with granuloma formation. Most forms of liver disease show increased serum immunoglobulin concentrations which may result from *de novo* synthesis within the liver, or from defective clearance of antigens by Kupffer cells. As with the gastrointestinal diseases, however, it is still unclear to what extent immunological events contribute to the pathogenesis of disease.

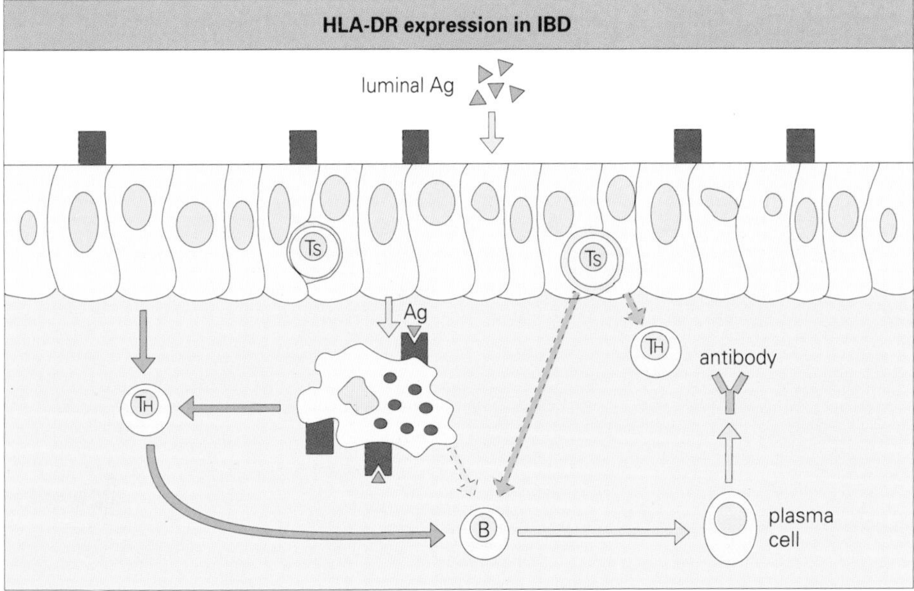

Fig. 10.16 Antigen presentation to TH cells in an inflamed mucosa may occur via epithelial cells or cells of the mononuclear phagocyte system (MPS). Continuing TH stimulation may lead to continuous B cell stimulation. Modulation of this by suppressor cells may be impaired.

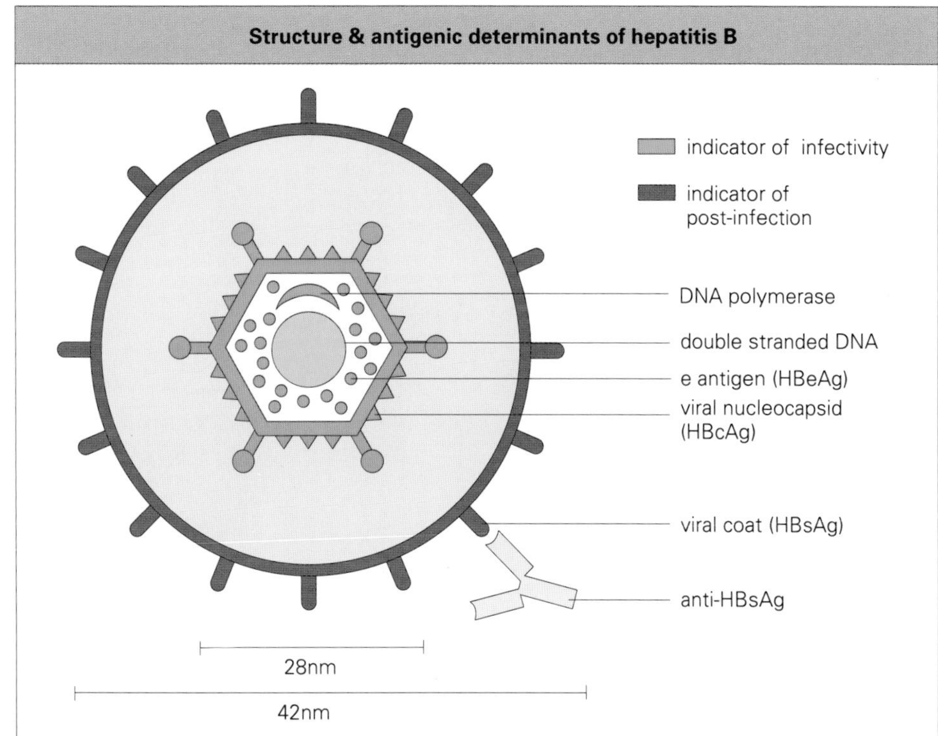

Fig. 10.17 Structure and antigenic determinants of the hepatitis B virus. The serological indicators of infectivity are shown.

HEPATITIS B

Hepatitis B virus (HBV)

The hepatitis B virion is seen on electron microscopy as the 'Dane particle', which has a diameter of 42nm. It consists of a central core, 28nm in diameter, containing subscripted DNA polymerase, the e antigen (HBeAg) and the core antigen (HBcAg) (Fig. 10.17). The surface coat contains the surface antigen (HBsAg) which was originally described as the 'Australia' antigen. The presence of Dane particles in serum, as seen by electron microscopy, is probably the best indicator of infectivity. Other markers of infectivity which are more readily measured are HBeAg, DNA polymerase and HBV DNA. Sera containing HBsAg alone have low infectivity. The presence of antibody to HBsAg and to HBcAg in serum indicates previous infection and, generally, immunity to HBV.

Hepatitis B is usually transmitted parenterally by blood or its products, by medical procedures, or by contaminated needles used by intravenous drug users or tattoo artists. Sexual transmission can also occur in both heterosexual and homosexual relationships. Oral transmission has been demonstrated and HBsAg has been found in saliva, semen and urine, but the infectivity of these has not been established. Once the virus has attached to the liver cell, viral DNA passes into the host cell nucleus and determines the production of core and surface components. Transcription by DNA polymerase will produce more viral DNA and, hence, more infective virions. During this phase of viral replication, surface, core and e antigens can be found in the blood (Fig. 10.18).

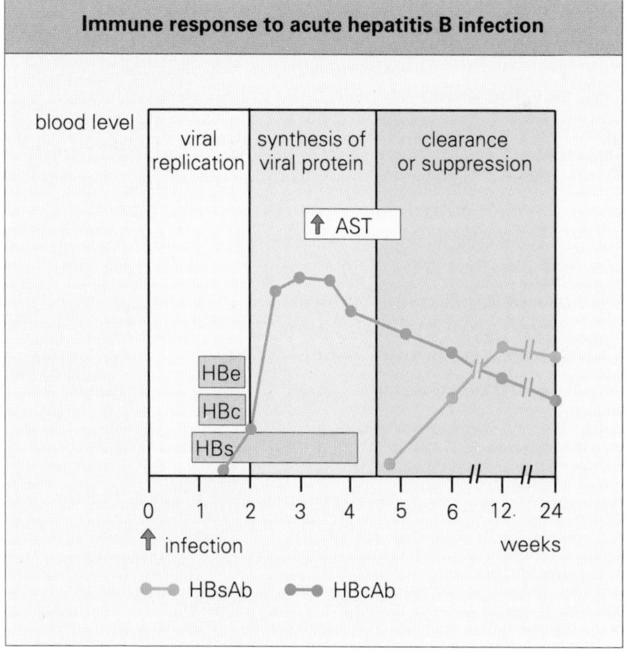

Fig. 10.18 For unknown reasons HBsAg is produced in excess of HBcAg and HBeAg, and may persist for several months. HBcAg and HbeAg are usually cleared in the prodromal period before there is a significant rise in aspartate transaminase (AST). Antibody to HBcAg is usually demonstrable soon after clinical hepatitis is recognized, but the antibody reponse to the surface antigen is delayed for several months, appearing after the surface antigen has been cleared.

Syndromes following acute hepatitis B

During the prodromal phase patients frequently complain of arthralgias and fever, and a vasculitis may occur. Circulating immune complexes have been demonstrated during this period, although there is little evidence that HBsAg is involved. The majority of patients with an acute attack of hepatitis B recover completely. Dane particles are cleared from the circulation very rapidly and long before HBsAg disappears, suggesting a specific immune response to the whole virus. Both humoral and cellular immune mechanisms are probably responsible for clearing the virus.

Less than 10% of patients with acute hepatitis B progress to chronic liver disease. Most of these will develop a chronic active hepatitis but a few will progress to a chronic persistent hepatitis. Some carriers of HBsAg with either normal liver histology or chronic persistent hepatitis may develop polyarteritis or a glomerulonephritis (Fig. 10.19). HBsAg-containing immune complexes may occur in the sera of patients with these two syndromes.

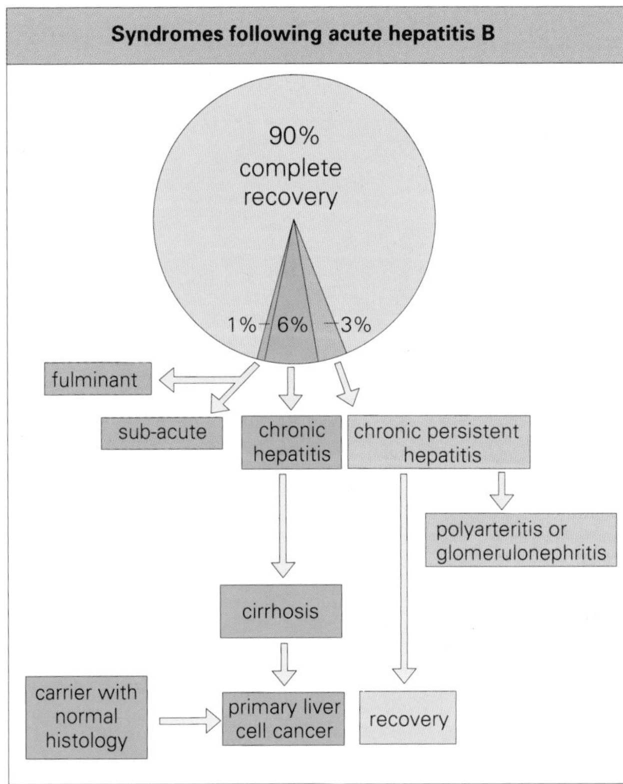

Fig. 10.19 Syndromes following acute hepatitis B.

Immunological mechanisms. A variety of immunological mechanisms have been proposed for the pathogenesis of chronic liver disease secondary to HBV. Inappropriately low serum concentrations and a reduced capacity to synthesize type 1 interferons (α, β interferons) have been shown in patients with HBsAg-positive chronic active hepatitis. This could lead to reduced expression of HLA class I molecules on the hepatocyte surface. Since the display of class I molecules on the surface of a virus-infected cell is essential for the recognition and lytic activity of a cytotoxic T cell, the failure to switch on class I expression (absent on normal hepatocytes) might lead to persistent infection. A reduced expression of HLA class I on liver cells has indeed been shown in chronic, but not acute, hepatitis B (Fig. 10.20) and treatment with IFNα has not only increased expression but has been associated with clearance of infected cells. The cytotoxic T cells appear to recognize nucleocapsid components of the virus (HBc, HBe) on the surface of the liver cell but the degree of cell lysis is probably modulated by serum antibody to these antigens since cytotoxicity *in vitro* can be blocked by antibody.

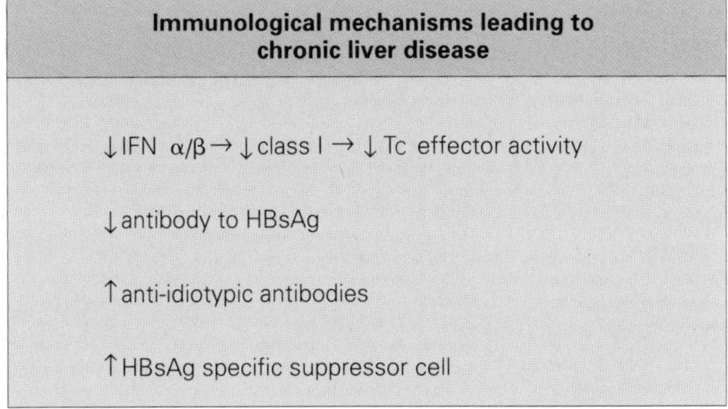

Fig. 10.20 Mechanisms causing chronic liver disease.

Failure to clear virus. The failure to mount an effective antibody response to HBsAg may also be a factor in the defective clearance of this antigen. A selective B cell defect in synthesizing anti-HBs, the presence of anti-idiotypic antibodies, and the existence of an HBsAg-specific suppressor T cell have all been described. A quite different mechanism favouring persistent infection is the existence of a receptor shared by the liver cell membrane and the HB virion (coded for by the pre-S region of the genome). This receptor reacts with polymeric serum albumin and it is possible that HBV bound to polymeric albumin is then able to bind to the receptor on the hepatocyte and gain entry into the cell (Fig. 10.21). Antibodies to the polymeric albumin could modulate this route of access. These antibodies are present in association with acute hepatitis B and appear to play a role in clearance of the virus. However, they are absent in patients with chronic hepatitis B and so continued infection may proceed unimpaired.

CHRONIC ACTIVE HEPATITIS

There are several causes of chronic active hepatitis:

- autoimmune hepatitis
- chronic hepatitis associated with HBsAg
- drugs
- α1-antitrypsin deficiency
- Wilson's disease.

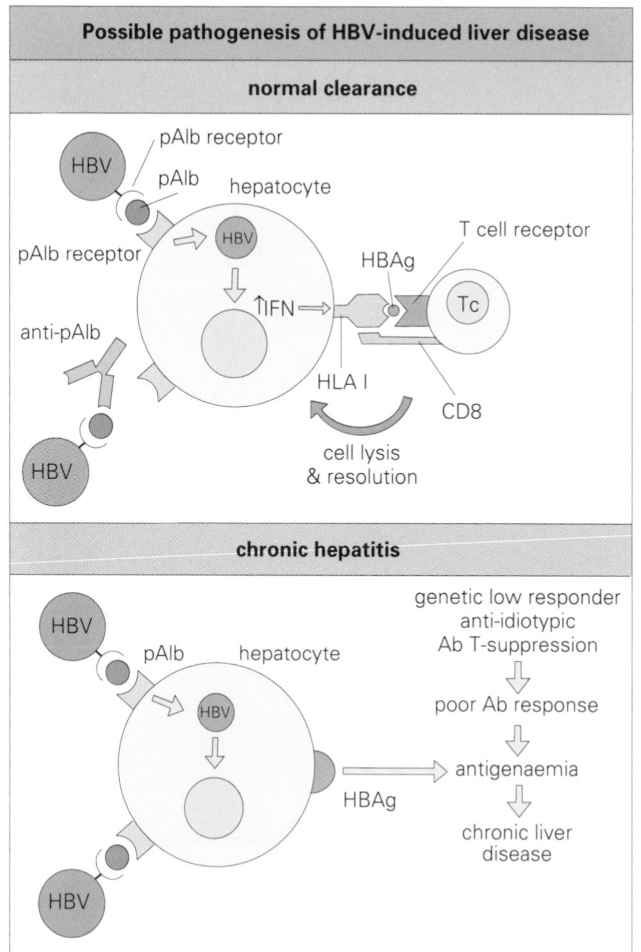

Fig. 10.21 Entry to the cell may be gained via a receptor shared by the virion and hepatocyte. The HBV receptor binds to polymeric serum albumin (pAlb) which can then bind to the hepatocyte receptor. Anti-pAlb would block this route of infection. If infection occurs, IFN-induced MHC class I may permit recognition of the infected cell by cytotoxic T cells. If however there is no recognition by cytotoxic cells, chronic antigenaemia results with reduced immunological functions

This section is concerned with autoimmune hepatitis, which occurs mainly in young women and is often associated with fever, arthralgias and skin rashes. There is a strong association with other autoimmune disorders and with the HLA-B8, DR3 haplotype. The majority of patients have circulating antibody titres to smooth muscle (mainly antibodies to actin) as well as other organ and non-organ specific autoantibodies (Fig. 10.22). Serum protein estimation shows a considerable rise in gammaglobulin. Histologically, there is a marked infiltration of the portal tracts with lymphocytes and plasma cells. The lymphocytes can be seen penetrating the liver parenchyma with liver cell death ('piecemeal necrosis') (Fig. 10.23). The inflammation and necrosis subsequently lead to fibrosis and cirrhosis.

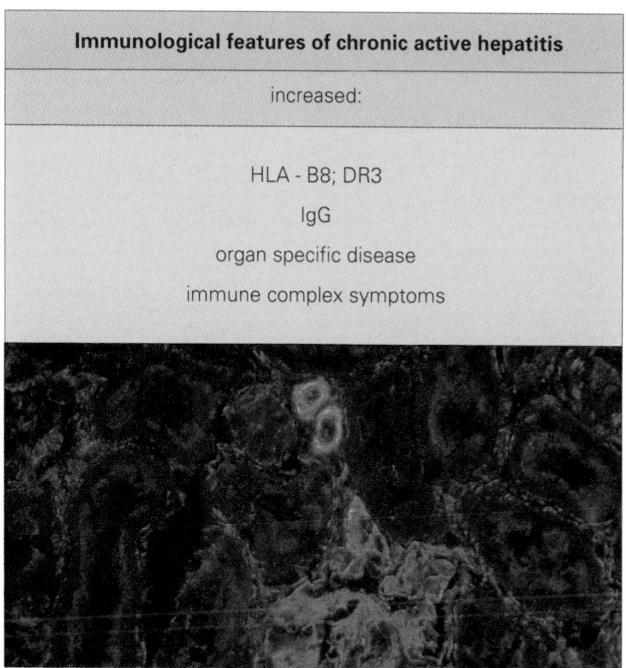

Immunological features of chronic active hepatitis
increased:
HLA - B8; DR3
IgG
organ specific disease
immune complex symptoms

Fig. 10.22 Immunological features of chronic active hepatitis include the appearance of smooth muscle antibodies seen here deposited in the arterial walls. x250.

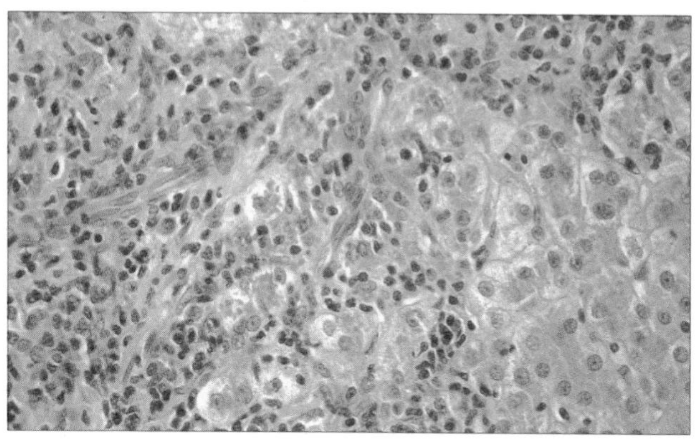

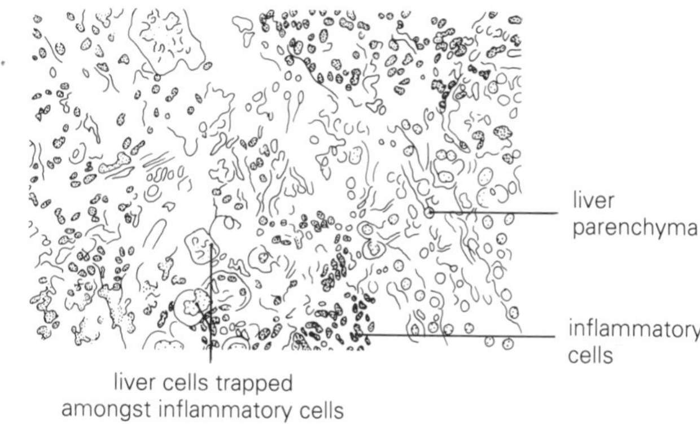

Fig. 10.23 Histological appearance of chronic active hepatitis, showing invasion of the liver parenchyma by inflammatory cells.

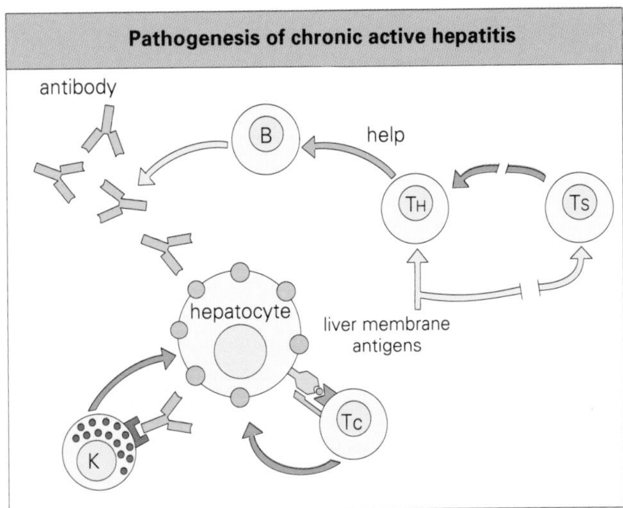

Fig. 10.24 Pathogenetic mechanisms in chronic active hepatitis. Hepatocytes may be killed by cytotoxic T cells specific for AGR, or K cells directed by antibody. Liver membrane antigens stimulate TH cells and may be involved in the reduction of TS activity.

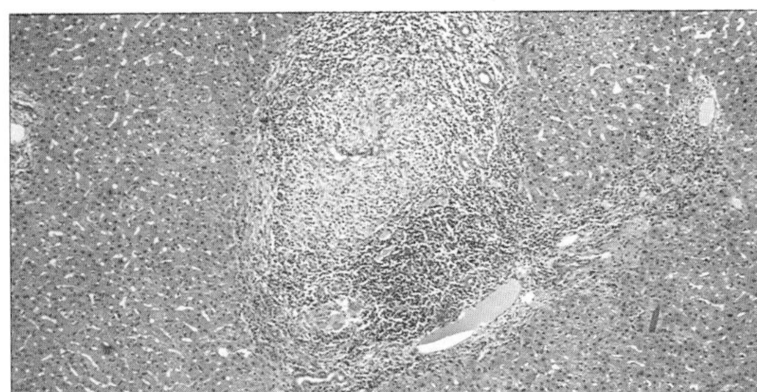

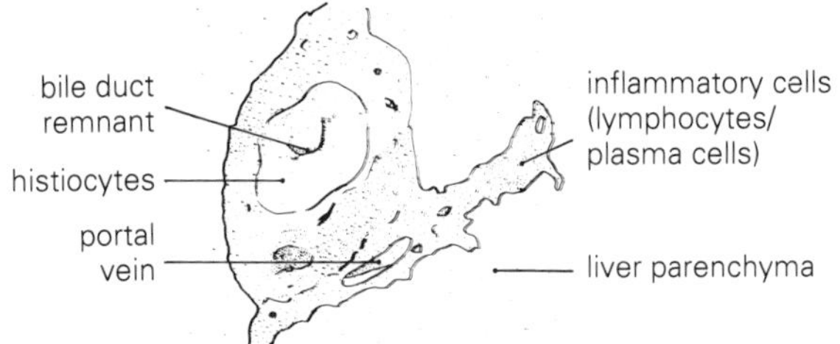

Fig. 10.25 Histological appearance of primary biliary cirrhosis, showing bile duct destruction and granuloma formation.

Pathogenetic mechanisms. The immunopathogenesis of autoimmune chronic hepatitis is complex but antibody, K cell cytotoxicity, and T cell responses to liver membrane antigens have been described. In addition, there may be an underlying disturbance in immunoregulatory control. Evidence for a lack of T suppressor activity has also been found, which may possibly explain the heightened immunological activity seen in these patients.

Liver-specific membrane lipoprotein. Initially, antibodies and specific T suppressor activity were described to a preparation of liver cell membrane known as liver-specific membrane lipoprotein (LSP). This is now known to contain many antigens, one of which is a receptor for asialoglycoprotein (AGR). T cell sensitization to this antigen is characteristic of all patients with chronic active hepatitis and is associated with a specific suppressor T cell defect for LSP. Thus it is proposed that if a T helper response to AGR or other liver membrane antigens is initiated in susceptible individuals, it will be perpetuated by the lack of antigen-specific suppression. This immunological activity might be amplified by a generalized defect in suppressor activity, as shown by impaired Con-A induced suppression, and contributed to by other mechanisms of immunological injury, such as K cell killing of liver cells to which antibodies against membrane components are bound (Fig. 10.24).

Genetic component. There is evidence for a familial predisposition to chronic active hepatitis. For example a proportion of first-degree relatives show T cell hypersensitivity to LSP (although not to AGR) as well as the antigen-specific suppressor cell defect. Spouses also commonly show T cell reactivity to LSP but rarely show the impairment of suppressor activity. Thus the genetic component may be a defect in LSP suppressor activity (now known to be mediated by a $CD4^+$ cell, hence reflecting an impaired suppressor-inducer sub-population). The environmental trigger may cause a TH response to liver membrane antigens which, in those with the genetically determined suppressor defect, may progress to a chronic inflammatory response.

PRIMARY BILIARY CIRRHOSIS

Primary biliary cirrhosis is a disease affecting primarily middle-aged women; men constitute less than 5% of all affected patients. The condition may be asymptomatic for many years, and is diagnosed increasingly by the finding of raised alkaline phosphatase on routine biochemical screening. It usually presents with pruritus and other features of cholestasis, but jaundice is usually a late feature. Histologically, there is a progressive destruction of bile ducts by lymphocytes and histiocytes, which frequently form granulomata (Fig. 10.25). The disease progresses slowly to a frank cirrhosis, although parenchymal function is usually well preserved until the later stages of the disease.

Anti-mitochondrial antibodies

The immunological diagnosis depends on the presence of the anti-mitochondrial antibody in the serum (Fig. 10.26) and an elevated serum concentration of IgM. The anti-mitochondrial antibody may be IgA or IgM, and the titre may increase as the disease progresses.

Mitochondrial antibody can be found in the sera of more than 95% of patients with primary biliary cirrhosis and is usually detected by immunofluorescence using rat kidney. The antigen (M2, now known to be a component

Immunological features of primary biliary cirrhosis	
increased	**decreased**
IgM (7s)	non-specific cellular responses
C1q, C3 metabolism	skin test reactions
immune complexes	lymphocyte function

Fig. 10.26 Immunological features of primary biliary cirrhosis include the presence of anti-mitochondrial antibodies in the serum, as shown here by immunofluorescence. x250.

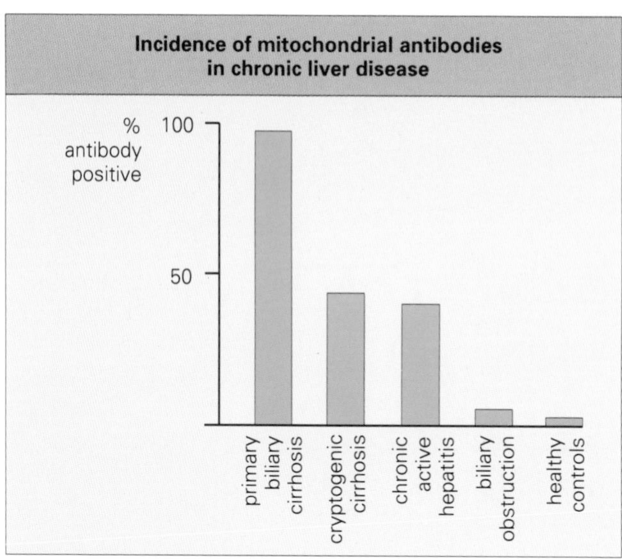

Fig. 10.27 Incidence of anti-mitochondrial antibodies in chronic liver disease.

of the pyruvate dehydrogenase complex) to which the antibody is directed is located in the inner membrane of mitochondria. These antibodies (anti-M2) are specific for primary biliary cirrhosis. The anti-mitochondrial antibodies which are often present in low titre in other diseases (Fig. 10.27), as detected by immunofluorescence, are directed towards mitochondrial antigens other than M2, with which they do not react. Hence, the most specific diagnostic test is an ELISA assay using purified M2 antigen, but this is not yet widely available, although the appropriate gene has been cloned.

Other autoantibodies. Patients with primary biliary cirrhosis also have a wide variety of circulating autoantibodies, including those directed against nuclear, cytoskeletal, bile canalicular, and liver membrane antigens, but they are not disease specific. In addition, antibodies to other mitochondrial antigens may be present but these are also not disease specific. However, the exact profile of anti-mitochondrial antibodies present in a patient with primary biliary cirrhosis, including anti-M2, has been shown to have prognostic significance with respect to progression of the disease to cirrhosis and mortality.

Circulating immune complexes have been described and mitochondrial and cytoplasmic antigens have been isolated from them by some, but not all, investigators. Metabolic studies have shown increased synthesis and catabolism of C1q and C3, suggesting complement activation by antigen-antibody complexes.

No direct pathogenetic role for anti-mitochondrial antibodies has been determined, but anti-M2 positive sera may cross-react with epitopes on micro-organisms, for example *E. coli*. This may merely reflect the known similarities between mitochondrial and bacterial membranes but could also have pathogenetic significance.

Lymphocytes

Patients with primary biliary cirrhosis have depressed T cell function, as shown by impaired delayed hypersensitivity skin tests and reduced lymphocyte proliferative responses to PPD and non-specific mitogens. Tests of non-specific suppressor T cell function have shown some impairment in patients and their relatives but helper T cell function is normal. The raised IgM concentrations in serum may be due to a specific defect in the suppression of IgM synthesis.

Within the liver, the lymphocytes in the portal tracts are predominantly T cells. $CD8^+$ cells are mainly associated with the liver cell plates, areas of piecemeal necrosis and injured bile ducts, whereas $CD4^+$ cells are found mainly in the centre of the portal tracts. B cells and plasma cells (containing IgA, IgG, and IgM) are present, but in lesser numbers than T cells. IgM plasma cells are particularly frequent in the inflammatory infiltrate around damaged bile ducts.

Bile duct epithelium and HLA

Normal bile duct epithelium does not express class II antigens but strong expression is seen on the epithelial cells of damaged ducts and of normal ducts within the same portal tract as the injured ones. The expression of class I is also increased. Thus, biliary epithelial cells may act as antigen-presenting cells and the increased class I expression may render the cells vulnerable to cytotoxic T cells. However, these changes in HLA expression are almost certainly secondary phenomena since class II molecules are not expressed on bile duct epithelium in portal tracts which are not inflamed, yet they are seen in other forms of biliary disease (for example, primary sclerosing cholangitis, extrahepatic obstruction) as well as in autoimmune and viral hepatitis.

FURTHER READING

Brandtzaeg P, Halstensen TS, Kett K, Krajci P, Kvale D, Rognum TO, Scott H, Sollid LM. Immunobiology and immunopathology of human gut mucosa: humoral immunity and intra-epithelial lymphocytes. *Gastroenterology* 1989; **97**:1562–1584.

Carman WF, Thomas HC. Hepatitis viruses. In: Ciclitira PJ, ed. *Clinical gastroenterology. Molecular biology and its impact on gastroenterology.* London: Baillière Tindall, 1990:201–232.

Ciclitira PJ, Hall MA. Coeliac disease. In: Ciclitira PJ, ed. *Clinical gastroenterology. Molecular biology and its impact on gastroenterology* . London: Baillière Tindall, 1990:43–59.

Jewell DP, ed. Gastrointestinal Immunology In: Miescher PA, Spiegelberg HL. *Springer Seminars in Immunopathology 12.* Springer International, 1990.

Rawcliffe PM, Priddle JD. Pathogenesis of coleliac disease. In: Jewell DP, Ireland A, eds. *Topics in gastroenterology 14.* Oxford: Blackwell Scientific Publications, 1986:23–34.

Wright R and Hodgson HJF, eds. *Clinical Gastroenterology. Gastrointestinal and liver immunology.* London: Baillière Tindall, 1987.

11

Cardiovascular Disorders

INTRODUCTION

Traditionally, immunological mechanisms have been thought to be less implicated in diseases of the heart and blood vessels than in many other organ systems, but this is probably untrue. Rheumatic fever and possibly post-cardiotomy syndrome are hypersensitivity disorders, with type II reactions predominating. Type III mechanisms are certainly relevant in bacterial endocarditis and in the vasculitides, and may also be of importance in atherosclerosis. Endomyocardial fibrosis is linked with activated eosinophils and damage from their mediators is a probable aetiological mechanism. The knowledge of transplantation antigens, immune rejection and its suppression have contributed to the success of cardiac transplantation.

RHEUMATIC HEART DISEASE

Clinical and pathological features

The symptoms and signs of acute rheumatic fever (RF) are encompassed by the modified Jones' criteria (Fig. 11.1). Carditis may affect the valves, usually causing mitral incompetence; aortic incompetence and a mid-diastolic (Carey-Coombs) murmur may also be heard. Myocarditis may be sub-clinical, or may lead to chamber dilatation and congestive cardiac failure. Pericarditis can occur with a characteristic rub and ECG changes, and sometimes an effusion.

Modified Jones' criteria	
Major criteria	**Minor criteria**
carditis polyarthritis chorea subcutaneous nodules erythema marginatum	fever arthralgia ↑ ESR or positive CRP prolonged PR interval past history of RF or RHD

Fig. 11.1 Two major or one major and two minor criteria indicate a diagnosis of RF if supported by evidence of preceding streptococcal infection.

Carditis. In this condition, all layers and structures of the heart are usually involved to a variable degree. Macroscopically, the pericardium appears thickened and covered with fibrinous exudate and there may be some pericardial fluid. Fibrosis and adhesions develop with healing and the pericardial space is totally or partially obliterated. The heart may appear dilated as a result of myocarditis. Microsopically, characteristic rheumatic granulomata, or Aschoff bodies (Fig. 11.2), are seen with a diffuse cellular infiltrate. Myofibres are damaged and may even be completely lost. In endocarditis verrucae of granular and acidophilic material develop on valves or chordae; as the condition progresses, the verrucae change to granulation tissue with vascularization and fibrosis affecting the valve cusps (Fig. 11.3), annulus and chordae. Arteritis also occurs but thrombosis of the large coronary vessels is very rare in this condition.

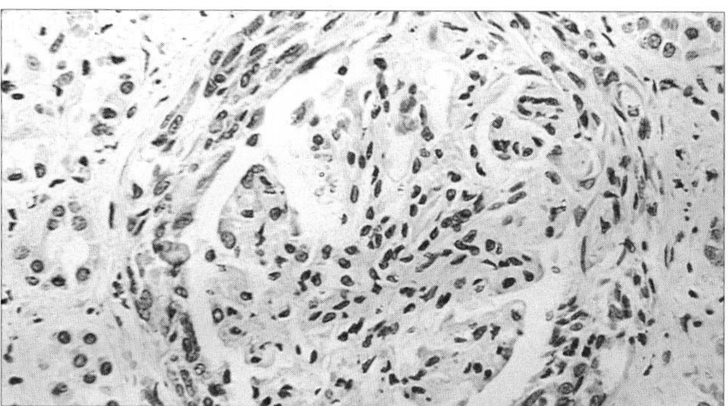

Fig. 11.2 Histological section of myocardium demonstrating a characteristic rheumatic granuloma — an Aschoff body — containing multinucleate giant cells. H & E stain.

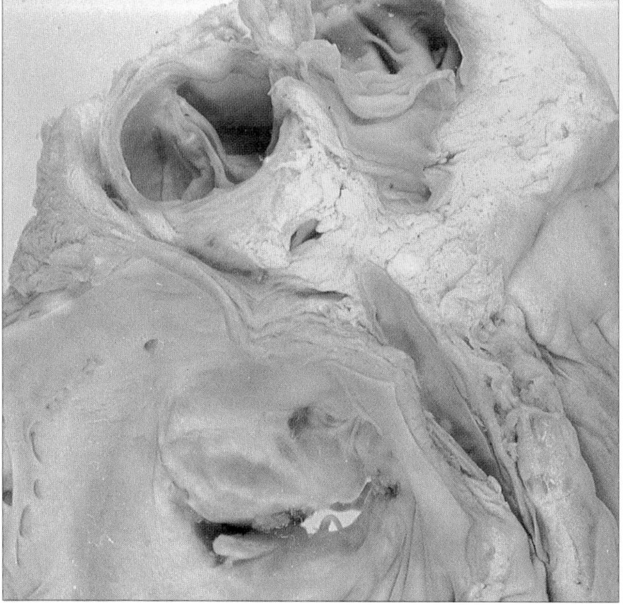

Fig. 11.3 Chronic rheumatic mitral valve disease. Looking from the left atrium into the mitral valve, the edges appear rolled, thickened and contracted.

Aetiology

The association between the streptococcus and acute rheumatic fever is well established. Usually acute rheumatic fever will follow two to three weeks after a streptococcal pharyngitis; however, not all streptococcal throat infections lead to rheumatic fever and not all cases of rheumatic fever have a history of a sore throat. Streptococcal antibodies are always detectable in acute rheumatic fever and it is accepted that the streptococcal infection is in some way responsible for its development.

Cross-reactivity between streptococcal antigens and human tissues

Streptococcal antigen	Human tissue antigen
M protein	sarcolemma & smooth muscle of vessels, probably against myosin heavy chain determinants
group A carbohydrate	heart valve glycoprotein
group A membranes	caudate nucleus of thalamus & sub-thalamic region of brain
group A (nephritogenic strains only) cell wall glycoprotein	glomerular basement membrane
hyaluronidase	synovium

Fig. 11.4 Certain anti-streptococcal antibodies will cross-react with human tissues, including the heart.

Anti-streptolysin O (ASO) titres are usually higher in patients with rheumatic fever than in those with uncomplicated streptococcal pharyngitis and there are certain anti-streptococcal antibodies which cross-react with extracts of human heart (Fig. 11.4). It is possible that such antibodies cause carditis by a type II hypersensitivity reaction. This theory is supported by the following findings:

- anti-heart antibody titres are higher in rheumatic fever than in simple streptococcal infections and decline slowly over a period of 2–3 years;
- anti-heart antibody titres are present before a recurrence of carditis in patients studied longitudinally (Fig. 11.5), in other words, these antibodies do not disappear between attacks of rheumatic carditis;
- bound imunoglobulin and complement have been demonstrated in rheumatic hearts at the sites of histological damage.

Passive transfer of anti-heart antibodies to animals has no effect on the heart, but it is possible that prior damage by streptococcal toxins is also necessary, or that the titre of antibody achieved was insufficient to cause damage. The rarity of rheumatic fever in children under four years of age suggests that repeated streptococcal infections may be necessary before this condition will develop.

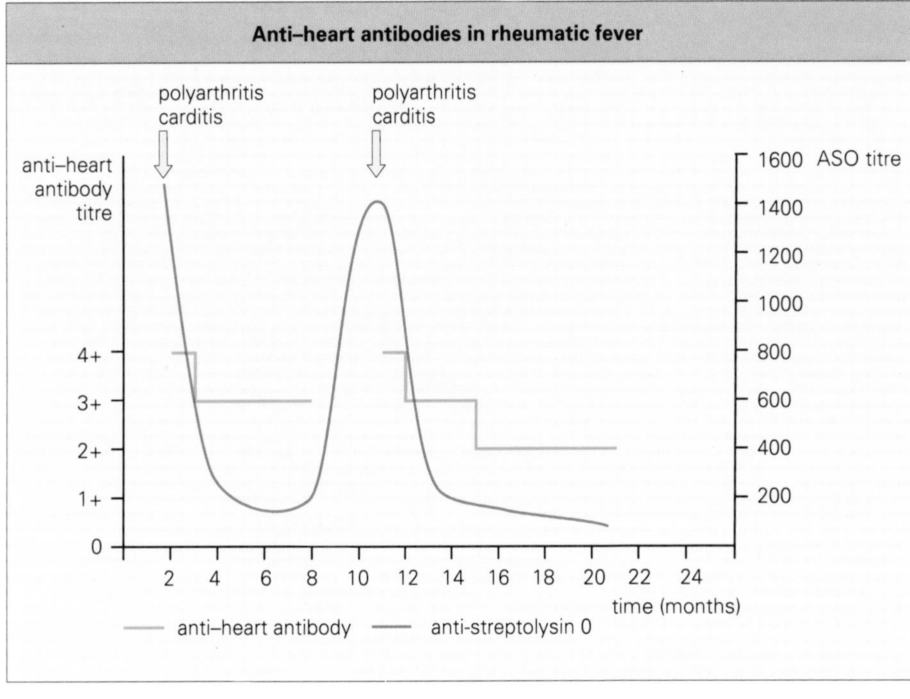

Fig. 11.5 This patient suffered recurrent attacks of rheumatic fever. The anti-heart antibodies persisted between attacks and were slow to decline. Modified from Zabriskie J B, Hsu K C & Segal BC (1970).

Exposure of new heart antigens. An alternative explanation is that streptococcal damage to the heart causes the exposure of new antigens, and hence antibody formation. Patients with valvular disease have higher titres of antibodies that bind the N-acetyl-glucosamine moiety of streptococcal group A carbohydrate than those without heart valve involvement, and these antibodies persist for years. Surgical replacement of affected valves often results in a fall of anti-group A carbohydrate levels to normal, suggesting that the slow and sustained release of valve cross-reactive glycoproteins perpetuates the valve damage long after the acute rheumatic phase has passed.

Immune complexes. Persistent high levels of circulating immune complexes have been noted in the sera of patients with the polyarthritis of rhematic fever. Antibodies to these complexes raised in rabbits react with extracellular products from group A streptococci; this pattern of reactivity is different from that seen with rabbit sera raised against immune complexes from patients with post-streptococcal glomerulonephritis. It is possible that the arthritis of RF is caused by a type III (serum sickness) reaction.

Cellular reactivity. Abnormalities of cellular reactivity also occur in rheumatic fever: marked hypersensitivity to group A streptococcal cell membranes persists for about five years. Patients with more severe cardiac damage show a greater response to streptococcal antigens and this correlates inversely with the C-reactive protein (CRP) level. However, the cellular response to a streptococcal extracellular antigen is reduced in rheumatic fever patients compared to normal subjects.

The role of the abnormalities of cellular immunity in rheumatic heart disease is not understood. Cytotoxic damage to cardiac fibres by mononuclear cells from patients with rheumatic fever has been reported but the significance of this is unknown. The foci of lymphocytic infiltration contain lymphocytes which are predominantly $CD4^+$ T cells; whether these secrete lymphokines or other factors which result in collagen synthesis and damage to heart valves is not known. There is evidence of persistent *in vitro* cell mediated activity to heart valve glycoproteins extracted by 8 molar urea, but not to acid extracts of heart muscle.

Sydenham's chorea (St Vitus' dance)

This neurological manifestation of chronic rheumatic fever consists of involuntary movements, muscular weakness and emotional disturbance. In all of five cases tested, a streptococcal antibody cross-reactive with the caudate nucleus was demonstrable.

Genetic predisposition

Rheumatic fever shows a tendency to run in families and an association with red hair has been noted. No major histocompatibility association has been found, but there is a B cell alloantigen (883) which is present in several ethnically distinct and genetically diverse populations of individuals who have had rheumatic fever. A monoclonal antibody to this antigen reacted with 100% of rheumatic fever patients from two different cities but only 4 of 40 controls (Fig. 11.6). This antigen was not detected on B cells from patients with post-streptococcal glomerulonephritis. An alternative theory suggests that the susceptibility to rheumatic fever is related to blood group secretor status genes.

Treatment

Any residual streptococci should be removed by antibiotics, usually penicillin. Bed-rest is essential where there is carditis. Aspirin relieves the symptoms in mild cases; more severe cases require oral corticosteroids but relapse may occur on withdrawal of treatment. Antibiotic cover should be given to previous sufferers before any procedure, such as dentistry, which is liable to cause bacteraemia.

Prevention of rheumatic fever by reducing the incidence of streptococcal throat infections has been achieved through socio-economic measures and the widespread use of antibiotics within communities, however, a recent resurgence of the disease in the United States has been noted. It is hoped that a vaccine might be produced which could confer streptococcal immunity without cardiac cross-reactivity.

BACTERIAL ENDOCARDITIS

Clinical and pathological features

Vegetations. Infection of the endocardium usually involves the valves of the heart, less often the endocardium of ventricles and atria, or the chordae tendinae and papillary muscles. The characteristic lesion is the vegetation, which consists initially of platelets and fibrin; this is followed by adherence and multiplication of organisms leading to

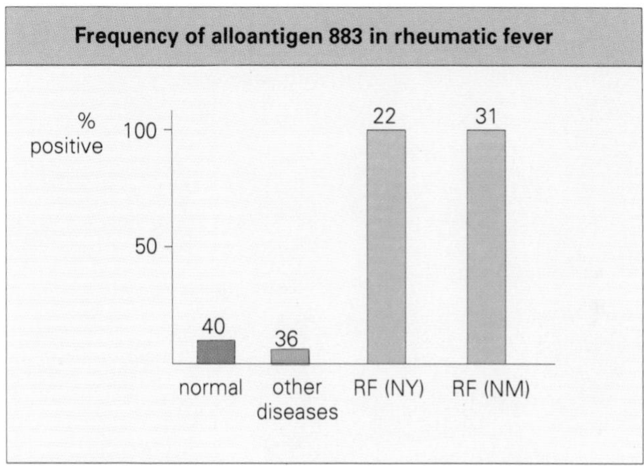

Fig. 11.6 Patients with rheumatic fever were studied separately in New York (NY) and New Mexico (NM). The category 'other diseases' includes multiple sclerosis, SLE and rheumatoid arthritis. The number at the top of each bar represents the number tested in each group.

growth of the vegetation (Fig. 11.7). It is friable and can embolize or it may invade locally causing abscess formation, conduction abnormalities, perforation of a valve cusp or an abnormal communication within the heart. Effective treatment results in shrinkage of the vegetations and endothelialization and organization, so that small, sterile, fibrotic, calcified nodules remain.

Clinical presentation. The patient presents with fever, malaise and non-specific symptoms of a chronic illness. On examination, heart murmurs are almost invariable, and the detection of changing murmurs is characteristic. The occurrence of congestive cardiac failure signifies important haemodynamic embarrassment due to valvular damage and may require prompt surgical intervention. Common extracardiac manifestations are as follows:

- splinter haemorrhages (Fig. 11.8 left)
- Janeway lesions (Fig. 11.8 middle)
- finger-tip gangrene (Fig. 11.8 right)
- Osler's nodes (transient, painful and erythematous; found on ends of fingers and toes)
- Roth spots (small, retinal haemorrhages with white centres)
- splenomegaly

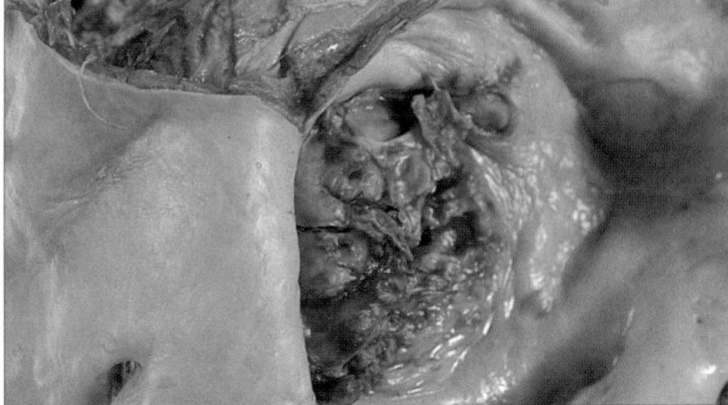

Fig. 11.7 Bacterial endocarditis. Macroscopic view of a prosthetic mitral valve covered with vegetations.

The patient will be anaemic and kidney involvement may cause proteinuria and haematuria. Other symptoms and signs may be caused by embolization to any part of the body. Detection of the causative organism in blood cultures is of primary importance, although this is not found in 10–20% of cases.

Immune response

The length of illness seems to determine the extent of the immune response. Apart from the specific antibody to the infecting organisms, chronic antigenaemia stimulates generalized hypergammaglobulinaemia so that after several weeks of infection, a variety of autoantibodies can be detected (Fig. 11.9).

Immune complex deposition may be the cause of the peripheral manifestations such as Roth spots, and Osler's nodes, but there is still uncertainty as to whether these are vasculitic lesions or microabscesses and microemboli. Certainly the immune complexes do cause nephritis: immunofluorescence has demonstrated immunoglobulin and complement deposition in irregular, granular deposits of the basement membrane of the kidney. Usually the damage is not severe and is reversible (see chapter 8). Immunoglobulin and complement deposits are found in the walls of capillaries, not only of the kidney, but also of the skin: this has been demonstrated both in normal skin and in the rather unusual vasculitic rash which can occur in endocarditis.

Aetiology

Streptococci are still responsible for the majority of cases of bacterial endocarditis; the second most common causative organisms are staphylococci. Endothelial damage is the primary event required in bacterial endocarditis; this is caused by abnormal haemodynamics due to regurgitant flow, pressure gradients or narrow orifices, and so usually occurs in the presence of heart disease. Once endothelial damage has occurred, platelet and fibrin deposition are followed by adherence and multiplication of organisms.

Why the heart develops endocarditis at a particular

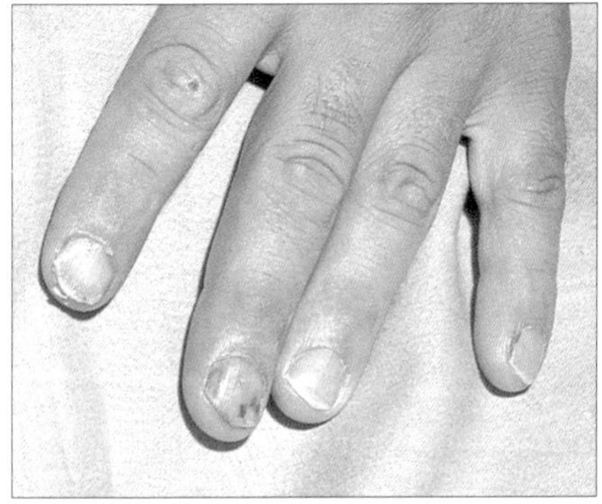

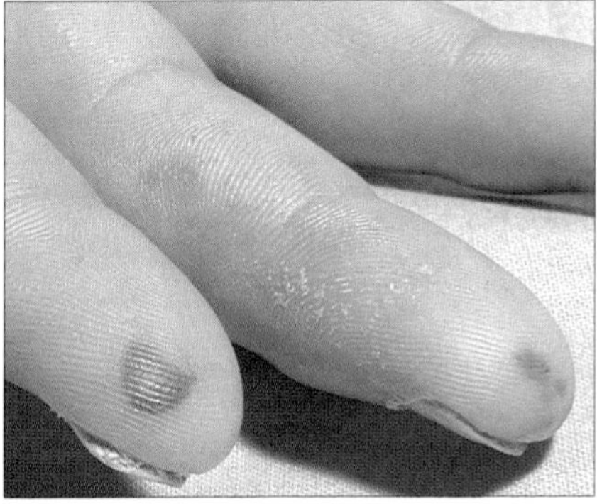

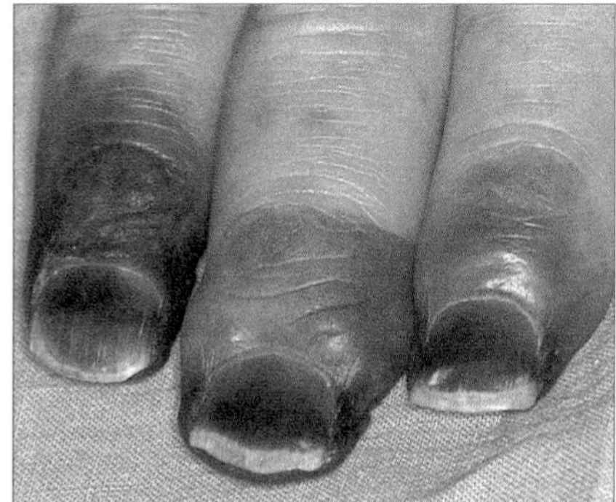

Fig. 11.8 Dermatological manifestations of bacterial endocarditis. Left: splinter haemorrhages on the finger nails. Middle: Janeway lesions. Right: vasculitic rash on the hands (not shown) and finger-tip gangrene due to showers of emboli from cardiac vegetations.

time when it is frequently exposed to transient bacteraemias is not known. It has been suggested that circulating agglutinating antibodies cause large numbers of bacteria to clump together, producing a large enough inoculum to sustain infection of a vegetation. However, it is not clear whether these antibodies are formed prior to infectious endocarditis or produced as a result. An alternative theory is that the organism itself produces a substance which encourages adherence to the vegetation, for example *Streptococcus sanguis* produces such a polysaccharide (dextran).

For most organisms, an underlying abnormality of the heart is a prerequisite for the production of disease; this is usually provided in the form of rheumatic or congenital heart disease. Prolapsed or prosthetic valves are also favourable targets for sepsis. In about 15% of cases, however, the valve is normal before the attack of endocarditis. Left-sided endocarditis is much more common than right-sided and the mitral valve is most often affected, then the aortic, and then both left-sided valves. Endocarditis is right-sided in about 5% of cases, although this figure is increasing because of escalation in intravenous drug abuse. Some organisms, such as *Staph. aureus*, are so virulent that they will attack a normal valve: these same organisms are often the cause of right-sided endocarditis and produce an acute illness rather than the usual subacute disease (Fig. 11.10).

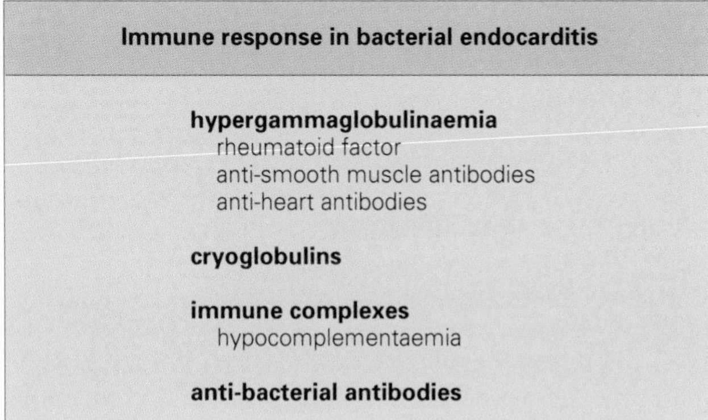

Fig. 11.9 Effective treatment results in reduction and eventually loss of these immunological abnormalities.

Treatment

Treatment involves effective and appropriate anti-microbial therapy with eradication of any persistent source of the organism. Surgery may be required where there is severe haemodynamic disturbance as a result of valvular damage, or for uncontrolled sepsis.

POST-CARDIOTOMY SYNDROME

Clinical presentation

Post-cardiotomy syndrome, post-myocardial infarction (Dressler's) syndrome and post-pericardial trauma syndrome are similar and are characterized by an illness which follows a latent period between insult and onset of

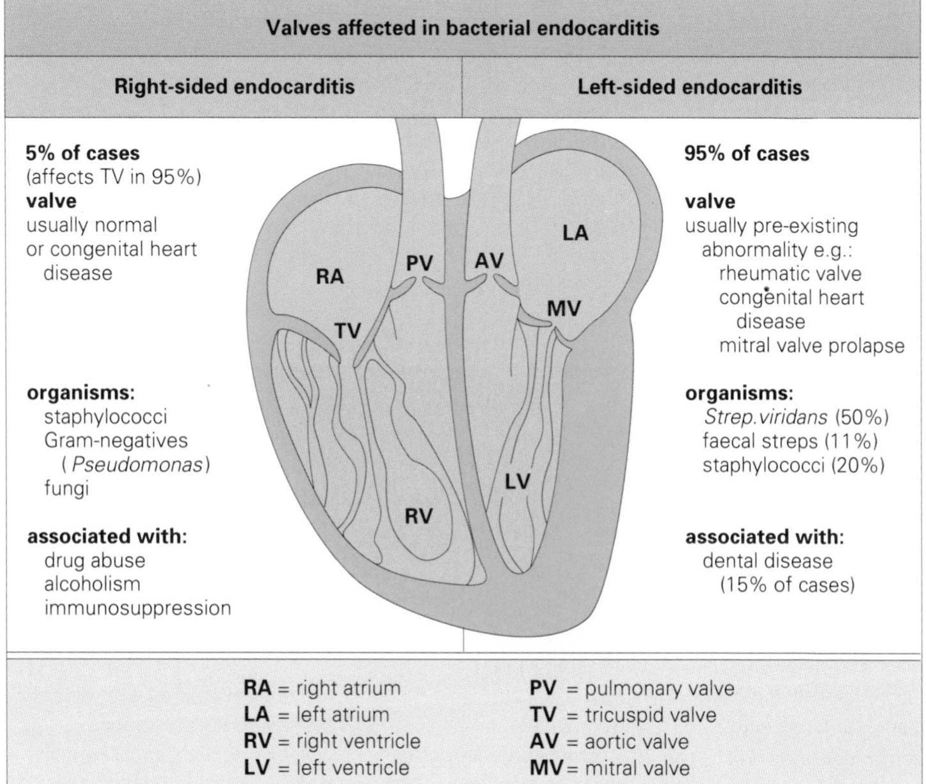

Valves affected in bacterial endocarditis
Right-sided endocarditis
Left-sided endocarditis
5% of cases
(affects TV in 95%)
valve
usually normal
or congenital heart disease
organisms:
staphylococci
Gram-negatives
(Pseudomonas)
fungi
associated with:
drug abuse
alcoholism
immunosuppression
RA
PV
AV
LA
TV
MV
LV
RV
95% of cases
valve
usually pre-existing abnormality e.g.:
rheumatic valve
congenital heart disease
mitral valve prolapse
organisms:
Strep.viridans (50%)
faecal streps (11%)
staphylococci (20%)
associated with:
dental disease
(15% of cases)
RA = right atrium
LA = left atrium
RV = right ventricle
LV = left ventricle
PV = pulmonary valve
TV = tricuspid valve
AV = aortic valve
MV = mitral valve

Fig. 11.10 Left-sided endocarditis due to staphylococci is usually found in association with a prosthetic valve or drug abuse.

symptoms. The latent period may be as short as ten days or as long as four weeks. It is characterized by a fever and symptoms and signs of pericarditis (Fig. 11.11). The histological findings are of non-specific inflammatory changes with fibrin deposition.

Immune response

The anti-heart antibodies that accompany these syndromes (Fig. 11.12) disappear on recovery or with steroid treatment and recur with relapses. Circulating immune complexes are also found and appear to correlate with the development of the syndrome.

Aetiology

An attractive hypothesis suggests that damage to the heart involving the pericardium results in the exposure of the new antigen to which autoantibodies are formed. However, these antibodies are also detectable when there is no syndrome and repeated surgical procedures on the heart do not result in a repeated, and more severe, post-pericardiotomy syndrome. The role of antibodies in the syndrome is not clear; cytotoxic reactions cannot be induced with these antibodies and their presence does not prove that they are primarily responsible for the illness.

The immune complexes found in association with anti-heart antibodies and the post-cardiotomy syndrome may be involved in the pathogenesis by the precipitation of circulating immune complexes in the pericardium. The similarity of the syndrome to viral pericarditis is striking. Elevated viral titres and seasonal variations suggesting a viral aetiology have been noted. This has led to an alternative hypothesis that the syndrome might be due to reactivation of a latent virus when the heart is traumatized. However, the literature on this aspect of the post-cardiotomy syndrome is contradictory. It has also been suggested that the syndromes might represent a hypersensitivity reaction to blood in the pericardial space.

Treatment

Initially, non-steroidal anti-inflammatory agents are used to relieve symptoms but steroids may be necessary if these are unsuccessful. The response to steroids is usually dramatic but there is a risk of relapse when the treatment is curtailed.

Presentation of post-cardiotomy syndrome		
Insult	**Illness**	**Signs**
cardiac surgery	post-cardiotomy syndrome	fever pericarditis pleurisy arthralgia pulmonary infiltration ↑ESR ↑WCC
myocardial infarction	post-myocardial infarction (Dressler's) syndrome	
pericardial trauma	post-pericardial trauma syndrome	

Fig. 11.11 Signs of pericarditis include pericardial and/or pleural effusions, pulmonary infiltration and arthralgia with a raised erythrocyte sedimentation rate (ESR) and white cell count (WCC).

CARDIOMYOPATHY

Cardiomyopathy is, by definition, heart muscle disease of unknown aetiology. There are three types:

- congestive
- hypertrophic
- restrictive

CONGESTIVE CARDIOMYOPATHY

Congestive cardiomyopathy is characterized by dilatation of the ventricles which overshadows any compensatory hypertrophy that might occur (Fig. 11.13). The diagnosis is made by exclusion of other causes of cardiac chamber enlargement with failure of systolic pump function, for example coronary disease, diabetes mellitus, hypertension, specific heart muscle disease and myocarditis.

Clinical presentation

Typically, patients present with symptoms of left and/or right heart failure; symptoms may be precipitated abruptly by an arrhythmia, commonly atrial fibrillation, but are usually insidious in onset. Embolic episodes, either systemic or venous, may occur as a result of mural thrombus on a hypokinetic cardiac surface, or through arrhythmias. Clinically, there are features of left and/or right heart failure, signs common to the many other causes of cardiomegaly and heart failure. The heart is enlarged and a

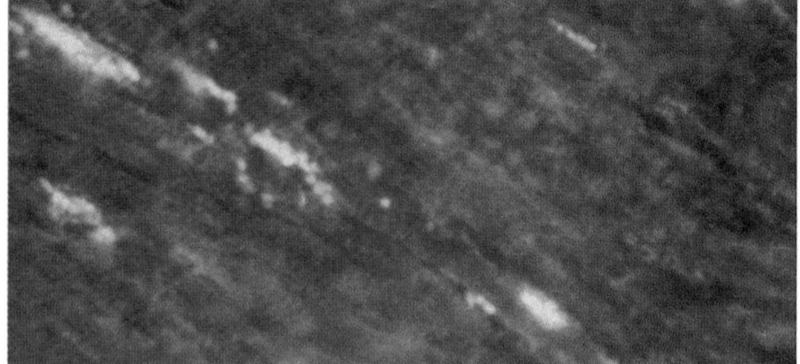

Fig. 11.12 Normal human myocardium stained with serum from a patient with Dressler's syndrome demonstrating positive immunofluorescence due to anti-heart antibody using a simple sandwich indirect immunofluorescence technique.

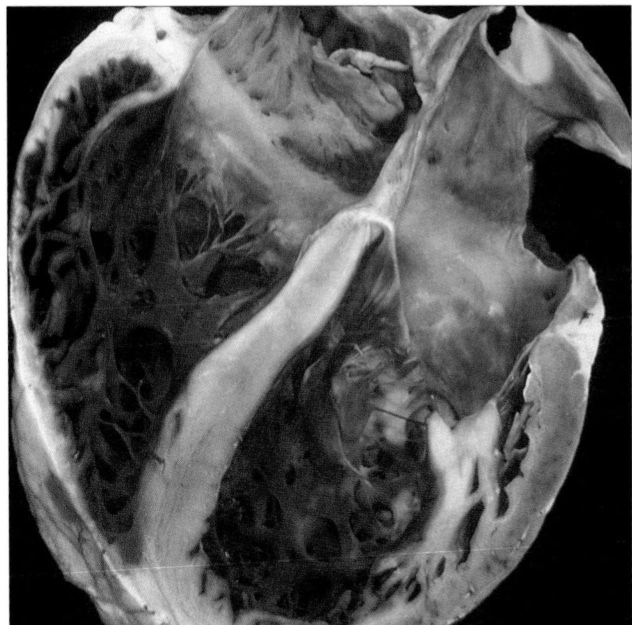

Fig. 11.13 Congestive cardiomyopathy. Note the gross dilatation of both ventricles. Courtesy of Professor R H Anderson and Professor A E Becker.

gallop rhythm is an early feature; later, tricuspid or mitral regurgitation may develop secondary to ventricular dilatation.

Autopsy

At autopsy the heart appears soft, flabby and pale, and there is usually dilatation of all chambers; the heart is heavier than normal but dilatation tends to mask the hypertrophy that is present. The endocardium is often thickened and mural thrombus is found in more than 60% of cases. Light and electron microscopy show abnormalities which are non-specific to congestive cardiomyopathy but which, if present, support the diagnosis. On light microscopy, there may be both hypertrophy and attenuation of myofibres, and nuclear changes associated with hypertrophy (Fig. 11.14). In areas, myofibres may be replaced by fibrous tissue and interstitial fibrous tissue is increased. Electron microscopy reveals degenerative changes in myocardial cells (Fig. 11.15), myofibrillar disarray, interstitial fibrosis and varying degrees of hypertrophy.

Immune response

Anti-heart antibodies to many different structures, for example anti-sarcolemmal and anti-mitochondrial, have been identified, but these are thought to be secondary to

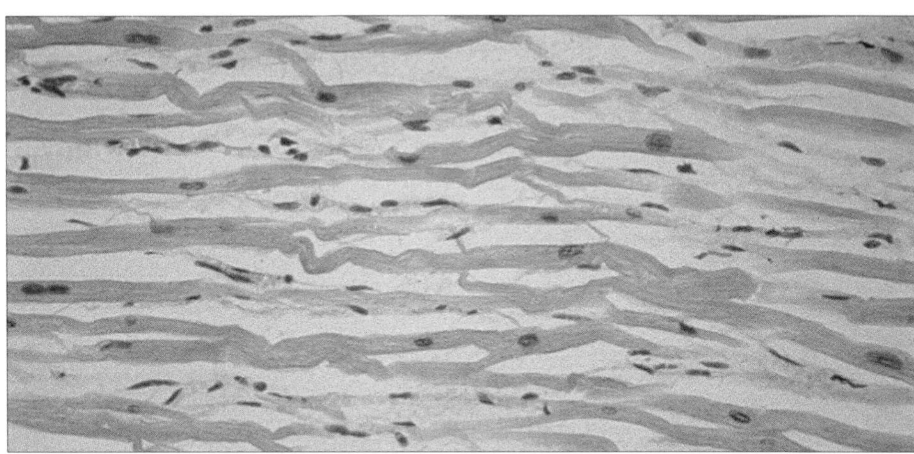

Fig. 11.14 Histological section of an endomyocardial biopsy from a patient with congestive cardiomyopathy showing myofibrillar degeneration and hypertrophic nuclei. Courtesy of Professor R H Anderson and Professor A E Becker.

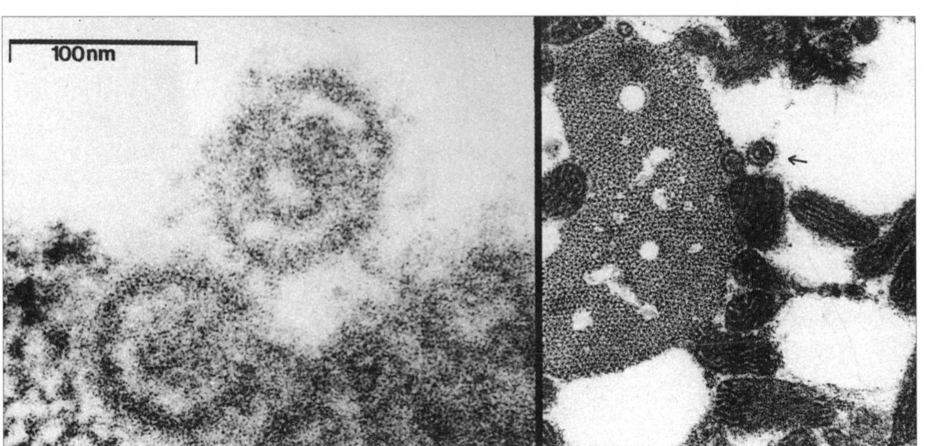

Fig. 11.15 EM of endomyocardial biopsy from a patient with cardiomyopathy. Left: virus-like particles of approximately 100nm diameter, with an outer coat and electron-dense core, and resembling viruses of the herpes group, were found in this case. Right: there is intracellular oedema, a little myofibrillar degeneration, increased numbers of mitochondria and mitochondrial pleomorphism.

myocardial damage. It has been difficult to demonstrate pathogenic organ- and disease-specific anti-heart antibody.

Reports of abnormalities of cellular immunity are contradictory. Depressed cell mediated immunity has been documented in some studies but not in others. A fairly constant finding, however, is that of a sub-group of patients with congestive cardiomyopathy who demonstrate sensitization to heart antigen using leucocyte migration inhibition. The significance of this may be clarified when the heart antigens can be purified and presented in a more appropriate form.

Impaired suppressor T lymphocyte activity has been reported in some patients with congestive cardiomyopathy; however other studies have failed to confirm this or suggest that reduced activity may occur in heart failure regardless of the cause. Work is hampered by the fact that patients with congestive cardiomyopathy are usually seen late in the course of the disease; there is possibly a transient abnormality detectable only at the early stages.

Aetiology

It is most likely that congestive cardiomyopathy is a final common pathway of myocardial damage due to different causes. The histological changes are non-specific and are seen in other conditions where the cause has been identified, for example hypertensive heart disease, toxic agents and coronary disease: it may simply be a matter of time before all cases of congestive cardiomyopathy can be assigned to a particular cause.

Pre-existing myocarditis. The possibility that congestive cardiomyopathy is the product of myocarditis has received much attention. Despite a great deal of work in this field, satisfactory evidence that myocarditis progresses to congestive cardiomyopathy has been hard to produce. However, evidence is accumulating from long-term biopsy follow-up of patients with myocarditis to show that some patients do progress to a picture of heart failure indistinguishable from congestive cardiomyopathy. The detection of virus particles within the myocardium in congestive cardiomyopathy (see Fig. 11.15) has been very unrewarding but virus genome has been demonstrated in myocardial biopsies in some patients with myocarditis and some with congestive cardiomyopathy (Fig. 11.16). The fact that many patients with myocarditis go undetected clinically, and that patients with congestive cardiomyopathy seem to present at a late stage of their illness, combined with the difficulties of diagnosis of both myocarditis and congestive cardiomyopathy even when endomyocardial biopsy is available, have made investigation of a link between myocarditis and at least some cases of congestive cardiomyopathy difficult.

The possibility that congestive cardiomyopathy might be an autoimmune disorder has been considered, but patients with cardiomyopathy do not have other features of autoimmune diseases and the immunological abnormalities demonstrated may be a result of the damage inflicted on the heart. Alcohol and pregnancy are also associated with congestive cardiomyopathy.

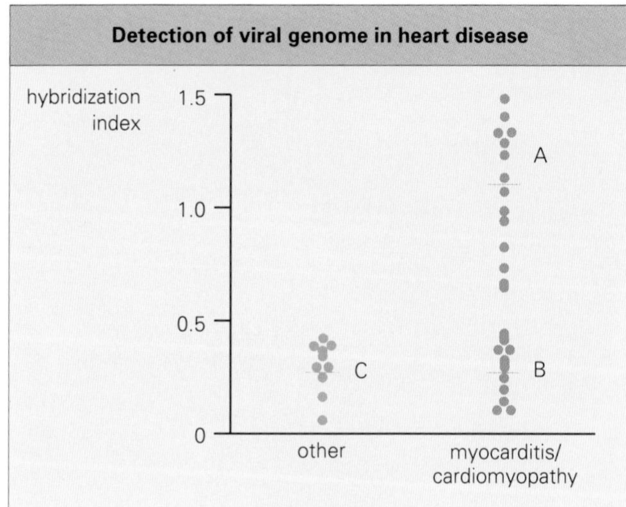

Fig. 11.16 Detection of Coxsackie B virus-specific RNA in endomyocardial biopsy samples. Groups A and B are patients with histologically proven myocarditis or dilated cardiomyopathy and are clinically similar but separated by the presence (group A) or absence (group B) of viral RNA. Group C consisits of patients with other specific heart disease without virus aetiology. Modified from Archard L C, Bowles N E, Olsen E G J & Richardson P J (1987).

Treatment

There is no specific treatment for congestive cardiomyopathy; immunosuppressives in particular have no place. Therapy is aimed at relieving heart failure and preventing arrhythmias and thromboembolic consequences. Cardiac transplantation is a successful option where pump failure is not controlled by medical therapy.

HYPERTROPHIC CARDIOMYOPATHY

Although anti-heart antibodies have been detected in some cases of hypertrophic cardiomyopathy, these are believed to be non-specific and the disease is not thought to be immunologically based.

RESTRICTIVE CARDIOMYOPATHY

Clinical features

Restriction may be due to either myocardial infiltration and/or endocardial fibrosis. The result is impaired diastolic filling and ventricular distensibility with normal systolic emptying. With progression of the disease, incompetence of the atrioventricular valves occurs and, with super-added thrombus, obliteration of a ventricular cavity may result. Symptoms and signs are those of heart failure relevant to the chamber involved. The main causes are amyloidosis (Fig. 11.17) and endomyocardial fibrosis (EMF); it is the latter which is of particular interest immunologically.

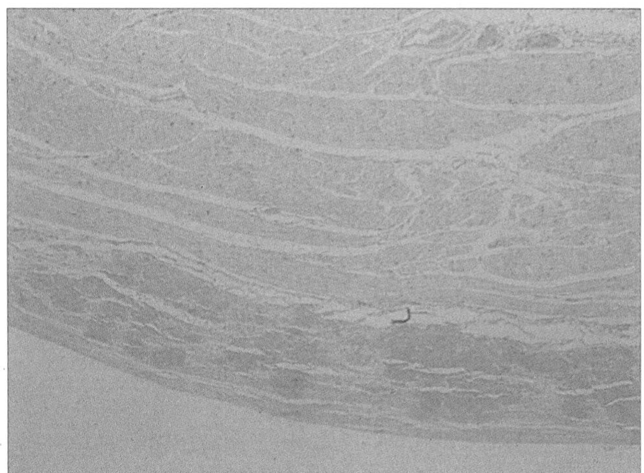

Fig. 11.17 Cardiac amyloidosis. Sub-endocardial amyloid deposits are visualized using Congo red stain. Courtesy of Professor R H Anderson & Professor A E Becker.

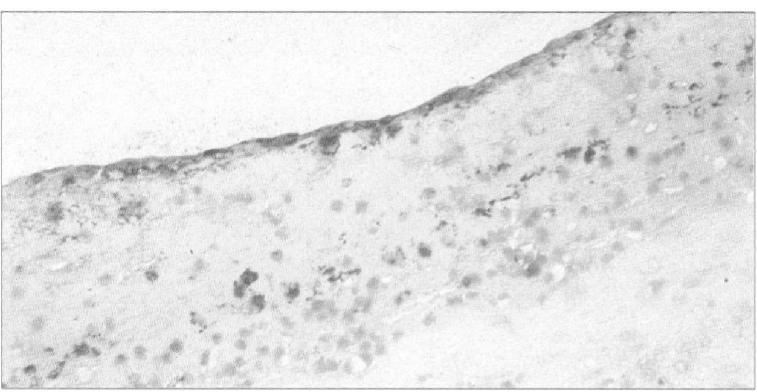

Fig. 11.18 Eosinophilic endomyocardial fibrosis (EMF). This section of endomyocardium, taken from a patient with early stage disease, was stained with antibody EG2, which binds to the secreted forms of ECP and to the eosinophil neurotoxin EDN. The presence of the alkaline phosphate-linked antibody was shown with fast red dye as a substrate. Courtesy of Professor C Spry.

Endomyocardial fibrosis

Initially, there is a myocarditis with acute necrotic lesions containing mainly eosinophils. This progresses over a period of months to a thrombotic stage and finally, over a period of months or years, to a fibrotic stage in which there is gross thickening of the endocardium of either or both ventricles, and which may involve the papillary muscles and chordae tendinae. Fibrous streaks may be seen penetrating the myocardium. Microscopically, collagenous tissue is seen beneath thrombus or fibrin, then a layer of granulation tissue containing vascular channels and varying numbers of inflammatory cells. Eosinophils may be seen and microthrombi are not uncommon.

Pathological features. EMF may occur with or without eosinophilia. In temperate climates it is usually associated with a marked eosinophilia; in about 50% of cases there is an associated condition, such as polyarteritis nodosa, tumour or parasites, giving rise to this; in the remainder, however, no cause is apparent (hypereosinophilic syndrome), although there may be features of a preceding parasitic or allergic disease. In tropical climates EMF is not associated with such an eosinophilic load, although repeated parasitic infections do give rise to a chronic hypereosinophilia. However, the pathological changes are very similar and it is thought that the temperate variety probably reflects a more virulent, rapidly progressive form compared with the tropical variety. In 85% of cases of EMF the hypereosinophilic syndrome occurs at some stage, suggesting that eosinophils may be responsible for endomyocardial damage.

Stimulus to eosinophil production. The initial stimulus to eosinophil production is unknown. Elevated IgE levels have been found in some cases suggesting that the hypereosinophilia might be an exaggerated response to an earlier, undetectable insult. The eosinophils in temperate EMF are abnormal in that they show degranulation. One of the proteins contained within the granules, eosinophilic cationic protein (ECP), has been shown to kill isolated rat heart cells. Monoclonal antibodies have been used to detect the presence of granule proteins in the endocardium of human hearts (Fig. 11.18). ECP has been demonstrated in both the endocardium and in areas of acute myocarditis in these patients. Release of ECP leads to inflammation, cell injury and death, and later fibrosis. Eosinophils also release factors which affect the coagulation system (Fig. 11.19) and this may account for the high incidence of thromboembolic complications, intraventricular thrombus and microthrombi.

Treatment

As the disease follows a periodic course of relapse and remission, treatment is instituted when there are symptoms and signs of active disease. The complications of the disease, such as heart failure and thromboembolism, are treated conventionally with the inclusion of dipyridamole to inhibit platelet activating factor (PAF) which is produced by eosinophils. Steroids and cytotoxic drugs aid recovery from relapse, but whether they can actually prevent the development of early endocardial lesions is not yet certain. Drugs which will prevent the release of eosinophil basic proteins are still awaited.

Reduction of eosinophil numbers has been achieved transiently using plasma exchange and leucopheresis. Surgical treatment involves valve replacement where haemodynamically indicated, and stripping of the fibrous layer in the ventricles.

ATHEROSCLEROSIS

Pathological features

Atherosclerosis is a generalized degenerative disease that affects large and medium-sized arteries. The atherosclerotic plaque has a white appearance until it

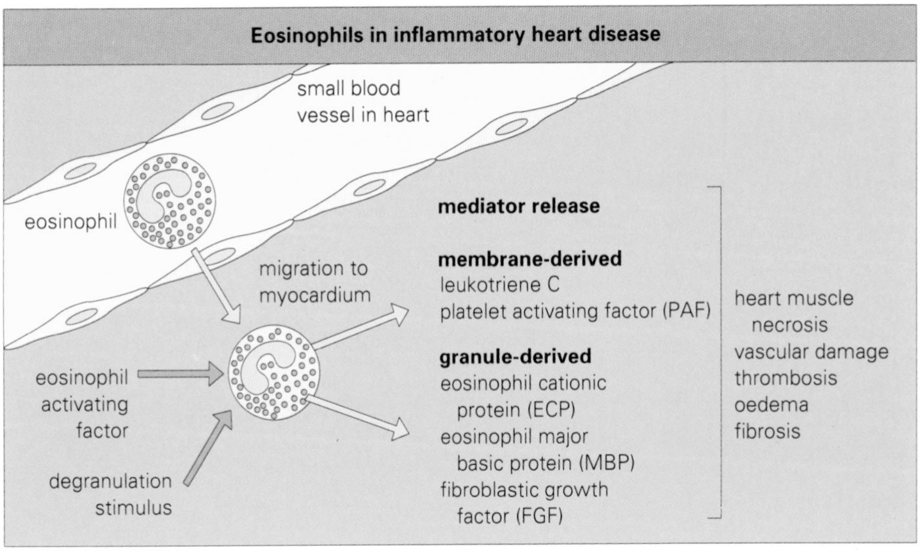

Eosinophils in inflammatory heart disease

small blood vessel in heart

eosinophil

migration to myocardium

eosinophil activating factor

degranulation stimulus

mediator release

membrane-derived
leukotriene C
platelet activating factor (PAF)

granule-derived
eosinophil cationic protein (ECP)
eosinophil major basic protein (MBP)
fibroblastic growth factor (FGF)

heart muscle necrosis
vascular damage
thrombosis
oedema
fibrosis

Fig. 11.19 Eosinophil mediators, which can be either membrane- or granule-derived, affect the coagulation system and may be involved in thromboembolic complications.

becomes complicated by thrombosis, calcification and ulceration. The plaque contains increased numbers of smooth muscle cells (which are also morphologically abnormal), increased connective tissue and lipid, mostly cholesterol (Fig. 11.20), which constitutes up to 50% by dry weight of the plaque. Monocyte-derived macrophages and lymphocytes are also found in the plaques.

Clinical features

The main clinical presentations are caused by:

- near-occlusion or occlusion of an artery giving rise to ischaemia or infarction of the tissue supplied;
- weakening of the arterial wall allowing aneurysmal dilatation, rupture or dissection.

The symptoms and signs will obviously depend on the site affected.

Immune response

Little in the way of immune response in atherosclerosis has been documented in man; this may be due to the difficulties encountered in studying plaques *in vitro* and relating this to the *in vivo* situations. However, complement components have been found and there is acceleration of atherosclerosis in heart and kidney transplant recipients. Animal experiments have yielded evidence of development of atheromatous plaques in response to immunological damage to vessels via a type III serum sickness mechanism, and in the environment of graft rejection. In hypercholesterolaemia atherosclerosis is accelerated.

Aetiology

Endothelial damage is believed to be the essential trigger for the development of atherosclerosis. Once injury to endothelium has occurred, platelets will adhere and aggregate, smooth muscle will proliferate, collagen and elastin will increase, and lipid is allowed to accumulate in the vessel wall via the area of increased permeability at the site of injury.

One cause of damage may be immunological. It is suggested that circulating complexes might penetrate even normal vessel walls and activate complement, which damages the vessel wall by releasing esterases and attracting polymorphs (type III hypersensitivity reaction). The vessel wall may be a direct target if it is seen to have antigen which is foreign, either because it has been damaged by chemicals, drugs or other environmental abnormalities in the bloodstream, or because of cross-reacting antibody (type II hypersensitivity reaction). Following transplantation, antibodies and sensitized T lymphocytes may damage the endothelium and allow atherosclerosis to proceed.

Treatment

Treatment is not aimed at immunologically mediated damage except in transplantation, where immunosuppression is required to suppress rejection (see chapters 3 & 27). Otherwise, treatment is aimed at preventing or alleviating factors which place arteries at risk, for example hypertension, smoking and hyperlipidaemia, by trying to prevent platelet adhesion and aggregation, and finally by relieving symptoms caused by atherosclerosis by surgical or medical means.

IMMUNOLOGICAL DISEASES

CONNECTIVE TISSUE DISEASES

The heart may be involved in many of the connective tissue diseases; this is often only appreciated at post-mortem when other organ involvement has proved fatal.

Rheumatoid arthritis

In rheumatoid arthritis (RA; see chapter 5) cardiac involvement is rare but severe and is associated with seropositive nodular disease. Pericarditis is the most common manifestation, with both pericardial layers becoming

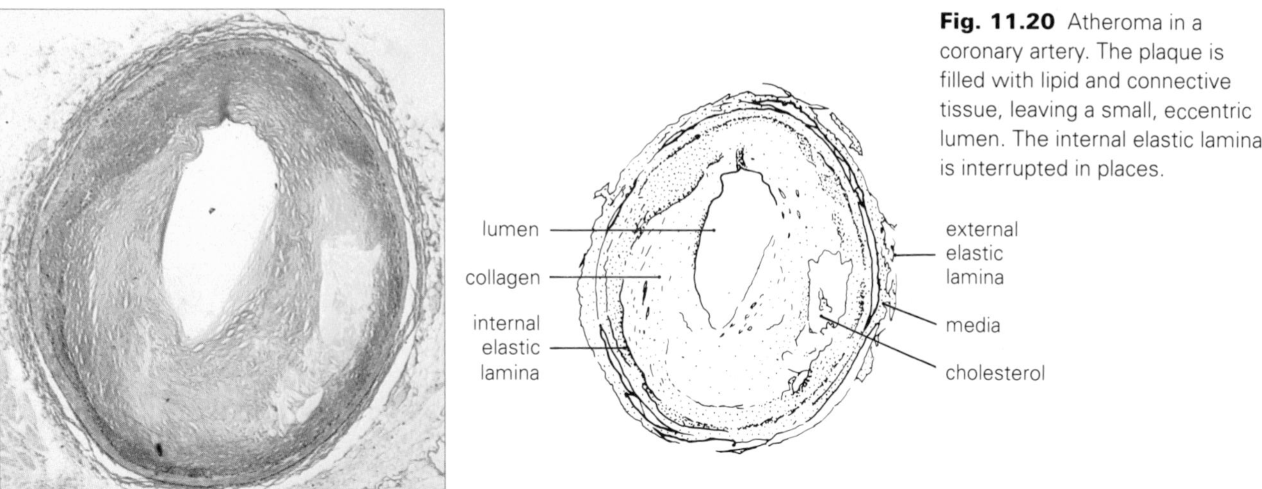

Fig. 11.20 Atheroma in a coronary artery. The plaque is filled with lipid and connective tissue, leaving a small, eccentric lumen. The internal elastic lamina is interrupted in places.

thickened, which can lead to constriction. Conduction abnormalities can occur from rheumatoid nodules, direct inflammation, or vasculitis affecting the specialized blood vessels of the conducting system.

Systemic lupus erythematosus (SLE)

In systemic lupus erythematosus (see chapter 6) pericardial inflammation is usually associated with pleurisy and is acute, less severe and short-lived, without serious sequelae. IgG, IgM and C3 have been demonstrated in pericardial tissue and, unlike RA, the blood glucose level of pericardial fluid is not low. Congenital heart block can occur in the children of mothers with SLE and is probably caused by transplacental passage of anti-Ro (SS-A) antibody.

Ischaemic heart disease is accelerated in SLE and shows a two-fold increase above the normal incidence in RA. Corticosteroid therapy may be partly responsible for this, but there may be additional factors, such as thrombosis, as a complication of anti-phospholipid antibodies in SLE and immune complex vasculitis.

Scleroderma and polymyositis

Cardiac involvement in scleroderma and polymyositis is usually insidious, but carries a poor prognosis. In scleroderma the myocardium can be primarily involved or secondarily, following pulmonary and systemic hypertension. Cardiac failure is the second most common cause of death. A rise in the cardiac isoenzyme (MB) or creatine phosphokinase (CPK) of more than 3% is a good indicator of cardiac involvement in polymyositis and suggests the need for aggressive therapy, including cytotoxic drugs.

Aortic incompetence is the most common valvular lesion in the connective tissue diseases, complicating any disease associated with aortitis (for example ankylosing spondylitis, Reiter's syndrome and giant cell arteritis) and those associated with valvulitis (such as RA, Still's disease and SLE). In HLA-B27-positive men, heart block is present in nearly half the patients with aortitis.

SYSTEMIC VASCULITIS

Clinical and pathological features

Vasculitis is the inflammation of blood vessels. The resulting clinical condition is determined by the size of the vessels which are inflamed, the severity of the inflammation and the organ(s) supplied (Fig. 11.21). Although in most cases no cause is found, some infectious agents, foreign

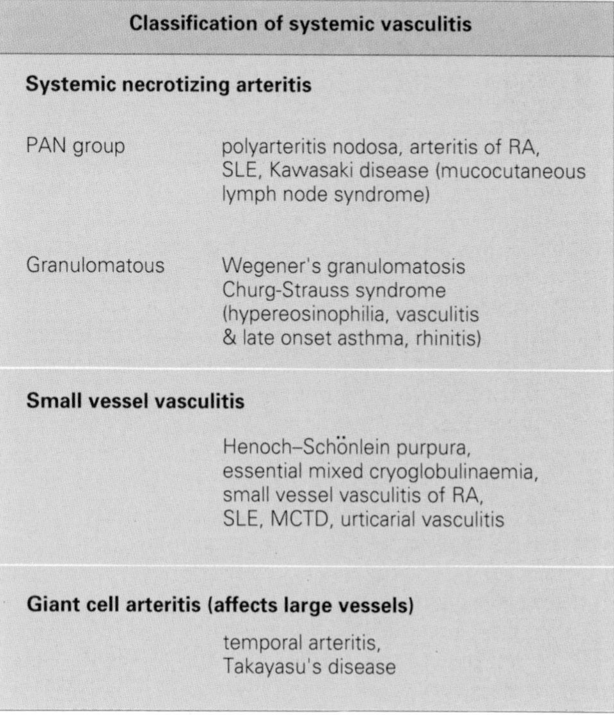

Classification of systemic vasculitis	
Systemic necrotizing arteritis	
PAN group	polyarteritis nodosa, arteritis of RA, SLE, Kawasaki disease (mucocutaneous lymph node syndrome)
Granulomatous	Wegener's granulomatosis Churg-Strauss syndrome (hypereosinophilia, vasculitis & late onset asthma, rhinitis)
Small vessel vasculitis	
	Henoch–Schönlein purpura, essential mixed cryoglobulinaemia, small vessel vasculitis of RA, SLE, MCTD, urticarial vasculitis
Giant cell arteritis (affects large vessels)	
	temporal arteritis, Takayasu's disease

Fig. 11.21 Systemic arteritis and giant cell arteritis are most likely to affect the heart; small vessel vasculitis usually causes skin disease. Other vasculitides are dealt with in the relevant organ chapter. MCTD=mixed connective tissue disease.

Agents implicated in vasculitis		
Infections	viral	hepatitis B EBV
	bacterial	bacterial endocarditis streptococci *Mycobacterium tuberculosis*
	rickettsial	dengue
Foreign protein	serum sickness	anti–tetanus antiserum, anti–lymphocyte globulin
Drugs	sulphonamides	
Autoantigens	SLE (nuclear antigens) RA, Wegener's granulomatosis ? neutrophil alkaline phosphatase	
Cryoglobulins	essential mixed cryoglobulinaemia	

Fig. 11.22 Although certain agents have been implicated in the aetiology of vasculitis, no cause is found in the majority of cases.

proteins and drugs have been implicated in the aetiology of this condition (Fig. 11.22).

Immune response

A type III hypersensitivity reaction, with the deposition of immune complexes in blood vessel walls, may be responsible. The antigen(s) involved are not completely eliminated (autoantigen, infection, repeated exposure) and thus chronic injury occurs. The site of deposition is probably determined by several factors, including previous damage to the vessel wall, which may be caused by mechanical factors or by turbulent flow, or immunological factors may be involved (type I or type IV reaction). Immune complexes are usually solubilized by complement and dealt with by the mononuclear phagocyte system, sometimes after transport on red blood cells which bear a CR1 receptor. Defects in various parts of this system, for example decreased CR1 or lack of C2 in SLE, would favour immune complex deposition.

Vasculitis affecting the heart

Coronary arteritis is dangerous in that it can lead to myocardial infarction and sudden death. Systemic necrotizing arteritis can involve these arteries directly, and large vessel giant cell aortitis may spread proximally to involve proximal coronary vessels. In this condition T cells dominate the inflammatory infiltrate, with $CD4^+$ T cells predominating in temporal arteritis, Takayasu's disease (Fig. 11.23) and Wegener's granulomatosis. Kawasaki disease is

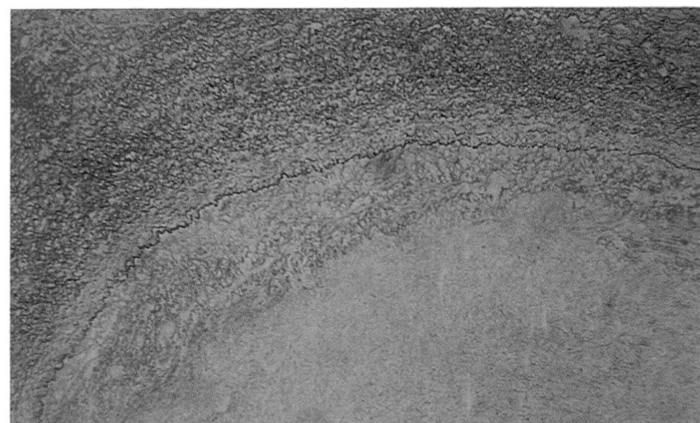

Fig. 11.23 Takayasu's disease. This section of artery shows a dense inflammatory infiltrate which consists predominantly of $CD4^+$ cells. Courtesy of Dr D Scott.

an acute febrile illness occurring in children with arteritis developing in the recovery phase. Two percent die suddenly from coronary arteritis and this occurs predominantly in those who have received steroids, which are therefore contraindicated. DNA studies suggest that a retroviral agent might cause Kawasaki disease.

Treatment

Cyclophosphamide is now used to treat many of the systemic vasculitides; if given intermittently together with prednisolone the side-effects are reduced.

CHAGAS' DISEASE

Chagas' disease is caused by infection with the protozoan *Trypanosoma cruzi* and is a major health problem in Central and South America. The infecting agent is transmitted to humans via the reduviid bug which excretes *T. cruzi* in its faeces, the parasite gaining entry through conjunctivae or abraded skin. Inoculation, multiplication and dissemination often occur unrecognized. The parasite favours myocytes for multiplication but also affects skeletal muscle, smooth muscle and glial cells.

Three phases are recognized in Chagas' disease: an acute phase, a latent phase and a chronic phase.

ACUTE PHASE

Few infected hosts exhibit this phase: in many it is subclinical. When apparent, fever, sweating and muscle pains are typical, and hepatosplenomegaly and lymph node enlargement may be present. Myocarditis, which may be fulminant, and meningoencephalitis may occur. Patients who die in the acute phase from myocarditis have *T. cruzi* parasites within myofibres; these can multiply and lead to myofibre rupture. There is a diffuse cellular infiltrate which tends to be more pronounced in areas of cell rupture and which leads to destruction of myofibres, the conducting system and autonomic cells. Involvement of the endocardium may lead to thrombus formation, whilst involvement of the pericardium may result in an effusion.

Immune response

There are antibodies to parasite membrane-bound antigenic determinants and to other intracellular antigens. These are found in both symptomatic and asymptomatic patients but there is no significant difference between the two groups; the significance of these antibodies is uncertain. There is a depression of cell mediated immunity in asymptomatic patients with acute Chagas' disease, demonstrated by the failure of leucocyte migration inhibition to occur in response to *T. cruzi* microsomal antigen; patients with symptoms do not show this immunosuppression. At what point this immunodepression begins, how long it lasts and its contribution in pathogenesis is not known.

The presence of *T. cruzi* parasites in myofibres seems to stimulate an intense inflammatory response which leads to damage of host cells. Myofibres and neurons not infected by *T. cruzi* may have parasite antigens on their surface, and the ensuing damage might be caused by cellular and/or humoral mechanisms.

LATENT PHASE

There appears to be a latent phase, when the patient is asymptomatic. This lasts for between 10 and 30 years, spanning the time of initial infection and the presentation of chronic Chagas' disease. It is assumed that there is a link between the two events, although there is no evidence to prove this.

CHRONIC PHASE

Cardiac abnormalities in chronic Chagas' disease range from asymptomatic patients with ECG abnormalities to severe congestive cardiac failure. Usually, there is cardiomegaly affecting all four chambers with symptoms and signs of congestive failure, although right-sided abnormalities may predominate. Tricuspid and mitral regurgitation are common findings and in 50% of affected hearts there is an apical pseudo-aneurysm. Patients may present with syncope or sudden death due to ventricular arrhythmia or conduction abnormalities. Although cardiac manifestations are common in the chronic phase, abnormalities of motor activity and coordination may predominate leading to dilatation of the oesophagus, stomach, colon (Fig. 11.24) or bronchi.

Microscopically the heart shows hypertrophy and focal myofibre degeneration and necrosis. There is extensive fibrosis with less cellular infiltrate than in the acute phase, and parasites are seldom seen. The conduction system is often damaged by infiltration or fibrosis and there is a reduction in the number of cardiac autonomic cells.

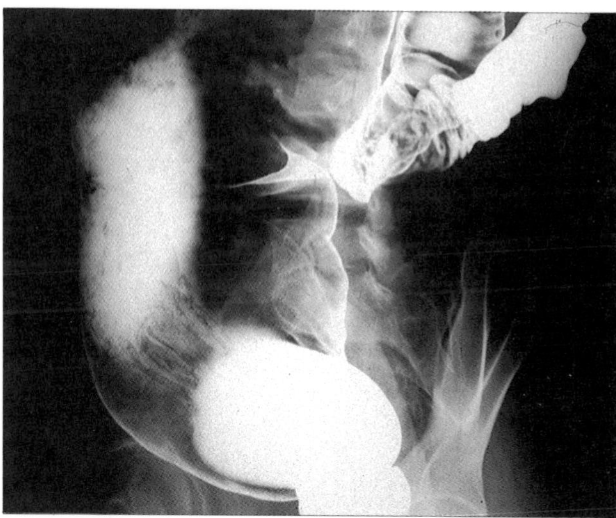

Fig. 11.24 Chagas' disease. Barium enema showing the typical appearance of megacolon. Courtesy of Dr A Habr-Gama.

Immunological abnormalities do occur in chronic Chagas' disease, which might explain why a disease occurring many years earlier might be involved in the pathogenesis of heart disease in later life.

Immune response

There is an autoantibody to endocardium, endothelium of vessels and interstitium of striated muscle (EVI antibody) which cross-reacts with antigen constituents of *T.cruzi* and which is found in the sera of 95% of patients with chronic Chagas' heart disease. This antibody may perpetuate damage to the heart long after the infecting agent has disappeared. However, it is not directed specifically at myofibres and may simply reflect tissue damage. IgG antibodies (and sometimes also IgA) are bound to neurons but, as with other antibodies found in this condition, they bear no relation to the degree of damage.

There are cytotoxic T cells sensitized to *T. cruzi* which will damage heart muscle cells: delayed hypersensitivity may have a role in causing cell destruction in chronic Chagas' disease.

Treatment

There is no specific treatment for Chagas' disease. Preventative measures involving improvement in housing and vector control are important.

RETROPERITONEAL FIBROSIS

Clinical and pathological features

Symptoms due to this condition are often non-specific. On examination 60% of patients will be hypertensive and may have signs of obstruction of the renal tract, gastrointestinal tract or vena cava. The ESR is usually elevated. A large retroperitoneal mass may be palpable. This is due to fibrosis of the retroperitoneal tissues, which macroscopically may appear as a uniform sheet or an irregular nodular mass. Microscopically the tissue may appear to be relatively avascular and fibrous, or it may be more vascular with foci of inflammatory cells.

Aetiology

Drugs, malignancy, radiotherapy and collagen diseases are believed to account for about a quarter of cases; in the rest the cause is unknown.

Immune response

Where there is severe atherosclerosis accompanied by a break in the wall of the aorta or an artery, insoluble lipid can leak through the wall into surrounding tissue and induce an immune reaction. IgG antibodies to insoluble lipid have been demonstrated.

Treatment

Treament is aimed at relieving obstruction which may be present or imminent. Steroids have been used, particularly postoperatively, to try to prevent further fibrosis.

FURTHER READING

Constantinides P, Pratesi F, Cavellero C, Di Perrit T. Immunity and atherosclerosis. In: *Proceedings of the Serono Symposia.* London: Academic Press, 1990.

Spry CJF. Eosinophilia and the heart. *Clin Immunol Allergy* 1987; **October**: 591–606.

Schultheiss HP, Bolte HD. Immunological analysis of autoantibodies against the adenine nucleotide translocator in dilated cardiomyopathy. 1985:**17**:603–617.

William Jr RC. Molecular mimicry and rheumatic fever. *Clinics in rheumatic diseases 11* (3). London: Baillière Tindall, 1985: 573–590.

12

Respiratory Disorders

INTRODUCTION

The respiratory tract, like the gastrointestinal tract (with which it shares a common embryological origin), is open to a wide variety of exogenous insults. At rest, more than 8500 litres of air daily traverse the conducting airways to reach the large area of gas exchanging alveolar surface. The inhaled air carries inorganic particles including smoke, dusts and fumes, and organic materials such as moulds, pollens and danders, viruses and bacteria. The conducting airways bear the brunt of these insults and are the sites of resultant diseases when the defence mechanisms are overwhelmed or overstimulated.

In numerical, morbidity and economic terms asthma, chronic bronchitis and bronchial carcinoma are a major health burden on the UK and other developed countries. Inhaled particulates and organisms that reach the terminal bronchioles and alveoli may initiate parenchymal diseases; of these, occupational lung disorders (see chapter 18) and, on a global basis, infectious diseases (especially tuberculosis) are of major importance. The lung is, however, also open to endogenous insults, as circulating toxins, antigens and immune complexes have ample opportunity to encounter the pulmonary vascular bed, which receives the entire cardiac output. Interstitial and drug-induced lung diseases, lung involvement in multi-system disorders, and acute lung injury may all be initiated via this route.

LUNG INJURY

Role of proteinases

Recognition of the role of phagocyte derived proteinases and reactive oxygen intermediates (ROIs) in causation of lung injury followed the observations that:

- pan acinar emphysema was associated with genetic deficiency of α1-anti-trypsin (α1-proteinase inhibitor — α1-Pi);
- intratracheal instillation of elastases caused emphysema to develop in animals.

The mechanisms of tissue injury have been most thoroughly explored with respect to emphysema and adult respiratory distress syndrome (ARDS), but similar reactions appear to operate in airway damage in bronchiectasis, lung damage in pneumonia and blood vessel damage in vasculitis.

Neutrophils, eosinophils and macrophages are rich sources of a wide range of proteinases. Although these are important for inactivation and degradation of ingested organisms and particulates within phagolysosomes, they are potent effectors of tissue damage when released into the external micro-environment. To prevent this, a wide range of proteinase inhibitors are present in the bronchial and alveolar secretions.

Usually, the proteinase inhibitors are available in excess, so proteolytic damage is prevented. However genetic deficiency, local inactivation or exclusion of proteinase inhibitors, and local excess of proteinases are all capable of adversely affecting the proteinase–anti-proteinase balance in favour of tissue destruction (Fig. 12.1).

Role of reactive oxygen intermediates (ROIs)

Superoxide (O_2), hydrogen peroxide (H_2O_2) and the hydroxyl radical (.OH) are ROIs generated by membrane bound NADPH-oxidase systems in neutrophils, eosinophils and macrophages. Like phagocyte proteinases, ROIs have important microbicidal functions, and can cause tissue damage in the cell's external micro-environment. This may be direct, for example, by lipid peroxidation of cell membranes, or indirect by oxidative inactivation of proteinase inhibitors, such as α1-Pi, which has a methionine residue within the enzyme's active site. Phagocytes are well protected against auto-oxidative damage

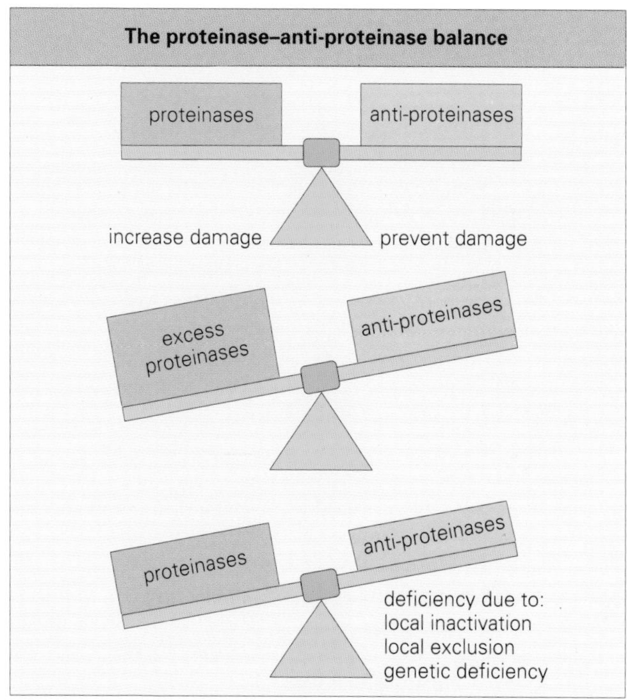

Fig 12.1 In the normal situation, a balance exists between proteinases and their inhibitors. Factors which increase the former or decrease the latter lead to lung damage.

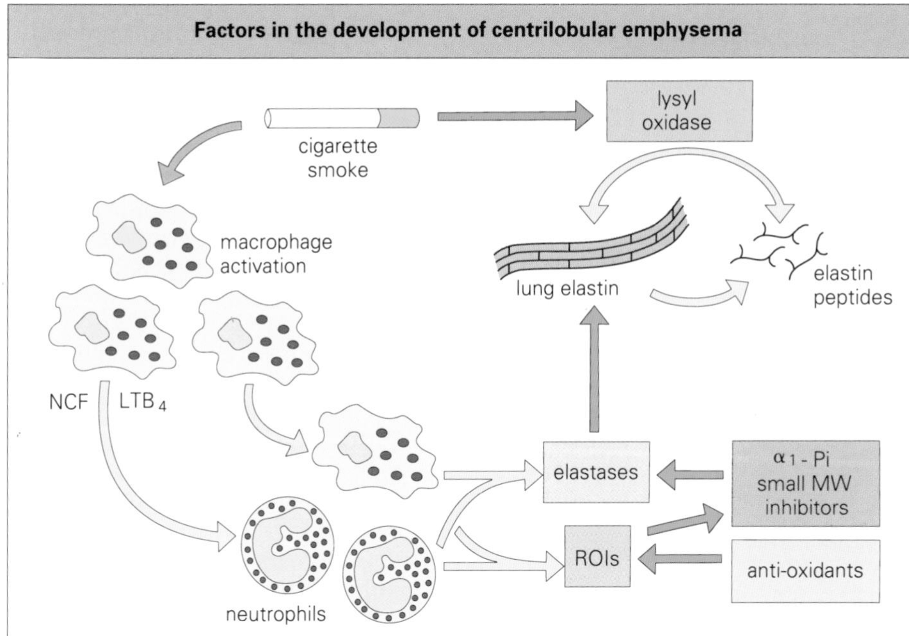

Fig. 12.2 Smoking results in increased numbers of macrophages in the terminal bronchioles. These generate chemotaxins for neutrophils (neutrophil chemotactic factor (NCF); leukotriene B_4(LTB4)); both cell types then release elastase and ROIs. Elastase cleaves interstitial elastin, but it is inhibited by α1-Pi and a number of small molecular weight serine elastase inhibitors. These may be inactivated by phagocyte derived ROIs, which in turn are inhibited by local anti-oxidants. Damaged interstitial elastin should be repaired with new elastin synthesis, but cigarette smoke can inhibit lysyl oxidase which is necessary for cross-linking of the elastin molecule.

by a wide range of intracellular anti-oxidants. Anti-oxidants are also readily found in the extracellular environment and a complex oxidant–anti-oxidant balance exists. Factors that favour uninhibited oxidant activity may promote tissue damage.

EMPHYSEMA

There is a strong association between cigarette smoking and development of emphysema. The relationship between the provocative actions of smoking and the host defence responses is complex and only a minority of smokers develop severe emphysema. Smoking is associated with substantial increases in numbers of pulmonary macrophages, which are primed for enhanced ROI release on stimulation, increased numbers of bronchoalveolar neutrophils, cigarette smoke derived free radicals, and reduced activity of lysyl oxidase (essential for cross-linking of elastin and hence its repair). All of these factors appear to be essential for the development of smoking related centrilobular emphysema (Fig.12.2).

Initial changes

The initial change in smokers is a clustering of macrophages in the terminal and respiratory bronchioles. Neutrophils are attracted and activated by a specific macrophage neutrophil chemotactic factor and arachidonic acid derivatives (LTB_4, 5-HETE). The subsequent release of neutrophil and macrophage proteinases and ROIs is responsible for elastin and connective tissue matrix damage if there are insufficient inhibitors. Although the level of proteinase inhibitors and anti-oxidants in the bronchoalveolar secretions may appear to be adequate, isolated micro-environments may occur when the phagocytes are 'adherent' to surfaces such that very localized inhibitor deficiencies may arise (Fig. 12.3).

Emphysema takes many years to develop, therefore repeated tissue damage associated with faulty repair mechanisms is probably essential in the aetiology. In this context, the effect of smoking on lysyl oxidase activity may be crucial.

ADULT RESPIRATORY DISTRESS SYNDROME (ARDS)

ARDS is a complex syndrome, giving rise to a non-cardiogenic pulmonary oedema with a mortality rate of 50–70%. In those who recover, pulmonary fibrosis may be prominent. Pathological features and the wide range of triggering factors are shown in Fig. 12.4.

Neutrophil involvement

The neutrophil is central to the pathogenesis of ARDS, sequestering in the pulmonary capillaries and passing into the alveoli, injuring the vessel wall and alveolar epithelium en route. The mechanisms of tissue damage appear to be a combination of proteolytic and oxidative processes, with neutrophil elastase making a major contribution. The initiators of neutrophil activation are not well defined. Endotoxin and complement activation are probably most important but macrophage, mast cell and platelet factors almost certainly contribute. Neutrophil proteinases promote a positive inflammatory cycle with further cleavage of complement components generating, for example, the potent anaphylatoxin, C5a. Also, proteolytic activation of

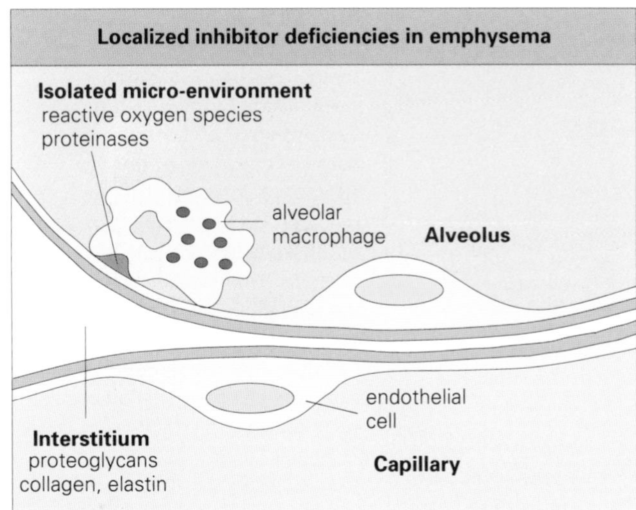

Fig. 12.3 When the phagocytes are closely adherent to epithelial surfaces or interstitial fibres, isolated 'pockets' can form between the surface and the ruffled cell membrane. Proteinase inhibitors and anti-oxidants present in adequate quantity in the alveolar/interstitial fluids may be excluded from these micro-environments, into which the cell may secrete proteinases and oxidants thus creating a local imbalance favouring proteolysis.

Pathological features & triggering factors of ARDS	
Triggering factors	**Pathological features**
septicaemia	oedema
trauma	haemorrhage
surgery	cell infiltration
infection	hyaline membrane
aspiration	thrombosis
drugs	fibrosis

Fig. 12.4 Pathological features and triggering factors of adult respiratory distress syndrome.

the kinin system generates bradykinin which exacerbates the microvascular leak.

Tumour necrosis factor

There is preliminary evidence that tumour necrosis factor (TNF) is raised in the broncho-alveolar lavage (BAL) of ARDS patients. It is known that TNF regulates adhesion molecules on capillary endothelium (ELAM and ICAM-1). If this mediator is one of the main provoking factors in ARDS, therapy with monoclonal antibodies against TNF may be helpful in the acute disease.

RESPIRATORY TRACT INFECTIONS

Infection of the respiratory tract can be considered according to the site involved in the infective process. Infection of the conducting airways (rhino-sinusitis, bronchitis) is far more common than infection of the alveolar spaces (pneumonia). The defences of the two sites are different and influence the various pathogenetic mechanisms involved.

Airway defence mechanisms

The linchpin for the protection of the bronchi against particulates (including micro-organisms) is the airway mucus and mucociliary clearance, but this is supplemented by specific and non-specific humoral and cellular immune mechanisms. The mucociliary system is non-specific, trapping and clearing inhaled particles. The speed of mucus transport is variable, being 4–10mm/min within the trachea, but slower in the more peripheral bronchi where the mucus layer is thinner.

The mucus around the cilia forms two layers: a lower, non-viscous periciliary (sol phase) fluid, and an upper visco-elastic (gel phase) mucus which is moved over the sol layer by the tips of the cilia during beating. The airway secretions contain lysozyme, lactoferrin and immunoglobulins, especially IgA, which all play an important role in mucosal protection.

Alveolar defence mechanisms

The alveolar defences are centred around cellular mechanisms. The alveolar macrophage is the resident defence cell and will remove small numbers of micro-organisms by phagocytosis. These cells may have microbicidal capacity, or may simply exert a bacteriostatic effect while additional defences are recruited. The macrophages are cleared from the alveolar space by migrating up the airway on to the mucociliary escalator, or exit via the lymphatics. Alveolar macrophage function is supported by an active humoral defence system, in which IgG is the predominant immunoglobulin. In the event of an overwhelming bacterial load, or infection with organisms the macrophage cannot readily kill, the resident alveolar macrophage plays an important role in cellular recruitment and inflammation, inducing influx of neutrophils and plasma exudation into the alveolar space (Fig. 12.5).

INFECTIVE RHINO-SINUSITIS

Chronic or recurrent rhino-sinusitis is a common problem in ENT practice and a proportion of patients undergo repeated operations without significant benefit. This group may include individuals with underlying predisposing conditions, some of which are correctable. These fall into three main groups: allergy, abnormalities of mucociliary transport and immune deficiency.

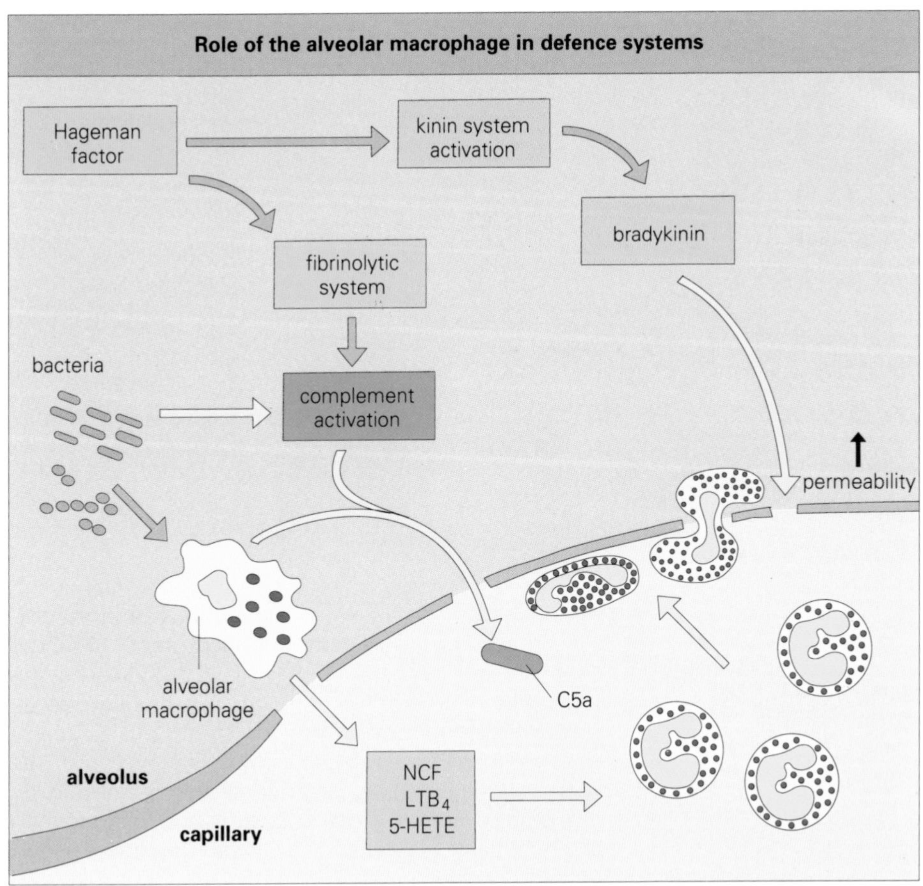

Fig. 12.5 Alveolar macrophage stimulation by bacteria results in the generation of factors chemotactic for neutrophils. Generation of C5a either by bacterial activation of the alternative pathway or by macrophage proteinase cleavage of C5, adds to the chemotactic stimulus. Neutrophils marginate in the pulmonary capillaries, attach to the endothelial cells and cross into the alveoli. Activation of the kinin system leads to increased capillary permeability.

Allergy

This is the most common predisposing cause, being present in nearly 60% of a recent series of patients.

The classical allergic nasal mucosa is swollen and boggy (see chapter 17), providing a suitable site for bacterial growth as well as reducing or obliterating the ostia which drain the sinuses. In addition, it has recently been shown that ciliary function is reduced during an allergic reaction.

When chronic allergic stimulation is present, symptoms such as sneezing and anterior rhinorrhoea are not marked; instead, the patients note nasal obstruction and post-nasal catarrh. Skin prick testing or nasal provocation will usually reveal the diagnosis; treatment of the allergic disease frequently prevents recurrence of sinusitis.

Abnormalities of mucociliary transport

Primary ciliary defects are inherited and rare, being associated in 50% of patients with situs inversus (Kartagener's syndrome). Genetic abnormalities of mucus also exist (Young's syndrome) and, like ciliary dyskinesia, occur together with bronchiectasis and infertility in most patients.

Secondary abnormalities of ciliary beating are now known to follow infection with certain organisms such as *Pseudomonas* and *Haemophilus influenzae*, being caused
12.4 by bacterial toxins. Leukotrienes decrease ciliary beat frequency *in vitro* and similar changes take place *in vivo* during an allergic reaction. Treatment is that of the underlying cause.

Immune deficiency

Hypogammaglobulinaemia (IgG <3g/litre) frequently presents with recurrent upper respiratory tract infections. Half of the individuals deficient in IgA are similarly affected. The remainder have secretory IgM which appears to be protective. IgG2-deficient persons account for some 5% of patients with chronic lower respiratory tract infections. In contrast, a recent series of chronic rhino-sinusitis patients had significantly reduced levels of IgG3 and IgG2 compared to normal controls, although no patients showed a complete lack of either subclass.

Surgery in chronic rhinosinusitis. The surgical approach to these patients now frequently involves exploration of the ostio-meatal complex of the ethmoid region, since infection of the remaining sinuses is thought to recur from inadequately treated disease there.

CHRONIC BRONCHITIS

Clinical definition

Chronic bronchitis is defined in terms of excessive mucus

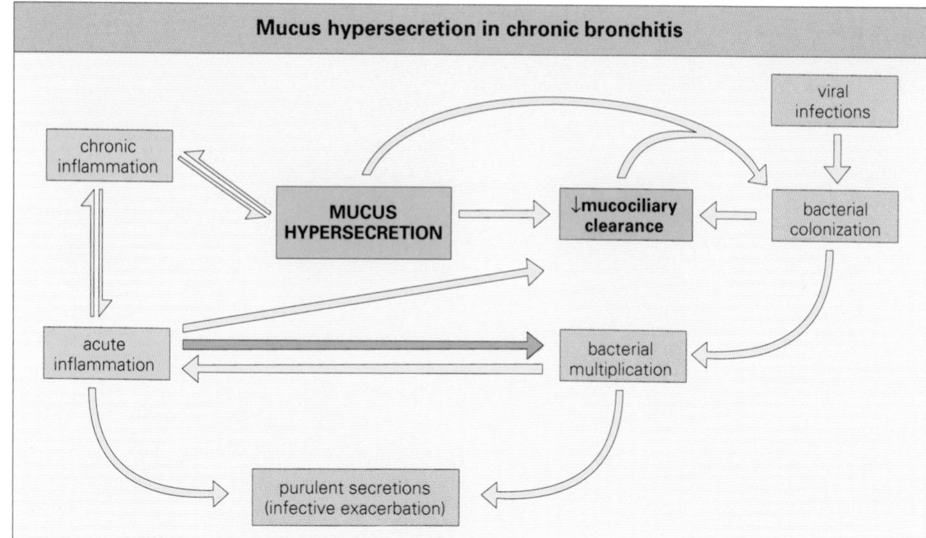

Fig. 12.6 Mucus hypersecretion slows mucociliary clearance, which predisposes to bacterial colonization of the airway epithelium. Cilio-inhibitory bacterial products further slow mucociliary clearance. Bacterial multiplication stimulates an acute inflammatory response with influx of neutrophils, which is manifest clinically as purulent sputum ('infective exacerbation') but inhibits bacterial multiplication. Simple bacterial colonization may be enough to provoke the chronic inflammatory state. Once established, however, chronic inflammation can stimulate mucus hypersecretion.

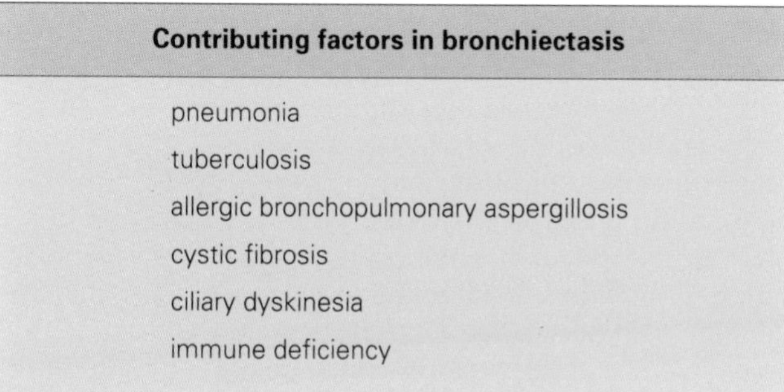

Contributing factors in bronchiectasis
pneumonia
tuberculosis
allergic bronchopulmonary aspergillosis
cystic fibrosis
ciliary dyskinesia
immune deficiency

Fig. 12.7 Contributing factors in bronchiectasis.

secretion in the bronchial tree. As a working definition, most clinicians accept a productive cough occurring on most days for at least three months in the year for a least two successive years. There is a strong association between chronic bronchitis and exposure to atmospheric pollutants, the most important in the UK being cigarette smoke. Only a minority of smokers develop significant bronchitis; on the other hand, very few chronic bronchitics are lifelong non-smokers. Chronic bronchitis is frequently associated with concomitant emphysema, but this is through the common aetiological factor of smoking.

Pathological changes

Substantial pathological changes may be seen in the airways of smokers:

- columnar epithelial cells are disorganized, with minor or gross changes to the cilia, which beat in an asynchronous fashion, or not at all;
- mucosal cells may be desquamated or replaced by squamous metaplastic epithelium;
- goblet cells are increased in number;
- submucosal glands are hyperplastic, occupying about a quarter of the bronchial wall, or occasionally almost half;
- in the absence of acute infection a chronic inflammatory infiltrate may be found within the bronchial wall.

The latter differs from the inflammation associated with asthma in that the majority of cells are lymphocytes and plasma cells. Lobectomy and pneumonectomy specimens from patients with clinical chronic bronchitis show greater inflammatory changes on mucosal surfaces of bronchi less than 2mm in diameter and around the glands and gland ducts in bronchi greater than 4mm in diameter, than from patients without bronchitis but with similar smoking histories and airflow obstruction. There appears, therefore, to be an association between mucus hypersecretion and airway inflammation (Fig. 12.6).

Bronchial mucus is approximately 95% water and 5% mucins; the latter consist of proteoglycans, lipids and glycoproteins. The cells responsible for its production are the serous and mucous cells of the submucosal glands, and the goblet and ciliated epithelial cells. Mucus secretion is markedly influenced by β-adrenoceptor agonists, vagal nerve activity, local release of neuropeptides, such as substance P and vasoactive intestinal peptide (VIP), bacterial products and neutrophil proteases.

Hypersecretion. Mucus hypersecretion and impaired mucociliary clearance allow bacteria, predominantly *H. influenzae* and *Strep. pneumoniae* to colonize the bronchi. *H. influenzae,* in particular, produces factors that further stimulate mucus secretion, induce ciliostasis and damage the mucosa, even at the stage of simple colonization of the mucosa.

BRONCHIECTASIS

Bronchiectasis is an abnormal widening of one or more branches of the bronchial tree. Usually there is no obvious precipitating event, although previous pneumonias or tuberculosis may be incriminated (Fig. 12.7). The damaged or diseased airway has impaired bacterial clearance and is predisposed to colonization by micro-organisms.

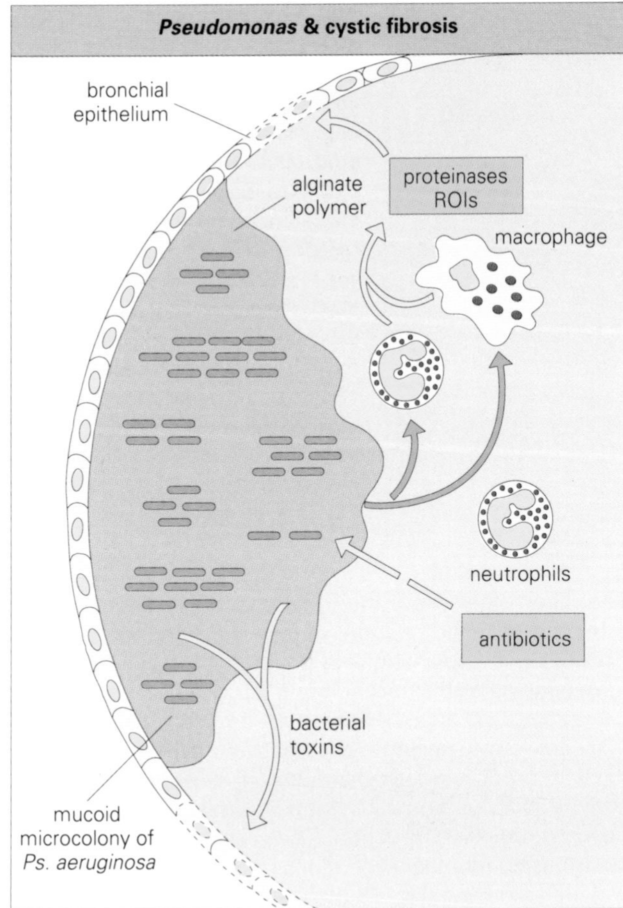

Fig. 12.8 Attachment of mucoid *Ps. aeruginosa* alginate to the bronchial mucosa allows the slow multiplication of organisms to proceed unhindered by phagocytosis. Phagocytes are activated, and release proteinases and oxidants locally, which further damage the bronchial epithelium but leave the bacteria relatively unscathed.

This triggers an inflammatory response in an attempt to eliminate the organisms.

Infectious agents

The principal organisms encountered in bronchiectasis are *Haemophilus influenzae, Staphylococcus aureus* and *Pseudomonas aeruginosa. Pseudomonas* produces a number of factors which can cause local damage. Metalloelastase is not inhibitied by α1-Pi and other serine elastase inhibitors. Pyocyanin inhibits ciliary function and disrupts epithelium, and l-hydroxyphenazine leads to rapid ciliary inhibition. Endotoxin from the Gram-negative organisms can also exert inflammatory effects, and contributes to macrophage and neutrophil activation and polyclonal elevation of immunoglobulins, which in turn favours immune complex formation.

Cystic fibrosis and *Pseudomonas*

The deleterious effect of *Pseudomonas* colonization in bronchiectasis is best exemplified by cystic fibrosis. Once colonization is established, the organism is never eliminated and significant clinical deterioration commences. Colonization of the airways is associated with mucoid transformation. These mucoid organisms establish microcolonies on the bronchial epithelium by production of an alginate-like polymer comprising homogenous or mixed blocks of mannuronic and glucuronic acids. This alginate inhibits antibiotic penetration to the organisms and is not amenable to phagocytosis by macrophages or neutrophils which, nevertheless, remain activated. The *Pseudomonas* toxins and enzymes continue to have access to the bronchial wall, which is further damaged (Fig. 12.8).

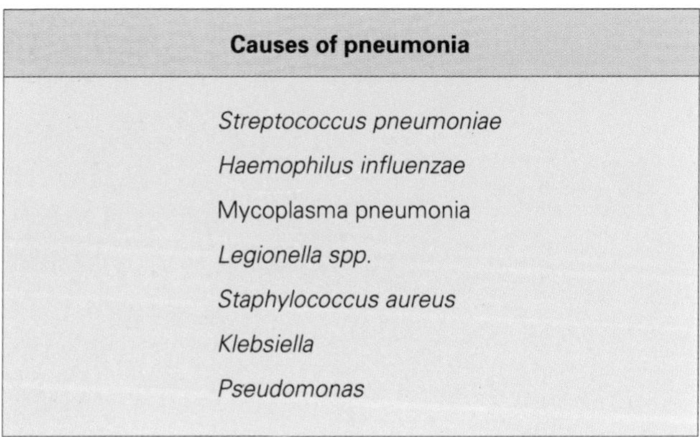

Causes of pneumonia
Streptococcus pneumoniae
Haemophilus influenzae
Mycoplasma pneumonia
Legionella spp.
Staphylococcus aureus
Klebsiella
Pseudomonas

Fig. 12.9 Causes of pneumonia.

PNEUMONIA

Pneumonia is a common cause of morbidity, hospital admission and death throughout the world. The alveolar macrophage provides the first line of defence against bacterial colonization of the alveoli, although neutrophil recruitment is necessary for the elimination of many species. The macrophage response will vary with the organism encountered. The principal causes of pneumonia are shown in Fig. 12.9. Other Gram-negative organisms rarely cause pneumonia, but are frequently encountered in the immunocompromised host.

Role of alveolar macrophages

The central role of the alveolar macrophage in co-ordinating the defences against bacterial pneumonia is illustrated in Fig. 12.10. The influx of neutrophils and the generation of toxic neutrophil and macrophage products provide the mechanisms for parenchymal lung damage, as they do in bronchiectasis. However, in pneumococcal lobar pneumonias there is frequently, but not always, an absence of tissue damage. This is due to the massive plasma exudation that occurs, providing an excess of proteinase inhibitors and anti-oxidants.

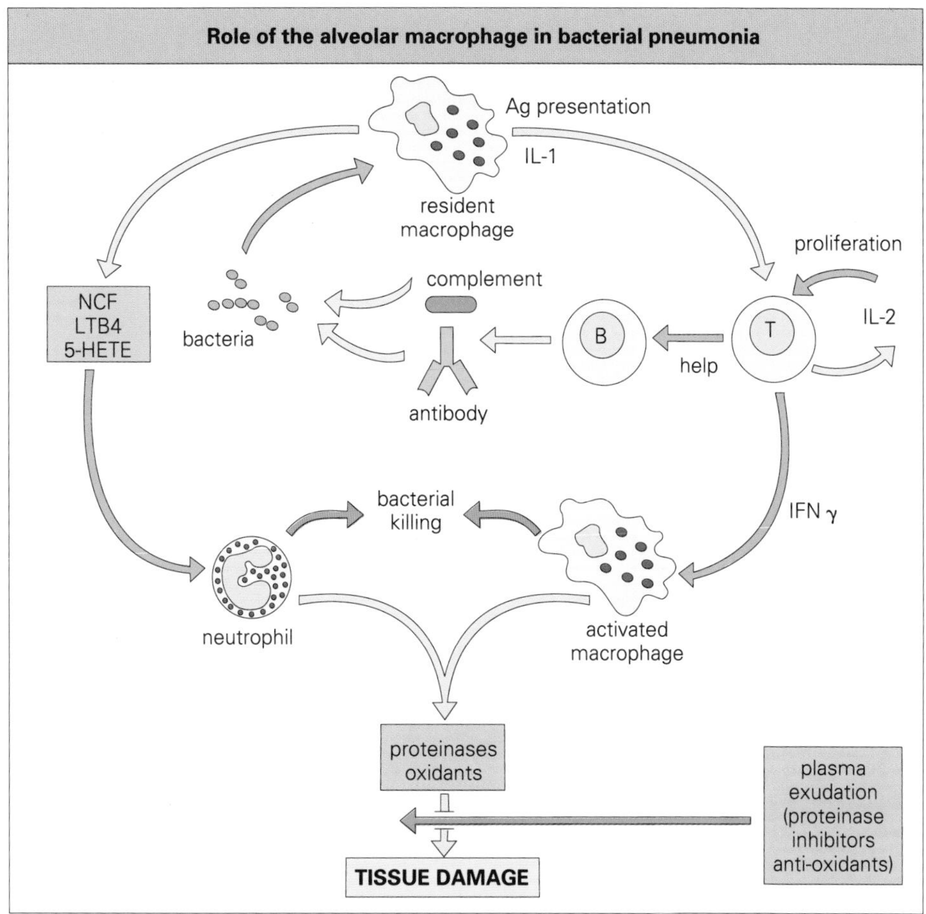

Fig. 12.10 On bacterial stimulation, the resident alveolar macrophage releases neutrophil chemotactic substances (NCF, LTB4, 5-HETE). Antigen presentation and IL-1 stimulate T cell proliferation. Local antibody synthesis, in conjunction with complement, provides opsonization of bacteria for phagocytosis by the neutrophils and macrophages which have been activated by interferon-γ (IFN_{γ}).

Causes of interstitial pulmonary fibrosis	
known aetiology	
	Cause
extrinsic allergic alveolitis	fungal spores avian proteins
pneumoconioses	asbestos silica talc ? cotton
drugs	nitrofurantoin bleomycin busulphan amiodarone
radiotherapy	ionizing radiation
berylliosis	beryllium
unknown aetiology	
pulmonary sarcoidosis histiocytosis X	cryptogenic fibrosing alveolitis

Fig. 12.11 Causes of interstitial pulmonary fibrosis.

BRONCHIAL ASTHMA

Asthma is discussed in detail in chapter 17. It is appropriate to emphasize here, however, the importance of airway inflammation in the pathogenesis of this disease. The mechanisms of the inflammatory response contrast with those operating in chronic bronchitis. The asthmatic airway is characterized by a luminal exudate, partial desquamation of the epithelium, increased proportions of goblet cells, submucosal oedema, smooth muscle hypertrophy, and an inflammatory cell infiltrate. The eosinophil is the most prominent cell type but mast cells, macrophages, lymphocytes and neutrophils are also present. The airflow obstruction is largely due to the exudate in the airway lumen and the submucosal oedema, and smooth muscle contraction adds the final insult.

INTERSTITIAL FIBROSING DISORDERS

Diagnosis

The interstitial fibrosing disorders are conditions in which fibrotic thickening of the alveolar walls occurs with little involvement of the conducting airways. There are numerous causes (Fig. 12.11), and the relative frequency of each

Disease associations in cryptogenic fibrosing alveolitis
rheumatoid arthritis
SLE
systemic sclerosis
mixed connective tissue disease
Sjögren's syndrome
polymyositis
chronic active hepatitis
ulcerative colitis

Fig. 12.12 Disease associations in cryptogenic fibrosing alveolitis/idiopathic pulmonary fibrosis (IPF).

Uses of bronchoalveolar lavage	
research tool	investigation of: cells, proteins & lipids
diagnostic tool	microbiological culture in: immunosuppressed patients possible TB
adjunct to diagnosis	study of BAL cells in: interstitial lung disease

Fig 12.13 Uses of bronchoalveolar lavage.

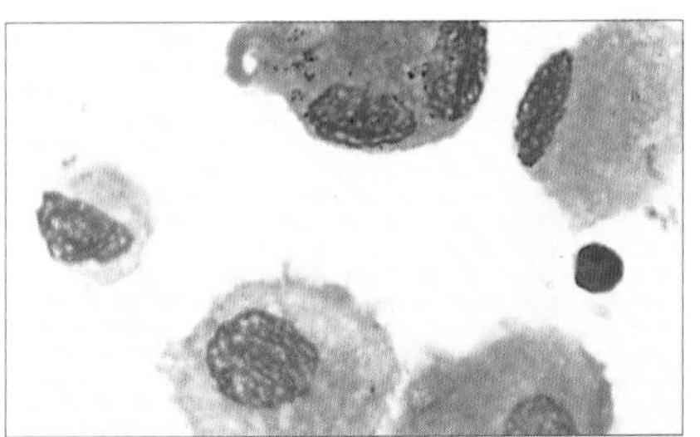
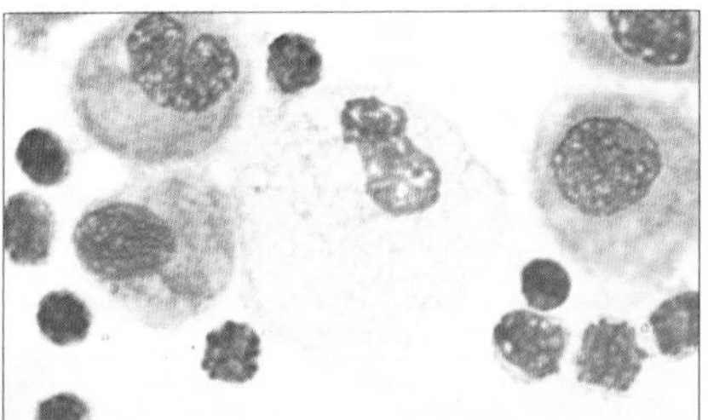
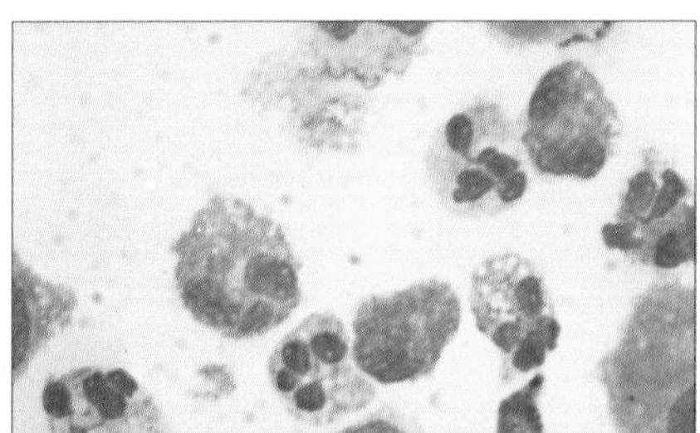

Fig. 12.14 Cytocentrifuge preparations of bronchoalveolar lavage cells. Left: normal subject (non-smoker). The majority of cells are alveolar macrophages with a smaller number of lymphocytes. Middle: sarcoidosis patient. There is a substantial increase in the proportion of lymphocytes. These are activated T cells. Most alveolar macrophages have a 'foamy' appearance. Right: fibrosing alveolitis patient. There are increased proportions of neutrophils and eosinophils. Often these cells are substantially degranulated.

disease varies with occupational exposure, geographical location, and area of interest in internal medicine. In many instances the provocative agent is readily identified and should be removed. In other cases a careful search of the patient's environment will yield the causative agent. Two important interstitial disorders, sarcoidosis and cryptogenic fibrosing alveolitis (CFA) are of unknown aetiology, although 20–30% of cases of CFA are associated with connective tissue or autoimmune diseases (Fig. 12.12).

Lung biopsy. Lung biopsy is an important investigation in most patients with interstitial disorders. For those in whom no aetiological agent is apparent, it may establish a diagnosis: even for those with an apparent aetiological agent it may allow clarification of differential diagnoses. For some disorders, transbronchial lung biopsy may yield diagnostic material (for example granulomata in patients with sarcoid or EAA), but for others open lung biopsy is necessary to obtain sufficient tissue for the pathologist (for example CFA). Differential counts of cells obtained by broncho-alveolar lavage act as a useful diagnostic adjunct in some cases.

Broncho-alveolar lavage. Broncho-alveolar lavage (BAL) is performed by wedging the tip of the fibreoptic bronchoscope in a segmental or sub-segmental bronchus. Aliquots of warmed, physiological saline are then instilled and aspirated via the biopsy channel. The recovered BAL fluid contains representative lipids, proteins and cells from the broncho-alveolar space of the lung segment lavaged. The uses of BAL are shown in Fig. 12.13. In the interstitial lung diseases abnormal patterns of BAL cells are seen; there are increased proportions of lymphocytes in sarcoidosis and EAA, and of neutrophils and eosinophils in CFA (Fig. 12.14).

Mechanisms of pulmonary fibrosis

Occurrence. Pulmonary fibrosis occurs in a wide variety of respiratory disorders. When associated with a relatively localized process such as infection (tuberculosis, pyogenic pneumonia) it has been viewed, perhaps naively, as a repair mechanism similar to scar formation after cutaneous injury. When it is part of a generalized lung disorder, such as fibrosing alveolitis, it is again following tissue injury, and so may be viewed as an aberrant repair mechanism. However, in these circumstances the fibrotic process is usually progressive and there is a concomitant, persisting lung inflammation and tissue injury. The generalized pulmonary fibrosis is then associated with several factors (Fig. 12.15).

Process of fibrosis. The process of fibrosis involves the lung interstitium, intercellular matrix and several cell types, but predominantly fibroblasts and macrophages. Neutrophils, eosinophils and lymphocytes may be vital components of the associated inflammatory process.

Fibronectin and macrophages. Alveolar macrophages, when appropriately activated, release fibronectin and alveolar macrophage derived growth factor (AMDGF). Fibronectin is chemotactic for fibroblasts and, in association with AMDGF, also causes fibroblasts to proliferate and produce collagen (Fig. 12.16). Fibronectin and platelet derived growth factor, provide competence signals to drive fibroblasts into the G1 phase of the cell cycle, and AMDGF the progression signal. Recent evidence suggests

Factors associated with pulmonary fibrosis

persistent antigen stimulation
- exogenous
- endogenous — autoimmune

inability to 'switch off' inflammation

inability to inhibit fibroblast stimulation

Fig. 12.15 Factors associated with pulmonary fibrosis.

that AMDGF reacts with the insulin growth factor (IGF-1) receptor and probably is IGF-1.

Fibroblasts and lymphokines. Fibroblasts are also subject to positive stimulation from macrophage cytokines IL-1 and TNFα and lymphocyte cytokines TNFβ and IFNγ. Synergistic effects occur between the various cytokines. Other macrophage products, PGE_2, LTB_4 and IFNα can provide inhibitory signals to the fibroblast. Thus, for individual patients the balance between stimulatory and inhibitory fibroblast signals may determine whether pulmonary fibrosis ensues.

Treatment

Present treatment is with the immunosuppressive agents prednisolone, azathioprine and cyclophosphamide and this underlines the importance of reducing the continuing inflammatory response that provides activation of the macrophages and fibroblasts. In fibrosing alveolitis there is sensitization of lymphocytes to collagen breakdown products and macrophage activation appears dependent on both T cell and immune complex stimulation (Fig. 12.17). The therapy is thus aimed at the macrophage–lymphocyte interactions.

EXTRINSIC ALLERGIC ALVEOLITIS

Classification

Extrinsic allergic alveolitis (hypersensitivity pneumonitis) is an inflammatory granulomatous response of the walls of the alveoli and terminal bronchioles to antigens in inhaled organic dusts. There is a wide range of causes of EAA (see

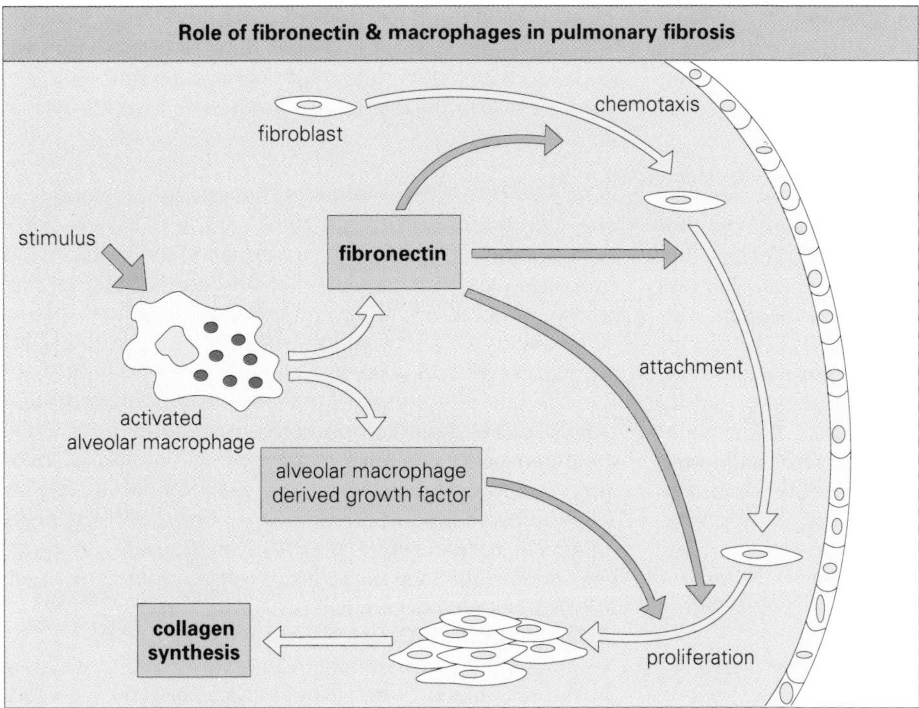

Fig. 12.16 Under the appropriate stimulation, activated alveolar macrophages secrete fibronectin and alveolar macrophage derived growth factor (AMDGF). Fibronectin induces fibroblast chemotaxis and attachment and, in conjunction with AMDGF, promotes fibroblast proliferation.

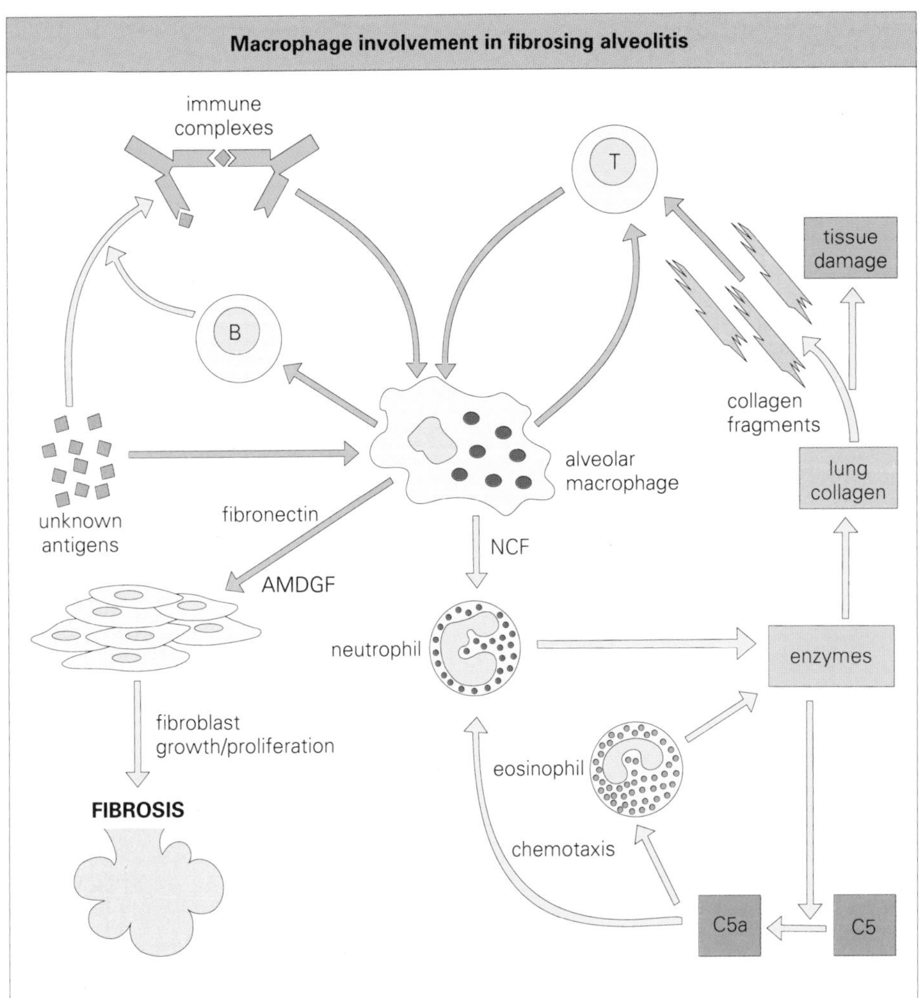

Fig. 12.17 The offending antigen(s) in CFA are unknown. They may form immune complexes with local antibodies. The complexes and T cell products (IFNγ) can then activate other macrophages, which release chemotactic factors for neutrophils and eosinophils. This is further enhanced by phagocyte enzymes generating C5a. Collagen fragments can be immunogenic and stimulate more T cells that, in turn, prime further macrophages. A positive inflammatory loop can thus be established even if the initiating, unknown antigens are no longer present.

chapter 18), the most common forms of which are farmer's lung and bird-fancier's lung (Fig.12.18). Clinically, three forms of allergic alveolitis are recognized (Fig. 12.19), but each may merge into the other.

Pathology

Pathologically there may be diffuse infiltrates of lymphocytes, plasma cells and macrophages in conjunction with rather poorly-formed granulomata. In the fibrotic stage, inflammatory infiltrates may be less pronounced. EAA was initially thought to be an immune complex disease, with serum precipitating antibodies a consistent feature. This concept was supported by the Arthus response seen when patients were skin tested with the relevant antigen, and by the onset of respiratory symptoms 4–6 hours after inhalational challenge. However, asymptomatic individuals with the relevant environmental exposure frequently have precipitating antibodies and vasculitis is an uncommon finding. This calls into question the importance of pulmonary immune complexes, especially as there is evidence of T cell, B cell and macrophage activation.

Acute illness. In the acute phase of the illness there are

(sometimes substantial) increases of T cell proportions in BAL with a relative increase in $CD8^+$ cells giving a reduced CD4:CD8 ratio. The picture is confused in that asymptomatic individuals with similar antigen exposure may demonstrate the same changes in lymphocytes in BAL fluid.

Funçtion of BAL lymphocytes. Functional assessment of the BAL lymphocytes can differentiate between symptomatic and asymptomatic individuals. For example, BAL lymphocytes from symptomatic pigeon breeders may show a marked increase in proliferation to both phytohaemagglutinin and pigeon serum compared with asymptomatic breeders. Also BAL T cells from asymptomatic individuals can suppress the proliferative response of autologous peripheral blood cells to pigeon serum, unlike the BAL cells from symptomatic patients. It appears, therefore, that symptomatic disease is associated with the loss of suppressor activity in the lungs, but the mechanisms involved are unclear.

ALLERGIC BRONCHOPULMONARY ASPERGILLOSIS

In the UK, allergic bronchopulmonary mycoses are best

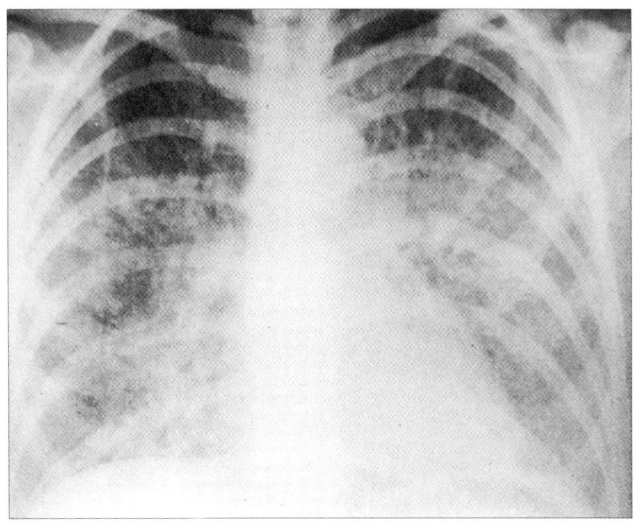

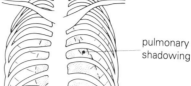

Fig. 12.18 Acute extrinsic allergic alveolitis in a bird fancier, characterized by widespread pulmonary shadowing. Courtesy of Dr A J Newman Taylor.

Clinical forms of allergic alveolitis			
Features	**Acute**	**Subacute**	**Chronic**
antigen exposure	short, heavy	low level	?
cough	+	+	+
breathlessness	+	+	+
fever	+	+	-
fatigue	-	±	±
weight loss	-	+	+
time	4 – 6 h	chronic	chronic
fibrosis	-	-	+
progression	-	-	+

Fig. 12.19 Clinical forms of allergic alveolitis. The chronic form is indistinguishable from other causes of diffuse pulmonary fibrosis and may progress after cessation of exposure to the antigen.

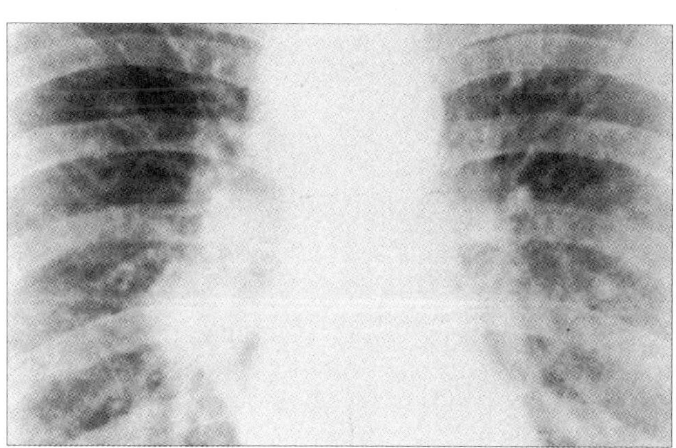

Fig. 12.20 Coccidioidomycosis. There is mottling throughout both lung fields (miliary dissemination) and right hilar lymphadenopathy. Courtesy of Dr I D Starke.

represented by allergic bronchopulmonary aspergillosis (ABPA). ABPA is almost always associated with asthma but usually develops some years after the asthma. The fleeting pulmonary infiltrates and elevated blood eosinophilia may or may not be associated with deterioration of the patient's asthma. ABPA favours the development of a proximal bronchiectasis and permanent radiological changes may occur relatively early in the disease. Once ABPA is recognized, regular oral steroid therapy of low to moderate dose is given in an attempt to control the inflammatory mechanisms responsible for the tissue damage and bronchiectasis.

Antibodies

Aspergillus-specific IgG and IgE may be markedly elevated, and the presence of precipitating antibodies is common. Circulating immune complexes may also be found. Lymphocytes of most ABPA patients are sensitized and will proliferate in response to *Aspergillus* antigens. However, neither these proliferative responses nor levels of precipitating antibodies correlate with disease activity. The mechanisms of tissue damage are uncertain but are probably eosinophil and neutrophil mediated.

Other fungal lung diseases

In the USA *Histoplasma capsulatum, Coccidioides imitis* and *Blastomyces dermatitidis* are the fungi responsible for many of the pulmonary infections.

The most common manifestation of primary coccidioidomycosis is cough and fever, sometimes with chest pain and less commonly with erythema nodosum. The chest X-ray shows patchy infiltrates with hilar lymphadenopathy in 20% of cases. Granuloma formation with fibrosis and calcification can occur. Miliary coccidioidomycosis is the result of haematogenous spread (Fig. 12.20).

Histoplasmosis arises as a result of spore inhalation. There is an influx of PMNs, followed by monocytes. The organism grows within these cells, stimulating a pneumonitis followed by fungaemia. With the development of cell-mediated immunity, an intense inflammatory response occurs at the initial site of infection in the lung and regional lymph nodes (Fig. 12.21).

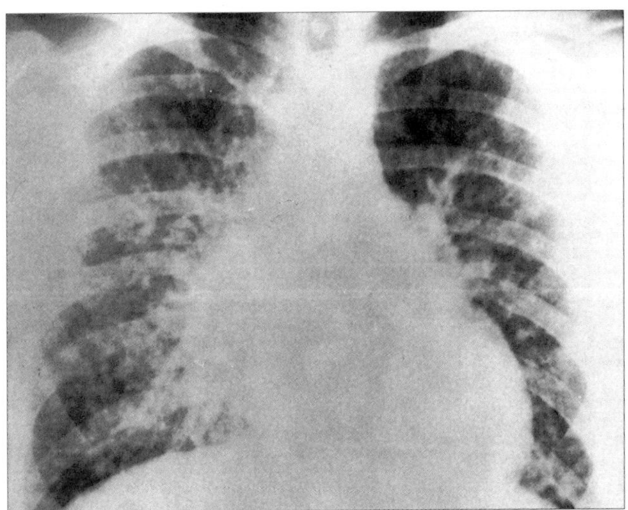

Fig. 12.21 *H. capsulatum* bronchopneumonia. Widespread, small nodular lesions are evident. This is the most common appearance of acute histoplasmosis at presentation. Courtesy of Dr I D Starke.

Classification & causes of granulomatous pulmonary disorders	
infectious	mycobacteria, fungi
unknown	sarcoidosis, histiocytosis X
extrinsic	allergic alveolitis
chemical	beryllium, talc
neoplasia	carcinoma, lymphoma
vasculitis	Wegener's, Churg-Strauss syndrome
genetic	chronic granulomatous disease

Fig. 12.22 Classification and causes of granulomatous pulmonary disorders.

GRANULOMATOUS PULMONARY DISORDERS

Occurrence

Granuloma formation may be seen in association with a wide variety of pulmonary disorders (Fig. 12.22). Such an inflammatory response may occur through a number of different mechanisms including exposure to organic, poorly degradable antigens (tuberculosis, EAA), large antigen–antibody complexes formed in antibody excess, inorganic particulates (talc), or as a consequence of a defect in phagocytic cell function (chronic granulomatous disease of childhood — CGDC).

For all these mechanisms some persistence of the initiating agent is required, but the type of granuloma varies with the nature of the agent. Thus an inert particle incites the formation of a granuloma consisting almost entirely of macrophages around it, whereas the majority of agents trigger a process characterized by an active cell-mediated immune amplification and specific macrophage activation. Tuberculosis and sarcoidosis provide good examples of the immunological processes involved.

Mechanisms of granuloma formation

Macrophage and T cell activation appear to be central to granuloma formation. In sarcoidosis, macrophages spontaneously release IL-1, and on stimulation release enhanced quantities of TNF and ROIs. T cells demonstrate active proliferation and spontaneous secretion of several cytokines such as IL-2, IFNγ , monocyte chemotactic factor, and macrophage migration inhibition factor. A likely sequence of events is shown in Fig. 12.23.

Vitamin D3. Recent data have also emphasized the role of

12.12 1,25-dihydroxyvitamin D_3 (1,25-$(OH)_2$ D_3 — calcitriol). Macrophages, probably under the influence of IFNγ acquire 25-hydroxyvitamin D_3, α1-hydroxylase activity. This accounts for the hypercalcaemia and hypercalciuria seen in sarcoidosis and, more rarely, in TB (a phenomenon encountered more frequently in the past when vitamin D was administered as part of the therapy!). The more important effects of calcitriol are local and immunoregulatory (Fig. 12.24).

Pulmonary fibrosis

The frequency of resolution of active pulmonary tuberculosis in the pre-chemotherapy era attests to the ability of the granulomatous inflammatory response to contain and kill *M. tuberculosis*, presumably through the mechanisms described above. However, this resolution was often at the expense of extensive tissue destruction. Pulmonary fibrosis at the site of disease activity (principally apical) in TB was found frequently, but is now much less common with the use of effective chemotherapy early in the disease. It is found in 10–20% of cases of pulmonary sarcoidosis, the exact incidence varying with the nature of the reporting centre (primary or secondary referral centre), and the racial origin of the patients; West Indians and North American Blacks have the most severe disease, followed by Celts. The development of fibrosis appears to rely upon specific macrophage activation.

Tuberculosis

The intensity of the granulomatous response in TB may not relate to the number of organisms present but to the degree of hypersensitivity to *M. tuberculosis* antigens. Thus in tuberculous lymphadenopathy or pleural effusion, organisms may be infrequent and indeed lymphadenopathy may worsen after therapy has started, suggesting that the death of organisms and release of antigens enhances

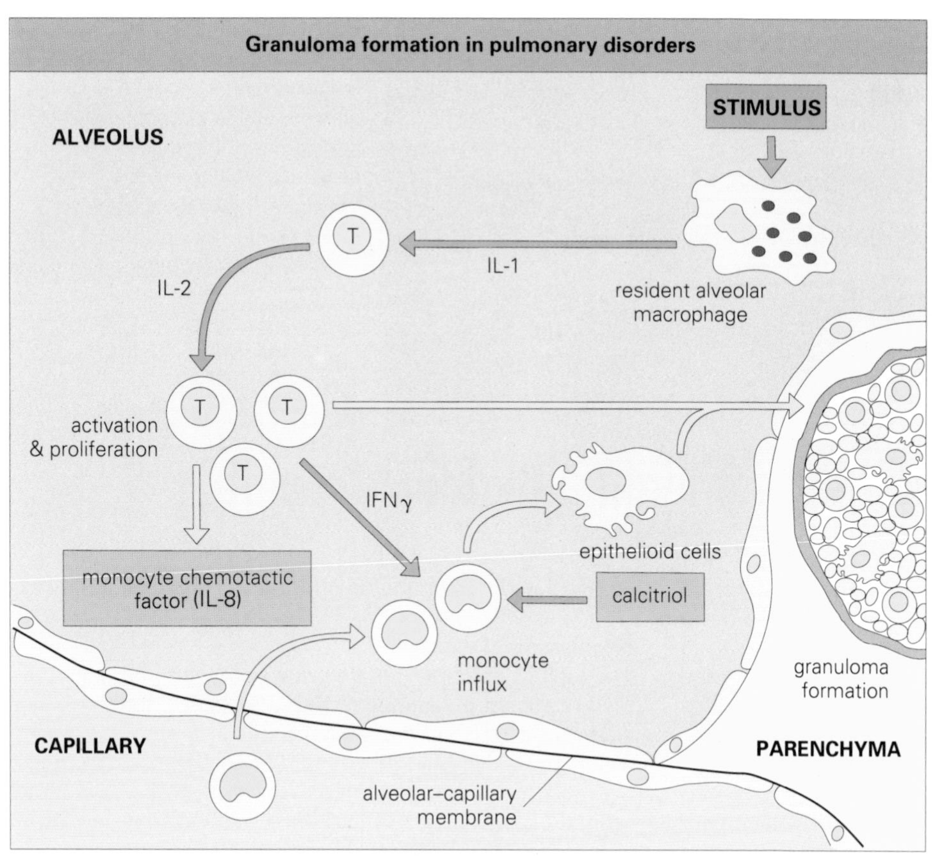

Fig. 12.23 Following stimulation of pulmonary macrophages there is an IL-1, IL-2 driven T cell activation and proliferation. Monocytes are attracted from the pulmonary circulation by monocyte chemotactic factor (IL-8). On activation by IFNγ, and under the influence of calcitriol, the monocytes differentiate to epithelioid cells and, in conjunction with T cells, form granulomata.

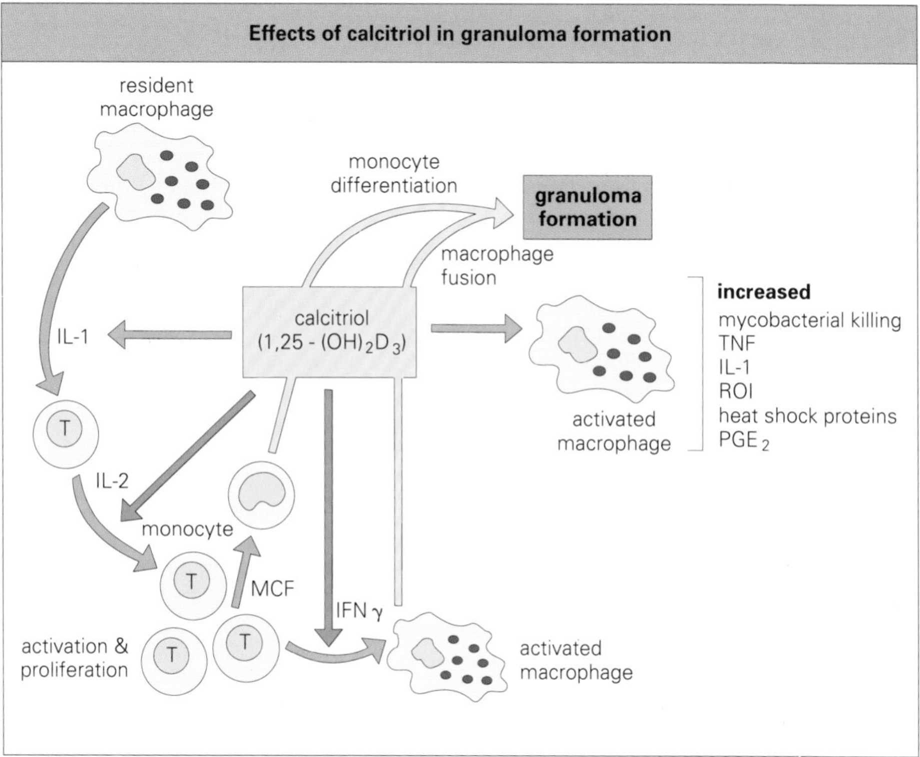

Fig. 12.24 Calcitriol is produced by virtue of specific macrophage activation in sarcoidosis and tuberculosis. It promotes monocyte differentiation and macrophage fusion, as well as enhancing a variety of macrophage functions, including mycobacterial killing. It also has an inhibitory effect on T cell cytokine release. MCF = monocyte chemotactic factor.

Classification of sarcoidosis		
Type I	**Type II**	**Type III**
hilar lymphadenopathy	hilar lymphadenopathy interstitial shadows	interstitial shadows fibrosis

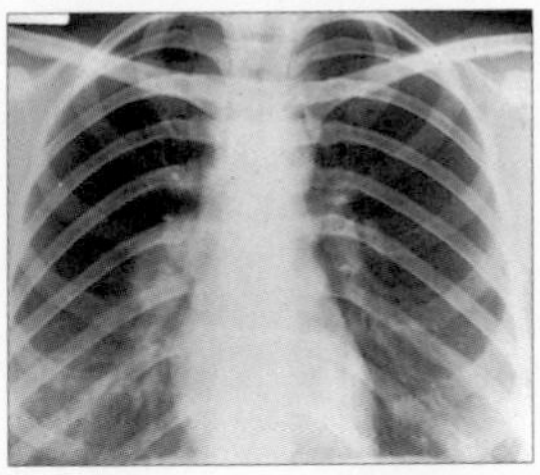

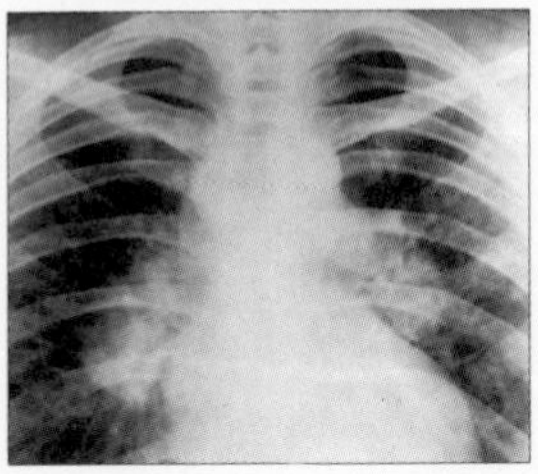

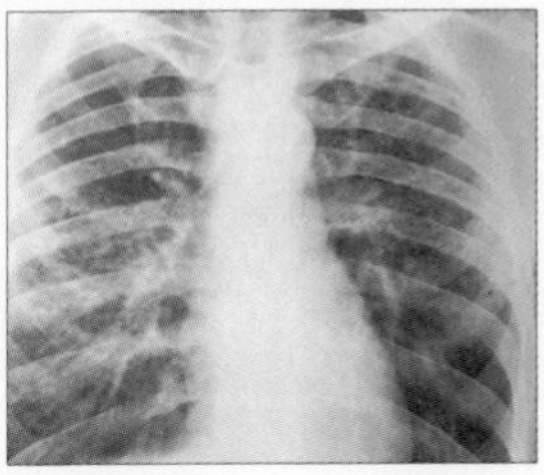

Fig. 12.25 Type I is characterized by hilar node enlargement, usually bilateral. Type II shows hilar gland enlargement with peripheral lung lesions. Type III is characterized by parenchymal lung lesions only. Courtesy of Professor M Turner-Warwick.

the hypersensitivity response. Extrapulmonary tuberculosis, predominantly TB lymphadenitis, is encountered in up to 40% of cases amongst the Asian immigrant population in the UK. Whether this reflects subtle differences in the antigenicity of the *M. tuberculosis* strains or of host immunity, or both, is unclear.

Sarcoidosis

Sarcoidosis is a generalized disorder although the major impact is usually on the lungs. Pulmonary sarcoidosis is conventionally classified by the radiological changes into types I, II, and III (Fig. 12.25). These have relevance in statistical prediction of spontaneous resolution of the disease, with some 90% of cases with type I disease resolving within two years, but only 60% of pulmonary infiltrates clearing in the same time period; however they do not reflect the immunological processes. For example, BAL reveals the presence of a lymphocytic (predominantly $CD4^+$ cell) alveolitis even in patients with no radiological evidence of pulmonary infiltrates.

Since the initiating factor(s) in sarcoidosis are unknown, specific treatment is not available. Non-specific therapy with corticosteroids is appropriate for relief of symptoms and is mandatory when hypercalcaemia and CNS disease is present, but there are no data to suggest that such treatment has any effect on established pulmonary fibrosis.

IMMUNE COMPLEX MEDIATED AND RELATED DISORDERS

The broad categorization of many pulmonary disorders by one of their prominent clinicopathological features sometimes obscures the immunopathological overlap between disease groupings. Immune complexes have important initiating or promoting roles in the pulmonary vasculitides, pulmonary eosinophilia, granulomatous diseases and the connective tissue disorders. Thus a single disease entity may display features of several conventional categories. For example, Churg-Strauss syndrome is a vasculitis which is associated with granuloma formation and eosinophilia.

Mechanisms of damage

The lung is, perhaps, uniquely susceptible to immune complex mediated inflammatory responses since antigens have access not only by the vascular but also by the inhaled route. There is local antibody formation particularly in relation to bronchial-associated lymphoid tissue and large numbers of alveolar and interstitial macrophages are available for immune complex activation. Airway immune complexes appear important for macrophage activation in allergic bronchopulmonary aspergillosis and possibly also in extrinsic allergic alveolitis (see chapter 18).

PULMONARY VASCULITIS

The pulmonary vasculitides are heterogeneous; the radiological appearance may be of infiltrates (fleeting or persistent) nodules, or cavitating lesions. Pathologically, necrosis, granulomata and haemorrhage are seen. They usually occur as part of a multi-organ disease, although Wegener's granulomatosis and Churg–Strauss syndrome may apparently be confined to the lung in some instances. Pulmonary involvement with polyarteritis nodosa is not infrequent but the major brunt of the disease is extra-pulmonary. Pulmonary involvement may occur in the hypersensitivity vasculitides (including Henoch-Schönlein purpura), but is uncommon. Behçet's disease is a leucocytoclastic vasculitis, like the hypersensitivity vasculitides and occasionally involves the pulmonary vessels including the arteries, leading to aneurysm formation.

Giant cell arteritis may involve the pulmonary vessels and although frequently not clinically recognized, pulmonary artery involvement in Takayasu's arteritis has been reported in as many as 50% of patients, giving rise to vessel stenosis and occlusion and pulmonary hypertension. The principal pulmonary vasculitides, however, are Wegener's granulomatosis and Churg-Strauss syndrome (allergic granulomatosis).

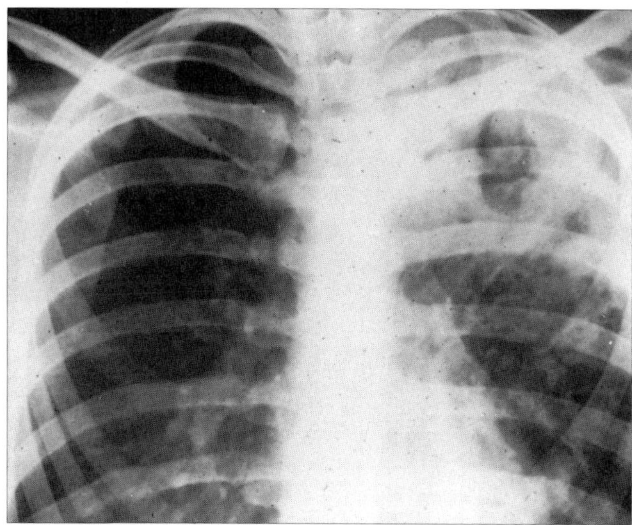

Fig. 12.26 Wegener's granulomatosis. A large lesion is present in the left apex, with extensive necrotic cavitation. Courtesy of Professor M Turner-Warwick.

Classification of pulmonary eosinophilia	
identifiable cause	
Allergic bronchopulmonary mycoses	
Aspergillus fumigatus	*Curvularia lunata*
Candida albicans	*Dreschlera hawaiiensis*
helminth infections	
Ascaris lumbricoides	*Schistosoma* spp.
microfilaria	*Toxocara canis*
drugs	
nitrofurantoin	penicillins
sodium aminosalicylate	tetracycline
sulphonamides (including sulphasalazine)	
unknown cause	
cryptogenic pulmonary eosinophilia	
allergic granulomatoses (Churg-Strauss syndrome)	

Fig. 12.27 Of the bronchopulmonary mycoses, *Aspergillus* is the most important.

Wegener's granulomatosis

The typical pulmonary findings are nodular infiltrates, which may be fleeting, and cavitating lesions (Fig. 12.26). Pathologically, there is a necrotizing granulomatous vasculitis with an infiltrate of neutrophils, lymphocytes (mainly T cells), plasma cells, macrophages and giant cells.

Diagnosis depends on lung biopsy although recent assessment of neutrophil anti-cytoplasmic antibody in the peripheral blood suggests that this is a relatively specific finding (see chapter 30). Diagnosis is important since immunosuppressive therapy with prednisolone and cyclophosphamide can induce complete remission in over 90% of patients, which contrasts markedly with a median survival time of five months in untreated patients.

Churg-Strauss syndrome

This is characterized by asthma, peripheral eosinophilia and systemic vasculitis, and radiologically by pulmonary infiltrates. It usually responds to corticosteroids alone, but evidence of vasculitis is essential to differentiate it from other causes of pulmonary eosinophilia. The prominence of necrotic lesions together with sparing of the kidneys and small vessel vasculitis distinguishes it from typical polyarteritis nodosa.

Immune alveolar haemorrhage

Immune alveolar haemorrhage is usually due to anti-basement membrane antibody disease (Goodpasture's syndrome), vasculitis (Wegener's, polyarteritis nodosa) or connective tissue disease, especially SLE, but may occur with idiopathic rapidly progressive glomerulonephritis and following certain drugs (*d*-penicillamine) or chemicals.

CONNECTIVE TISSUE DISORDERS

Pulmonary involvement in the connective tissue disorders (see chapter 6) is not uncommon and may take a variety of forms. Immunofluorescent studies of lung biopsies demonstrate deposits of IgG and IgM in fibrosing alveolitis and immune complexes can be detected in BAL fluid, so immune complex macrophage activation may have an important role.

Fibrosing alveolitis and rheumatoid arthritis

Fibrosing alveolitis is found in association with rheumatoid arthritis (see chapter 5) SLE, systemic sclerosis, Sjögren's syndrome and polymyositis. The pattern of non-organ-specific autoantibody is no different to that occuring in the same disease without lung involvement. Fibrosing alveolitis in association with rheumatoid arthritis may precede or follow the development of arthritis, but generally the two processes are relatively close temporally. Pathologically there is the same variability as with cryptogenic fibrosing alveolitis, ranging from an intense lymphocytic inflammatory infiltrate to fibrosis with destroyed alveolar architecture and honeycombing.

PULMONARY EOSINOPHILIA

The term 'pulmonary eosinophilia' is used to describe a group of diseases characterized by infiltration of the parenchyma with eosinophils, usually manifest as fleeting infiltrates on the chest X-ray, and characteristically associated with a raised blood eosinophil count. The classification is based on aetiology which determines treatment, but in several instances the cause is unknown (Fig. 12.27).

PATHOGENESIS

The immunopathological response depends on the route by which the aetiological agent reaches the lungs. Thus inhaled fungal spores give rise to a bronchocentric response and drugs or helminths entering via the pulmonary circulation give an angiocentric response. The degree of blood eosinophilia varies with the cause and with the total serum IgE. In general, IgE and the eosinophil count are elevated proprotionately in helminth infections, the IgE disproportionately elevated in allergic bronchopulmonary mycoses and the eosinophil count disproportionately elevated in cryptogenic pulmonary eosinophilia.

Tropical eosinophilia

On a worldwide basis, tropical eosinophilia is the most important type of pulmonary eosinophilia. It is helminth induced and presents as a syndrome of malaise, weight loss, fever, cough and breathlessness. The microfilariae within the pulmonary parenchyma stimulate the production of specific IgE. Subsequently microfilarial antigens reacting with IgE release mast cell derived chemotactic factors for eosinophils. In addition some helminthic products are specifically chemotactic for eosinophils. The mechanisms of drug hypersensitivity which induce blood and tissue eosinophilia are less clear, but immune complex mediated complement activation, producing C3a and C5a, and subsequent mast cell degranulation may be relevant.

Eosinophilic pneumonia

With eosinophilic pneumonia the degree of eosinophilia may be marked and its onset is often accompanied by non-specific systemic symptoms such as anorexia, malaise and fever. More than half the patients have, or develop, asthma. X-ray changes may be those of pulmonary oedema or of confluent, non-segmental peripheral shadowing, particularly in the upper zones, when it may be mistaken for TB. BAL has shown:

- the presence of eosinophils in radiologically unaffected parts of the lung;
- increased numbers of neutrophils and lymphocytes in addition to eosinophils.

The pathogenetic mechanisms are far from clear but clinically there is a good response to relatively low dose steroids. Maintenance immunosuppression is required until spontaneous remission occurs.

FURTHER READING

Brewis RAL, Gibson GJ, Geddes DM, eds. *Respiratory medicine.* London: Baillière Tindall, 1990.

Hoiby N, Koch C. *Pseudomonas aeruginosa* infection in cystic fibrosis and its management. *Thorax.* 1990; **45**: 881–884.

Kelley J. Cytokines of the lung. *Am Rev Respir Dis.* 1990; **141**: 765–788.

Kunkel SL, Chensue SW, Streiter RM, Lynch JP, Remick DG. Cellular and molecular aspects of granulomatous inflammation. *Am J Respir Cell Mol Biol.* 1989; **1**: 439–447.

Sarosi GA, Davies SF, eds. *Fungal diseases of the lung.* Orlando: Grune & Stratton, 1986.

Sibille Y, Reynolds HY. Macrophages and polymorphonuclear neutrophils in lung defense and injury. *Am Rev Respir Dis.* 1990; **141**: 471–501.

Vaillet J, Minna JD. Dominant oncogenes and tumour suppresor genes in the pathogenesis of lung cancer. *Am J Respir Cell Mol Biol.* 1990; **2**: 225–232.

13

Ophthalmic disorders

INTRODUCTION

The exposed nature of the eye and the transparency of the cornea, lens and vitreous make the eye a unique model for observing the natural history of disease processes. Many ocular diseases are poorly described in immunopathological terms, particularly in the earlier stages of the disease. This is because only a limited number of ocular sites may be biopsied without potentially serious problems.

A variety of characteristics make the eye immunologically special:

- there is no lymphatic drainage apart from the conjunctiva ;
- the normal cornea is an immunologically privileged site, but this privilege is lost when the cornea is vascularized;
- several antigens isolated from the normal eye are capable of inducing disease;
- anterior chamber associated immune deviation occurs, the significance of which is uncertain;
- although intraocular components are protected from the bloodstream by blood vitreous and blood aqueous barriers, the choroidal system is exposed by virtue of its capillaries with wide fenestrations;
- retinal components are of neural origin and consequently neurotrophic processes often have retinal manifestations.

PROTECTION OF THE EYE

Physical, innate and immunological factors are involved in the protection of the eye.

PHYSICAL FACTORS

The major importance of the physical protective factors is frequently not appreciated until there is a defect in the system. The orbital bony structure, the lids, tears, corneal epithelium, and the tight endothelial junctions of the intraocular retinal vasculature and retinal pigment epithelium contribute to the exclusion of noxious agents (Fig. 13.1).

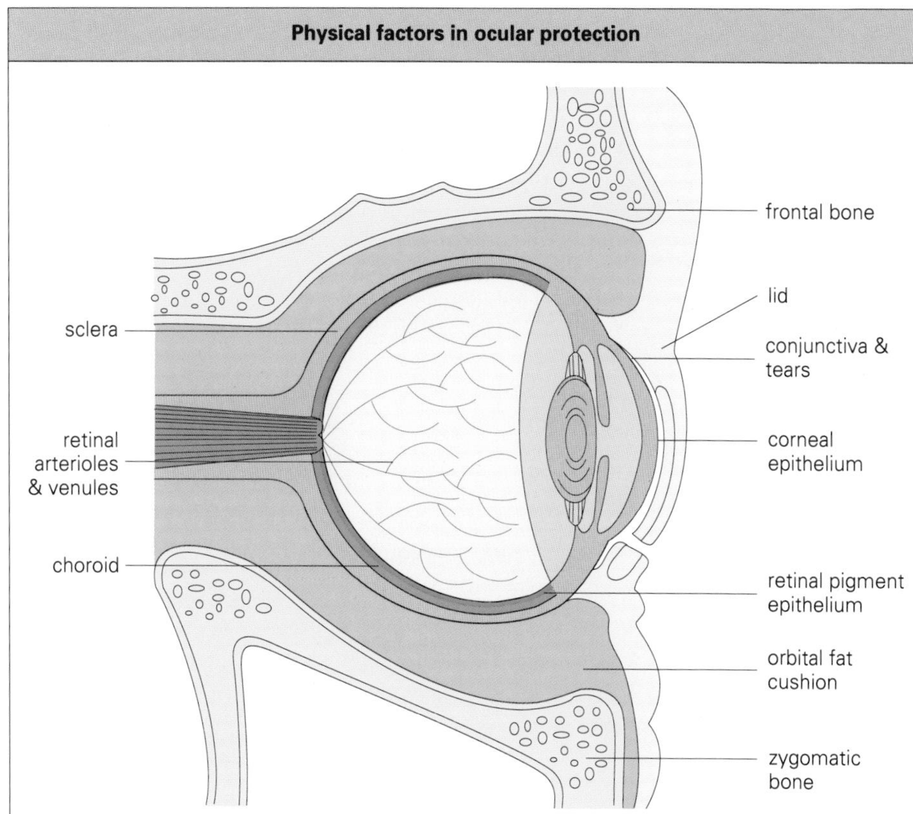

Fig. 13.1 The strong periorbital rim and weaker orbital walls of the bony structure allow blow-out fractures to occur before rupture of the eye. The corneal epithelium, lids and tears are barriers to direct trauma, whilst the tight junctions of the vascular and pigment epithelia prevent entry of circulatory factors.

IMMUNE FEATURES: ANTERIOR SEGMENT

Conjunctiva and tears

Profound alteration in the calibre and permeability of conjunctival blood vessels may occur in response to injury, resulting in exudation of immunoglobulins and cellular immune factors into the tears from the bloodstream. Dendritic antigen presenting cells (Langerhans' cells) are normally resident in the conjunctiva (Fig. 13.2) and are capable of presenting antigen to conjunctival lymphocytes. They do not reside in the normal central corneal epithelium but do infiltrate it during corneal inflammation.

The structure and components of tears are complex and can alter as part of a local immune reaction under pathological conditions (Fig. 13.3). The tear constituents may be permanently altered by disease processes (Fig. 13.4). Immunoglobulins probably form an important aspect of the defence system: IgA is found in the highest concentrations, but IgG, IgE and sometimes IgM may also be detected.

Alterations of tear components in disease		
Tear component (origin)	**Pathology**	**Result**
aqueous (lacrimal & accessory glands)	lacrimal gland infiltration conjunctival cicatrization	↓volume
mucus (goblet cells)	Stevens–Johnson syndrome pemphigoid chemical injury ↓vitamin A	↓spreadability
lipid (meibomian glands)	meibomitis blepharitis	↑evaporation of aqueous

Fig. 13.4 Inadequacy in any one of the tear components results in a poor tear film and therefore a compromised defence.

IMMUNE FEATURES: CORNEA

The cornea is avascular but does contain immunoglobulins and complement components. The avascularity, lack of antigen presenting cells (APCs) and effector cells in the normal cornea are thought to be the reasons for the excellent survival of corneal transplants. This immunological privilege is lost when the cornea is vascularized.

IgG is resident throughout the stroma and IgM is present in the peripheral cornea. The C1 component of complement is present only in the peripheral corneal stroma, whilst the other components are found throughout. It is probable that these diffuse from the limbal blood vessels and consequently alter in health and disease, reflecting the levels of immunoglobulin found in the bloodstream.

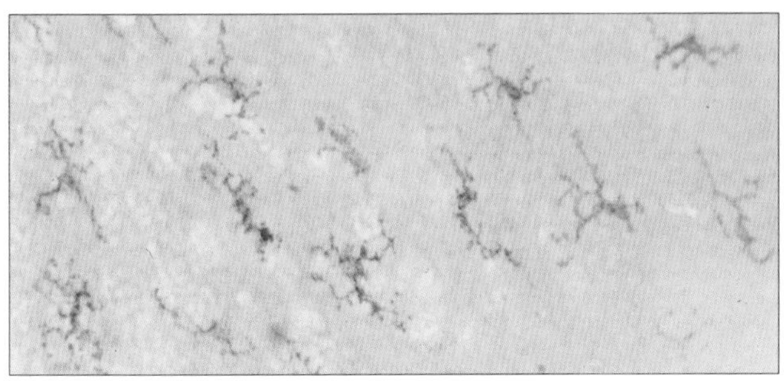

Fig. 13.2 Conjunctival Langerhans' cells show the typical appearance of dendritic antigen presenting cells, with long cytoplasmic processes extending out from the centre of the cell.

Antigen presenting cells and effector cells infiltrate the cornea during keratitis, perhaps due to a protruding suture from a corneal transplant or to herpes simplex keratitis, and contribute to the erosion of corneal privilege.

Anterior chamber associated immune deviation (ACAID)

An unusual and unique pattern of immune responses occurs when antigen is introduced primarily into the anterior chamber:

- antibodies to intraocular antigen are detectable;
- Tc and antigen-specific Ts cells are found in the spleen;
- delayed hypersensitivity is abrogated.

Tear immunoglobulins in health & disease				
Ocular disease	**IgA (mg/ml)**	**IgG (mg/ml)**	**IgE (ng/ml)**	**IgM (mg/ml)**
normal	16	1	1	absent
allergic	normal	slight ↑	slight ↑	absent
vernal	normal	↑	↑	↑
GPC	normal	↑	↑	↑
bacterial infection	↑	slight ↑	normal	↑/normal
graft rejection	↑	↑/normal	normal	↑/normal

Fig. 13.3 The elevation of tear immunoglobulins during disease is partly due to local production and also to transudation. This occurs in conditions such as herpes simplex keratitis and chlamydial conjunctivitis, but the role of tear immunoglobulins in local control of infection is uncertain. Vernal = vernal kerato-conjunctivitis; GPC = giant papillary conjunctivitis.

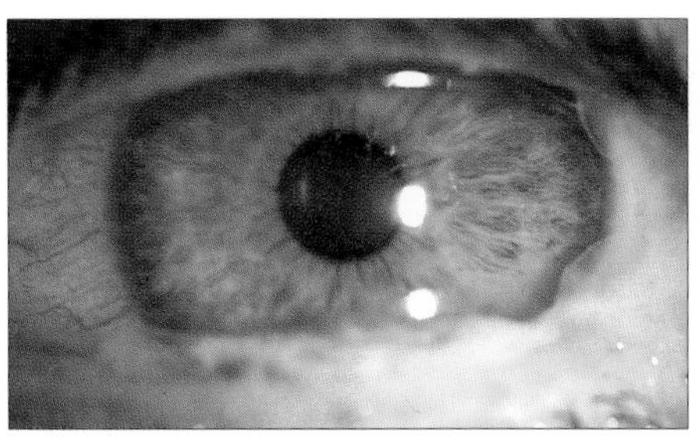

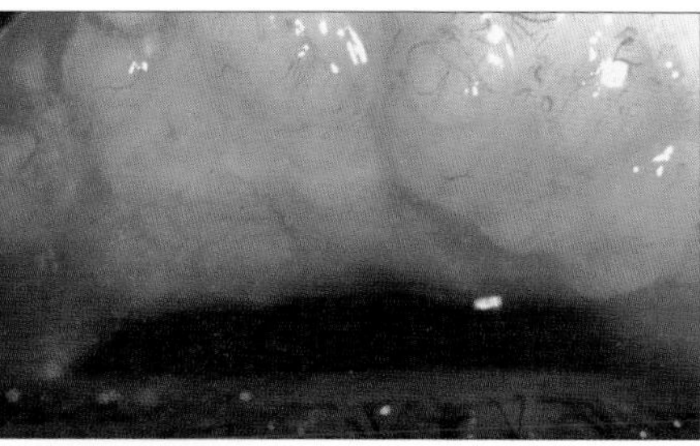

Fig. 13.5 Acute conjunctivitis. Left: bacterial conjunctivitis is characteristically red with a purulent discharge. Right: conjunctival follicles due to *Chlamydia trachomatis* infection are evident.

The slow drainage of antigen through the trabecular meshwork directly into the venous system is likely to contribute to the phenomenon of ACAID. The clinical importance of ACAID is uncertain; it may partly account for the relative rarity of diseases such as lens-induced uveitis following extracapsular cataract extraction and sympathetic uveitis following intraocular surgery.

MANIFESTATIONS OF OCULAR DISEASE

Conjunctivitis

This may be acute or chronic, each type having quite different manifestations. The former is characterized by a red eye with a purulent or watery discharge; conjunctival follicles (Fig. 13.5) tend to occur if the cause is chlamydial or viral. Features of chronic conjunctivitis are variable because of the many different causes.

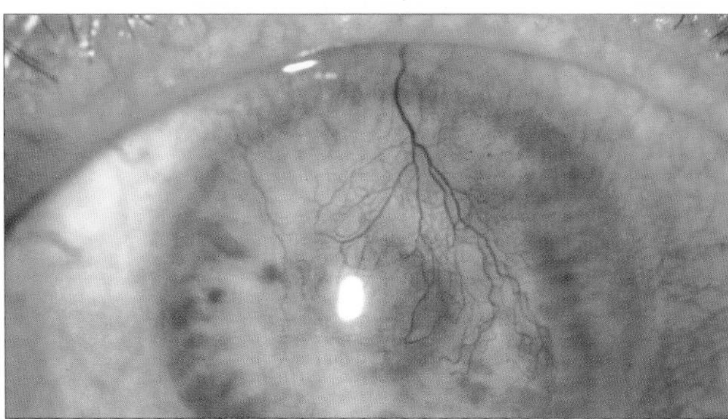

Fig. 13.6 Corneal disease. Vascularization and stromal scarring caused by old episodes of keratitis are evident. Small blood vessels are prominent on the nasal side of the eye, indicating the presence of active disease.

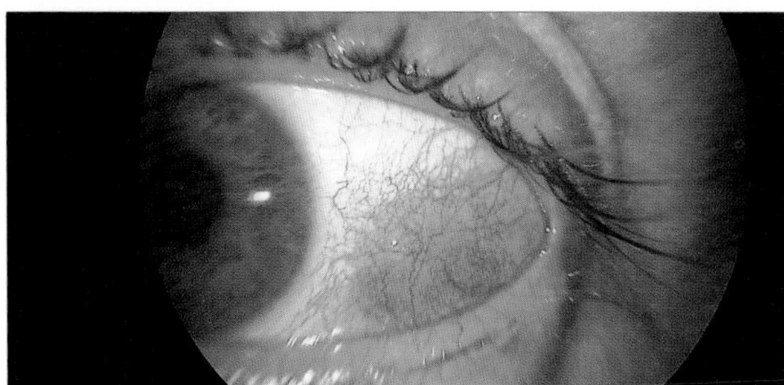

Fig. 13.7 Episcleritis. This condition is characterized by bright red, localized, non-tender injection of the episcleral blood vessels.

Corneal inflammation

A variety of insults result in corneal inflammation, and examination may reveal features of active or old keratitis, or both (Fig. 13.6). In active disease there is limbal injection and white infiltrates (of leucocytes) may appear in the corneal stroma. Neovascularization, oedema of the cornea and keratitic precipitates (leucocyte aggregates on the endothelium) may also be apparent. Inactive disease is characterized by scarring, thinning and the appearance of dilated or ghost vessels in the cornea. Band keratopathy and intrastromal lipid deposition may also occur.

Episcleritis

This is a self-limiting, frequently recurring inflammation of the episclera (Fig. 13.7), which is packed with lymphocytes. It is found principally in young adults: 70% of cases are idiopathic and the remaining 30% are associated with generalized conditions such as connective tissue disorders or herpes zoster infection.

Scleritis

This is a serious destructive inflammation of the sclera. It may be associated with an increase in blood flow, or a decrease caused by occlusive vasculitis, which may result in scleral infarction. There are a variety of presentations (Fig. 13.8). Anterior segment scleritis may be diffuse, nodular, or necrotizing (with or without inflammation); in the latter case, the condition is known as scleromalacia perforans. Posterior segment scleritis presents with a variety of inflammatory features which may or may not include pain, proptosis and retinal detachment.

Scleritis may be associated with connective tissue disorders and some infectious conditions (Fig. 13.9). Immune complexes may be precipitated in and around the inflamed area, resulting in activation of complement and infiltration of PMNs, leading to further inflammation and possible autoimmunization. In those cases in which histopathological investigation is possible, a granulomatous lesion of the sclera is evident and the surrounding blood vessels show perivascular cuffing with lymphocytes and medial necrosis.

Urgent treatment is required to prevent the destructive consequences which include scleral perforation, keratitis, uveitis, glaucoma and cataract.

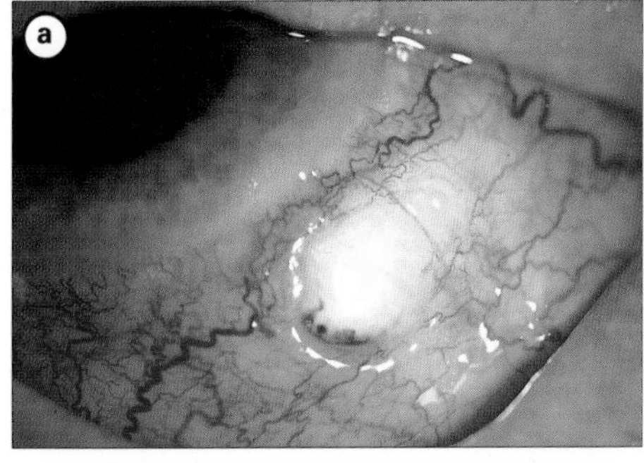

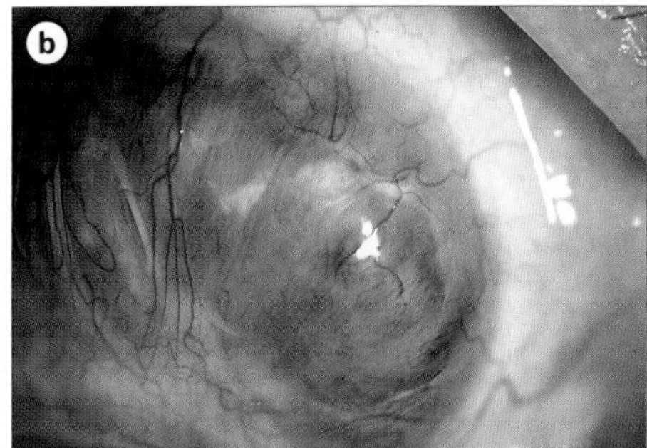

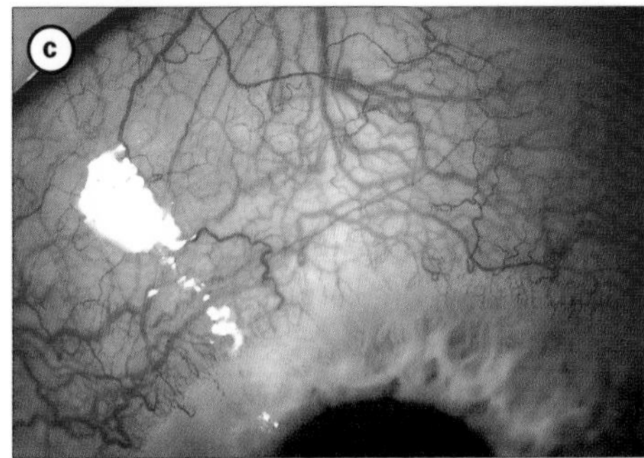

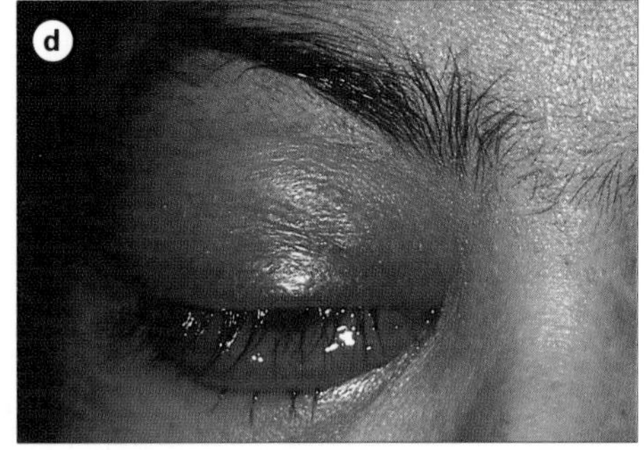

Fig. 13.8 Types of scleritis. a) necrotizing anterior scleritis with inflammation. The eye is painful, red and tender. The white area represents scleral infarction. b) necrotizing anterior scleritis without inflammation (scleromalacia perforans). The eye is not injected and not painful. The choroid (blue) is bulging forward with overlying thin sclera. c) diffuse anterior scleritis without occlusive vasculitis. The eye is painful and tender. d) posterior scleritis presenting as painful proptosis and masquerading as an orbital cellulitis. A CT scan of the orbit showed marked scleral thickening.

Diseases associated with scleritis		
Autoimmune/connective tissue disorders	**Infections**	**Metabolic**
rheumatoid arthritis PAN/Wegener's/ giant cell arteritis relapsing polychondritis SLE	viruses (herpes zoster & simplex) bacterial (TB, syphilis) fungi (*Aspergillus*)	gout cystinosis porphyria

Fig. 13.9 Diseases associated with scleritis. PAN = polyarteritis nodosa.

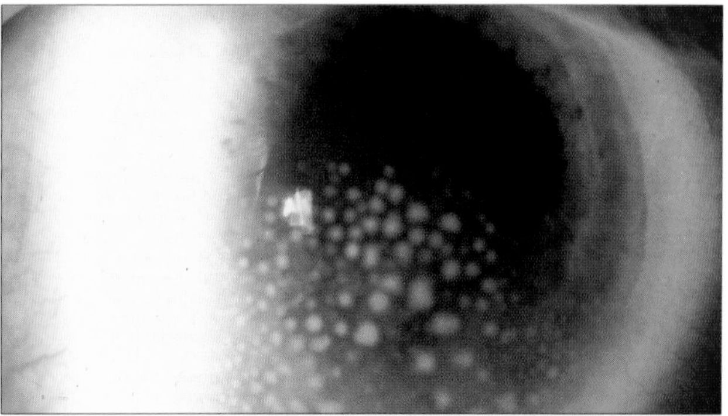

Fig. 13.10 Anterior uveitis. Keratitic precipitates are visible on the corneal endothelium.

Uveitis

Uveitis refers to inflammation of the uveal tract, which is composed of three parts: the iris, the ciliary body, and the choroid. It tends to affect predominantly either the anterior (Fig. 13.10) or the posterior uvea, but occasionally both may be involved (pan uveitis). In posterior uveitis the retina is frequently affected (chorioretinitis).

It is useful to think of ocular inflammation at a cellular level and in terms of the permanent structural alterations that may occur (Fig. 13.11). A stimulus results in accumulation of inflammatory cells at a particular site, and release of mediators which amplify the inflammation and recruit other cells. The nature of the stimulus in most forms of uveitis is uncertain, but it may be associated with viral, bacterial, fungal and helminthic diseases and with non-infectious entities. The uveitis may have the appearance of a type IV hypersensitivity granulomatous reaction (nodular collections of epithelioid and giant cells surrounded by lymphocytes), a non-granulomatous reaction which may result from immune complex deposition (type III hypersensitivity), or a mixture of both.

The severity of the uveitis varies with different conditions. It tends to be acute and aggressive in onset in ankylosing spondylitis and Behçet's disease, often with hypopyon formation (pus in the anterior chamber), but is usually mild in Reiter's disease and chronic in sarcoidosis, juvenile rheumatoid arthritis and heterochromic cyclitis.

Retinal vasculitis

Predominant involvement of the retinal vasculature occurs in a variety of diseases:

- sarcoidosis
- Behçet's disease
- systemic lupus erythematosus
- polyarteritis nodosa
- Whipple's disease
- Crohn's disease
- viral diseases

The inflammation may involve predominantly arteries (as in Behçet's disease), the venous system (as in sarcoidosis), or it may be mixed. Some cases of retinal perivasculitis are secondary to primary choroidal inflammation.

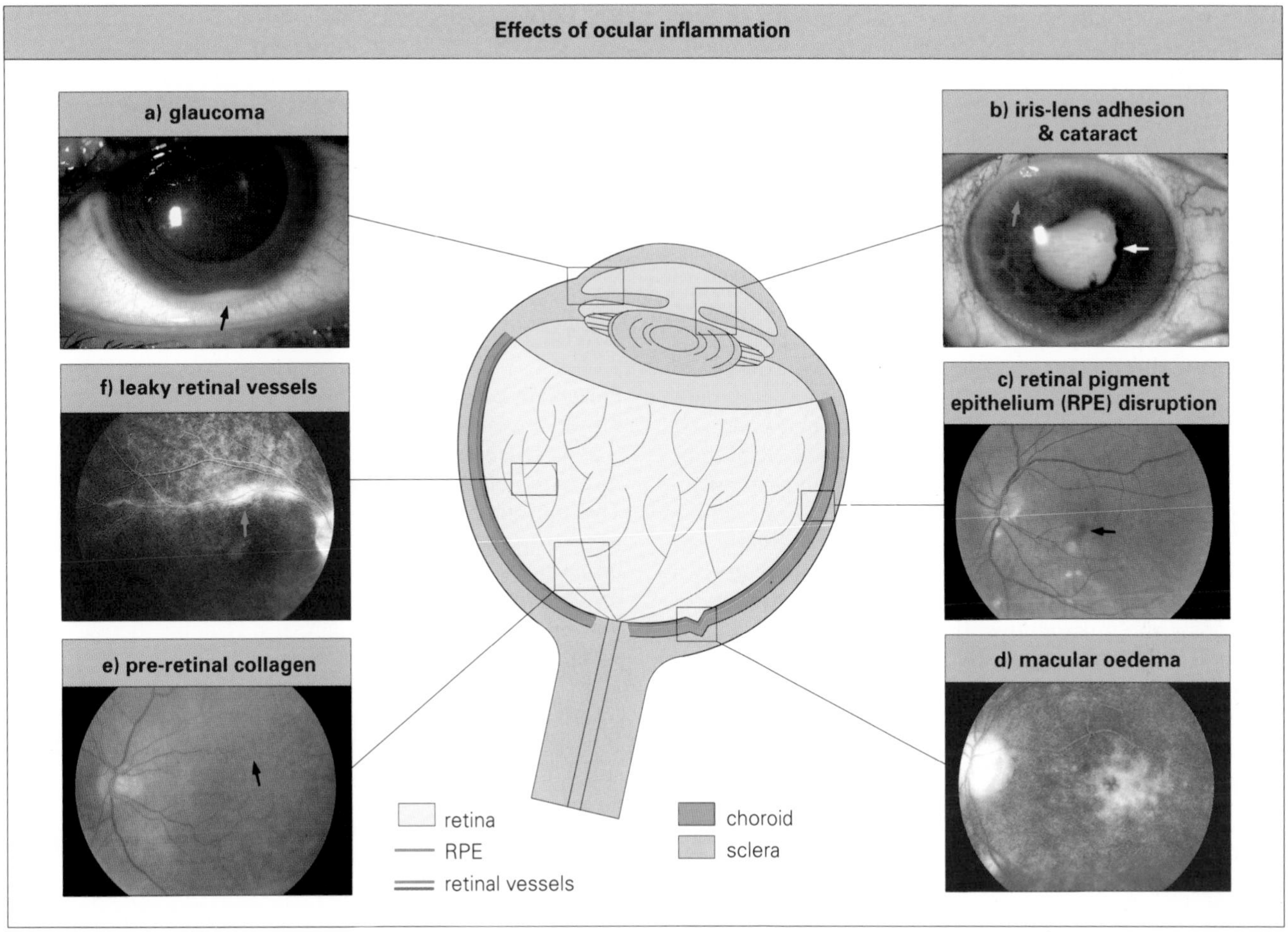

Effects of ocular inflammation

a) glaucoma

b) iris-lens adhesion & cataract

f) leaky retinal vessels

c) retinal pigment epithelium (RPE) disruption

e) pre-retinal collagen

d) macular oedema

retina

RPE

retinal vessels

choroid

sclera

Fig. 13.11 a) secondary glaucoma due to accumulation of white blood cells in the anterior chamber, forming a hypopyon (arrow), and obstructing aqueous outflow. b) iris lens adhesions (white arrow) causing iris bombé and secondary angle closure glaucoma, requiring peripheral iridectomy (blue arrow). The lens is cloudy due to cataract. c) disruption of RPE and secondary growth of a sub-retinal neovascular membrane which has bled (arrow). Pale lesions are seen, presumably due to old histoplasmosis choroiditis. d) macular oedema: fluorescein dye has leaked at the macula (arrow).
e) pre-retinal collagen causes tangential traction on the retina, seen as tortuous small macular blood vessels (arrowed).
f) fluorescein dye leaking from retinal blood vessels (arrowed) with disturbed endothelial junctions.

ALLERGIC DISORDERS

Hay fever conjunctivitis

The prominent feature of this process is rapid, non-injected conjunctival chemosis in a patient who experiences hay fever. The allergens involved are the pollens of grass, trees, weeds and ragweed. It appears that the allergen dissolves in the tear film, penetrates the conjunctiva and elicits a type I hypersensitivity reaction (see chapter 17).

VERNAL EYE DISEASE

This disease is predominantly a bilateral inflammation of the conjunctiva, thought to be a response to external allergens.It is distinguished by giant papillae of the upper tarsal conjunctiva or limbal papillary hypertrophy (Fig. 13.12);

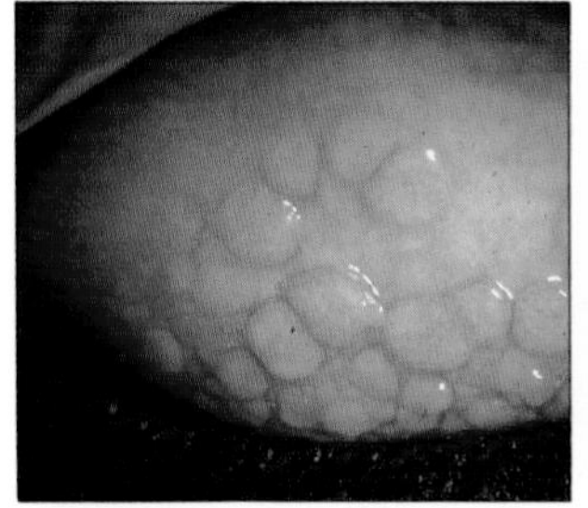

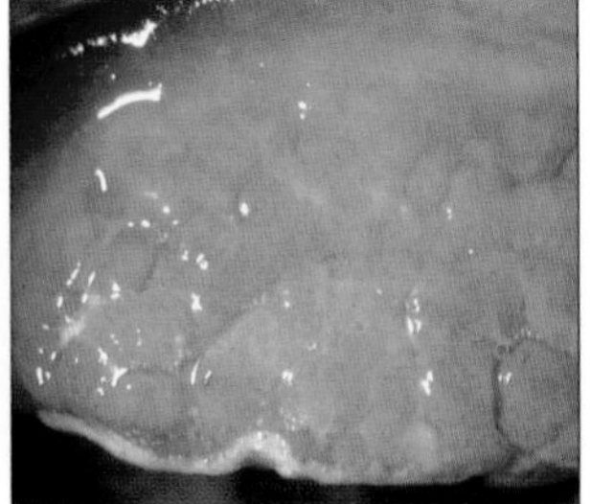

Fig. 13.12 Vernal keratoconjunctivitis. Left: the everted upper tarsal plate in a patient with inactive disease showing cobblestone papillae. Right: in active disease, the papillae are swollen and hyperaemic and there is a stringy mucous discharge.

other signs include ptosis, superficial punctate corneal erosions and plaque-like corneal ulcers with adherent mucus. The principle problems associated with vernal eye disease are the marked degree of symptoms (itchiness, photophobia, tearing and a stringy discharge), the chronic course and the secondary corneal injury, which may result in scarring and loss of visual acuity.

There is a variety of evidence to suggest that this disease is an allergic conjunctivitis. Most cases relapse during the spring and summer months and many patients can relate exacerbations to high pollen counts; three-quarters have other atopic diseases such as asthma, atopic eczema or allergic rhinitis. The conjunctiva of patients with vernal eye disease contains eosinophils, basophils and mast cells (the normal conjunctiva contains only mast cells) and tear (and sometimes serum) IgE levels are elevated. Symptoms and signs improve with mast cell stabilisers and steroids.

The exact nature, interplay and extent of immediate and delayed immune factors involved in this disease has not been elucidated. Certainly it appears that there is a type I hypersensitivity component. However, in view of the considerable tissue growth due to collagen manufacture and new blood vessel formation and the presence of a basophil infiltrate, a delayed hypersensitivity response, possibly related to the cutaneous basophil hypersensitivity, has been implicated.

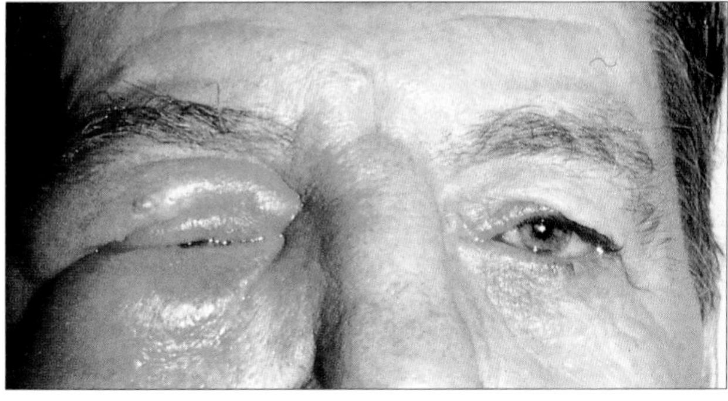

Fig. 13.13 Eye drop allergy showing periorbital lid swelling.

EYE DROP ALLERGY

This differs considerably from hay fever conjunctivitis in clinical appearance and in immunological mechanisms. The typical reaction occurs after about one week of use of a new drop, or within hours in a previously sensitized person. The lids become red, swollen, wrinkled and scaly (Fig. 13.13). The conjuctiva is injected and there is mild to moderate chemosis.

CONTACT LENS RELATED ALLERGIES

Preservative allergies

Preservative allergies usually produce a less dramatic clinical picture than eye drop allergy, but a secondary response may cause a reaction which is rapid and severe. The patient usually experiences discomfort following insertion of the contact lens which has just been immersed in a cleaning solution containing the offending preservative, for example thiomersal, but the symptoms may subside as the day progresses. Usually, there is a fine papillary reaction of the upper tarsal plate and there may also be a keratopathy of varying severity; this often involves mainly the superior cornea with associated corneal vascularization (Fig. 13.14). The disease process subsides with removal of the offending agent from the cleaning solution.

Giant papillary conjunctivitis (GPC)

This condition occurs not just in contact lens wearers but also in patients wearing an artificial eye (a keratoprosthesis), and in those with a nylon suture protruding from the cornea (Fig. 13.15). The papillary conjunctivitis in GPC is less severe than that of vernal eye disease, being less extensive with less prominent papillae. The symptoms are of mild itching, discomfort and increased conjunctival mucus. Giant papillae of the upper tarsal plate are the pathognomonic sign. Although trauma may be involved in the aetiology of this condition, it is thought to be predominantly an immunological reaction to the cells, protein, mucus and bacteria which adhere firmly to contact lenses.

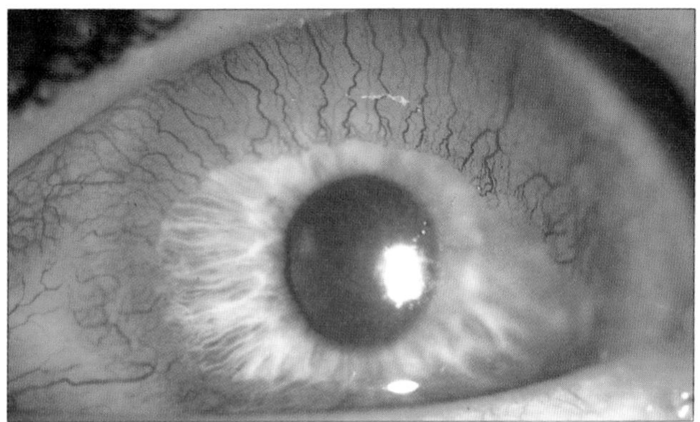

Fig. 13.14 Thiomersal hypersensitivity showing superior corneal vascularization.

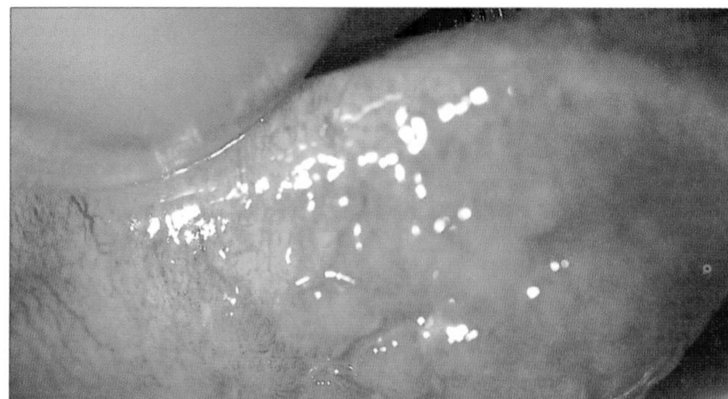

Fig. 13.15 Giant papillary conjunctivitis. The everted upper lid shows nasally located giant papillae caused by a protruding suture.

ISOLATED OCULAR IMMUNE DISEASE

Ocular disease may occur in association with disease of other systems and may precede the onset of systemic disease. However, ocular immune processes can occasionally occur in isolation, for example corneal graft rejection (see chapter 3). Other examples are discussed below.

Phlyctenular keratoconjunctivitis

This is a manifestation of a delayed type hypersensitivity reaction to a variety of microbial proteins (for example *Staph. aureus, M. tuberculosis, Candida albicans, Chlamydia*). The lesion is found most frequently near the limbus. The small, pink-white nodule represents a focal sub-epithelial infiltration of lymphocytes, histiocytes and plasma cells. In cases with associated cell death and ulceration, polymorphonuclear leucocytes are also found.

Corneal immune rings

Discrete rings of immune origin may occur in the cornea (Fig. 13.16). It is likely that these represent a similar process to that seen in 1911 by Wessely, who noted that when antigen is injected into the cornea a white precipitin ring appears in the periphery and then moves to the centre. This ring has been found to contain antigen–antibody complexes. It is thought that the antigen–antibody reaction activates complement, with a resultant chemotactic effect on neutrophils.

Ocular-induced autoreactivity

Some of the protein constituents of the eye are not in contact with the immune system. The enveloping capsule of the crystalline lens develops early in embryogenesis, and prevents lens proteins from being exposed to the immune system, and thus from being recognized as self antigens. Although very small quantities of these proteins may normally leak through the lens capsule throughout life, damage to this structure results in exposure of large quantities of antigens with a resultant inflammatory response. Some retinal and uveal antigens may be exposed as autoantigenic following perforating injury. Some of the retinal specific antigens are as follows:

- soluble (S) antigen surrounding photoreceptor cells;
- particulate (P) antigen is rhodopsin in the outer segments of the rods;
- insoluble (U) antigen at the choroidal base of retinal pigment epithelium (RPE).

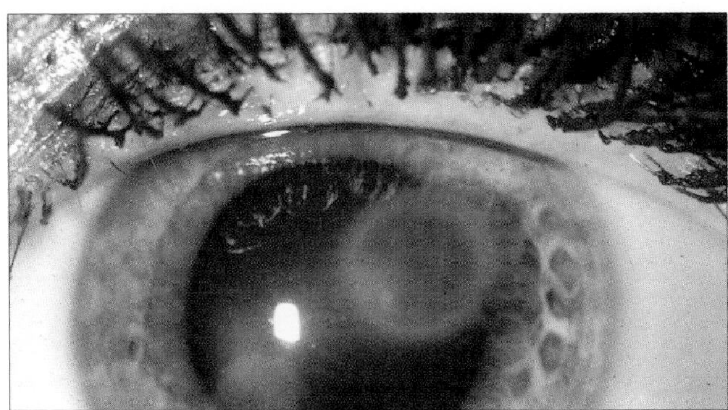

Fig. 13.16 Immune ring in the cornea of a patient with stromal herpes simplex keratitis.

Sympathetic uveitis (SU)

This disease refers to a bilateral granulomatous uveitis which occurs following penetrating trauma to one eye. The second eye becomes involved after a variable period of time, usually 1–2 months after the injury. It is thought not to occur if the injured eye is removed within 10 days of injury. Once the uveitis is established in the second eye, enucleation should not be performed on a seeing existing eye, as it may have the best long-term visual potential. Modern surgical techniques, involving rapid closure of penetrating eye injuries and avoidance of incarceration of uveal and retinal tissue in wounds probably contributes to the rarity of this disease.

Sympathetic uveitis probably occurs due to sensitization to an intraocular antigen which is presented to the immune system as foreign (possibly due to virus induced alterations). It appears that the protein must be presented in a highly immunogenic form. There may also be disturbances of the normal immunoregulatory mechanisms, for example loss of generation of normal suppressive immunological factors. Certain individuals may be genetically predisposed to the development of such autoreactive mechanisms.

Histopathology of human eyes with SU reveals a diffuse choroidal infiltrate, predominantly of T cells (Fig. 13.17). T helper cells invade the eye during the initial

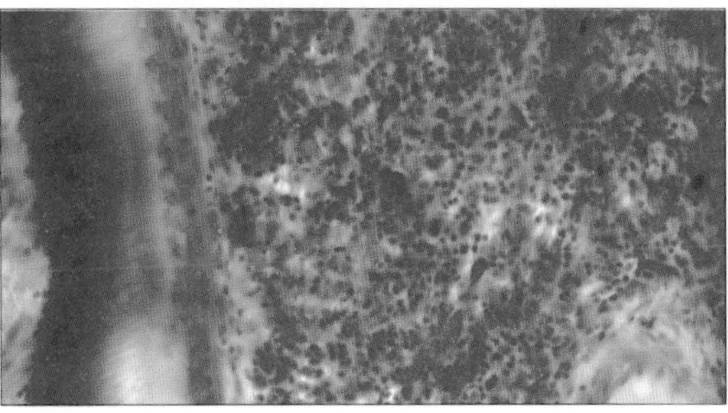

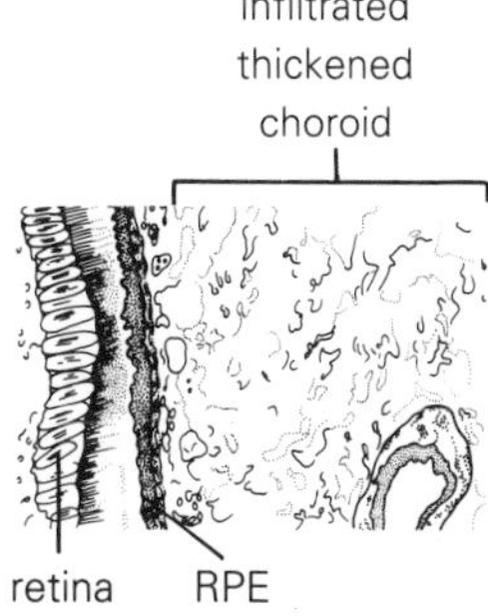

Fig. 13.17 Histology of sympathetic uveitis. There is diffuse infiltration of the choroid by lymphocytes. RPE = retinal pigment epithelium.

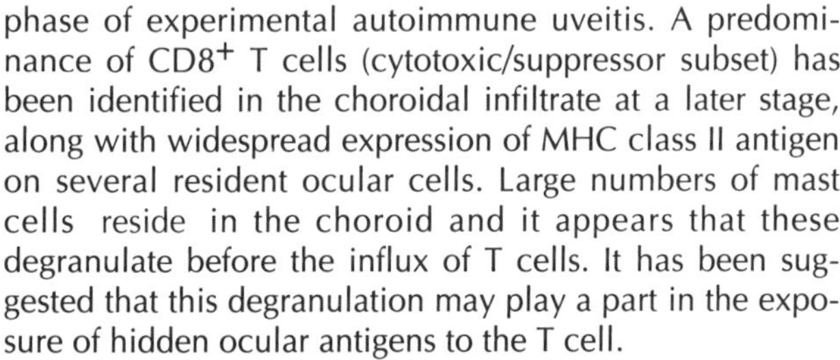

Diseases associated with PCM	
Systemic disease	**Local ocular disease**
rheumatoid arthritis	staphylococcal infiltrates
polyarteritis nodosa	silk sutures at limbus
Wegener's granulomatosis	herpes zoster keratitis
SLE	scleritis
graft–versus–host disease	cicatricial conjunctivitis

Fig. 13.18 Diseases associated with peripheral corneal melting (PCM).

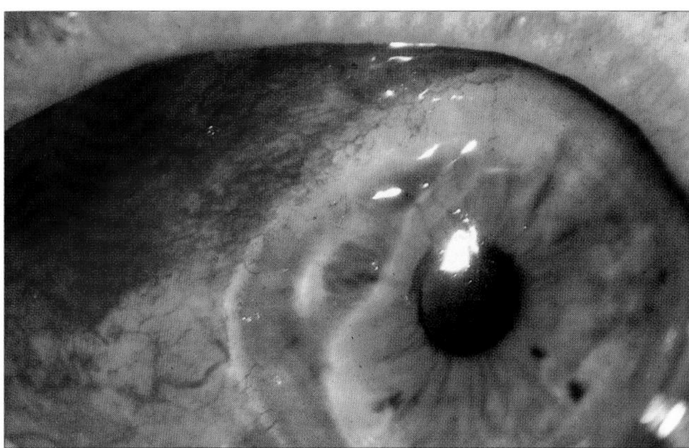

Fig. 13.19 Peripheral corneal melting.

phase of experimental autoimmune uveitis. A predominance of $CD8^+$ T cells (cytotoxic/suppressor subset) has been identified in the choroidal infiltrate at a later stage, along with widespread expression of MHC class II antigen on several resident ocular cells. Large numbers of mast cells reside in the choroid and it appears that these degranulate before the influx of T cells. It has been suggested that this degranulation may play a part in the exposure of hidden ocular antigens to the T cell.

Although the specific human antigens involved in SU have not been identified, retinal S antigen can induce an experimental uveitis in animals. In some patients a delayed hypersensitivity reaction to melanin-containing structures appears to play a part in the pathogenesis of SU. This reaction is manifested as the development of vitiligo, poliosis, hearing defects and meningitis. It is therefore possible that SU represents a cell-mediated response to surface antigens shared by photoreceptors, retinal pigment epithelium and choroidal melanocytes, all of which are derived from neuroectoderm.

In vitro studies evaluating cell-mediated responses have indicated the importance of uvea and uveoretinal tissue as causative factors in sympathetic uveitis. However, studies on circulating T and B cells have failed to show specific abnormalities in sympathetic uveitis compared to non-granulomatous uveitis.

Lens-induced uveitis

Clinical and experimental evidence has shown that immunological mechanisms are involved in many of the reactions directed against solubilized lens proteins. A spectrum of clinical disease exists and the individual type of reaction appears to be determined by multiple factors, for example type of trauma, amount and period of antigen liberation, composition of the lens, and genetic and individual factors such as age. The immunological reaction in certain types of lens-induced uveitis appears to be antibody mediated and complement dependent; in other types, a granulomatous reaction occurs. Although cortical lens protein remnants are frequently left in the eye following extracapsular cataract extraction, lens-induced uveitis is a rare occurrence in this situation.

Peripheral corneal melting (PCM) with ulceration

When this condition occurs as an isolated ocular phenomenon and in the absence of apparent local precipitating factors it is known as Mooren's ulcer. It may also occur in association with a mixed group of diseases (Fig. 13.18). The most common presentation is of variably progressive ulceration and destruction of the peripheral cornea with remissions (Fig. 13.19). In some cases, there is evidence to support an autoimmune process to an antigenically altered cornea: in others, evidence suggests that the process may be an immune complex type disease. It may be that this is a mixed group of diseases with different basic mechanisms producing a similar clinical picture.

Heterochromic cyclitis

This is usually a unilateral, frequently asymptomatic chronic uveitis of adults. Pathologically, there is moderate atrophy of the iris and ciliary body, patchy depigmentation of the iris and a diffuse infiltration of lymphocytes and plasma cells. It is suggested that the iris plasma cells form antibodies, which in turn form antigen–antibody complexes. These may be associated with an occlusive vasculitis in the iris, resulting in atrophy. Immune complexes have also been identified in the aqueous humour of these patients.

SYSTEMIC DISEASES WITH OCULAR MANIFESTATIONS

The most common ocular manifestations of systemic disease are the dry eye, uveitis, scleritis and retinal vasculitis.

Sarcoidosis

This infiltrative, granulomatous, multi-system disease is associated with substantial ocular involvement and induces pathology, not only within the eye itself, but also

Ocular manifestations of sarcoidosis		
uveitis (anterior/posterior)		
calcium deposition in conjunctiva		
band keratopathy		
retinal phlebitis	→	↓ visual acuity & floaters
lacrimal gland infiltration	→	dry eye
conjunctival infiltration	→	conjunctival nodules
lid skin infiltration	→	skin nodules
optic nerve infiltration	→	visual loss
cranial nerve infiltration	→	diplopia
7th nerve palsy	→	exposure keratitis

Fig. 13.20 Ocular manifestations of sarcoidosis. The uveitis is usually granulomatous and bilateral. Conjunctival calcium deposition and band keratopathy are due to hypercalcaemia; the latter may also be caused by chronic uveitis.

Features of acute and chronic uveitis with JRA	acute	chronic
eye	red (unilateral)	white (bilateral)
pain	+	–
glaucoma	–	+
cataract	–	+
macular oedema	–	+
band keratopathy	–	+
iris adhesions	+	+
visual acuity	normal/↓	↓
sex	male (HLA-B27)	female (HLA-Dw5)

Fig. 13.21 Unlike chronic uveitis, the acute form is usually treated early in the course of the disease because of the pain.

involves the surrounding tissues and nerves. Ophthalmic involvement occurs in about 30% of cases. The systemic and ocular manifestations are varied (Fig. 13.20). There is a defect in T cell function but B cell responses are said to be normal. Frequently there is an exaggerated IgG peak on electrophoresis.

Many cases of isolated granulomatous uveitis are probably sarcoidosis but it may be difficult to establish the diagnosis, which is usually confirmed by the multi-system involvement. Occasionally conjunctival nodules are present, and these may be biopsied to confirm the diagnosis; other sites of biopsy are the liver, scalene lymph node and bronchus.

RHEUMATOID DISORDERS

Rheumatoid arthritis

Dry eye. This results from infiltration of the lacrimal gland with lymphocytes and histiocytes and from the associated gland destruction and scarring. The majority of the lymphocytes are $CD4^+$ T cells and the leucocyte migration inhibition test is positive in many cases using parotid gland extracts as the challenge antigen. Antibodies to salivary duct antigens have been detected in this condition, the significance of which is uncertain; it has been suggested that they protect certain receptor sites in the lacrimal gland.

The mildly dry eye may be easily managed with artificial tear drops, but the treatment of the severe form is difficult and may require permanent occlusion of the lacrimal drainage system. There may be a filamentary keratitis (filaments of mucus attached to the disturbed dry corneal surface), and the condition potentiates the severity of the corneal melting that may accompany rheumatoid arthritis.

Scleritis. Diffuse anterior scleritis and scleromalacia perforans are particuarly associated with rheumatoid arthritis. The destruction of the sclera may be so severe that uveal tissue bulges through (see Fig. 13.8).

Juvenile rheumatoid arthritis (JRA)

Uveitis. The pauciarticular forms of JRA account for almost all the cases of uveitis, which may be acute or chronic (Fig. 13.21). Chronic uveitis has a variable prognosis, even with treatment, and about 25% of patients do not improve. It is frequently asymptomatic and the patient presents late. The pathogenesis of the uveitis is uncertain. A weakly penetrant polygenic genetic component in conjunction with an exogenous trigger factor, for example viral infection, are likely to be important in the pathogenesis. Granuloma formation in the uveal tract has been noted and numerous plasma cells and Russell bodies have been found in uveal tissue. Sarcoidosis may have a similar ocular clinical presentation and must be excluded.

Patients with pauciarticular arthritis who are ANA-positive should be screened every three months for the development of chronic uveitis.

Reiter's syndrome

The ocular disease in Reiter's syndrome usually runs a benign course, and has a characteristic presentation:

- acute anterior uveitis;
- papillary conjunctivitis ± mucopurulent discharge;
- keratitis, with punctate, epithelial or sub-epithelial infiltrates.

A susceptible immunogenetic constitution (particularly HLA-B27) in conjunction with an exogenous factor (*Chlamydia, Salmonella, Mycoplasma* or *Yersinia*) have been implicated as important predisposing factors. Immune complexes may trigger the clinical disease.

Ankylosing spondylitis

This important cause of anterior uveitis again underlines the association of genetic constitution (in this case HLA-B27) as a risk factor in the development of uveitis. These patients develop recurrent episodes of unilateral or bilateral acute anterior uveitis which may occur in the absence of back symptoms. Iris–lens adhesions are common but other complications are rare if adequate steroid treatment is given during acute attacks.

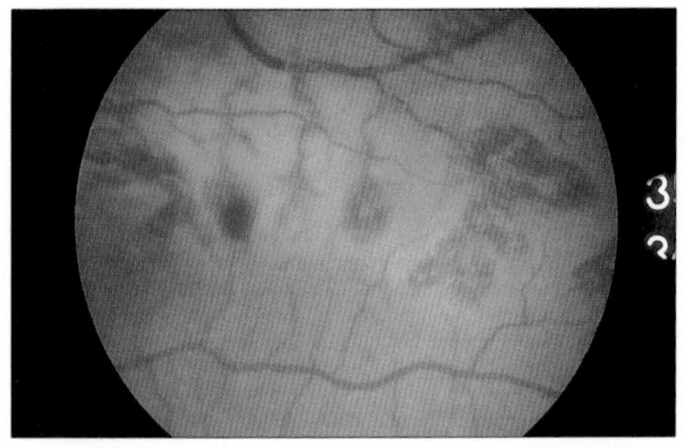
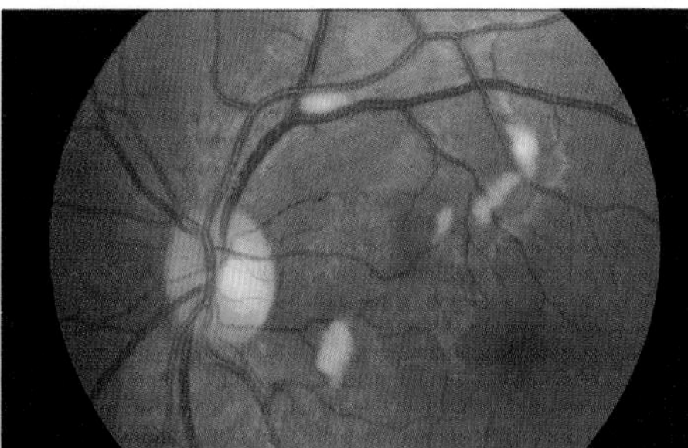

Fig. 13.22 Retinal vasculitis in a patient with SLE. Left: ischaemic retina (pale) and haemorrhages. Right: cotton wool spots. Other ocular manifestations of the disease include hypertensive retinopathy, proliferative retinopathy, Sjögren's syndrome, keratitis, scleritis and optic neuropathy.

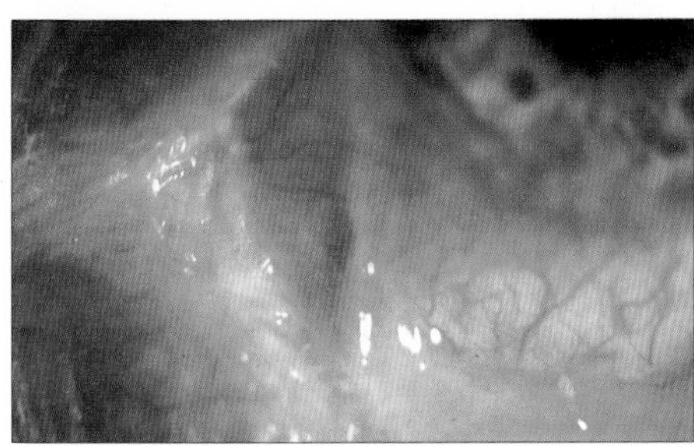
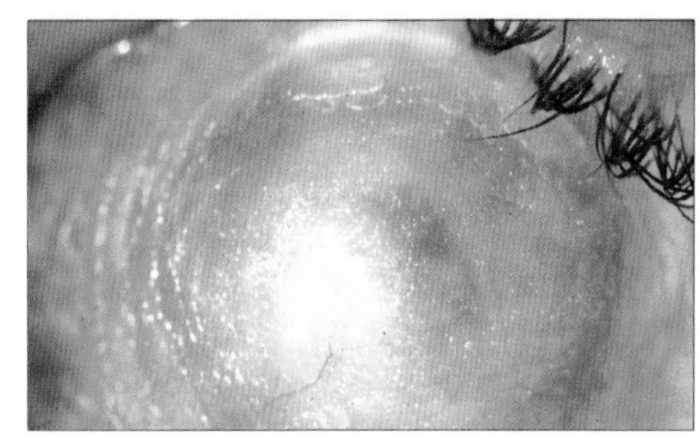

Fig. 13.23 Cicatricial pemphigoid. Left: destruction and shrinkage of the conjunctiva. Right: this results in secondary damage to the cornea.

CONNECTIVE TISSUE DISORDERS

Systemic lupus erythematosus (SLE)

The ocular complications of SLE (see chapter 6) usually manifest as a retinal vasculitis. This appears as cotton wool spots, retinal haemorrhages, retinal and optic nerve head oedema and proliferative retinopathy (Fig. 13.22). The cotton wool spots are thought to represent sites of infarction in the nerve fibre layer, where deposition of antigen–antibody complexes and complement has taken place in the capillaries. It is important to exclude hypertension in SLE patients who present with this retinal picture. It is unusual for anterior uveitis to occur in this condition.

Polyarteritis nodosa (PAN) & Wegener's granulomatosus

PAN is a disease of medium and small sized arteries and may involve almost any tissue of the eye. The scleritis tends to occur as the necrotizing variety, and may be associated with peripheral corneal ulceration and melting.

The most common ocular complication of Wegener's granulomatosus is orbital involvment. Indeed, the first presentation of the disease may be ocular, particularly proptosis or scleritis.

Giant cell arteritis

Patients with this type of arteritis usually present to the ophthalmologist with acute painless loss of vision due to ischaemic optic neuropathy, caused by occlusion of the posterior ciliary artery which supplies the optic nerve head. Clinically the optic disk is swollen but pale, unlike the hyperaemic optic nerve head swelling associated with papilloedema. Occasionally the visual loss is due to central retinal artery occlusion. A typical history of temporal arteritis is characterized by the following:

- ≥50 years old
- malaise and weight loss
- temporal headaches & tenderness over superficial temporal artery
- jaw claudication
- polymyalgia
- ↑ ESR

This history is not, however, always present. In cases of doubt, a superficial temporal artery biopsy is a reliable diagnostic investigation. A positive biopsy reveals a granulomatous arteritis with prominent giant cells involving the vessel wall, fragmentation of the internal elastic lamina, intimal thickening and a varying degree of luminal occlusion.

MUCOCUTANEOUS DISORDERS

Pemphigus and pemphigoid

Pemphigus rarely affects the eyes. The conjunctival involvement usually manifests in a purulent form but does not result in the progressive scarring associated with cicatricial pemphigoid.

Cicatricial pemphigoid frequently affects the eyes. Ocular involvement may precede or occur after other mucous membrane or skin involvement. Sub-epithelial vesicle formation heals with scarring, shrinkage and destruction of the conjunctiva and secondary damage to the corneal epithelium (Fig. 13.23). The immunopathological mechanism involved appears to be a type II antibody dependent cytotoxic hypersensitivity initiated by an insoluble antigen attached to the basement membrane of the epithelium. The extent to which the tissue destruction is phagocyte induced or antibody-dependent, cell-mediated is unclear.

Clinical ocular features of Behçet's disease		
acute anterior uveitis	→	hypopyon formation
occlusive retinal vasculitis	→	retinal ischaemia & neovascularization
choroiditis (occasionally)	→	chorioretinal degeneration
vitreous inflammation	→	cells & floaters in vitreous
optic neuropathy	→	optic atrophy

Fig. 13.24 Clinical features of ocular Behçet's disease.

Stevens-Johnson syndrome

Stevens-Johnson syndrome (erythema multiforme with bullous mucosal involvement) has been associated with a variety of triggering factors including infection, vaccination and drug ingestion. It is assumed that the trigger alters autologous protein in such a way that it is recognized as foreign. Antibody formation is stimulated, with subsequent deposition of immune complexes in the microvasculature of the skin and mucous membranes, followed by microthrombosis and necrosis. There is a mononuclear cell infiltrate rather than PMN infiltration.

The severity of the disease varies considerably. The clinical appearance is of conjunctival blisters which later rupture: as such, the condition is similar to cicatricial pemphigoid but it is not progressive.

Vogt-Koyanagi-Harada syndrome

This is a uvea-meningitis involving ocular structures (including the choroid, optic nerve and retina), the central nervous system, the cochlea and skin. The disease has a variable course and is most common in the Far East, where 40% of patients with the disease have the HLA-B22 genotype.

The histological picture has similarities to that of sympathetic uveitis but the plasma cell infiltration seen in VKH syndrome is not present in SU.

Behçet's disease

There are a variety of types of Behçet's disease, which is likely to be an immune complex disorder occurring in a genetically susceptible individual exposed to an exogenous trigger factor. The result is an occlusive vasculitis. It is also suggested that TH cells play a role in the underlying mechanism. The basement membrane of the blood vessel seems to be the main target of attack, resulting in small vessel infarction with perivascular infiltration of lymphocytes. In ocular Behçet's disease, which is associated with HLA-B5, a complex of IgG, C3 and C5 releases a chemotactic factor for polymorphonuclear leucocytes with resultant hypopyon formation. A reduction in the level of serum complement components has been detected prior to exacerbation of the condition. The clinical features of the ocular disease are outlined in Fig. 13.24.

GASTROINTESTINAL DISORDERS

Ulcerative colitis, Crohn's disease and Whipple's disease all have ocular manifestations (Fig. 13.25). It is suggested that a partial disruption of a section of the gastrointestinal mucosa allows antigen to enter the systemic circulation. In a genetically predisposed individual, it appears that this antigen is capable of binding to the basement membrane of the uvea and episcleral vessels. In ulcerative colitis it is suggested that the membrane-bound antigen may be attacked by antibody and cytotoxic lymphocytes, leading to complement pathway activation and an associated acute inflammatory cell infiltrate.

Ocular disease associated with GI disorders	
Ulcerative colitis/Crohn's	**Whipple's disease**
anterior uveitis episcleritis & scleritis keratoconjunctivitis sicca sub-epithelial keratitis optic neuritis	bilateral retinal inflammation retinal haemorrhages vitreous cells ophthalmoparesis

Fig. 13.25 The ophthalmoparesis in Whipple's disease is predominantly vertical and is due to CNS involvement.

Clinical features of idiopathic orbital inflammation	
Cardinal signs	**Associated signs**
pain proptosis	swollen lids blood vessel engorgement limitation of ocular movement visual loss papilloedema

Fig. 13.26 Major clinical features of idiopathic orbital inflammation.

ORBITAL DISORDERS

These include thyroid eye disease (see chapter 7), idiopathic orbital inflammations (pseudotumour of the orbit) and Wegener's granulomatosis.

Idiopathic orbital inflammations (pseudotumour)

This is a group of diseases of uncertain aetiology in which there is orbital inflammation ranging from the granulomatous form to vasculitis; pure granulomatous or vasculitic lesions are rare. There is usually a non-specific polymorphous infiltrate of inflammatory cells involving lymphocytes, plasma cells and macrophages. There may be variable involvement of different orbital tissues. The inflammation may be localized and resemble a tumour, or it may be diffuse in its orbital involvement.

The symptoms and signs will depend on the type of orbital involvement; the most important clinical aspects are outlined in Fig. 13.26. The course of this group of diseases is very variable; they may be chronic or may settle

Ocular manifestations of congenital immunodeficiency states		
IgA deficiency	**Mucocutaneous candidiasis**	**Chediak-Higashi syndrome**
vernal atopic disease conjunctival nodules keratoconus corneal abscesses nasolacrimal infections	keratitis: peripheral cornea punctate epithelial disease corneal vascularization stromal oedema & scarring	oculocutaneous albinism nystagmus skin infections (including lids) corneal infections
Ataxia telangiectasia		**Keratitis, icthyosis, deafness (Kid) syndrome**
conjunctival telangiectasia nystagmus		chronic blepharitis corneal plaques of epithelial hyperplasia

Fig. 13.27 Ocular manifestations of congenital immunodeficiency states.

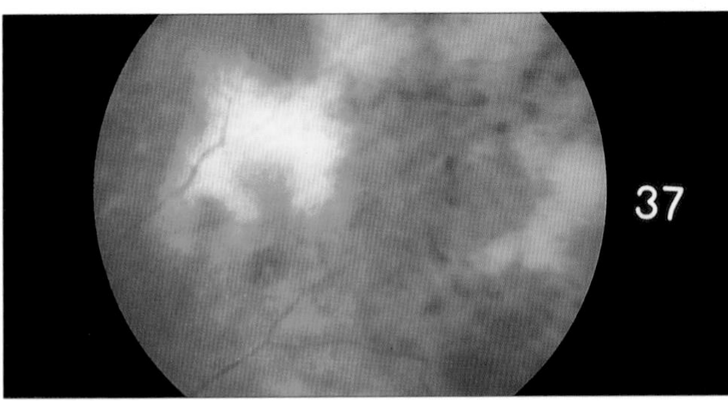

Fig. 13.28 Ocular manifestations of AIDS. CMV retinopathy showing areas of retinal infarction (pale) and retinal pigment epithelium disturbance.

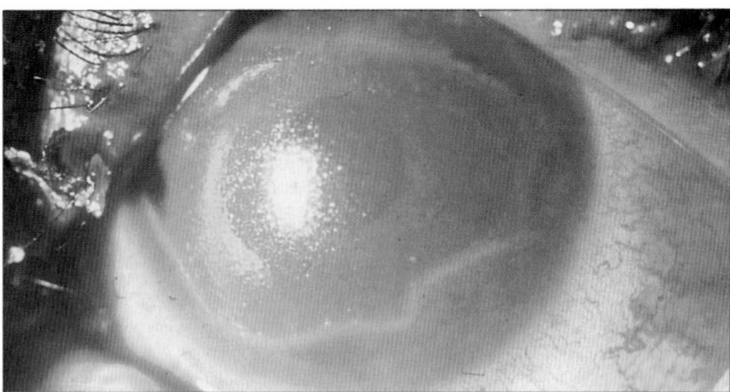

Fig. 13.29 Fluorescein staining of a large amoeboid herpetic corneal ulcer in a child with measles and malnutrition. This can also be caused by topical corticosteroids.

spontaneously. The differential diagnoses to be considered include thyroid eye disease, scleritis, orbital cellulitis and tumours (usually secondaries).

Interpretation of the pathology of the disease is difficult, as the pathological appearance varies with the site biopsied and the histology may vary at different stages of the disease. Orbital biopsy is, however, an important investigation to consider. If the inflammatory infiltrate is polymorphous the diagnosis of pseudotumour may be made with relative certainty: when a monomorphous pure lymphocytic infiltrate is identified, considerable problems may arise in distinguishing a pseudotumour from a lymphoma.

IMMUNODEFICIENCY STATES

Congenital immunodeficiency (see chapter 23) may have ocular manifestations (Fig. 13.27), but the most common immunodeficiency states which involve the eyes are acquired.

Virus induced immune deficiency

AIDS (see chapter 24) is associated with ocular opportunistic infections such as CMV, varicella-zoster, cryptococcal choroiditis, toxoplasma chorio-retinitis and *Pneumocystis carinii* choroiditis. Kaposi's sarcoma of the lids and conjunctiva and neuro-ophthalmic lesions are also found in this syndrome. It is these opportunistic insults related to the immunosuppression that produce the ocular manifestations (Fig. 13.28).

Measles infection is capable of suppressing the normal immune response. This is frequently not significant but if the patient is already immunocompromised, for example because of malnutrition or drug-induced immunosuppression, the effects may be serious (Fig. 13.29).

Iatrogenically induced immune deficiency

Drugs, steroids and cytotoxic agents are the most common forms of iatrogenically induced immune suppression. Although serious ocular complications in association with

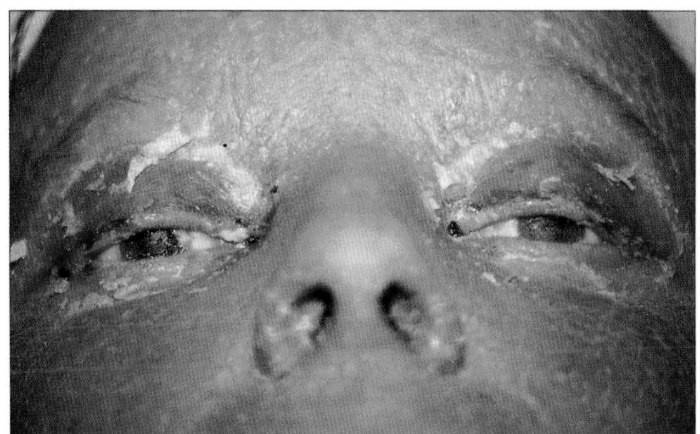

Fig. 13.30 Acute graft-versus-host disease. Exfoliation of epithelial surfaces, including the eye. Loss of tears has resulted in dry eyes and loss of corneal clarity.

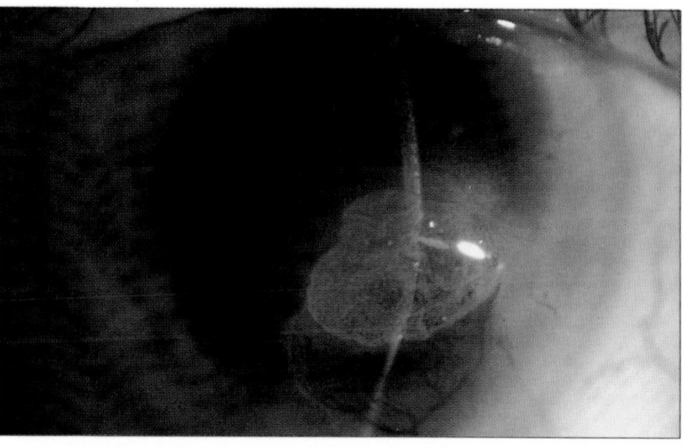

Fig. 13.31 Chronic graft-versus-host disease. Corneal perforation in a dry eye, sealed temporarily with histoacrylate ('Super') glue. The patient required corneal transplantation.

graft-versus-host disease are not common, they do occur and pose particular problems for the ophthalmologist.

Graft-versus-host disease (GVHD)

This disease occurs following the transfusion of white blood cells into an immunosuppressed patient. The degree of antigenic disparity between donor and recipient, the number of lymphocytes transfused, the age of the recipient, bacterial microflora and viral infection are some of the factors associated with the development of GVHD. The type of reaction (acute, chronic or mixed) which results is variable.

In some acute forms there is a toxic epidermal necrolysis affecting skin and mucous membranes, including the conjunctiva, bladder and gut epithelium. There is an associated generalized exfoliation of all epithelial surfaces, with loss of conjunctiva and corneal epithelium. The eye is dry, the cornea cloudy and the lids adhere to the globe (Fig. 13.30). Maintenance of the lid fornices and copious lubrication to the eye are important palliative measures.

In chronic GVHD, which typically occurs about 30 days after bone marrow transplantation, there is a rash which may be accompanied by mouth lesions. The patient develops sicca syndrome which is usually mild and controlled with artificial tear drops. Occasionally, it may be more severe and associated with corneal melting and perforation (Fig. 13.31).

The depression of cell mediated immunity and immunoglobulin production may result in reactivation of viruses such as herpes simplex, varicella and cytomegalovirus. The clinical manifestations of these diseases will be altered in the immunocompromised evironment.

Drug induced immunosuppression is associated with reactivation of latent viruses (HSV and VZV). The clinical disease is altered for the worse. In herpetic keratitis dendritic ulcers become amoeboid, and there is an increased incidence of secondary bacterial and fungal keratitis in patients on topical corticosteroids.

FURTHER READING

Friedman MG. Antibodies in human tears during and after infection. *Survey Ophthalmol* 1990; **35(2)**:151–157.

Kanski JJ. *Clinical Ophthalmology (2E)*. London: Butterworth's 1989.

Lightman S, ed. *Immunology of Eye Disease*. Place: Kluwer Academic Publishers, 1989.

Lucas DR. *Greer's Ocular Pahtology (4E)*. Oxford: Blackwell Scientific Publishing, 1989.

Streilein JW. Anterior chamber associated immune deviation: The privilege of immunity in the eye. *Surgery Ophthalmol* 1990; **35(1)**:67–73.

14

Skin Disorders

INTRODUCTION

There are over 700 skin diseases, many of which show immunological reaction patterns with infiltration of the dermis and epidermis by lymphocytes, macrophages, dendritic cells, granulocytes and mast cells. The majority are poorly understood, but in some disorders the mechanisms involved have been elucidated. This chapter concentrates on those which follow well recognized immunological mechanisms such as hypersensitivity and immunodeficiency, and on those related to connective tissue diseases and neoplasia.

Hypersensitivity can be defined according to the Coombs and Gell classification. There are many examples in skin disease, the most important of which are shown in Fig. 14.1.

DISEASES CAUSED BY TYPE I HYPERSENSITIVITY

URTICARIA

Urticaria is a transient eruption characterized by erythematous or oedematous swelling of the dermis or subcutaneous tissue (Fig. 14.2 left). Angioedema (giant urticaria) is a variant which involves mainly the subcutaneous tissues and commonly affects the face and lips (Fig. 14.2 right). In both disorders the lesions characteristically fade within 24 hours but in many cases new lesions subsequently appear.

Urticaria is common, occurring in about 15% of the population at some time. It is due to increased permeability of capillaries or other small vessels and the resulting transudation of fluid. The underlying mechanism involves several chemical mediators, of which histamine is the best

Hypersensitivity reactions of the skin	
Type I anaphylactic	urticaria
Type II cytolytic/cytotoxic	pemphigus pemphigoid
Type III immune complex	allergic vasculitis urticarial vasculitis erythema nodosum leprosum erythema induratum erythema multiforme ? dermatitis herpetiformis
Type IV delayed	allergic contact dermatitis ? atopic eczema borderline leprosy reactions

Fig. 14.1 Skin diseases associated with hypersensitivity.

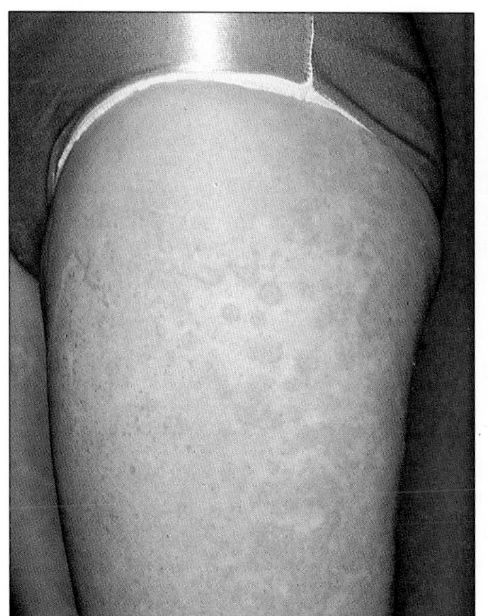

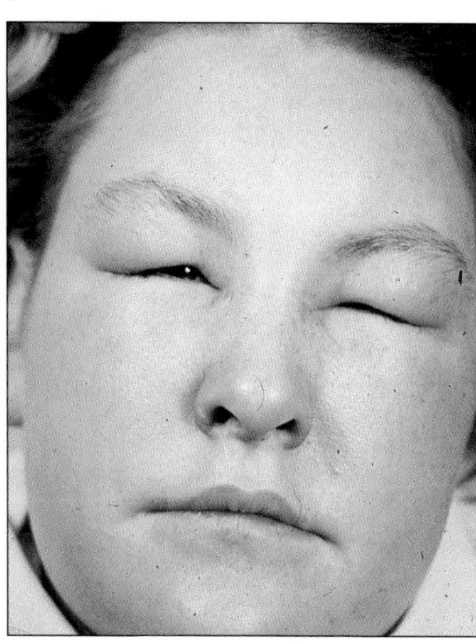

Fig. 14.2 Left: urticarial weals on the thigh. Right: angioedema of the face with swelling of the mouth and eyelids.

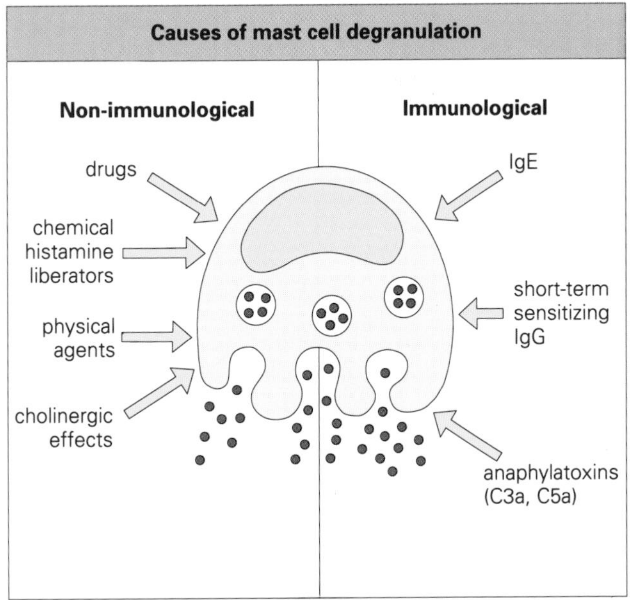

Fig. 14.3 Imunological and non-immunological causes of mast cell degranulation.

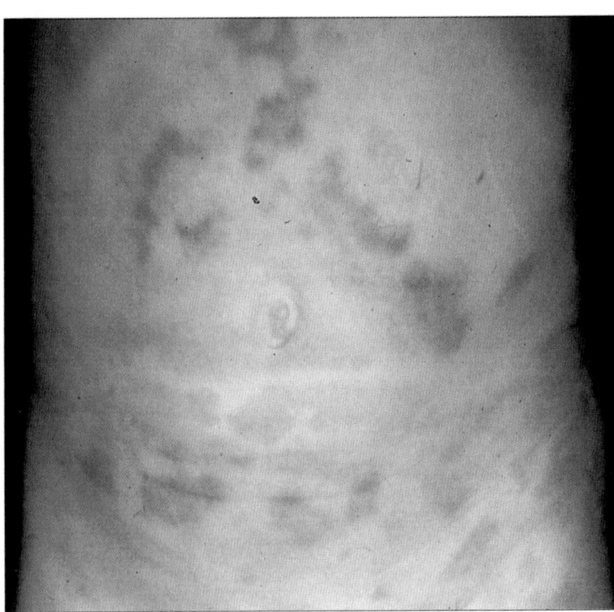

Fig. 14.4 Urticarial vasculitis presenting with weals and extensive bruising. Courtesy of Dr R P Warin.

known: fibrin degradation products, complement and leukotrienes are also involved. The release of histamine and other mediators follows degranulation of mast cells, which are found in the dermis at a density of around $7000/mm^3$. Mast cell degranulation results from both immune and non-immune mechanisms (Fig. 14.3).

IgE-mediated urticaria and angioedema

The appearance of urticaria or angioedema following ingestion of food allergens is relatively common in atopics, especially children, and is usually IgE mediated. Swelling of the lips and tongue develop immediately after eating the food, and vomiting may occur if it is ingested. Contact urticaria may occur if the allergen is splashed onto the skin. Generalized urticaria may then develop due to intestinal absorption of the food. The symptoms usually last for a few hours, and the cause is often obvious to both the patient and parent because the interval between eating the food and the appearance of symptoms is short. Common allergens include cows' milk, hens' eggs, fish and nuts, and certain drugs such as penicillin. This type of food allergy is not restricted to children; it may develop for the first time later in life, for example during pregnancy or following a viral infection.

Type I hypersensitivity can be demonstrated by skin prick tests, the antigen in question producing a weal and flare response: radio-allergosorbent testing of the serum will also confirm the diagnosis.

Urticaria due to ingestion of foods (or drugs) can also be caused by non-IgE-mediated mechanisms; immune complex deposition, for example, activates complement
14.2 leading to release of anaphylatoxins which are potent mast cell degranulators. Urticaria may also be caused by foods (for example smoked mackerel) containing histidine, which can be converted to histamine. Other foods (for example tomatoes and strawberries) may act as non-specific histamine release agents by directly affecting mast cells in the skin.

Urticaria may occur as part of a generalized anaphylactic reaction following injection of an allergen such as penicillin; similar reactions can follow insect stings, for example by bees or wasps, where the subject has been sensitized to the venom.

Immune complex-mediated urticaria (urticarial vasculitis)

Although it is not due to type I hypersensitivity, this form of urticaria can be confused with that produced via IgE mechanisms. Immune complex disease affecting the skin usually causes a vasculitis, but a serum sickness type reaction may produce urticaria with associated arthralgia and fever. Causes of this syndrome include drugs, especially penicillin, and infection, such as hepatitis B. The weals usually last longer than in other urticarias, and there may be associated bruising and purpura (Fig. 14.4).

OTHER CAUSES OF URTICARIA

Hereditary angioedema

This results from a genetically determined (autosomal dominant) absence of C1 esterase inhibitor or the presence of a dysfunctional protein. Attacks of angioedema are associated with activation of C1, consumption of C4

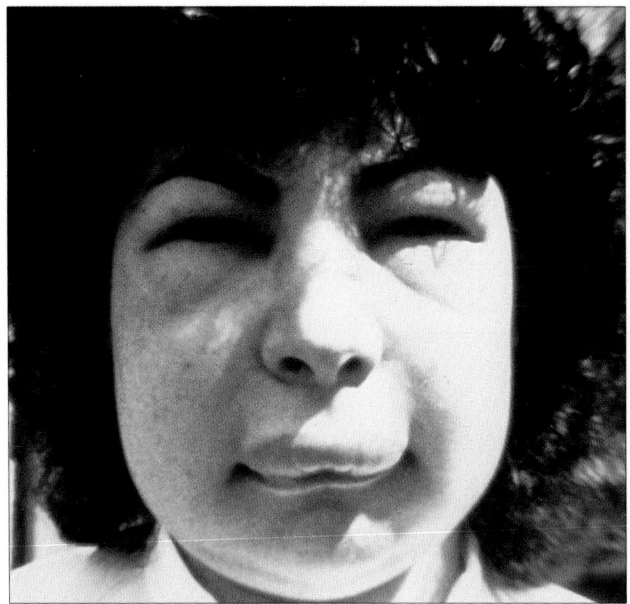

Fig. 14.5 Hereditary angioedema with marked swelling of the upper lip. Courtesy of Dr R P Warin.

and C2, and production of a vasoactive kinin-like polypeptide. Patients present with recurrent episodes of facial angioedema (Fig. 14.5), often with glottal oedema and abdominal pain due to gastrointestinal involvement.

Severe acute attacks should be treated by infusion of fresh frozen plasma (which contains C1 esterase inhibitor) or purified protein, which has only recently become available. Prophylactic treatment using danazol, an inhibitor of pituitary gonadotrophin which has little androgenic effect, may induce the required increase in C1 esterase inhibitor levels, and C4 levels may return to normal. In women of child-bearing age, tranexamic acid, an anti-fibrinolytic, is also effective when used prophylactically.

Physical urticarias

These are a heterogeneous group of disorders in which weals and erythema result from physical agents, which presumably have a direct effect on mast cells. There is no evidence at present that they are IgE- or immune complex-mediated.

Dermographism, in which weals develop within minutes of scratch trauma, is present in about 5% of the normal population and may represent a physiological variant. In some subjects, usually young adults, a severe form of dermographism may develop; this often occurs quite suddenly, sometimes following a virus infection.

Cold urticaria results in wealing on exposure to cold. The rare autosomal dominant form presents soon after birth, and is associated with malaise and arthralgia, but most cases develop in early adult life. On exposure to cold, often in the form of a cold wind or cold water, urticaria develops within minutes and lasts for up to 24 hours. Mostly, no underlying cause is found, but some patients have cryoglobulins, cold agglutinins or cryofibrinogens in their blood. The diagnosis is confirmed by applying an ice-cube to the forearm for 5 minutes: weals form on rewarming. A number of cases have been reported in which cold urticaria has been transferred to normal skin by administration of serum, suggesting the possibility of an IgE-mediated mechanism in some subjects.

Solar urticaria represents a cutaneous response to solar irradiation, often within the ultraviolet wavelengths. H1 antihistamines may reduce symptoms, whilst exposure to artificial ultraviolet radiation can induce tolerance.

Cholinergic urticaria is a distinctive condition in which widespread small papular weals with variable erythema develop after stimuli such as exercise, emotional stress, or heat, for example from a hot bath. It usually affects young adults and presents as intense pruritus lasting for 15 to 60 minutes, after which the weals disappear. Extensive involvement may induce syncope. Cholinergic urticaria appears to result from local release of acetylcholine in the skin, with subsequent liberation of histamine. The condition usually settles after a few years.

Aquagenic urticaria is induced by contact with water irrespective of its temperature. H1 antihistamines reduce symptoms.

Deep pressure urticaria is characterized by swelling which appears after 4 to 6 hours of sustained pressure, for example from the seat of a chair, and lasts for 6 to 48 hours. Indurated itchy or painful swellings develop and can, if extensive, be accompanied by arthralgia and malaise. The cause of this condition is not known, but in view of the time delay it cannot be due to histamine release alone.

Chronic idiopathic urticaria. Patients often present with urticaria and angioedema for which no cause is found, despite extensive investigations, although it may occur after a viral infection. The condition usually remits spontaneously within two years.

DISEASES CAUSED BY TYPE II (CYTOTOXIC/CYTOLYTIC) HYPERSENSITIVITY

A number of important bullous diseases, including pemphigus and pemphigoid, are caused by type II hypersensitivity reactions. Both are organ-specific autoimmune diseases: they are potentially fatal and characterized by widespread blistering. In the case of pemphigus, drugs and, in one variant, infection may play a precipitating role. Both pemphigus and pemphigoid present in a similar way.

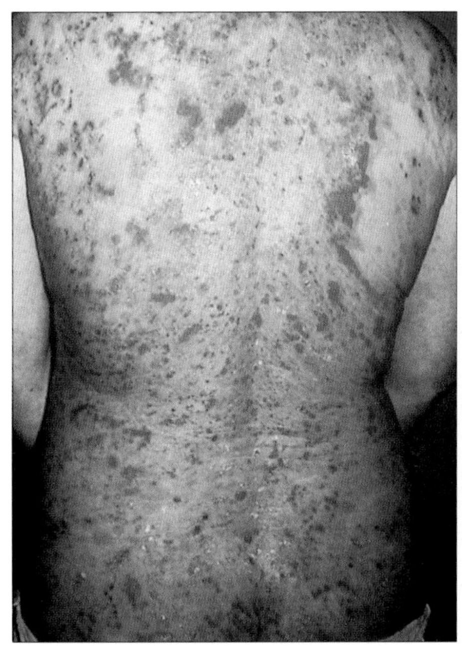

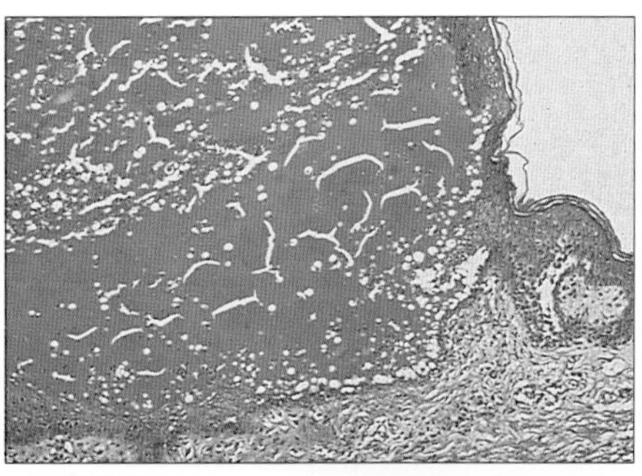

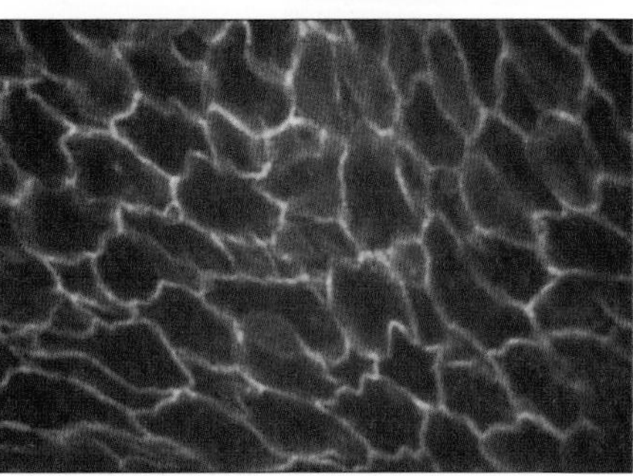

Fig. 14.6 Pemphigus vulgaris.
Left: the clinical appearance is typified by extensive blistering and erosions.
Upper right: histological examination shows a characteristic intra-epidermal blister.
Lower right: immunoflourescence reveals IgG in an intercellular distribution.

PEMPHIGUS

Pemphigus is a rare disease in Britain, occurring mainly in middle-aged subjects. It is more common in some tropical countries, where it is found in adolescents and children. Prior to the availability of corticosteroids, pemphigus was often fatal. Clinical variants include pemphigus vulgaris (Fig. 14.6 left), characterized by fragile blisters which break to leave denuded skin and often with associated oral lesions, and pemphigus foliaceus, which often starts on the head or chest with scaling and crusting rather than obvious bullae. All variants show an intraepidermal bulla on histological examination (Fig. 14.6 upper right).

Autoantibodies

Direct immunofluorescence of the perilesional skin shows intercellular IgG within the epidermis (Fig. 14.6 lower right); indirect immunofluorescence reveals circulating IgG autoantibodies in the patient's blood, the antibody titre being proportional to the disease activity. Exactly how the autoantibodies induce acantholysis and blister formation is unclear, but it is known that both proteolytic enzymes and the complement system are involved. Pemphigus is thus a true autoimmune disease, a fact which is reflected in its association with myasthenia gravis and thymoma, and lupus erythematosus.

Aetiology

The cause of pemphigus is not known, but some cases are drug related. Penicillamine, ampicillin, rifampicin, captopril and piroxicam can all induce this condition and presumably do so by a subtle alteration in the mechanisms controlling recognition of self-antigen. Fogo selvagem is
 an interesting variant of pemphigus foliaceus which affects children and young adults in Brazil: epidemiological work indicates that it is due to an infective agent spread by an arthropod vector.

Treatment

The treatment of pemphigus requires high doses of corticosteroids; 180–360mg/day of prednisolone may be necessary to control the disease. Unresponsive cases are sometimes helped by plasma exchange in conjunction with high-dose corticosteroids. Pemphigus is occasionally self-limiting, although to a lesser extent than pemphigoid.

PEMPHIGOID

Pemphigoid is relatively common in Britain, mainly affecting people over the age of 60 years. The most common subtype is bullous pemphigoid (Fig. 14.7 left); other subtypes include mucous membrane pemphigoid which causes scarring, principally of the conjunctivae and other mucosae, and cicatricial pemphigoid in which scarring lesions occur, often on the scalp. Pemphigoid (herpes) gestationis is a rare variant which occurs during pregnancy, apparently as an 'autoimmune' reaction to fetal antigens. In bullous pemphigoid subepidermal bullae form (Fig. 14.7 upper right), often on an erythematous or urticarial background. They usually appear first on the limbs and then spread to involve the trunk; oral involvement occurs in about 10% of cases. Before corticosteroids became available, pemphigoid was fatal in one- third of subjects.

Autoantibodies

Patients with bullous pemphigoid have circulating autoantibodies, usually IgG, to an antigen in the lamina lucida of

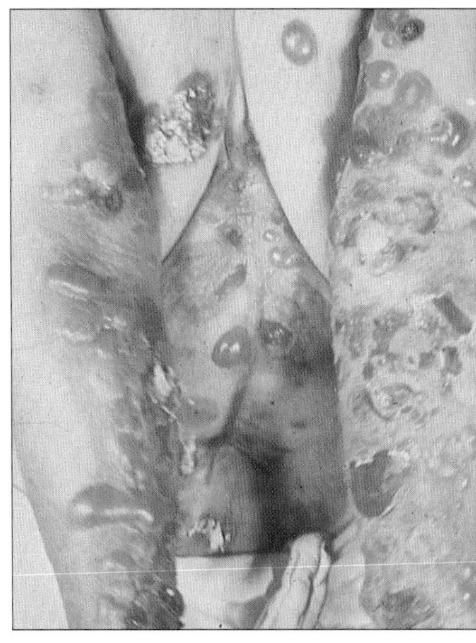

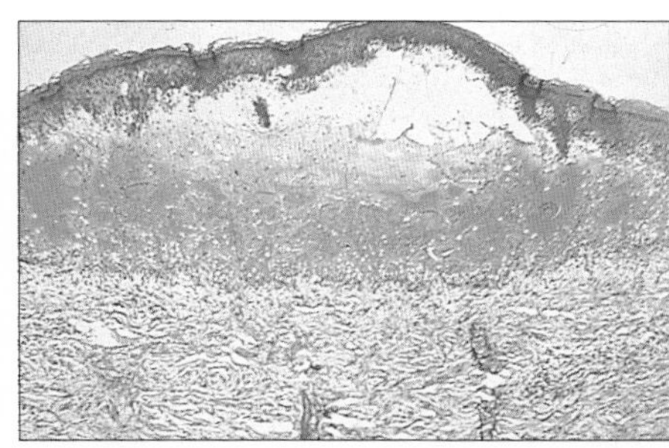

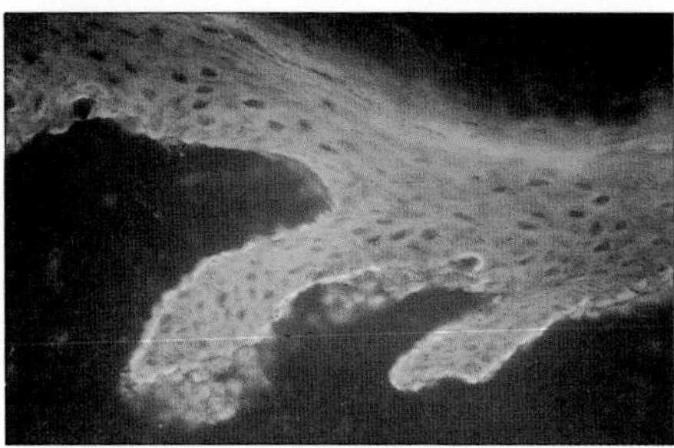

Fig. 14.7 Bullous pemphigoid. Left: clinically, the condition presents with extensive bullae and erosions. Upper right: typical histological appearance showing a subepidermal blister. Lower right: direct immunofluorescence reveals IgG antibodies at the basement membrane. Courtesy of Dr C Harrington.

Bullous disorders		
Feature	**Pemphigus**	**Pemphigoid**
bullous lesion	intra-epidermal	sub-epidermal
auto-antigen	intercellular substance (of epidermal pickle cells)	basement membrane (at dermo-epidermal junction)
mouth involvement	>90%	<10%
HLA association	A10, B13	none
antibody titre	proportional to disease	no relationship
IgE	normal	raised in 50%

Fig. 14.8 Features of bullous disorders.

the basement membrane at the dermo-epidermal junction (Fig. 14.7 lower right). This antigen is synthesized by the basal keratinocytes of the epidermis. It is different from the antigens in pemphigoid gestationis and cicatricial pemphigoid, although the latter two are also found in the lamina lucida. The titre of circulating autoantibodies in pemphigoid does not correlate with disease activity, unlike in pemphigus. Patients may be split at presentation into two groups: those with high, and those with low autoantibody titres. Some with low titres have active disease whereas others continue to have high titres but are disease free. Direct immunofluorescence of perilesional skin shows IgG antibody, and sometimes C3, deposited in a linear fashion at the dermo-epidermal junction. The mechanism of bulla formation is thought to involve interaction between the antigen and autoantibodies, complement and leucocytes.

Aetiology

The cause of pemphigoid is unclear; a few cases have followed drug ingestion, for example furosemide, or ultraviolet or X-irradiation. Overall, there is no increase in the prevalence of malignancy in bullous pemphigoid, although patients who present with a figurate erythema may have an underlying neoplasm.

Treatment

Pemphigoid is treated with systemic corticosteroids, although in much more modest doses than those used for pemphigus: 40mg/day of prednisolone is usually sufficient. Spontaneous remission is more common than in pemphigus: in about half the patients with bullous pemphigoid, steroids can be discontinued after two years without recurrence. A comparison of the major features of pemphigus and pemphigoid is shown in Fig. 14.8.

DISEASES CAUSED BY TYPE III HYPERSENSITIVITY (IMMUNE COMPLEX DISEASE)

Immune complexes are usually cleared by the mononuclear phagocyte system, but sometimes result in disease. Most diseases of this type that affect the skin result from complex deposition in vessel walls of the dermis and

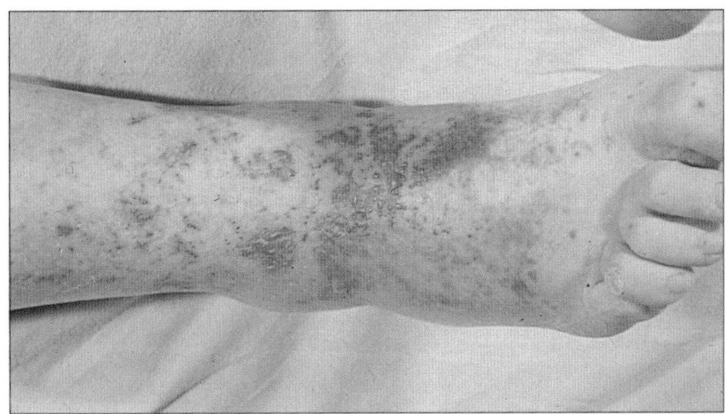

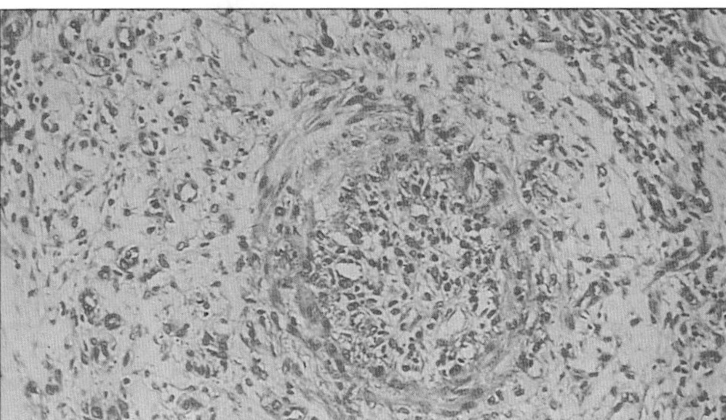

Fig. 14.9 Allergic vasculitis. Left: marked purpuric rash on the lower leg. Right: histological examination shows a thrombosed vessel with fibrinoid change and polymorphic infiltration.

subcutaneous fat, although some (notably erythema nodosum leprosum in leprosy) are caused by extravascular complex formation.

Circulating immune complexes are believed to localize at a specific vessel site because of the action of vasoactive amines, which alter vascular permeability; endothelial cell surface receptors are probably also important, and in some diseases clearing of complexes by the mononuclear phagocyte system may be defective. The complexes cause vasoactive amine release, either via C3a and C5a which act on basophils, or by directly stimulating basophils and platelets. When in the vessel wall, complexes induce platelet aggregation (which may form microthrombi) and complement activation. The chemical mediators produced attract polymorphs, lymphocytes and macrophages. Polymorphs may be unable to phagocytose the fixed complexes, and thus release lysosomal enzymes and generate oxygen-derived free radicals. These events result in damage to the vessel wall, producing the clinical picture of vasculitis. This takes a variable form in the skin and depends on a number of factors:

- site of vessel involved
- size & solubility of immune complexes
- antibody class
- local production of immune complexes
- deposition from distant source
- chronicity (of immune complex formation)

Other organs are frequently involved in the disease process. Symptoms relating to kidney, gut, joint or neurological involvement may have more serious consequences than those related to the skin changes.

ALLERGIC VASCULITIS (LEUCOCYTOCLASTIC VASCULITIS)

14.6 This is a common condition, characterized clinically by the development of a purpuric rash over the lower limbs (Fig. 14.9 left), buttocks and forearms, which may lead to ulceration. Other organs involved include the joints and kidneys, which may be involved to the extent that the patient proceeds to renal failure. Histological examination shows a prominent vasculitis (Fig. 14.9 right); there is endothelial swelling, intense polymorph and lymphocyte infiltration, and disintegration of the polymorphs (leucocytoclasis) resulting in nuclear 'dust'. The vessels may be thrombosed, with fibrinoid change and epidermal necrosis.

Henoch-Schönlein purpura is an important example of this type of vasculitis, affecting both children and adults. It usually follows a virus infection, or respiratory infection with *Streptococcus pyogenes*. The purpura is accompanied by proteinuria and haematuria, gastrointestinal haemorrhage and arthralgia.

The course of allergic vasculitis is variable: it may last for 2–3 weeks or several years. It usually follows infection, but may also be caused by drugs such as thiazides and phenylbutazone.

URTICARIAL VASCULITIS

This is a variant of allergic vasculitis, in which the urticarial weals are prominent presumably due to anaphylatoxin release or complement activation by deposited immune complexes. The weals differ from those in 'classical' urticaria in that they may last for several days and tend to become purpuric. Arthralgia and hypocomplementaemia are common, and histological examination of the skin reveals a leucocytoclastic vasculitis. The condition may follow drug ingestion or infection, or it may be a feature of systemic lupus erythematosus.

ERYTHEMA NODOSUM

Erythema nodosum is a common condition, characterized clinically by tender, erythematous nodules on the shins (Fig. 14.10 left) and, less commonly, on the thighs and forearms. The lesions tend to resolve after six weeks. On

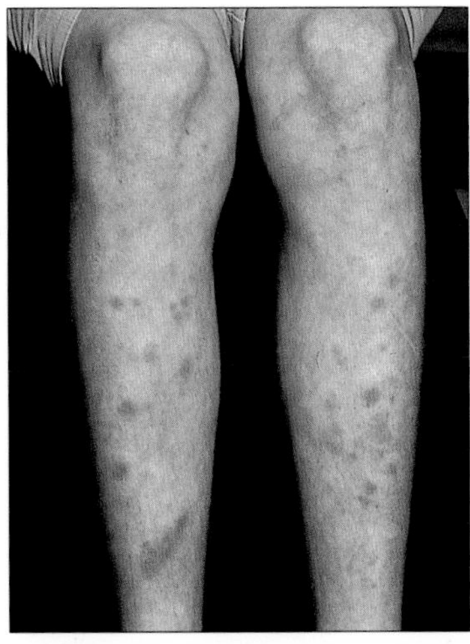

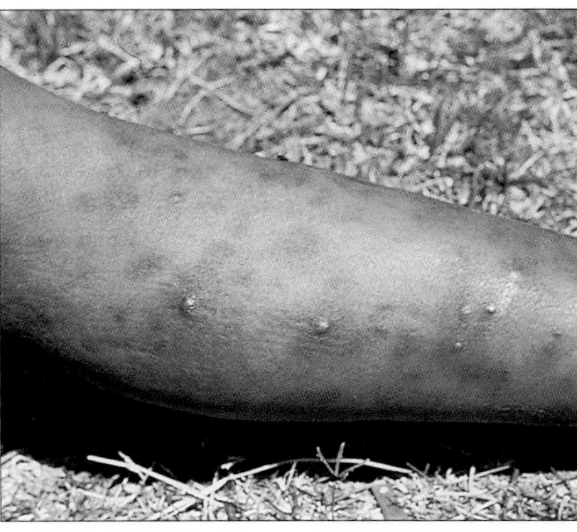

Fig. 14.10 Left: erythema nodosum, presenting as red, tender nodules on the shins. Right: erythema nodosum leprosum is characterized by red indurated areas, seen here on the leg, with pustule formation.

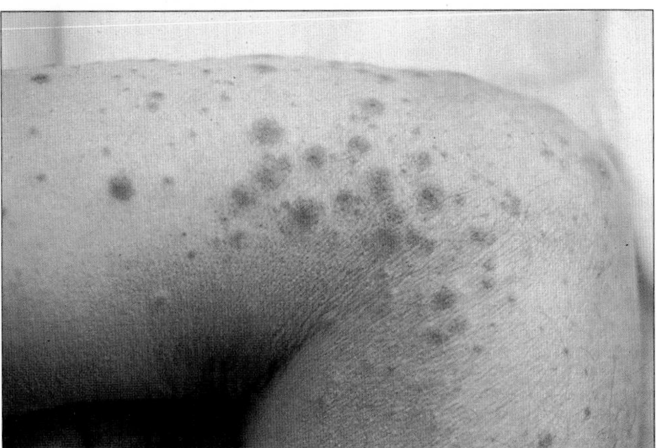

Fig. 14.11 Polyarteritis nodosa with palpable purpura on the thigh.

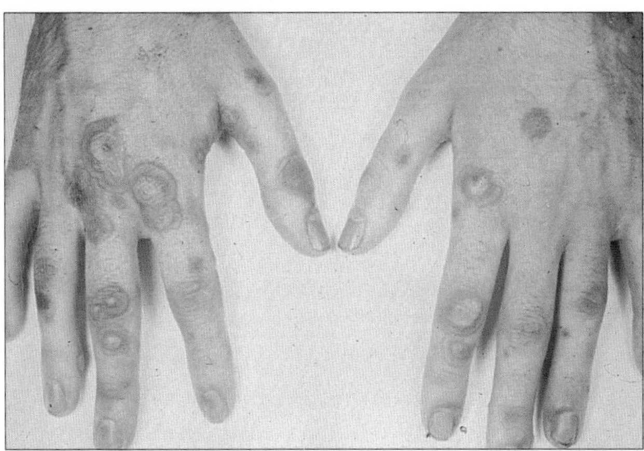

Fig. 14.12 Erythema multiforme with target lesions on the dorsa of the hands.

histological examination there is evidence of vasculitis but, unlike allergic vasculitis, the vessels involved are in the subcutaneous fat and hence the different clinical picture. The most common causes are streptococcal infections, sarcoidosis, tuberculosis, pregnancy and drugs such as sulphonamides

ERYTHEMA NODOSUM LEPROSUM

This usually occurs during the first two years of treatment in lepromatous leprosy patients. The condition differs from classical erythema nodosum in that the erythematous nodules last only for about a week, and are as common on the face and arms (Fig. 14.10 right) as on the legs. There is associated fever, malaise, neuralgia and arthralgia. Renal amyloid may eventually develop from glomerulonephritis.

On histological examination there is little evidence of vasculitis, and the lesions are thought to be due to extravascular complex formation. This is not surprising as the antigen (*M. leprae*) is already in the skin. Thus the situation is somewhat different from the other types of dermatological immune complex disease.

POLYARTERITIS NODOSA

This is an important disease because it is often fatal. Renal and cardiac involvement are common, but there is a benign form, confined to the skin, which is known as 'cutaneous polyarteritis nodosa'. Small and medium sized arteries in the dermis are involved, leading to a nodular vasculitis in the skin (Fig. 14.11).

The cause of the disease is unknown, although hepatitis B virus is involved in 25% of patients. Whereas the disease process in other types of vasculitis is self-limiting, in polyarteritis nodosa it tends to be progressive.

ERYTHEMA MULTIFORME

This condition is easy to recognize because of the characteristic target lesions on the arms (Fig. 14.12) and legs,

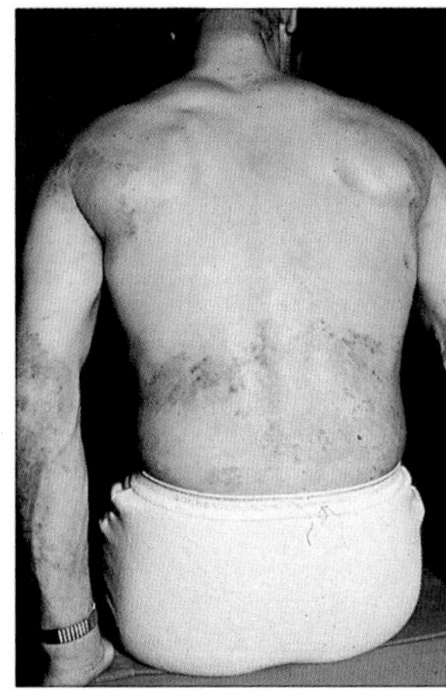

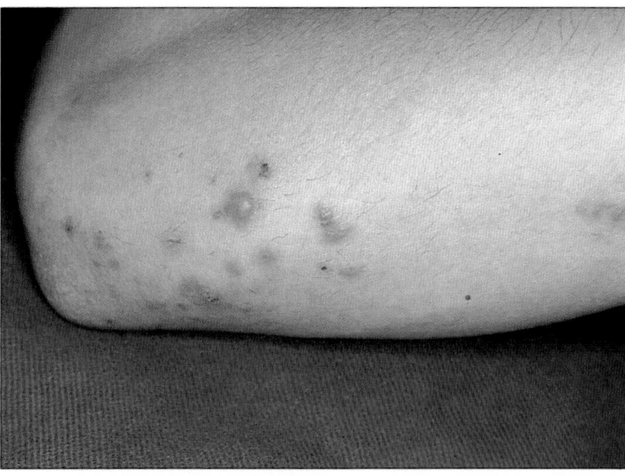

Fig. 14.13 Dermatitis herpetiformis, showing characteristic distribution of small blisters on the shoulders, lower back and elbows.

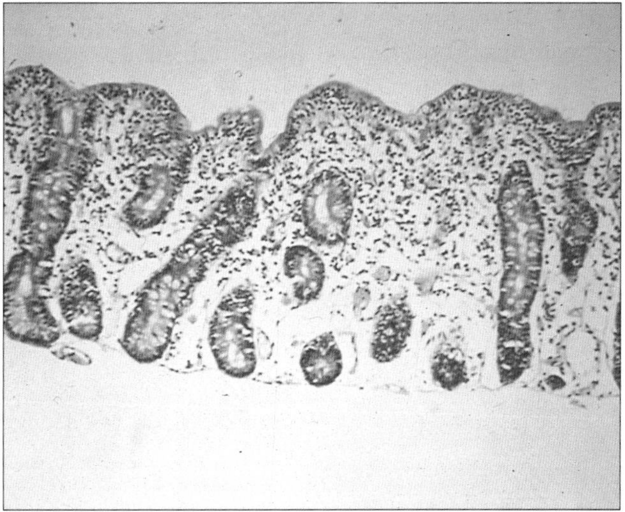

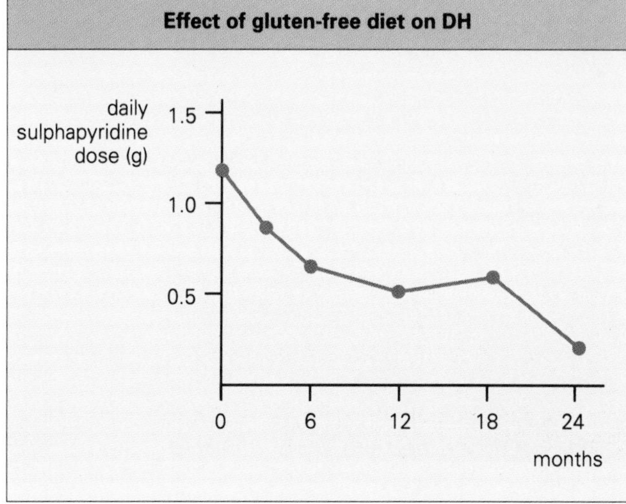

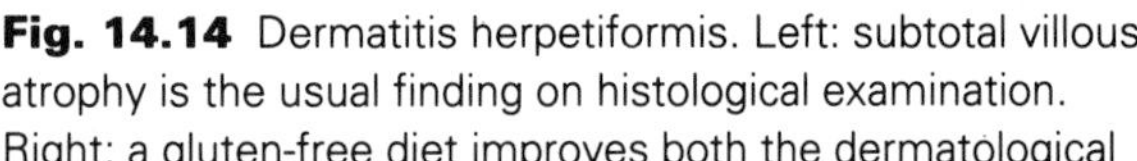

Fig. 14.14 Dermatitis herpetiformis. Left: subtotal villous atrophy is the usual finding on histological examination. Right: a gluten-free diet improves both the dermatological and gastrointestinal manifestations of the disease, as indicated here by the reduced daily sulphapyridine requirements of 10 patients.

which present in association with stomatitis, iritis, and malaise. There is vasculitis on histological examination, and IgM has been demonstrated in the vessels but the evidence for the condition being due to immune complex deposition is still largely circumstantial. It usually follows herpes simplex or *Mycoplasma pneumoniae* infection or sulphonamide ingestion.

DERMATITIS HERPETIFORMIS (DH)

Intensely itchy blisters appearing on the extensor aspects of the limbs, shoulders, buttocks and scalp, characterize the clinical picture of DH (Fig. 14.13). The blisters are subepidermal: polymorphs and occasional eosinophils accumulate in the papillary dermis and blister cavity. In most patients DH is associated with the villous atrophy of coeliac disease, and both the gut lesion and the skin changes will respond to a gluten-free diet (Fig. 14.14). Dapsone will suppress the skin lesions, possibly by blocking release of neutrophil chemotactic factors. Evidence to support circulating immune complexes as the cause of DH is as follows:

- All patients have IgA deposited in a granular pattern in the dermal papillae of perilesional skin (Fig. 14.15), binding to the dermal microfibrillar bundles. C3 and C5 are sometimes also found.
- IgA anti-gluten antibodies have been found in some patients, but these have not been related to the deposition of immunoglobulin in the skin.
- Circulating immune complexes have been detected in the serum of 30–40% of DH patients. They are primarily IgA , but occasionally contain IgG or IgM. The level of these complexes increases about two hours after ingestion of wheat.

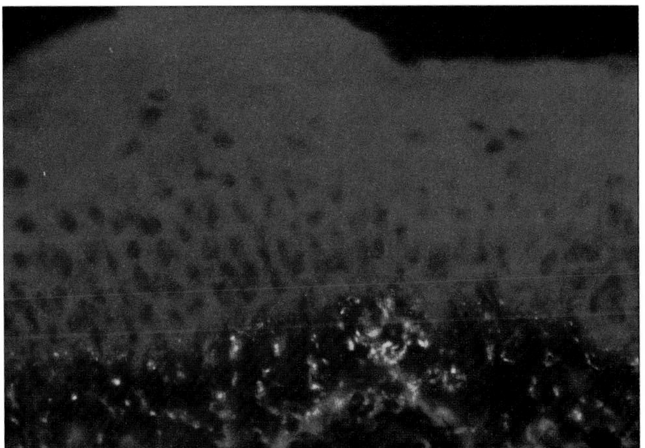

Fig. 14.15 Immunofluorescent staining of skin taken from a patient with dermatitis herpetiformis shows granular deposits of IgA in the subepidermal region. Rhodamine stain.

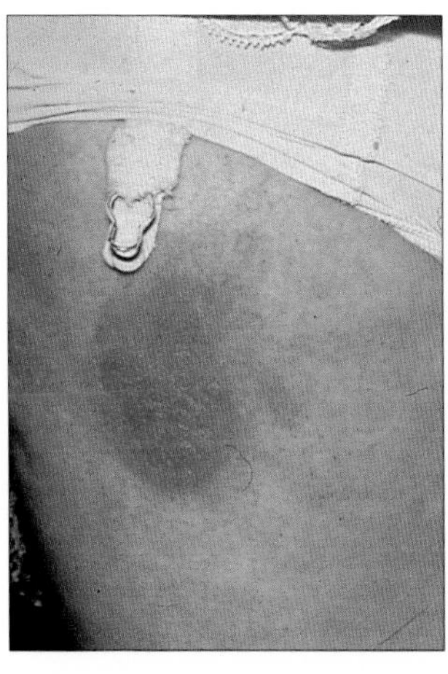

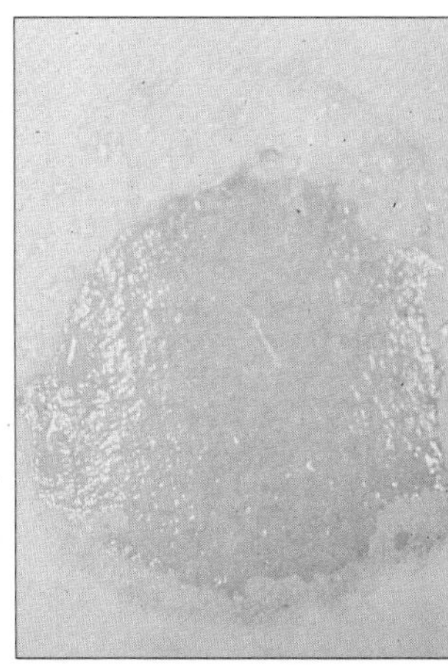

Fig. 14.16 Allergic contact dermatitis. Left: in this case the reaction was caused by the rubber component in the patient's suspenders. Right: the suspected allergen can be identified by applying it to the skin as a patch test. An eczematous reaction, as seen here, appearing between 48 and 72 hours after application confirms the diagnosis.

These observations suggest that the allergen, gluten, can stimulate an immune complex response in DH patients. It is presumed that the IgA-containing immune complexes lodge in the skin, activate the alternative complement pathway and generate the cascade of inflammation which results in blistering, although direct evidence for this is lacking at present.

DISEASES CAUSED BY TYPE IV (DELAYED) HYPERSENSITIVITY

Allergic contact dermatitis (Fig. 14.16) is the main example of type IV hypersensitivity in the skin, although it differs slightly from the classical model of delayed hypersensitivity, the tuberculin reaction, because the antigen is applied epicutaneously and not intradermally. Atopic eczema is also discussed in this section, although the evidence for the role of delayed hypersensitivity in its aetiology is still debatable. The borderline leprosy reaction is an excellent example of granulomatous hypersensitivity in the skin.

ALLERGIC CONTACT DERMATITIS

Allergic contact dermatitis has been the subject of much research by immunologists over the last 60 years. The evidence for it being due to cell-mediated immunity may be summarized as follows:

- Lymphatic continuity with the body is required for sensitization through the skin.
- Sensitivity can be passively transferred to a naive animal by the injection of peritoneal exudate cells from a sensitized animal.
- Challenge to a skin site attached by the vascular supply will elicit a response only after sensitization at a distant site.
- Sensitivity can be transferred by intraperitoneal grafting of a draining lymph node from a sensitized animal.
- Following application of a chemical to the skin of a sensitized animal, the number of veiled cells (like Langerhans' cells but without Birbeck granules) is greatly increased in the draining lymph and there is a several-fold increase in the number of Langerhans' cells and interdigitating reticulum cells in the paracortical areas of regional lymph nodes.
- Epidermal Langerhans' cells can act as antigen-presenting cells *in vitro* for the T lymphocytes of sensitized subjects.

Pathogenesis

In a sensitized subject, an epicutaneously applied chemical (usually a hapten) combines with epidermal proteins to form an antigen; this is taken up by epidermal Langerhans' cells which carry it via the lymphatic channels to the regional lymph nodes. There they present the antigen to T lymphocytes, although peripheral antigen presentation may also occur. Recognition of the antigenic determinants on the Langerhans' cell by specific delayed hypersensitivity T cells stimulates the antigen-presenting cell to release interleukin-1, which in turn stimulates the lymphocyte to release cytokines including interleukin-2. Clonal expansion of T cells follows and the specific T lymphocytes migrate to the skin via efferent lymphatics,

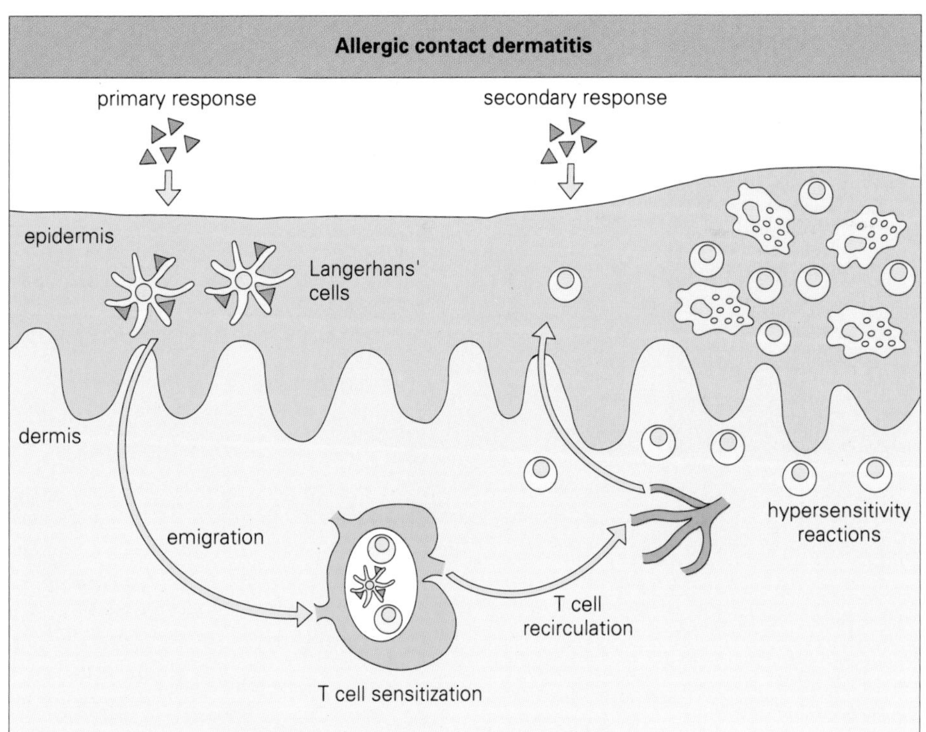

Fig. 14.17 Proposed mechanism for allergic contact dermatitis. Antigen entering the skin is taken up by Langerhans' cells which migrate to the lymph nodes, appearing as veiled cells; these then present antigen to TH cells within the T cell area of the lymph node. Sensitized T cells recirculate and enter the skin through the dermal capillaries. If they then encounter immunogenic antigen they are activated, release cytokines, recruit further inflammatory cells and initiate the typical reactions of delayed hypersensitivity.

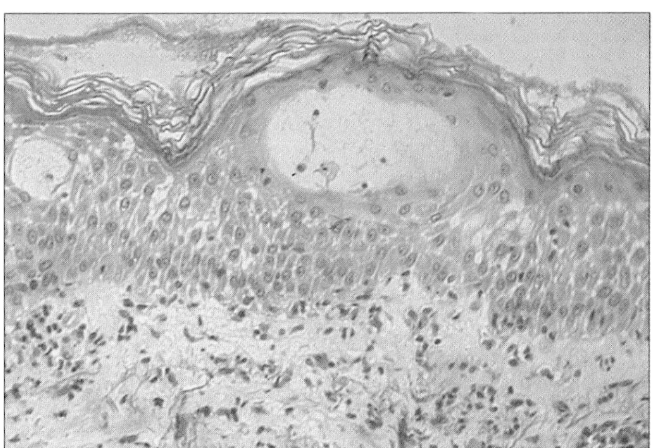

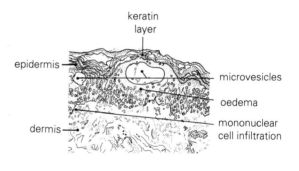

Fig. 14.18 Histological appearance of lesion in contact hypersensitivity. There is infiltration of the epidermis (which is pushed outwards) by mononuclear cells, and microvesicle formation with oedema. The dermis is also infiltrated by mononuclear cells. H & E stain, x130.

where they recognize the antigen and initiate a cascade of events that produces inflammation and dermatitis (Fig.14.17).

Histology

At the challenge site, helper ($CD4^+$) T cells begin to enter the skin after four hours and gradually increase in number, in both dermis and epidermis, up to 48 hours after challenge (Fig. 14.18). Suppressor/cytotoxic ($CD8^+$) T cells infiltrate the skin, but in lesser numbers, and the number of Langerhans' cells in the dermis also increases over the first 24 hours. Keratinocytes express MHC class II antigens at 24 and 48 hours after application of the antigen, although the exact significance of this is unclear.

Clinical reaction

Allergic contact dermatitis develops as an idiosyncratic reaction to an allergen, and is characterized clinically by erythema and small blisters developing at the site of contact. Some chemicals, for example 2,4–dinitrochlorobenzene, will sensitize almost everyone, but in many cases it is not easy to predict the development of contact allergy in an individual. Only a fraction of those occupationally exposed to an antigen will develop sensitivity and the

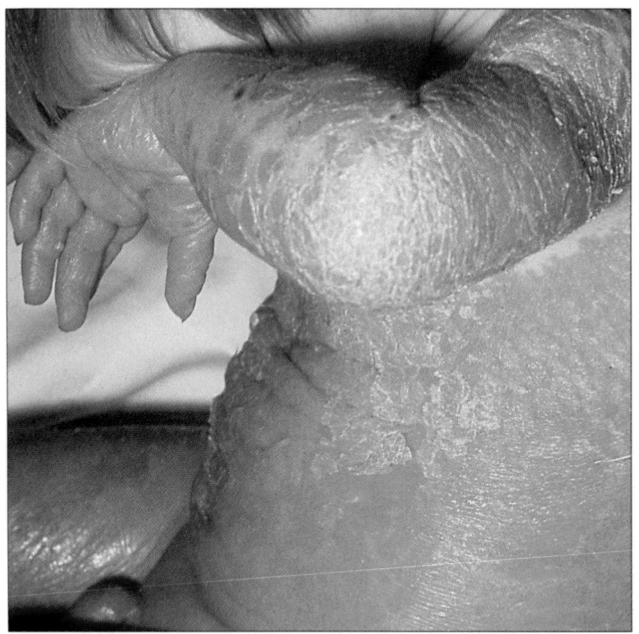

Fig. 14.19 Extensive atopic eczema. Courtesy of Dr D Sharvill.

time taken for it to develop varies according to the antigen. For example, bricklayers exposed to chromium in cement develop sensitivity on average after 10 or more years in the trade, whereas hairdressers exposed to nickel often develop sensitivity within a few months of starting work.

Identification of allergen

Identification of the allergen is vital. The history and examination may suggest certain substances which can be confirmed by epicutaneous patch testing. This involves the occlusive application, in relevant concentrations, of a series of at least 22 common allergens on small aluminium discs (Finn chambers) to the back of the subject, where they are secured with adhesive tape. The patches are left in place for 48 hours, removed, and then read. A further reading is done 48 hours later. Interpretation requires expertise, as not all reactions are necessarily specific delayed hypersensitivity reactions.

Effect of ultraviolet radiation

Ultraviolet (UV) radiation is able to modify the immunological function of the skin. In mice, UVB (wavelength 290–320nm) can induce unresponsiveness to contact allergens and enhance systemic susceptibility to UV-induced tumours, both effects being due to the generation of specific T suppressor cells.

Epidermal Langerhans' cells are obvious potential targets for the effects of UV. Treatment with UVB, and with psoralens (a photosensitizer) plus UVA (PUVA) produce a reduction in epidermal Langerhans' cell numbers in mice and humans as judged by different types of marker, although the cells may still be identifiable ultrastructurally. *In vitro,* UVB irradiation of Langerhans' cells reduces their ability to present antigen to lymphocytes. Clinically, impaired contact hypersensitivity to dinitrochlorobenzene has been noted in PUVA-treated patients. Keratinocytes are another possible target for UV as they produce IL-1.

This ability to alter the immune state of the skin with UV has therapeutic potential although clinical experience is limited. Single doses of PUVA or UVB have no effect on the allergic nickel patch test reaction but UVB may help patients with chronic allergic contact dermatitis of the hands.

ATOPIC ECZEMA

Atopic eczema (Fig. 14.19) is an enigma. On histological examination, the skin changes are very similar to those in allergic contact eczema, with microvesiculation in the epidermis, and an infiltrate of lymphocytes and macrophages within the dermis, infiltrating into the epidermis. The appearance is therefore quite unlike that seen in IgE-mediated hypersensitivity. Despite this 80% of patients have raised concentrations of IgE (up to 50,000ng/ml) with positive skin prick tests to inhalants and, in some, to foods.

The role of delayed hypersensitivity in atopic eczema is at present open to question. In patients with house dust mite allergy (which is the case in most atopic eczema patients), it has been shown that a patch test applied for 48 hours on abraded skin will produce an inflammatory reaction resembling eczema. Lymphoproliferative responses to house dust mite are positive in these patients, confirming that they are able to mount a delayed hypersensitivity reaction to this allergen. However, not all atopic eczema patients are allergic to the house dust mite, indeed some show no evidence of IgE-mediated allergy to any antigen. This suggests that, in such patients, IgE-mediated and delayed hypersensitivity reactions may be complicating factors rather than primary aetiological factors.

Certain patients (usually children) with IgE-mediated food allergy (to cow's milk, egg, fish, nuts) show exacerbated atopic eczema following ingestion of the food. They may develop angioedema, contact urticaria and widespread urticaria, and it seems likely that the latter then leads on to the eczematous process, although the mechanisms involved are still unclear. There is often a history of seasonal exacerbation of atopic eczema, which is associated with high levels of grass pollen or house dust mite.

When patients outgrow their atopic eczema, which often occurs at puberty and sometimes around the menopause in females, the total and specific IgE concentrations fall, but the other symptoms such as asthma and food allergy may continue. This seems to suggest that T cell regulation is important in both the IgE production,

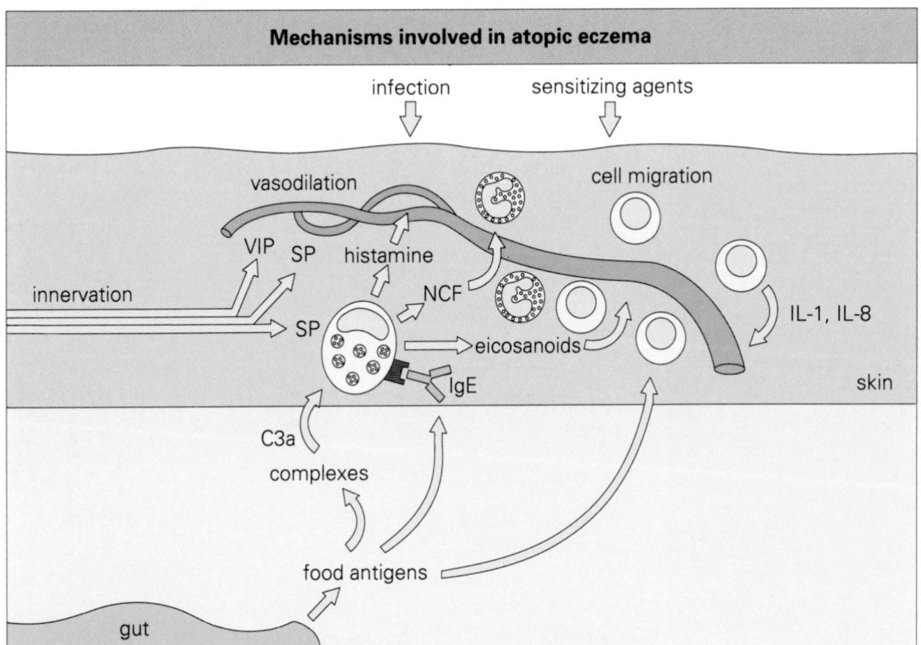

Fig. 14. 20 Food antigens can trigger mast cells via their surface IgE, or indirectly by the formation of immune complexes and activation of complement. Mediators including histamine are vasodilatory, and substance P (SP) and vasoactive intestinal peptide (VIP) can also cause cutaneous vasodilation. Nervous control may be mediated via the mast cells which are triggered to release eicosanoids by SP. Chemotactic factors including leukotriene B4 and neutrophil chemotactic factor (NCF) signal cellular infiltration and activated cells can cause further cell migration by releasing IL-8 and IL-1 which act on endothelium.

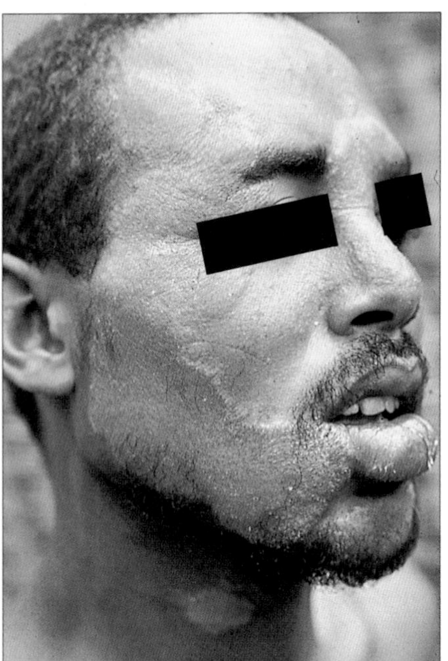

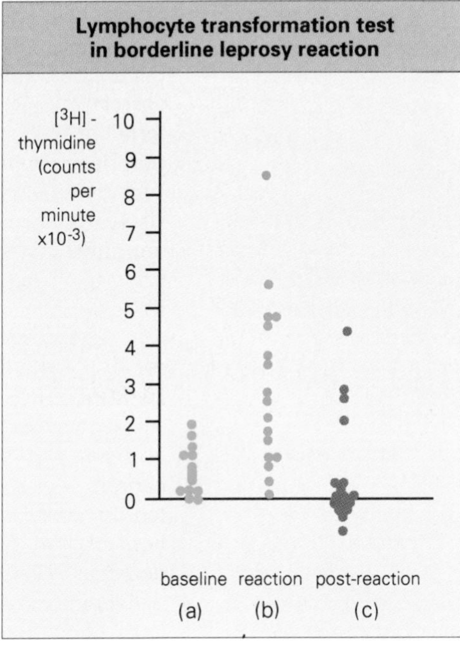

Fig. 14.21 Left: These previously hypopigmented skin lesions have become swollen and inflamed. Right: during the reaction the lymphocyte transformation response to *M. leprae* rises and then falls when the reaction is successfully treated with oral steroids.The lymphocyte transformation responses (uptake of [^{3}H]-thymidine) to sonicated *M. leprae* are shown for 17 patients who developed such reactions: (a) before starting leprosy treatment (baseline); (b) during the reaction; and (c) on cessation of steroids.

and the eczema. A summary of the mechanisms involved in atopic eczema is shown in Fig. 14. 20.

BORDERLINE LEPROSY REACTION

In leprosy, protective immunity depends on cell-mediated factors, and humoral immunity has no apparent role. The spectrum of disease depends on the competence of the host immune response to the organism: tuberculoid leprosy develops in those with good responsiveness, whereas lepromatous follows in those with little or no response. Borderline leprosy occurs in those whose immunity lies between these two extremes.

Borderline reactions are a dramatic example of delayed hypersensitivity, with greatly increased lymphocyte proliferative responses to *M. leprae* (Fig. 14.21). This can occur naturally or following drug treatment. The affected skin

Eczema herpeticum
Patients with atopic eczema often get widespread herpes simplex infections (Fig. 14.25), with marked fever and malaise. In a child, the condition may be fatal.

Hyperimmunoglobulinaemia E (Staphylococcal abscess syndrome)
This is a rare condition, in which patients with atopic eczema and markedly raised concentrations of serum IgE develop staphylococcal abscesses in the skin and lungs. IgE antibodies to staphylococcus are found in the majority of cases, some of whom also show evidence of a defect in neutrophil function.

GENERALIZED HERPES ZOSTER INFECTIONS.

Varicella-zoster virus is the cause of chickenpox and shingles. Patients with lymphoma and consequent immunodeficiency may develop a generalized 'shingles' infection and are covered in blisters containing the virus.

IMMUNODEFICIENCY AND PAPILLOMA (WART) VIRUSES

Epidermodysplasia verruciformis is a rare familial condition in which patients develop widespread warty lesions due to infection with a number of papilloma viruses, particularly human types 5 and 8. These may progress to squamous cell carcinoma (SCC).

Patients who have had renal transplants and who are receiving immunosuppressive therapy are liable to develop extensive wart infections (Fig. 14.26), particularly in the perineum. These are very difficult to treat, and may also progress to SCC.

ACQUIRED IMMUNODEFICIENCY SYNDROME (AIDS)

Seborrhoeic eczema
AIDS patients are prone to develop seborrhoeic eczema, which is thought to result from colonization of the skin by *Pityrosporum*; the infection clears with anti-yeast treatment.

Kaposi's sarcoma
Kaposi's sarcoma is a multicentric angiomatous neoplasm which is commonly seen in homosexual men with AIDS. It is suggested that this results from a defect in immune surveillance (see chapter 24).

CONNECTIVE TISSUE DISEASES

The connective tissue diseases are an important group of disorders which are covered in chapter 6. Lupus erythematosus and scleroderma have a form which is confined to the skin, and it is probable that there is a spectrum of disease in each case.

LUPUS ERYTHEMATOSUS (LE)

Chronic discoid LE
This form is confined to the skin, occurring on sun-exposed areas, and is exacerbated by sunlight. Red plaques appear on the face (Fig. 14.27) and scalp, and lead to scarring. Immunofluorescence of the involved skin shows granular IgG (or IgM) deposition at the basement membrane zone of the epidermis. Whilst the disease remains confined to the skin in most patients, 5% progress to systemic LE.

Subacute cutaneous LE
In this form, the cutaneous involvement is more extensive than in discoid LE. Annular or papulo-squamous eruptions are present and may be accompanied by manifestations of systemic LE, such as arthralgia, fever, anaemia, leucopenia, thrombocytopenia and circulating anti-nuclear antibodies: renal involvment is rare. Antibodies to the Ro and La cytoplasmic antigens are often detected. Subacute cutaneous LE may occur half way through a spectrum of disease which has chronic discoid LE and systemic LE at opposite ends.

Systemic LE
The many manifestations of systemic LE include a number of skin signs, such as a butterfly rash, chronic discoid plaques, chilblain-like plaques on the fingers and capillary dilatation at the nail folds. Patients often have IgG (or IgM) deposits in the skin of both involved and uninvolved sites.

SCLERODERMA

The aetiology of this spectrum of diseases remains uncertain, but the similarity of the skin to that seen in graft-versus-host disease suggests a common pathogenesis. In the majority of cases, endothelial cell destruction is prominent and this has led to the theory that ischaemia may also be important.

Morphoea
Morphoea is characterized by localized sclerosis of the skin, presenting with a bluish plaque which becomes indurated and later develops an ivory colour. The plaque may appear anywhere on the body but is most commonly found on the trunk, thighs and upper arms. Scarring is evident on histological examination, and IgM and C3 may be found at the basement membrane and in blood vessels of the skin. There are no serological abnormalities.

Generalized morphoea
Plaques of skin sclerosis start on the trunk and gradually coalesce with new plaques to become generalized. There may also be spindling of the fingers, as in systemic sclerosis. Raynaud's phenomenon occasionally occurs, and joint pains are reported in 40% of patients. Examination of the blood may reveal a raised ESR, anti-nuclear

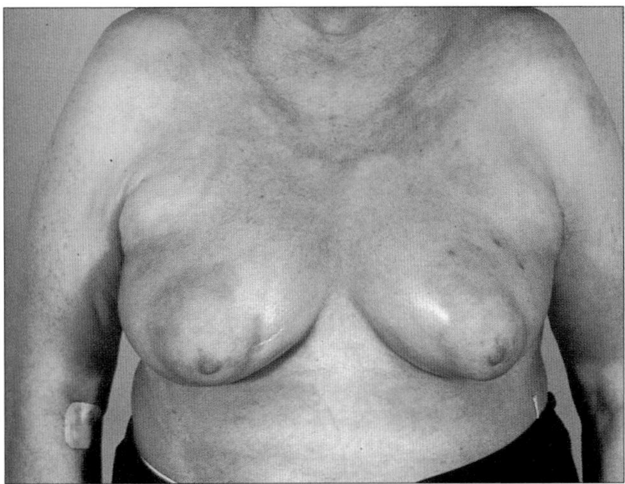

Fig. 14.28 Generalized morphoea, showing large, confluent plaques affecting the breasts and trunk.

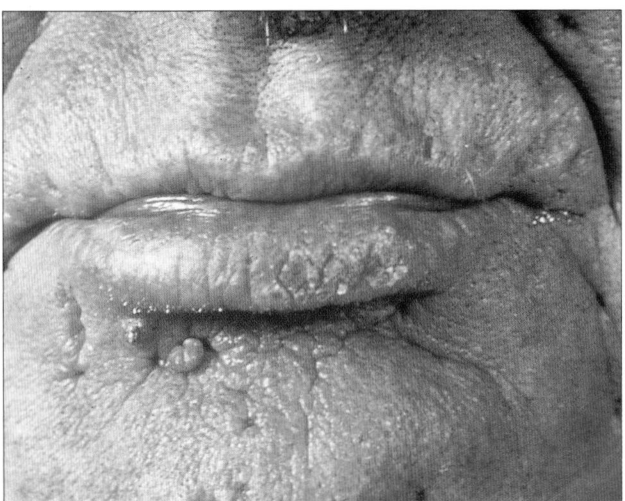

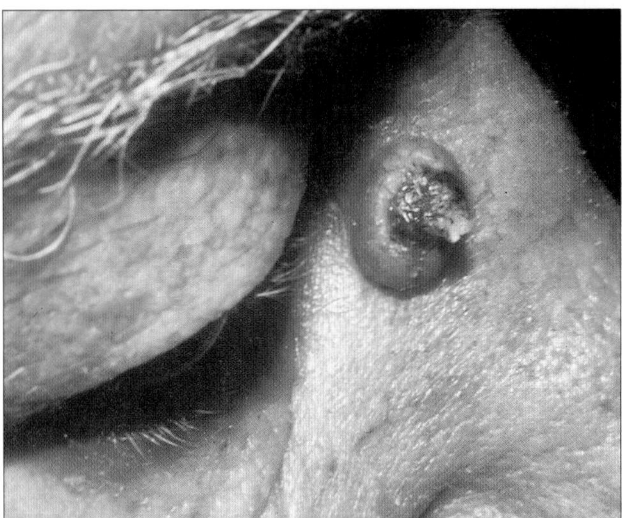

Fig. 14. 29 Squamous cell carcinoma. Upper: self-healing epithelioma on the chin of a patient with familial disease. Lower: keratoacanthoma with characteristic keratin plug.

antibodies, and eosinophilia. Immunofluorescence of the skin may show IgM and C3 in the basement membrane and in the blood vessels of the dermis. The characteristic clinical appearance is shown in Fig. 14.28.

Systemic sclerosis

Systemic sclerosis differs from morphoea in that it is not confined to the skin. The skin changes usually affect the limbs and face, and Raynaud's phenomenon is the most common presenting feature. This is followed by sclerosis of the skin of the fingers, calcinosis and gangrene, together with oesophageal stricture, disorders of the colonic motility, pulmonary fibrosis and renal dysfunction. Antinuclear (anti-centromere and anti-Scl 70) antibodies are almost invariably found.

NEOPLASIA

BASAL CELL CARCINOMA

Basal cell carcinoma (BCC) is common in patients with white skins, usually resulting from sun exposure. A shiny nodule develops, which then ulcerates and locally invades the surrounding tissues (hence the name rodent ulcer). Despite this, it hardly ever metastasizes, the reason for which is unclear.

SQUAMOUS CELL CARCINOMA

Squamous cell carcinoma (SCC) occurs in skin damaged by various factors such as sunlight, irradiation, chronic irritation, or contact with chrome. The tumours desquamate and ulcerate early, but metastasize late. There are two variants which resolve spontaneously:

- Familial self-healing epithelioma (of Ferguson-Smith) (Fig. 14.29 upper). There is a hereditary tendency to develop SCC from a young age, but these resolve spontaneously.
- Keratoacanthoma is an SCC with a central keratin plug which gives it a characteristic appearance (Fig. 14.29 lower). It develops within a few weeks and then, despite its malignant histology, resolves spontaneously, to leave a cratered scar.

MALIGNANT MELANOMA

This is a much feared skin tumour derived from melanocytes, which metastasizes very early. By the time the nodular tumour reaches the size of a lentil, the 5-year survival prospect is grim: it is thus arguably the most malignant tumour afflicting man. There is as yet no effective treatment for advanced disease, although total surgical excision of early lesions is curative. Primary malignant melanomas do sometimes resolve, leaving secondary melanomas in the lymph nodes or elsewhere.

SKIN LYMPHOMAS

Lymphomas of the skin are rare and may be T cell or, less commonly, B cell derived. The most widely known type is mycosis fungoides, which has three phases:

1. premycotic, which may last for 30 years before progression;
2. infiltrative, which may last for several years;
3. tumourous, by which time the prognosis is poor.

Unfortunately chemotherapy, which used to be administered in the premycotic phase in an attempt to abort the process, tends to aid progression of the disease.

KAPOSI'S SARCOMA

There are three types of Kaposi's sarcoma, classified according to patient group:

- Classical Kaposi's occurs in elderly men, often of Jewish origin, who have relatively benign angiomas on the legs.
- African Kaposi's is a multicentric tumour affecting skin, bones and internal viscera. It has a variable prognosis.
- AIDS-related Kaposi's is confined to the skin but may be widespread (see chapter 24).

FURTHER READING

Barnetson RStC. Allergy and the skin. In: Lessof TH, Lee TH, Kemeny MH. *Allergy: An international textbook.* Chichester: Wiley, 1987.

Beutner EH, Chorzelski TP, Kumar V, eds. *Immunopathology of the skin* (3E). New York: Wiley, 1987.

Boss JD, Kapsenberg ML. The skin immune system: Its cellular constituents and their interactions. *Immunol Today*; 1986;**7**:235–240.

Dahl MV. *Clinical immunodermatology* (2E). Chicago: Year Book Medical Publishers Inc, 1987.

Kripke ML, Morison WL. Studies on the mechanism of systemic suppression of contact hypersensitivity by UVB radiation. II. Differences in the suppression of delayed and contact hypersensitivity in mice. *J Invest Dermatol* 1986;**86**:593–599.

Mackie RM, ed. *Current perspectives in immunodermatology.* Edinburgh: Churchill Livingstone, 1984.

Thiers BH, Dobson RL, eds. *Pathogenesis of skin disease.* New York: Churchill Livingstone, 1986.

15

Oral Disorders

INTRODUCTION

The major difference between the mouth and the tissue lining the remainder of the gastrointestinal tract is the presence of teeth. The junction between the teeth and mucosa not only allows a greater access of serum proteins to the mucosal surface, but also results in exposure of the unique junctional epithelium to microbial challenge. If breached, this permits access, via the periodontal membrane, to the alveolus of maxilla and mandible (Fig. 15.1).

As in other parts of the mucosal system, the oral mucosa is exposed to both the systemic and secretory immune systems. There are some aspects of immunity which are qualitatively or quantitatively unique to the oral cavity and these will be discussed.

THE SECRETORY IMMUNE SYSTEM

Many of the mucous membranes of the body are constantly exposed to micro-organisms, and the secretions bathing epithelial surfaces play a major role in the local defence against infection. The secretory immune system is one of local immunity which protects mucosal surfaces by mucosal-associated lymphoid tissue (MALT) and which can be stimulated independently of systemic immunity.

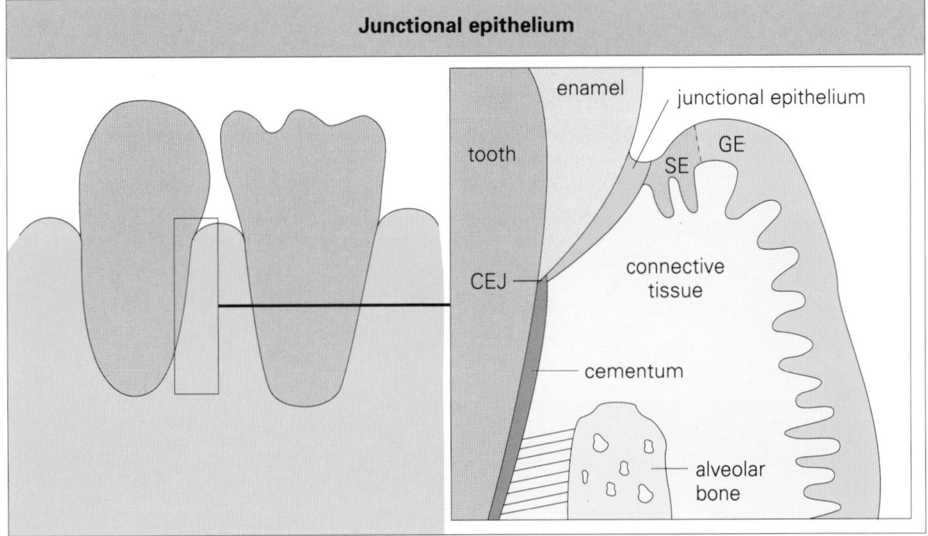

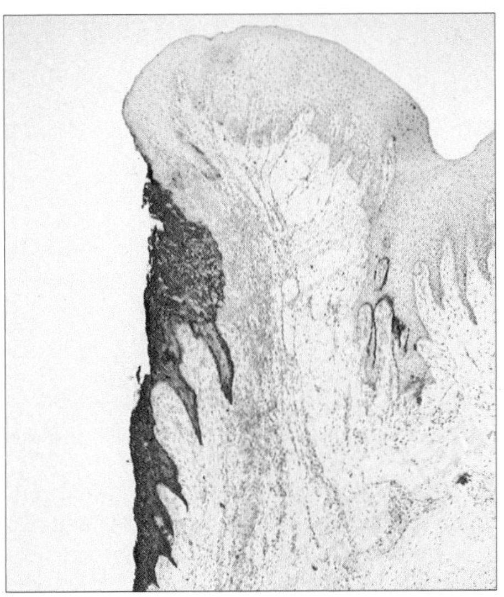

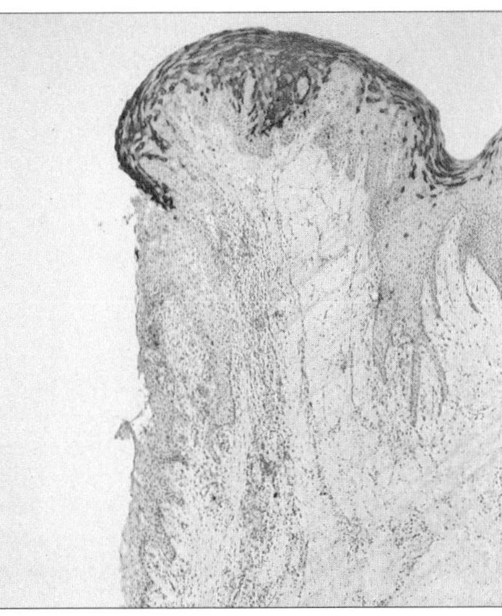

Fig. 15.1 Upper: relationship between the tooth and the junctional and gingival epithelia. Sulcular epithelium is transitional and between the other two types. GE = gingival epithelium; SE = sulcular epithelium; CEJ = cementum–enamel junction. Lower left: section of gingiva stained with monoclonal antibody to keratin 19, which reveals junctional but not gingival epithelium. Lower right: section of the same gingiva stained with monclonal antibodies to keratin 4 distinguishes the gingival from the junctional epithelium. Courtesy of Dr P Morgan.

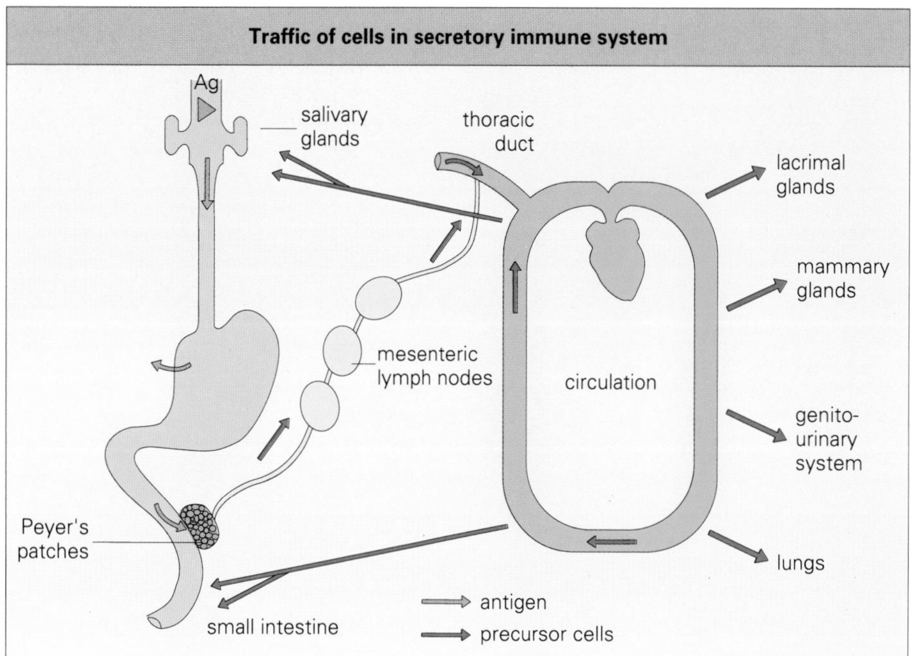

Fig. 15.2 Antigen in the gut stimulates the release of IgA precursor cells from Peyer's patches. These cells then migrate to all secretory tissues.

The system comprises the secretions bathing the mucous membranes of the body and their associated glands. The organs involved include the eye, middle ear, salivary glands, lungs, gastrointestinal tract, genito-urinary tract and the mammary glands. There is specialized lymphoid tissue associated with the secretory system in the gut (gut-associated lymphoid tissue, or GALT) and in the lungs (bronchial-associated lymphoid tissue, or BALT).

STIMULATION OF THE SECRETORY IMMUNE SYSTEM

Antibodies can be induced in secretions by local immunization, or by stimulation of GALT; the latter results from either ingestion or deposition of antigen in the small bowel. This leads to the release from Peyer's patches of IgA precursor cells, which selectively migrate to (or are selectively retained in) mucosal tissues. The cells are released into the local lymphatics and migrate sequentially to the mesenteric lymph nodes, to the thoracic duct and into the bloodstream before migrating to the lamina propria of the gut and other secretory tissues, including the mammary glands (Fig. 15.2). Local immunization leads to proliferation of these cells, recruitment of others and an enhanced local secretory IgA response.

Plasma cells in the lamina propria (the connective tissues adjacent to the epithelium) secrete dimeric IgA, which includes one unit of J chain. This molecule binds to the poly-Ig receptor which is produced by epithelial cells and found on their cell membranes (Fig. 15.3). The whole complex is taken up into the cells and secreted into the lumen of the gland as secretory IgA (sIgA) by cleavage of the receptor, leaving secretory component attached to the secreted IgA. The secretory component presumably acts by covering sites attacked by proteolytic enzymes.

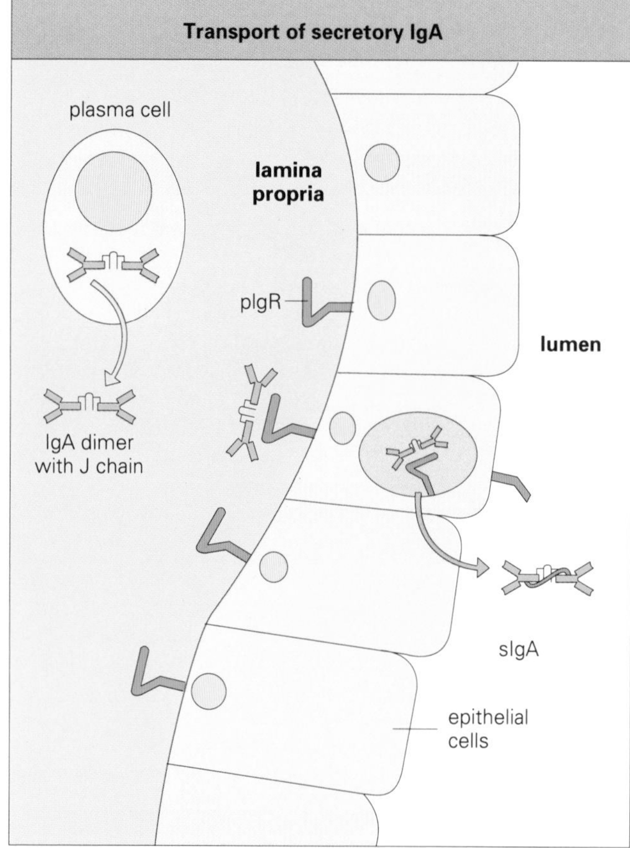

Fig. 15.3 Plasma cells in the lamina propria secrete dimeric IgA, which binds to the poly-Ig receptor (pIgR) on the surface of epithelial cells. The sIgA is internalized, transported across the cell and secreted into the ducts. The precursor of the plasma cell may have originated in GALT.

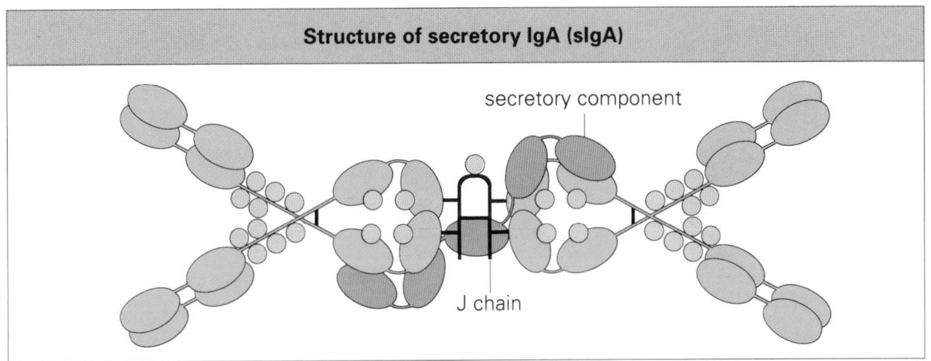

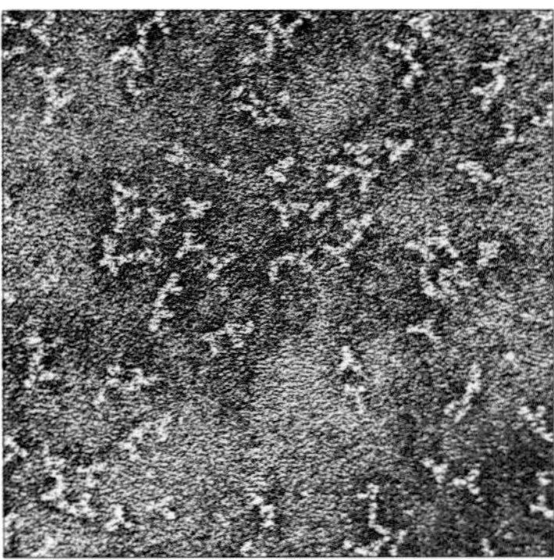

Fig. 15.4 Left: structure of a secretory IgA molecule showing the J chain and secretory component. Right: electron micrograph of human dimeric IgA showing monomeric sub-units linked end to end. Courtesy of Dr R Dourmashkin.

Main functions of secretory IgA
inhibition of microbial adherence
antigen exclusion
virus neutralization
modulation of enzyme activity
toxin neutralization

Fig. 15.5 sIgA does not rely on opsonization or complement fixation for its biological activity, as neither complement components nor phagocytes are normally found in abundance in secretions. An example of the importance of antigen exclusion is the finding that IgA-deficient children have serum antibodies to cow's milk protein, unlike normal children.

Possible causes of immunologically mediated mucosal damage
antigens: local microbial flora or food
accumulation of circulating antigen
B cell mitogens: micro-organisms & food
mitogenic complement split products
blastogenic factors from locally activated T and B cells
lymphostimulatory factors from macrophages and neutrophils
altered autologous IgG — immune complexes
endogenous tissue antigens cross-reacting with microbial components

Fig. 15.6 The oral mucosa is constantly bathed in antigens and any deficiency in the surface mucosal systems, for example following trauma or inflammation, may result in increased antigen access.

Secretory IgA (sIgA)

Secretory IgA (Fig. 15.4) differs from serum IgA in that the molecules are almost entirely dimeric and are independent of monomeric serum IgA. SIgA antibodies form a sort of paint, and are found in the secretions covering mucosal surfaces including gastric, bronchial and nasal secretions, colostrum, milk, tears and saliva (partly bound to high molecular weight mucins).

The concentration of sIgA differs in various secretions but is always greater than that of IgG. In whole saliva the concentrations of sIgA, IgA and IgM are approximately 20, 0.1 and 0.1mg/100ml respectively. In serum, the ratio of IgA1 to IgA2 is approximately 75:25 but in secretions there is less IgA1 and more IgA2 (40:60). The main functions of sIgA are shown in Fig. 15.5.

Oral lymphoid aggregates

The oral cavity is rich in lymphoid aggregates, which are similar to Peyer's patches in that they are not encapsulated and have no afferent lymph supply. These exist in addition to the normal lymphatic drainage. It is not clear what their role is or whether they are functionally linked to just the secretory system or to both the secretory and systemic immune systems.

Salivary gland lymphoid tissue, particularly that surrounding the ducts of minor salivary glands, is thought to play a role in local production of secretory antibody. Minor salivary glands contribute only about 10% of the total volume of saliva, but the sIgA content is much greater than that found in the main salivary glands, and may account for up to 25% of the total salivary IgA. Bacteria have been observed in duct-associated lymphoid tissue and it is possible that direct access of antigens to lymphoid aggregates in the oral cavity occurs via the short ducts of the minor salivary glands.

Mechanisms of damage to oral mucosa

Various cellular or humoral mechanisms, including cellular cytotoxicity, immune complexes or direct antibody damage may be involved in different mucosal diseases such as gingivitis or oral ulceration, and they can be activated by a number of antigens and factors, some of which are listed in Fig. 15.6. As well as antigens, micro-organisms may contain adjuvant and non-specific B cell mitogens, and this has been demonstrated with the polysaccharide components of some fungi and bacteria in plaque.

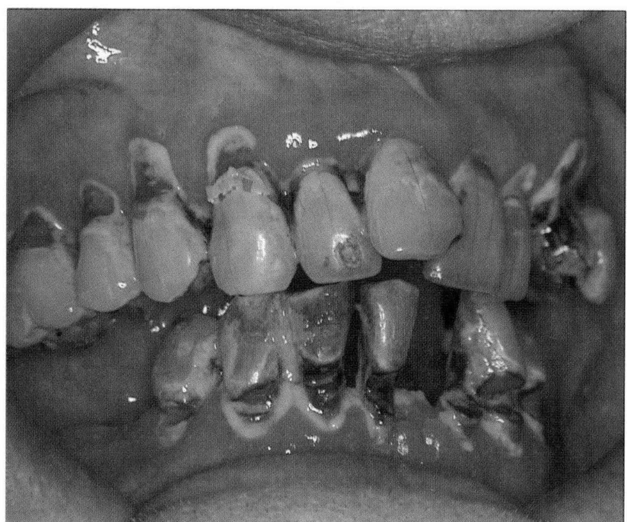

Fig. 15.7 Extensive dental caries, mainly cervical, in a 32-year-old male.

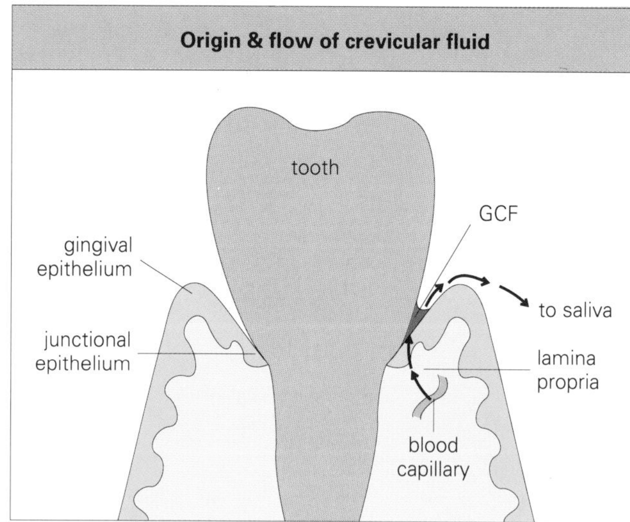

Fig. 15.8 Crevicular fluid is derived mainly from tissue fluids in blood capillaries. It flows into the lamina propria, through the junctional epithelium and into the gingival crevicular fluid (GCF). It then passes into saliva at a rate of about 0.3 μl/tooth/hour.

It is believed that the pathogenesis of some mucosal diseases is related to the fact that tissue antigens of the host cross-react with microbial components and stimulation of a normal immune response results in host damage. If antigen is not cleared from the mucosal site or if further antigen gains access, then locally activated T and B cells may release various blastogenic and lymphostimulatory factors from associated macrophages and neutrophils, resulting in localized inflammatory reactions which also cause damage to the host.

SPECIFIC ORAL DISEASES

DENTAL CARIES

Dental caries is one of the most prevalent diseases of man; it still affects 95% of the population in the developed world, and is increasing in developing countries. Dental disease is probably the most expensive bacterial infection to treat and also results in considerable loss of working time and productivity.

Dental caries may be defined as the localized destruction of tooth tissue by bacterial action. Dissolution of hydroxyapatite crystals precedes the loss of organic components of both enamel and dentine; this demineralization is thought to be caused by acids resulting from the bacterial fermentation of dietary carbohydrates. Not all surfaces of the tooth are equally afflicted: areas which are protected from cleansing, such as the fissures and areas between the teeth, are much more susceptible to decay (Fig. 15.7). The damage caused by caries is irreversible and thus the number of restorations and missing teeth due to the disease provides a record of the total caries experience.

Immunity to caries

The concept of immunity to caries depends on the demonstration that the disease is an infection. Although vaccination was attempted in the 1930s, the real impetus for development came with the demonstration, using germ-free animals, that caries could not occur in the absence of bacteria whatever the diet, and that specific bacteria were needed.

The tooth sits in a unique position between the secretory and systemic immune systems. The majority of the tooth surface is accessible to saliva, although the most caries-susceptible sites around the gingival margin and between the teeth (approximally) are bathed in crevicular fluid which is derived from serum (Fig. 15.8).

Antibodies in crevicular fluid are largely serum-derived, although there is a local contribution, particularly of IgG. Thus either serum or salivary antibodies could play a role in protection against caries, and both mechanisms have been examined for natural immunity in man, and for protective effects in vaccination experiments in animal models. To achieve 100% protection by immunological methods, effective induction of antibodies in both systems would probably be necessary.

Causative bacteria

Streptococci, lactobacilli, and *Actinomyces* species are all capable of causing caries in animal models. In humans the strongest association is with *Streptococcus mutans*, which is acidogenic and can produce copious amounts of extracellular polysaccharide from sucrose, much of which is insoluble in saliva.

Many studies have shown that the number of *S. mutans* in plaque over carious lesions is far greater than that found in plaque over sound surfaces. However, some caries can apparently develop in the absence of

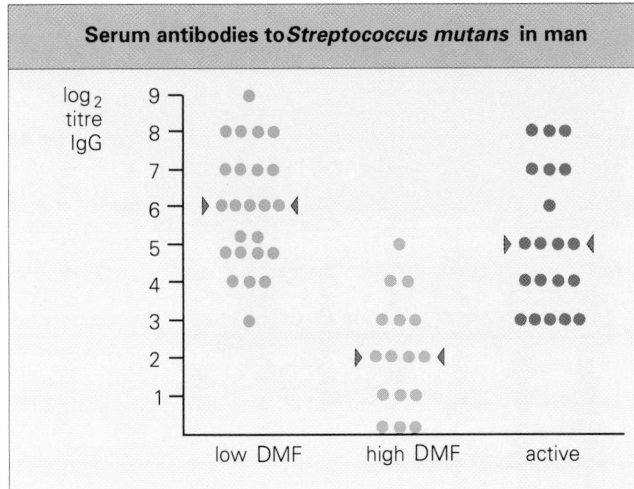

Fig. 15.9 DMF = index of decayed, missing or filled teeth; active = high DMF group with one or more carious lesions. Serum IgM antibodies followed a similar but less significant pattern.

S. mutans, particularly in fissures, and large numbers of the bacterium can sometimes be found in plaque which does not progress to caries.

Relationship of serum antibody to caries

When subjects with carious lesions are excluded, it has been found that subjects of low caries experience have significantly raised serum IgG antibody titres against whole cells of *S. mutans* and its antigen I/II compared with subjects of high caries experience (Fig. 15.9). This relationship is specific to *S. mutans* and has not been found with strains of *S. sanguis*, *S. salivarius*, *L. casei*, *L. acidophilus*, or *Actinomyces viscosus*. However, subjects with active carious lesions have levels of antibody as high as those with low caries experience. These studies strongly suggest that serum IgG contributes to protection against caries in man and that infection with *S. mutans* and the development of carious lesions is associated with a rise in antibody titre, as in most infectious diseases. Topical application to teeth of monoclonal antibody against antigen I/II can inhibit colonization by *S. mutans*.

Protein antigen I/II has been used to immunize animals; inhibition studies indicate that this is a major antigenic component of the *S. mutans* cell wall. IgG antibodies to antigen I/II are mainly of the IgG1 sub-class, whereas those to whole cells of *S. mutans* are mainly IgG1 and IgG2.

Relationship of salivary antibodies to caries

No consistent patterns have emerged and raised levels of salivary IgA to *S. mutans* have not been found in subjects of low caries experience. In fact salivary IgA levels may increase with the degree of caries experience, and may reflect cumulative caries experience.

Genetic factors

Using streptococcal antigen (SA) I/II, it was found that specific helper factor was optimally released from lymphocytes by a dosage of 1–10ng of SA I/II in low caries subjects but that the optimal for caries-prone subjects was 1000ng. This marked difference in response supports the suggestion that caries-resistant and caries-prone subjects differ in their ability to mount and maintain serum antibody responses to *S. mutans*. Using SA I/II, HLA-DRw6-positive subjects generally showed an optimal response at a low dose, whereas HLA-DRw6-negative subjects showed maximal response with high antigen dose.

These findings suggest that the ability to respond to very small amounts of streptococcal antigens may be the reason for the high antibody levels to *S. mutans* in low caries subjects. However, the immunoregulation of such responses is complex and this is an area requiring further study.

Immunization against dental caries

Successful immunization against dental caries in monkeys was first reported in 1969. In early experiments animals were immunized subcutaneously with whole cells of *S. mutans* in Freund's incomplete adjuvant, and a 75–80% reduction in caries, which correlated with serum antibodies to *S. mutans*, was seen. Passive transfer experiments in monkeys have confirmed that serum IgG antibodies may be the class effective in reducing caries. In contrast, experiments in rats have shown that the induction of salivary antibodies can lead to a reduction in caries, suggesting species differences.

Purified antigens are also effective in reduction of caries in the monkey (Fig. 15.10). A single subcutaneous injection of 1mg of antigen I/II in aluminium hydroxide elicits serum IgG antibodies, skin delayed hypersensitivity and a reduction of caries equivalent to that seen with immunization with whole cells of *S. mutans*. A low molecular weight protein (3.8 kDa) derived from antigen I/II has now been shown to be effective in reducing experimental dental caries, raising the possibility of vaccination in man.

PERIODONTAL DISEASES

Periodontal diseases can be divided into at least four clinical entities, each of which is associated with different causative organisms:

- gingivitis —may be associated with many bacterial species;
- acute necrotizing ulcerative gingivitis (ANUG) — spirochaetes, *Bacteroides intermedius*;
- adult periodontitis (AP) — *Bacteroides* (*Porphyromonas*) *gingivalis*;
- juvenile periodontitis (JP) — *Actinobacillus actinomycetem-comitans*.

Gingivitis

Gingivitis is a reversible inflammation of the gingivae and

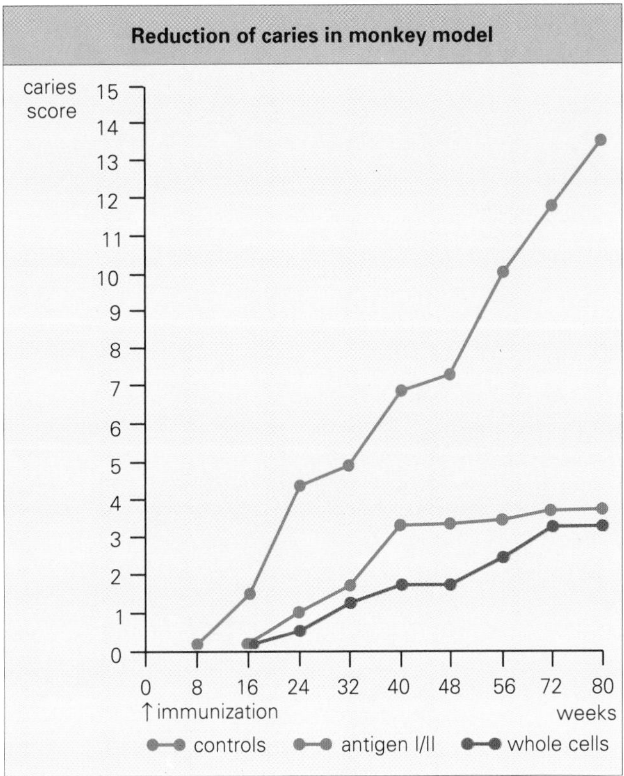

Fig. 15.10 Immunization against dental caries in rhesus monkeys. Immunization was subcutaneous with whole cells of *S. mutans* or with purified protein antigen. A similar reduction in dental caries was found with both antigen preparations examined. Modified from Challacombe S J (1988).

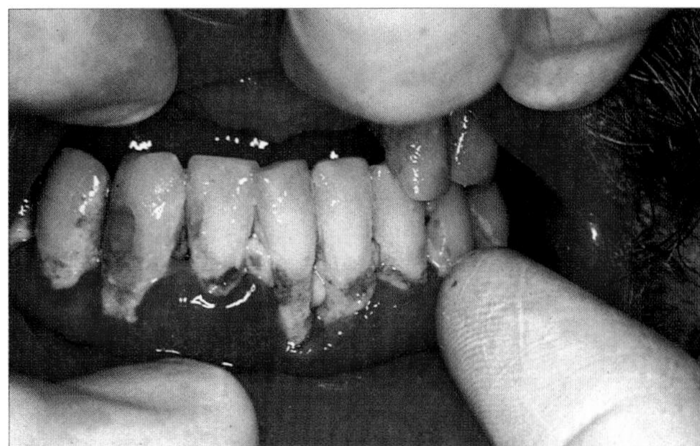

Fig. 15.11 Severe periodontal disease (adult periodontitis) in a 30-year-old male. Note the gingival swelling and detachment overlying probable extensive loss of alveolar bone.

can be considered as an inflammatory reaction to the presence of plaque. Plaque contains many bacterial species, and this represents a non-specific response to bacterial toxins and antigens. Only 10–15% of subjects with gingivitis go on to develop severe periodontal disease (Fig. 15.11). This clearly suggests the role of host factors in the progression of periodontal diseases.

Adult periodontitis

Gingivitis always precedes periodontal disease. There appear to be four stages in the development of periodontal lesions, based mainly on the histopathological findings (Fig. 15.12).

Initial lesions. This is essentially gingivitis and is reversible. Histologically it is characterized by a polymorphonuclear leucocyte (PMN) infiltration in response to plaque, and is largely acute inflammatory in nature. The infiltrate develops within 2–4 days of plaque accumulation and the lesions are localized to the gingival sulcus. Since serum antibodies to a variety of plaque bacteria can be detected, this initial lesion could be caused by complement activation either by plaque components through the alternative pathway, or by antibodies via the classical pathway.

Early lesion. This is still essentially reversible and is characterized by a replacement of the polymorphonuclear infiltrate with lymphocytes, which may constitute some 75% of the cellular infiltration, but with few plasma cells. Most of the lymphocytes are T cells with a small proportion of B cells.

Established lesion. Two or three weeks after plaque accumulation the lesion is established, with a predominantly plasma cell infiltrate. It is assumed that many of the B cells seen in the early lesion have been transformed by plaque antigens. Most of the plasma cells are of the IgG isotype. At this stage the junctional epithelium may extend apically into the connective tissue with an associated loss of collagen. Pocket formation occurs by a deepening of the gingival sulcus and circulating systemic lymphocytes sensitized to plaque bacteria can be detected.

Advanced lesion. This marks the transformation from a chronic established lesion into a destructive state. Recent evidence suggests that this stage of the disease is specific and associated with *Bacteroides gingivalis.* Undoubtedly, the host immune response also plays a critical role. Histopathological features include pocket formation, ulceration of the pocket epithelium, destruction of the collagenous periodontal ligament and significantly, bone resorption. These are the features which lead eventually to loosening and loss of teeth. The dense infiltration of plasma cells, lymphocytes and macrophages now extends apically and is progressive.

Host responses to bacteria may play a role in several stages in the pathogenesis of periodontal disease and are summarized in Fig. 15.13. Several studies have found raised antibodies to *B. gingivalis* in patients with AP in comparison with controls. *Bacteroides intermedius* has not been associated immunologically with AP, but has been implicated in ANUG.

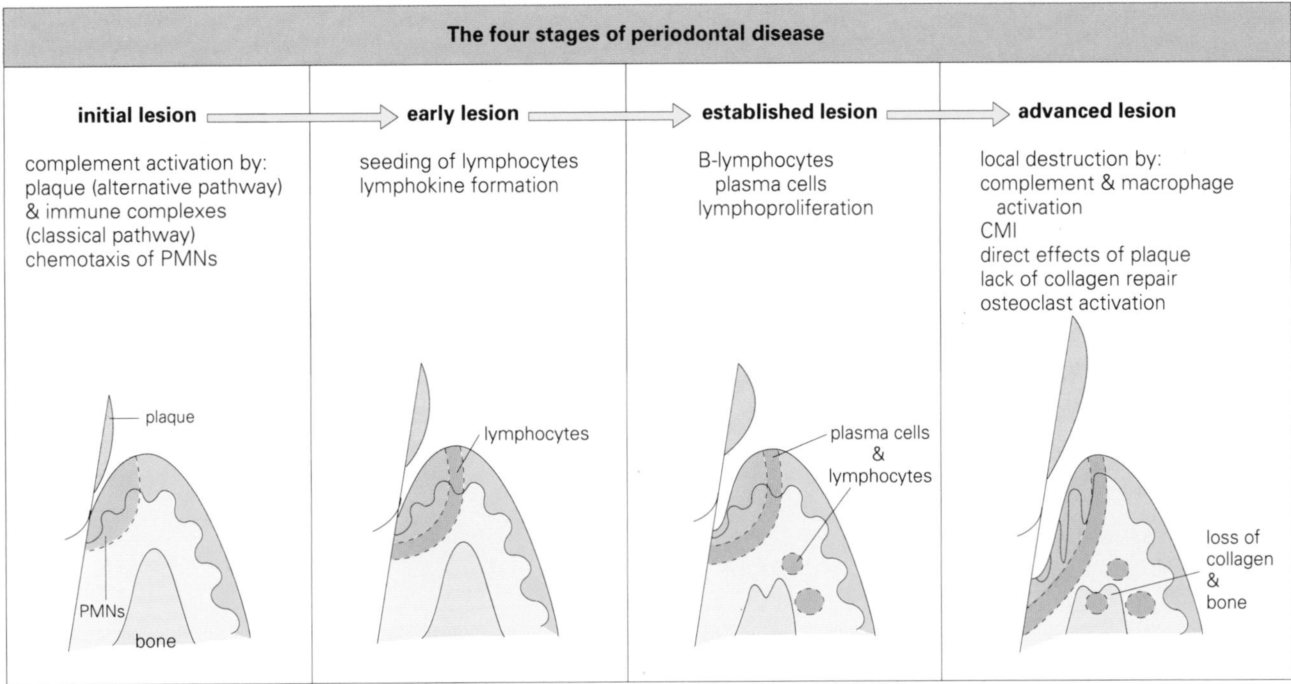

Fig. 15.12 The four stages of development of periodontal disease and their immunopathological features.

Host responses in periodontal diseases

Stage of disease	Damage	Protection
bacterial colonization	plaque	inhibition of adherence by Ab
bacterial invasion	direct effects of invasion, toxins & immune response	toxin neutralization by Ab, complement lysis
tissue destruction	damaging effects of cells, cell products & toxins	toxin neutralization by Ab,
healing & fibrosis	gum recession	lymphocytes produce fibroblast activating factor → repair, phagocytic removal of bacteria

Fig. 15.13 Host responses in periodontal diseases.

Juvenile periodontitis (JP)

This disease is strongly associated with the bacterium *Actinobacillus actinomycetem-comitans* (Aa), and antibodies to Aa have been found in all patients with JP at levels significantly greater than in controls (Fig. 15.14). Aa produces a powerful leucotoxin, and neutralizing activity against the toxin is present in the serum of these patients, who also have depressed neutrophil chemotaxis, phagocytosis and migration. Some 75% of patients with the classical localized JP appear to suffer from a peripheral blood neutrophil chemotactic abnormality. These findings suggest a role for neutrophils in normal protection, and indicate that in JP this function is depressed, allowing for the overgrowth of organisms, particularly those such as Aa which produce leucotoxic factors.

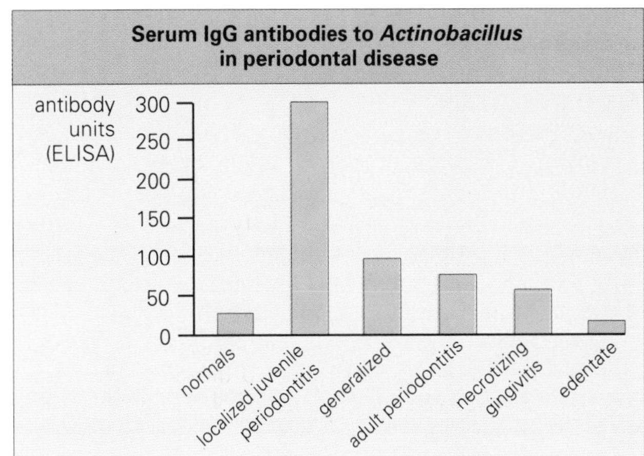

Fig. 15.14 Antibodies to *Actinobacillus actinomycetem-comitans* in different types of periodontal disease.

Characteristics of different types of RAS			
	major (MaAU)	**minor (MiAU)**	**herpetiform (HU)**
Sex ratio (F:M)	1.5:1	2:1	2:1
Peak age of onset	10–19	0–19	20–29
Number of ulcers	1–5	1–10	10–100
Size	>10mm	<10mm	1–2mm
Duration	10–30 days	4–14 days	7–14 days
Recurrence	1–4 months	monthly	monthly
Sites	non-keratinized mucosa (lips, cheeks, sides of tongue)	lips, cheeks, palate, dorsum of tongue, pharynx	as MiAu, & floor of mouth & gums
Healing by scar	no	yes	some

Fig. 15.15 Characteristics of the three different types of recurrent aphthous stomatitis (RAS).

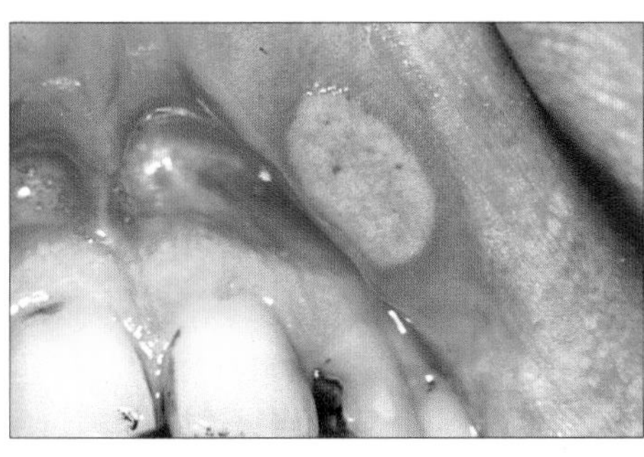

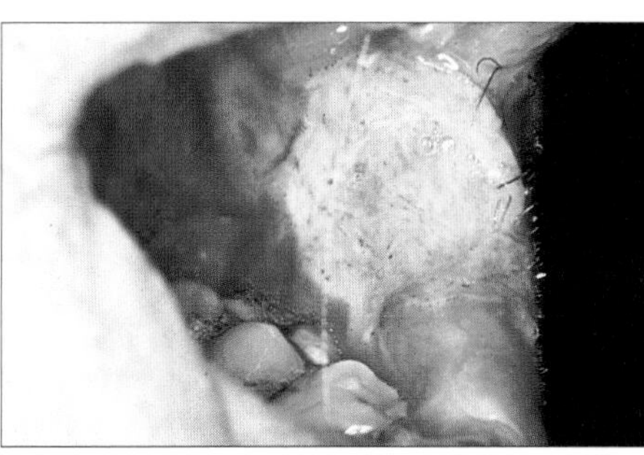

Fig. 15.16 Aphthous ulcers. Left: minor aphthous ulceration. Note the ellipitical shape and defined peri-ulcer erythema. This condition usually affects non-keratinized mucosa. Right: major aphthous ulceration in the left buccal mucosa. These ulcers may grow to over 2cm in diameter.

Some types of oral ulceration	
May mimic RAS	**Do not usually mimic RAS**
Behçet's syndrome Cyclical neutropenia Coeliac disease Iron deficiency Folate deficiency Ulcerative colitis	Pemphigus Mucous membrane pemphigoid Erythema multiforme Erosive lichen planus Crohn's disease Wegener's granulomatosis Carcinoma Leukaemia

Fig. 15.17 Some types of oral ulceration. RAS = recurrent aphthous stomatitis.

APHTHOUS ULCERS

Characterization

Recurrent aphthous stomatitis (RAS), or recurrent oral ulceration (ROU) is characterized by oral ulcers, occurring singly or in crops, which usually last for 7–21 days before healing spontaneously. These ulcers recur after a variable period of time which may be a few days or several weeks. RAS can be separated clinically into three types: minor aphthous ulcers (MiAU), major aphthous ulcers (MaAU) and herpetiform ulcers (HU) (Figs 15.15 & 15.16). There has been a tendency for clinicians to describe any ulcer occurring in the mouth as aphthous. However, aphthous ulcers have been carefully defined to allow differentiation from the many other types of ulcers occurring in the oral cavity.

The prevalence of RAS is about 10% of the population with a wide range reported in the literature; 85% of patients develop these ulcers in the first three decades.

Genetic aspects

A family history of ulcers is found in approximately 40% of patients; the highest incidence occurs in siblings of parents both of whom have experienced RAS. Identical twins show a 90% concordance, implicating a genetic component and this has been confirmed by HLA studies which show a relationship with A2 and B12 (B44).

Aetiology

Many factors have been implicated in RAS, although it is likely that many influence the nature of the disease rather than cause it. These include hereditary factors as discussed above, hypersensitivity predisposition, socio-economic status, psychological factors, endocrine factors, microbial agents and chemicals in foods. There is no evidence that food allergy is causative in the majority of cases, but it is likely that food allergy or intolerance can initiate some cases of oral ulceration. It is not clear whether these can be distinguished clinically from the majority of cases of RAS.

Haematological deficiencies may cause some types of oral ulceration and influence susceptibility to others. Lesions clinically consistent with RAS are found in association with some multi-system illnesses (Fig. 15.17). There is little evidence for a viral aetiology for RAS.

Pathogenesis

A currently accepted hypothesis of RAS is that patients are exposed to an unidentified infective agent which, in susceptible patients, triggers an autoimmune response against oral mucosa. The agent is thus either in, or cross-reacts with, oral mucosa in these patients. Autoantibodies, cytotoxic lymphocytes and circulating lymphocytes sensitized to oral mucosa can be demonstrated in RAS patients (Fig. 15.18). In the majority, anti-epithelial antibodies which are cytotoxic to oral epithelial cells can also be found.

Management

Since there are at least 40 different types of oral ulceration, many of them reflecting systemic disease, correct diagnosis is imperative. A full medical history should be taken, with particular emphasis on the possibility of multifocal involvement (Behçet's syndrome). In patients with anaemia or malabsorption states, the history or clinical presentation may be atypical, for example ulcers presenting later in life.

Treatment

Treatment is directed at healing current ulcers and preventing the formation of new ones. The duration of ulcers in RAS is largely attributable to secondary infection and mouthwashes of chlorhexidine or tetracycline may aid healing, but will not prevent the appearance of new ulcers. Prevention is best attempted with local topical steroids or systemic corticosteroids for severe MaAU.

BEHÇET'S SYNDROME

Recurrent oral ulceration (ROU), genital ulcers (Fig. 15.19) and uveitis are the major features of Behçet's syndrome (BS), but cutaneous, vascular, arthritic, neurological and gastrointestinal manifestations may also occur. BS is uncommon in the United Kingdom but prevalent in Japan and the Eastern Mediterranean. Haematological abnormalities may be found, particularly sideropenia or low serum ferritin. Patients may suffer a variety of manifestations and only some may have the classical triad of ROU, genital ulcers and iridocyclitis, but involvement of a minimum of two of the major sites is sufficient for diagnosis. BS can be separated on clinical and prognostic grounds into three main types:

- mucocutaneous (type 1), involving the mouth, genitals, skin and conjunctiva;
- arthritic (type 2), involving one or more of the large joints in addition to one or more of the mucocutaneous manifestations;
- neuro-ocular (type 3), which shows ocular and/or neurological involvement in addition to any of the mucocutaneous or arthritic features. 92% of those with neurological manifestations show ocular involvement (usually anterior chamber).

In the UK, 80% of Behçet's cases are type 1, 10% type 2, and 10% type 3. Behçet proposed a viral aetiology, but

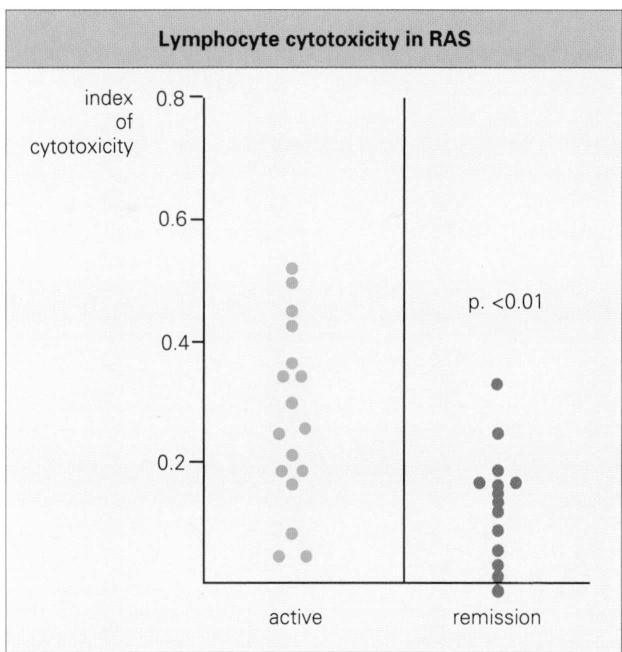

Fig. 15.18 Cytotoxicity of lymphocytes from patients with recurrent aphthous stomatitis (RAS) for cultured oral epithelial cells. Patients with active disease show significantly greater cytotoxicity. Modified from Thomas *et al.* (1989).

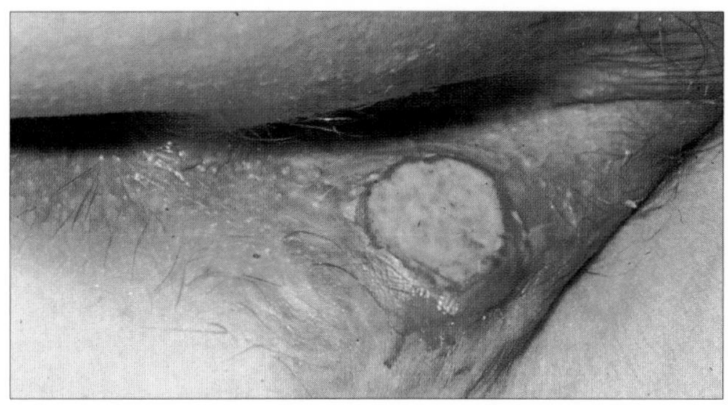

Fig. 15.19 Vaginal ulceration in Behçet's syndrome. The ulcer has a typically regular margin and resembles an aphthous ulcer (see Fig. 15.16).

attempts to isolate viruses have been largely unsuccessful; however, recent studies using DNA hybridization support viral involvement. Histopathological examination shows an early intense mononuclear cell infiltrate, prominent vascular lesions, endarteritis obliterans, fibrinoid necrosis and thromboses. The basic underlying histopathological lesion is thus consistent with a vasculitis.

Immunological findings

Humoral immunity. There is no obvious association with classical autoimmune disease. Haemagglutinating antibodies to fetal oral mucosal homogenates are found in the majority of patients, and antibodies against PMNs and increased leucocyte chemotaxis have been reported.

Serum C9 may be increased. Serum C2, C3 and C4 levels may be depressed before an attack of uveitis, indicating activation of the classical pathway of complement. Immune complexes have been detected in the serum of 60% of patients, especially those with active neuro-ocular and arthritic disease.

The abnormalities in the complement components and the clinical manifestations of uveitis, arthritis and erythema nodosum suggest that such immune complexes may play a role in the pathogenesis of BS. The size and nature of the immune complexes may differ in the different types of the syndrome.

Cellular immunity. Lymphocytes from patients with BS may show proliferation to homogenates of fetal oral mucosa. Intradermal injection of homogenates from non-ulcerative scrotal lesions of BS induces delayed hypersensitivity skin reactions.

HLA in ROU and Behçet's syndrome

The class I gene product HLA-B51 (B5) is raised in all ethnic groups with BS so far studied. The class II products DRw52 and DR7 also have raised prevalences, although this might be due to linkage disequilibrium with class I genes.

ORAL MANIFESTATIONS OF SYSTEMIC IMMUNOLOGICAL DISEASES

GASTROINTESTINAL DISEASES

Coeliac disease, ulcerative colitis and Crohn's disease are discussed in chapter 10. Each of these gastroenteropathies can be associated with oral ulceration.

Coeliac disease

About 25% of patients with coeliac disease give a history of oral ulceration, but the incidence of coeliac disease in patients presenting with recurrent aphthous stomatitis is only 2–4%. The oral ulcers of coeliac disease are probably due to the associated nutritional deficiencies (and respond to supplementation), rather than a direct response of the oral mucosa to the allergen. Oral signs and symptoms such as ulceration and macroglossia accompanied by varying abdominal problems can be associated with gluten sensitivity in the absence of coeliac disease.

Crohn's disease

Crohn's disease in the mouth may present either as thickened rubbery lips and cheeks with deep fissures and enlarged gingiva, or as ulcers and epithelial tags in the buccal sulcus in the absence of gastrointestinal disease (Fig. 15.20). In both types, biopsy of the affected areas will show granulomata. A number of cases of swollen lips without any intraoral signs have been reported and these have also been classified as oral Crohn's by some workers, although the term cheilitis granulomatosa would be more appropriate. The role of allergy to food or other substances has not been fully investigated.

Ulcerative colitis

Oral ulceration is frequently associated with ulcerative colitis occurring in 20% of patients, and may be one of at least four types: aphthous (Fig. 15 21), pyostomatitis necrotica, pyostomatitis vegetans, or haemorrhagic. The oral ulcers in the latter three are readily distinguishable

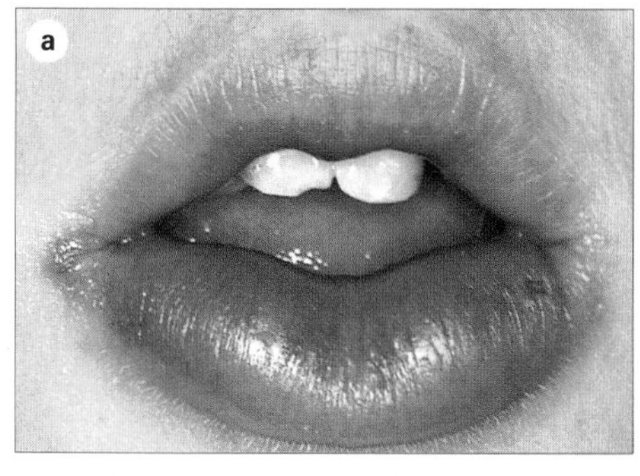

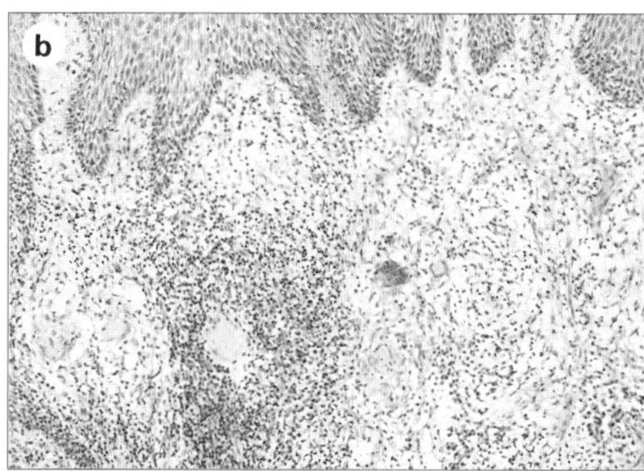

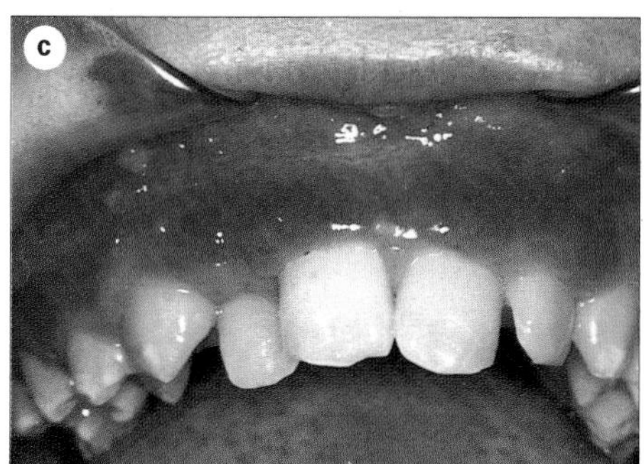

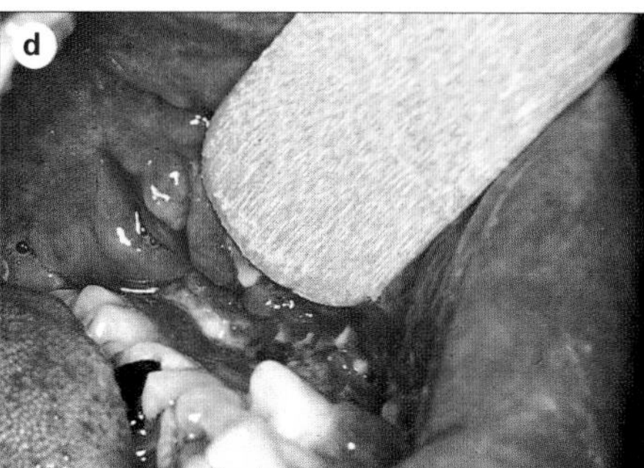

Fig. 15.20 Crohn's disease. a) Cheilitis granulomatosa of oral Crohn's disease. The lower lip is enlarged, giving a firm 'rubbery' appearance. Angular cheilitis is also evident. b) Histological examination shows multinucleate giant cells in the connective tissue beneath the epithelium and a marked chronic inflammatory infiltrate. H & E stain. c) Gingival enlargement. d) Oral Crohn's disease in a 21-year-old male showing firm, rubbery enlargement of the left cheek and several epithelial tags, as well as linear ulceration.

from the more common types of aphthous ulceration and unlike Crohn's disease, do not occur in the absence of bowel symptoms.

Food allergy and oral disease

Allergies to foods may be manifest in the oral cavity. They may present with a variety of oral signs and symptoms including a perioral rash, swelling of the lips, oral pruritus, fissuring of the tongue or oral ulceration. Aphthous ulceration affects approximately 10% of the population but it is unlikely that food allergy or intolerance is responsible for more than a very small proportion of these cases, perhaps less than 1%. Overall, oral symptoms are most likely to be found in the atopic patient and in these subjects allergy to foods should be entertained as a possible diagnosis, even in the absence of disease elsewhere.

DERMATOLOGICAL DISEASES

Lichen planus

Lichen planus is a distinctive mucocutaneous disease which commonly presents in the mouth as bilateral symmetrical white patches or striae on the mucosa, but may present as a bullous, erosive, or ulcerative condition, or even as desquamation of the gingivae (Fig. 15.22). The most common form is a reticular pattern with a network of white striae, principally on the buccal mucosa (Wickham's striae). The lesions sometimes appear as white plaques on the mucosa or tongue, but these are often associated with radiating peripheral white striae. Desquamative gingivitis is essentially an atrophic form of lichen planus. About 10% of patients presenting with oral lesions have cutaneous manifestations which appear as a papular rash, predominantly affecting the flexor surfaces of the arms. It is a common condition with a peak incidence in middle age, and the lesions of the mucosa may persist for several years.

Lichenoid drug eruptions, which closely resemble lichen planus, can be precipitated by a number of drugs including methyldopa, beta-blockers, non-steroidal anti-inflammatories, and some anti-malarials. It is difficult to distinguish clinically and histologically between true lichen planus and lichenoid reactions.

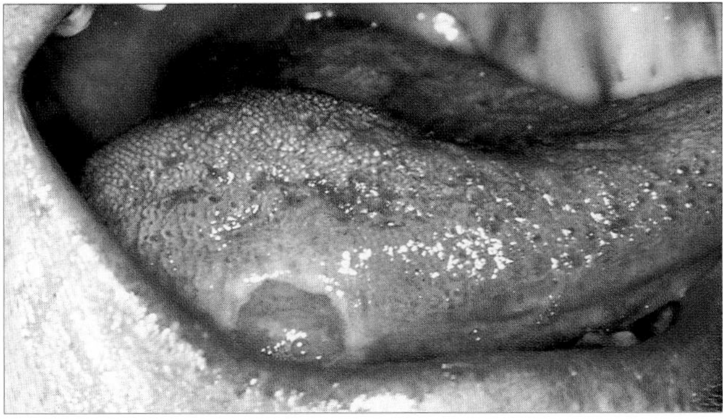

Fig. 15.21 Lingual ulceration in ulcerative colitis, producing a leathery appearance with little erythema. The condition is usually bilateral.

Immunological findings. An intense lymphocytic infiltrate and degeneration of the basal cell layer suggests that immunological mechanisms may be of major importance.

Among the early changes are increased numbers of Langerhan's cells in the epithelium. There is also HLA-DR expression by keratinocytes, providing a possible mechanism by which epithelial-associated antigen could be presented to the lymphocytic infiltrate. However HLA-DR expression could be switched on by IFNγ from infiltrating lymphocytes, and thus occur secondary to inflammation rather than being a primary event.

The lymphocytic infiltrate consists almost entirely of DR antigen-positive, activated T cells, predominantly of the $CD8^+$ (suppressor/cytotoxic) phenotype in oral mucosa, in contrast to cutaneous lesions in which CD4 cells predominate.

Pemphigus

This potentially lethal chronic bullous disease of the stratified squamous mucosa and skin (see chapter 14) can also affect the oral cavity (Fig. 15.23), often without skin involvement.

Benign mucous membrane pemphigoid (BMMP)

This cicatricial or ocular pemphigoid gives rise to bullous lesions involving predominantly the mucous membranes. Most cases are detected in the fourth decade and the

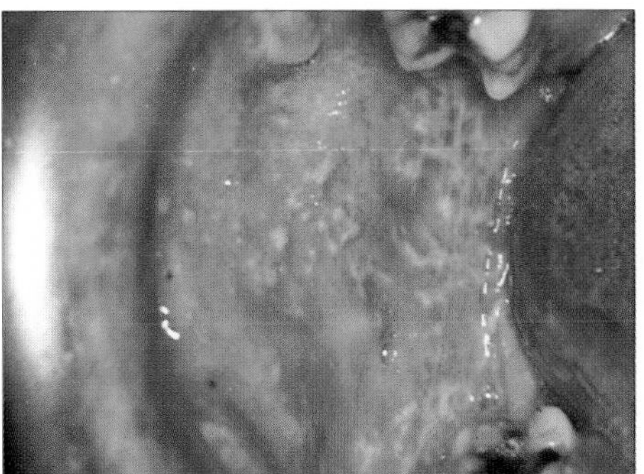

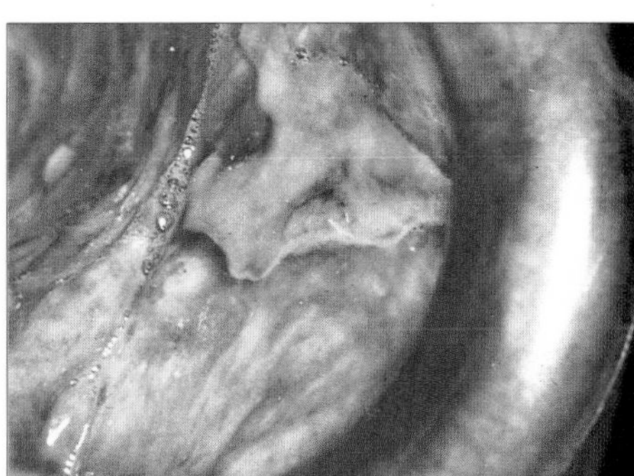

Fig. 15.22 Lichen planus. This is nearly always bilateral and usually symmetrical. Left: reticular form in the right buccal mucosa with papules anteriorly and striae distally. Right: ulcerative form in the left buccal mucosa of a 57-year-old male.

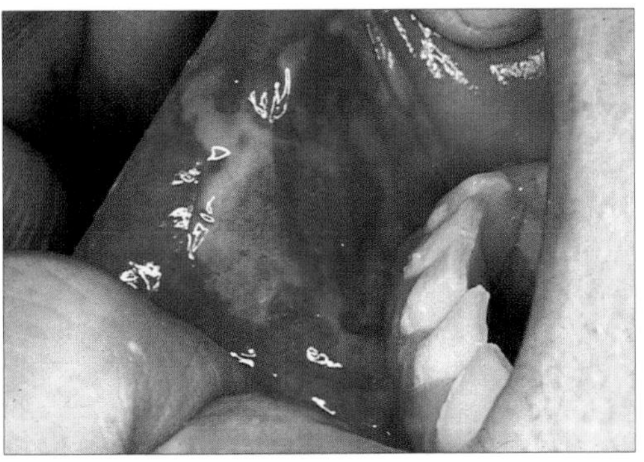
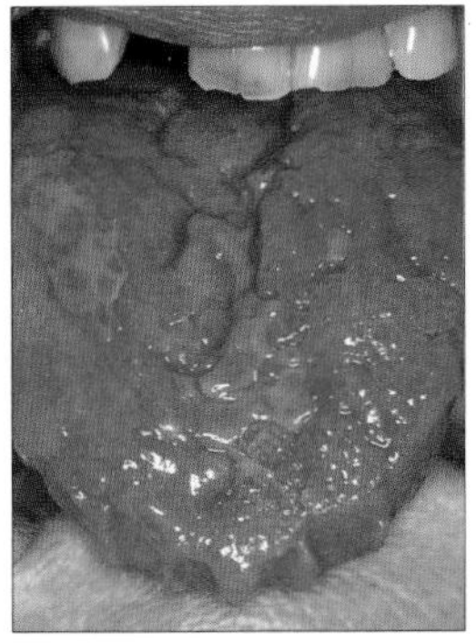
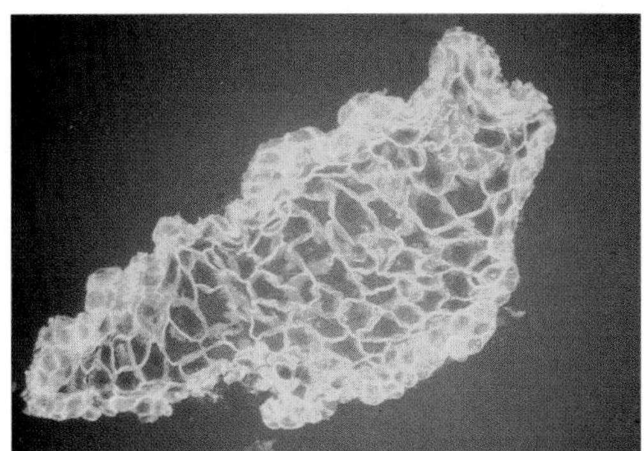

Fig. 15.23 Pemphigus. Left: shallow but extensive ulceration with irregular margins. Middle: marked ulceration of the dorsum of the tongue. Note the indentation marks at the tip, caused by the teeth pressing on the swollen tongue. Right: immunofluorescence of epithelial fragment showing strong staining of intercellular substance, giving a fish-net appearance.

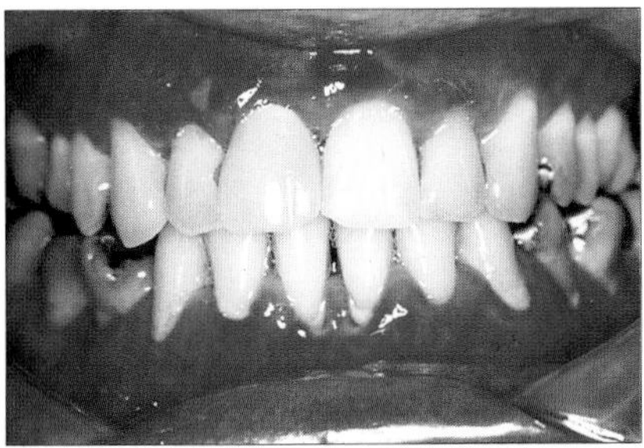
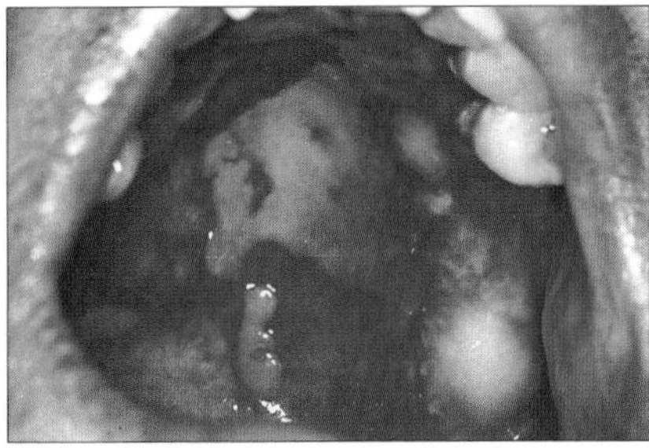
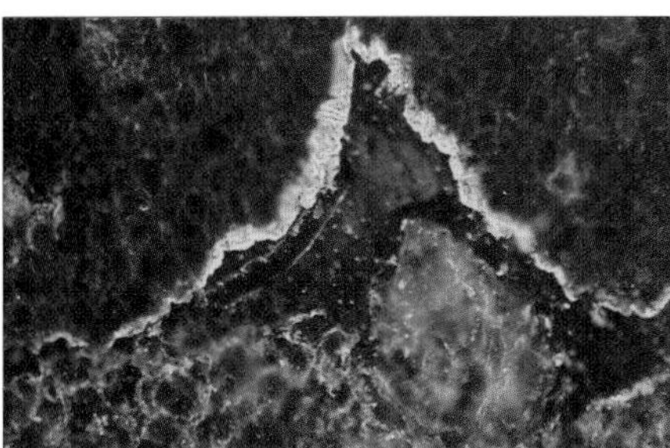

Fig. 15.24 Benign mucous membrane pemphigoid. Left: desquamatous gingivitis with marked erythema away from the gingival margins and small erosions. Middle: irregular ulcers on the palate of a 54-year-old female. Right: immunofluorescence showing IgG deposition along the basement membrane of the mucosal epithelium.

disease is more frequent in females. In the UK it is the most common bullous disorder of the mouth. In contrast to bullous pemphigoid, serum autoantibodies to epithelial basement membrane are rare. There are two intra-oral variants: bullous lesions involving much of the non-keratinized mucosa, or a desquamative gingivitis involving the gingivae of both maxilla and mandible (Fig. 15.24). Small bullae may be formed in protected areas around the teeth. It is possible that antibodies to a basement membrane zone antigen result in loss of anchoring fibrils from the epithelial cells to the connective tissue.

Erythema multiforme

This mucocutaneous disease characterized by typical target skin lesions (see chapter 14) frequently affects the oral cavity, often without skin involvement (Fig. 15.25).

CONNECTIVE TISSUE DISEASES

Sjögren's syndrome

Secondary Sjögren's syndrome is characterized by a triad of dry eyes (keratoconjunctivitis sicca), dry mouth (xerostomia) (Fig. 15.26) and a connective tissue disease (see chapter 6).

Wegener's granulomatosis

Wegener's granulomatosis (see chapter 12) is an uncommon disease characterized by necrotizing giant cell granulomatous lesions and a generalized necrotizing vasculitis. Oral manifestations are found in 50% of patients, and may be the first indication of the disease (Fig. 15.27).

Malignant midline granuloma (Stewart's granuloma)

Midline granuloma differs from Wegener's granulomatosis in the absence of arteritis, pulmonary lesions and glomerulonephritis and may well be a form of histiocytic lymphoma. Spread to lymph nodes, skin, liver, spleen and bones may occur. Most patients have nasal symptoms but occasionally the lesion presents orally. Antral involvement can cause toothache, and extractions may result in delayed socket healing. The hard palate is often invaded, with the formation of large rapidly progressing perforating ulcers. These lesions are fatal if untreated.

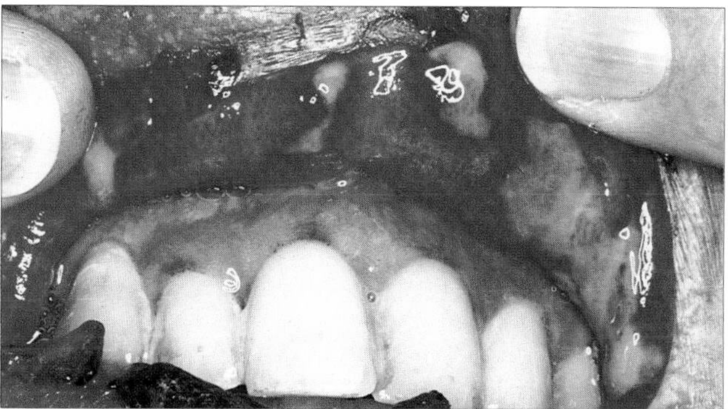

Fig. 15.25 Erythema multiforme of lupus showing irregular ulceration and crusting of haemorrhagic areas. This often occurs in the oral cavity without skin involvement.

Classification of oral candidal infections	
Type	**Synonym**
Acute pseudomembranous candidiasis (APC)	thrush
Acute atrophic candidiasis (AAC)	antibiotic sore tongue
Chronic hyperplastic candidiasis (CHC)	candidal leucoplakia
Chronic atrophic candidiasis (CAC)	denture sore mouth
Chronic erythematous candidiasis (CEC)	

Fig. 15.28 Classification of oral candidal infections. AAC often occurs during antibiotic therapy, hence its pseudonym.

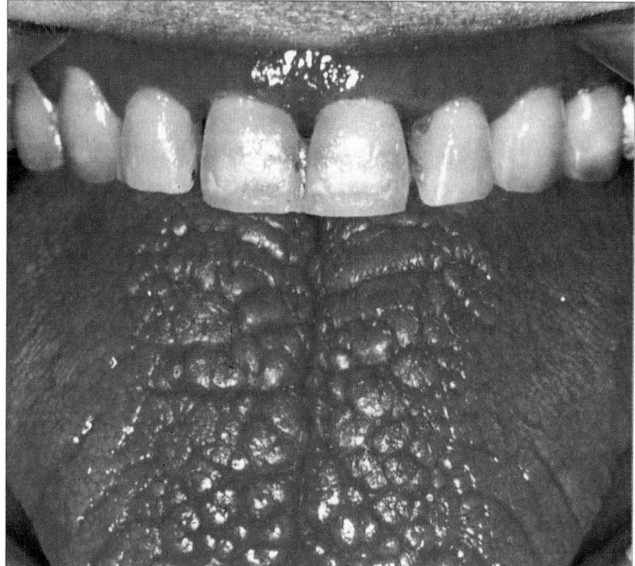

Fig. 15.26 Sjögren's syndrome. Dry tongue is a common problem. Note the lobulated 'crocodile skin' appearance and erythematous gingivae.

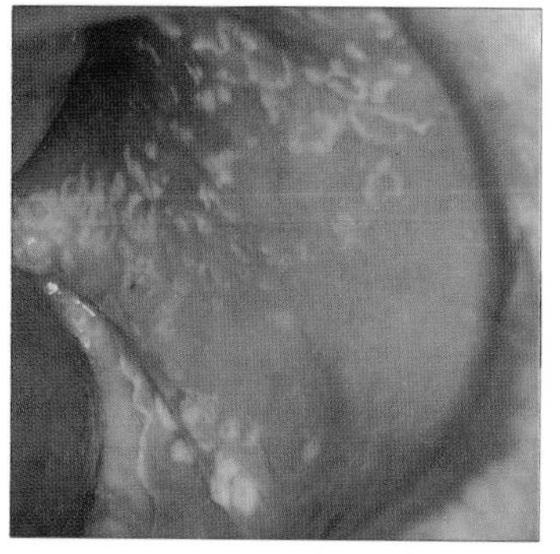

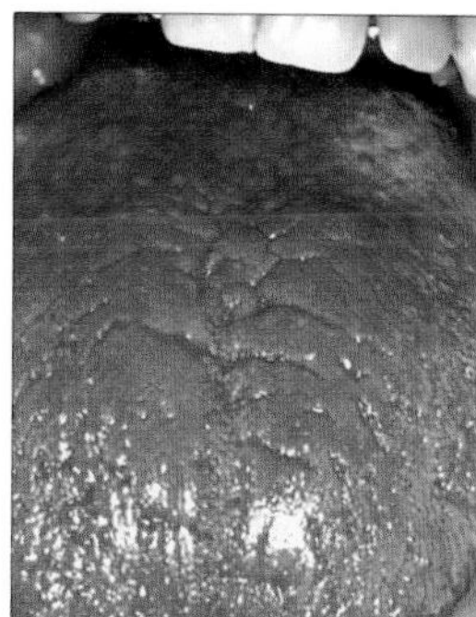

Fig. 15.29 Acute candidiasis. Left: acute pseudomembranous candidiasis (thrush). There are detachable white plaques on the buccal mucosa which contain fungal hyphae, epithelial cells and polymorphs. Right: acute atrophic candidiasis showing erythema and partial atrophy of the lingual papillae.

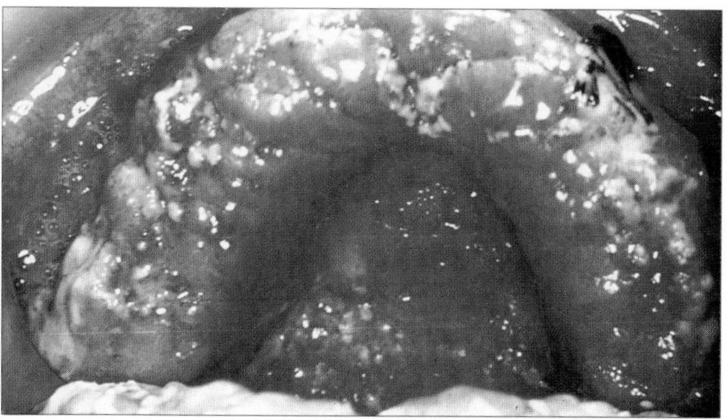

Fig. 15.27 Wegener's granulomatosis. Granulomatous lesions affecting most of the upper alveolar ridge and palate, which has the characteristic strawberry appearance. There is often destruction of the alveolar bone.

CANDIDA INFECTIONS

Species of *Candida* can be found in the mouths of 40% of normal subjects in amounts up to approximately 800 colony-forming units/ml of whole saliva. However, in patients with the various forms of candidiasis these are greatly increased and counts of greater than 10^4 may be found. A classification of candidal infections is shown in Fig. 15.28. Acute pseudomembranous candidiasis (thrush) (Fig. 15.29 left) is a common infection in the young, and in elderly or debilitated people.

Atrophic candidiasis

Acute. This is a response to the suppression of the normal bacterial flora and there is a widespread erythematous stomatitis with accompanying depapillation of the tongue (Fig.15.29 right).

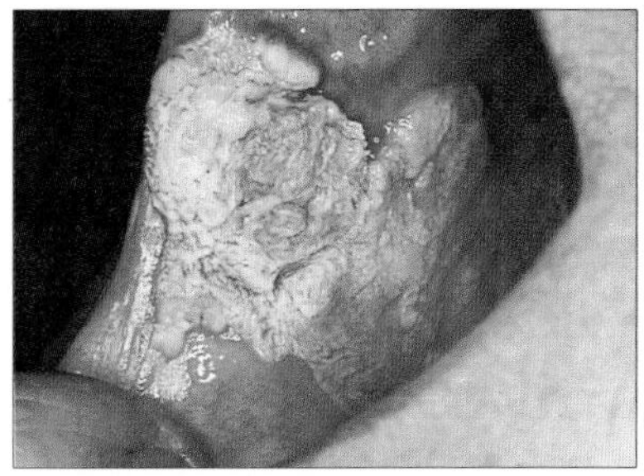

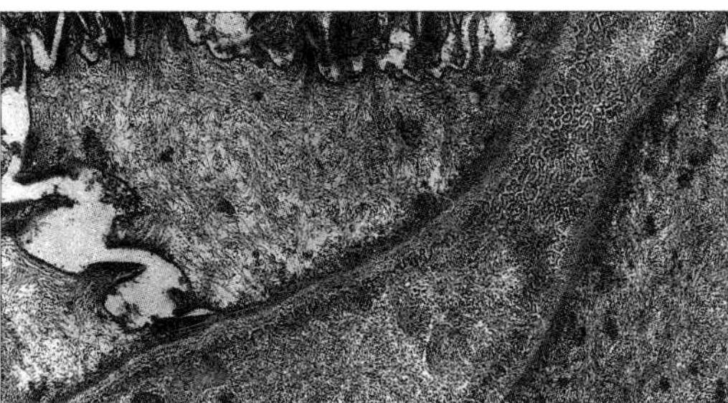

Fig. 15.30 Chronic candidiasis. Left: chronic hyperplastic candidiasis in the right commissure region. The condition commonly occurs at this site and is usually bilateral. Right: transmission EM of *Candida albicans* showing hyphae driving through the epithelial cells in chronic hyperplastic candidiasis. x 27,000.

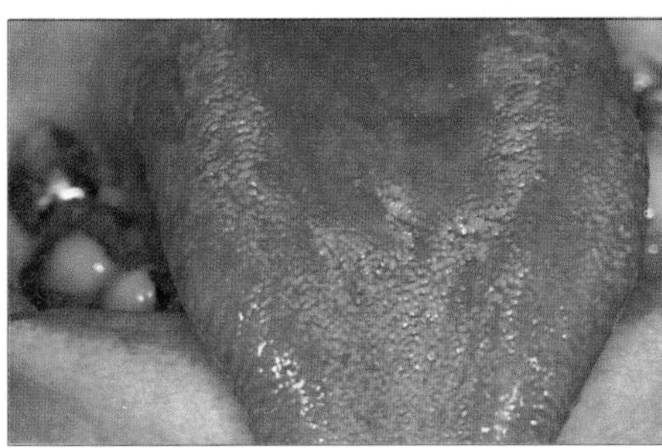

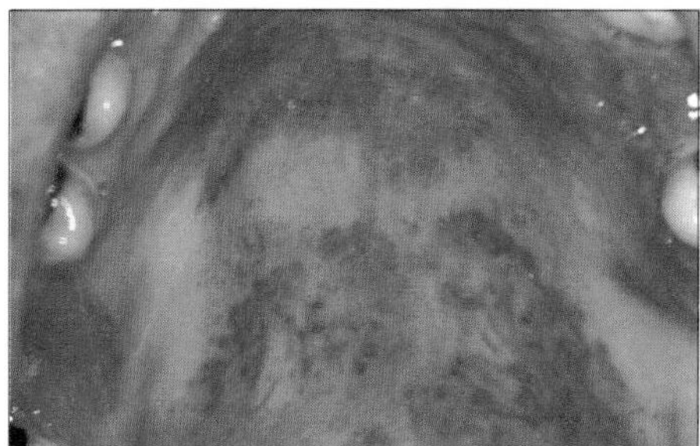

Fig. 15.31 Chronic erythematous candidiasis. Left: HIV-positive patient showing a central area of depapillation on the dorsum of the tongue. Right: HIV antibody-positive patient showing central palatal erythema.

Chronic. This is also known as denture sore mouth and presents as a relatively asymptomatic confluent erythema and inflammation of the entire denture-bearing mucosa of the palate. This results from candidal colonization of the surface of the denture, usually in patients who wear their prosthesis continuously. It is the most common candidal infection in the UK.

Chronic hyperplastic candidiasis

This speckled or nodular chronic leucoplakia (Fig. 15.30) is usually found in middle-aged or elderly patients and carries a significant risk of malignant transformation.

Chronic mucocutaneous candidiasis (CMCC)

A wide spectrum of immune abnormalities has been reported, ranging from lowered serum IgM and IgG to defects in lymphocyte transformation and mitogen stimulation in the most severe types. It is not clear, however, whether these immune defects are primary to the disease or secondary. A number of studies have shown restoration of immune functions once *Candida* has been cleared by anti-fungal therapy.

Mucosal protection

Theoretically, it might be expected that both secretory IgA and cellular immunity might play a role in the protection of mucosal surfaces against candidal infections. Animal studies using the azathioprine-treated rhesus monkey have emphasized the role of cellular immunity in chronic oral candidal infections.

Candida infection is not a noted feature of selective IgA deficiency, although in patients with chronic mucocutaneous candidiasis over 50% appear to have reduced salivary IgA antibodies. Although serum IgA antibodies to *Candida* can readily be detected in man, sero-diagnosis of infections is inconsistent.

T cell immunodeficiency

Infection with *Candida albicans* is an almost universal finding in patients with severe T cell immunodeficiency but is not seen in patients with purely B cell defects. *Candida* infections are found in nearly all patients who suffer from AIDS. This is usually either pseudomembranous (thrush) or erythematous, affecting the palate or buccal mucosa (Fig. 15.31). This has been termed chronic erythematous candidiasis.

FURTHER READING

Jones HJ, Mason DK, eds. *Oral manifestations of systemic disease* (2E). London: Baillière Tindall, 1990.

Lehner T. Regulation of immune responses to streptococcal protein antigens in dental caries. *Immunol Today* 1982;**3**:73–77.

Samaranayake LP, MacFarlane TW, eds. *Oral candidosis*. London: Wright (Butterworth Scientific), 1990.

Smith C, Pindborg JJ, Bunnie WH, eds. *Oral cancer. Epidemiology, etiology and pathology*. New York: Hemisphere Publishing Corporation, 1990.

 Van der Waal I, ed. *The burning mouth syndrome*. Copenhagen: Munksgaard, 1990.

16

Immunohaematology

Immunohaematology is primarily concerned with blood transfusion and the diagnosis, investigation and management of alloimmune, autoimmune and drug-induced immune cytopenias (haemolytic anaemia, thrombocytopenia and neutropenia). Immune mechanisms may affect bone marrow precursor cells as well as mature circulating cells resulting in, for example, some cases of pure red cell aplasia, agranulocytosis and aplastic anaemia. These aspects of immunohaematology will be discussed in this chapter; other special aspects, including bone marrow transplantation and neoplasms of the immune system are described elsewhere.

Immunohaematology has evolved from red cell serology. Landsteiner's discovery in 1900 of the ABO blood group system of red cells initiated the concept of polymorphic antigen systems on blood cells. This marked the beginning of modern blood transfusion practice. The next major contribution to red cell serology, and immunology in general, was the introduction of the antihuman globulin technique by Coombs, Mourant and Race in 1945, for the detection of 'incomplete' (non-agglutinating) antibodies. In addition to its application to the problems of alloimmunization associated with blood transfusion and pregnancy, the Coombs' technique opened the way for the investigation and diagnosis of autoimmune haemolytic anaemia.

Platelet and leucocyte serology progressed more slowly than red cell serology. These cells are more difficult to work with than red cells, and modified methodology had to be developed. While lymphocyte immunology is well established (and will be discussed elsewhere in this book), methods for studying platelet and neutrophil immunohaematology are far from standardized. In spite of the limitations of methodology, antigen systems on platelets and neutrophils have been defined, and the clinical significance of platelet and neutrophil antibodies can now be studied.

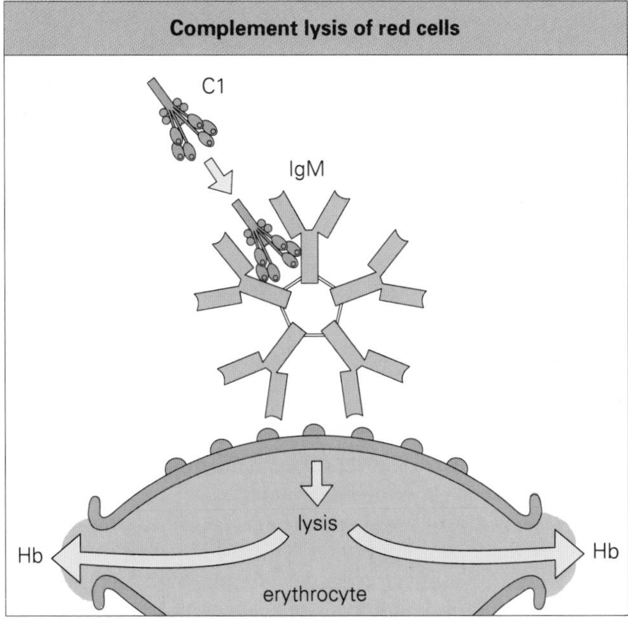

Fig. 16.1 The pentameric structure of IgM allows it to make a firm bond with C1q. In the case of IgG, two molecules are required to bind C1q and these must be in close proximity (within 20–30nm) on the cell membrane. With full activation of the classical pathway, the membrane attack complex (C5b–9) punctures the red cell membrane leading to osmotic lysis.

MECHANISMS OF IMMUNE DESTRUCTION OF BLOOD CELLS

Immune haemolysis will be used as a model to illustrate the mechanisms of immune destruction of blood cells. Immune haemolysis depends on:

- the Ig class of the antibody — both IgM and IgG antibodies are involved;
- the ability of the antibody to activate complement;
- interaction with the mononuclear-phagocyte (MP) system: the most important phagocyte participating in immune haemolysis is the macrophage, acting predominantly in the spleen.

The mechanism of immune haemolysis determines the site of haemolysis.

INTRAVASCULAR HAEMOLYSIS

Intravascular haemolysis is due to complement lysis, and is characteristic of IgM antibodies (Fig. 16.1); some IgG antibodies (notably IgG3 and IgG1 subclasses) are also haemolysins. Red cells are typically destroyed by intravascular complement lysis in ABO incompatible transfusion reactions (see page 16.8). Most other alloimmune red cell destruction occurs by extravascular phagocytosis.

Red cell autoantibodies may cause intravascular haemolysis, especially the IgG autoantibody of paroxysmal cold haemoglobinuria (PCH) and some IgM autoantibodies of cold haemagglutinin syndrome. Complement-mediated intravascular haemolysis also occurs in drug-induced immune haemolysis of the immune complex type (see page 16.18).

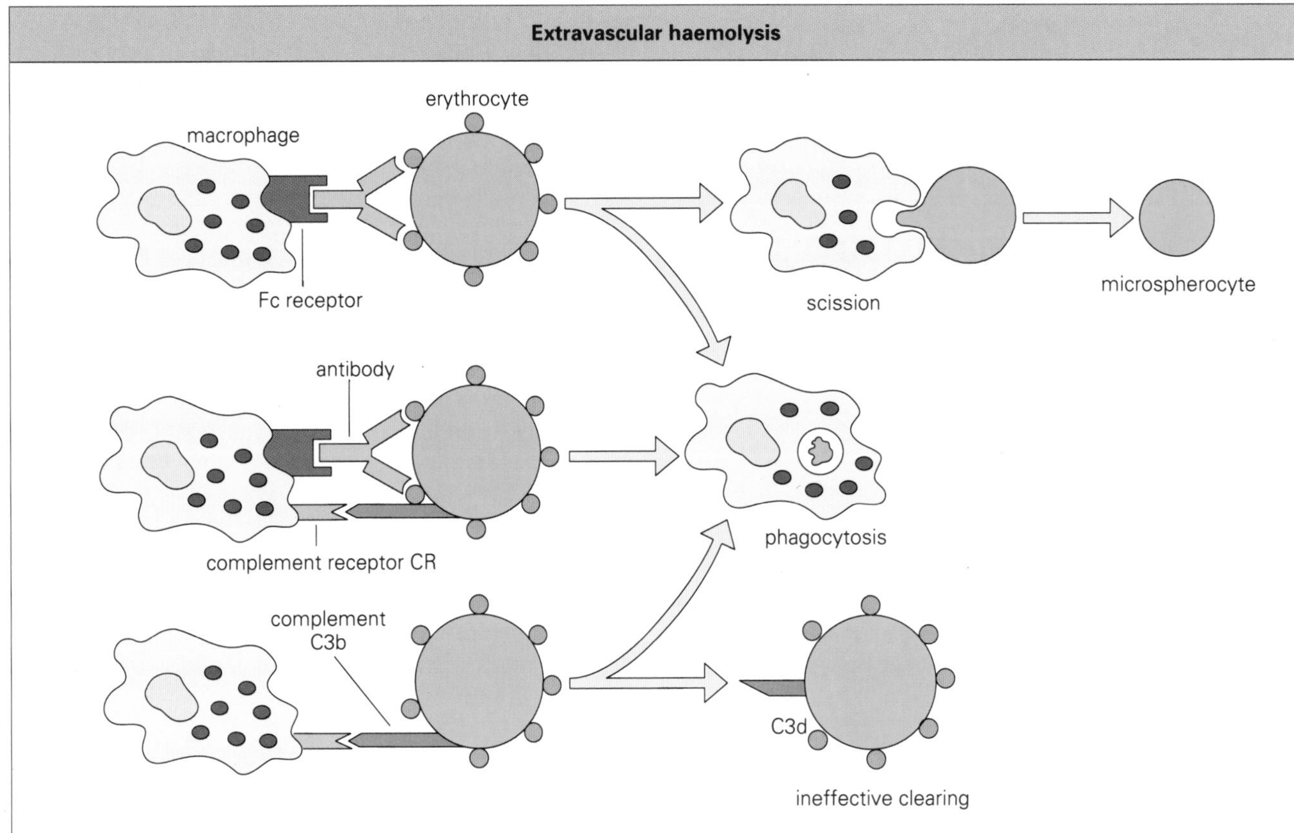

Fig.16.2 This is caused by interaction of antibody coated cells with the mononuclear-phagocyte system (MPS). Partial membrane loss ('scission') leads to spherocytosis. The combination of IgG and C3b on the cell surface enhances phagocytosis,which occurs in both liver and spleen. C3b alone is a poor stimulus for phagocytosis and is converted by plasma enzymes to C3d. Red cells bearing the 'inactive' C3d form are ineffectively cleared by the MPS and persist in the circulation.

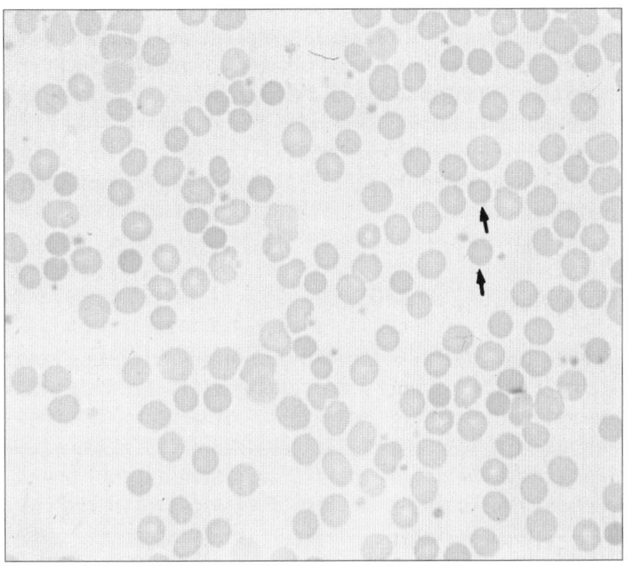

Fig.16.3 Peripheral blood film of patient with autoimmune haemolytic anaemia showing spherocytosis (arrows) due to immune red cell damage. The direct antiglobulin test was positive with anti-IgG.

Extravascular haemolysis

Extravascular haemolysis is caused by interaction between red cells and cells of the MP system, and occurs within tissues (Fig. 16.2). It is characteristic of IgG antibodies and occurs predominantly in the spleen, where the relatively slow-moving bloodstream encourages more intimate contact with the lining macrophages, which have Fc receptors for cell-bound IgG.

The sensitized red cell is either wholly phagocytosed or loses part of its membrane ('scission') and returns to the circulation as a microspherocyte (Fig. 16.3). Spherocytes are less easily deformed than normal discoid cells and tend to be trapped in the spleen, thus shortening their life span.

In addition to Fc receptor-mediated phagocytosis, it is now thought that antibody-dependent cell-mediated cytotoxicity (ADCC) may also contribute to cell damage during the phase of close contact with splenic macrophages. The contribution of lymphocyte (K cell)-mediated ADCC to *in vivo* immune haemolysis remains to be determined.

Complement components

Complement components may also enhance red cell destruction. Complement activation by some IgM and most IgG red cell antibodies is not always completed, but stops at the C3 stage, thus allowing the red cell to escape intravascular haemolysis.

Cells with active C3b on their surface adhere to mononuclear phagocytes (monocytes, macrophages), which have corresponding membrane receptors (CR1). C3b-sensitized cells are mainly sequestered in the liver because of the bulk of phagocytic (Kupffer) cells and large blood flow in this organ. C3b alone is a poor stimulus for phagocytosis; it is rapidly converted by a plasma enzyme to C3d. Red cells bearing C3d are not effectively cleared by the MP system and persist in the circulation. However, when IgG is also present on the cell surface, C3b enhances phagocytosis (see Fig. 16.2), and under these circumstances both liver and spleen are important sites of extravascular haemolysis.

Macrophage activity

A number of factors may affect interaction between cell-bound IgG and macrophage Fc receptors:

Fluid-phase IgG. Plasma IgG is a major determinant of Fc-dependent MP function. Normal levels of IgG will block the adherence of sensitized red cells to monocyte Fc receptors (FcR) *in vitro.* Haemoconcentration in the splenic sinusoids is probably a major factor in minimizing this effect *in vivo.* For this reason, the spleen is about one hundred times more efficient at removing IgG-sensitized red cells than the liver, in spite of the greater macrophage mass and higher blood flow in the latter.

Patients with high plasma concentrations of IgG have a slower rate of clearance of IgG-sensitized red cells because of more effective competition for macrophage FcγR. High dose intravenous IgG can produce acute macrophage blockade by blocking the FcγR. This reduces the immune clearance of antibody-coated cells and has a therapeutic application in the management of immune cytopenias, especially autoimmune thrombocytopenia and post-transfusion purpura.

IgG subclass. IgG1 and IgG3 have a higher binding affinity for mononuclear Fcγ receptors than IgG2 and IgG4.

Steroids. These depress macrophage activity through their effect either on phagocytosis or on extravascular cytotoxicity, and are used in first-line treatment of immune cytopenias. A satisfactory response to steroids is indicated by a prompt increase in the peripheral cell count, even though antibodies can still be detected on circulating cells.

Infection. This may increase macrophage phagocytic activity through the induction of increased FcγR activity by IFNγ.

The rate of immune cell destruction is therefore determined by antibody characteristics and MP function. The severity of the resultant cytopenia is a balance between cell destruction and the compensatory capacity of the bone marrow to increase cell production.

CLASSIFICATION OF BLOOD CELL ANTIBODIES

These may conveniently be classified as alloantibodies, autoantibodies and drug-induced antibodies. The specificity of the antibody determines the target cell involved. Similar conditions affect red cells, platelets and neutrophils, and the corresponding clinical presentations are discussed in the following sections.

BLOOD TRANSFUSION

The cells and proteins of the blood carry antigenic determinants which are the product of polymorphic genes, that is, some antigens are present in some individuals but not in others. A blood transfusion may immunize the recipient against donor antigens that the patient lacks — a process known as alloimmunization; repeated transfusions increase the chance of this happening. Similarly, the transplacental passage of fetal blood cells during pregnancy may alloimmunize the mother against incompatible fetal antigens inherited from the father.

BLOOD GROUP SYSTEMS

The red cell antigens are arranged into blood group systems, the most important of which are the ABO, Rh, Lewis, Kell and Duffy systems. Almost all blood group genes are expressed as codominant antigens so that, with the exception of 'silent' alleles, both genes are expressed in the heterozygote.

The importance of a blood group antigen in blood transfusion practice depends on the frequency of occurrence of the corresponding antibody and its ability to haemolyse red cells *in vivo.* Based on these criteria, the ABO system is the most important, followed by the Rh system, in which the D antigen is a strong immunogen.

ABO system

This is defined by the allelic genes A, B and O, on chromosome 9, which are inherited in pairs as Mendelian dominants (Fig. 16.4). An H gene (with a silent allele, h) at a separate locus codes for H substance, which is converted by enzymes encoded by the A and B genes to A and B antigens respectively. The O allele is silent, and H substance persists unchanged as the H antigen in group O persons. In those rare individuals who do not inherit an H gene (hh) no H substance is produced, and A and B antigens cannot be expressed, even though the corresponding genes are present. They are said to have the Bombay phenotype (Oh).

The ABO antigens are widely distributed on body tissues and are important histocompatibility antigens. They are also present in water-soluble form in most body fluids in those (about 80% of the population) who have inherited the secretor gene (Se).

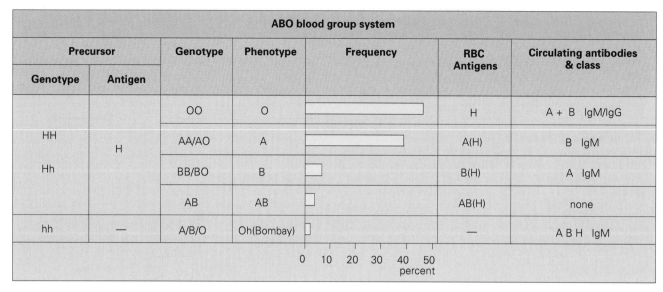

ABO blood group system						
Precursor		**Genotype**	**Phenotype**	**Frequency**	**RBC Antigens**	**Circulating antibodies & class**
Genotype	**Antigen**					
HH Hh	H	OO	O		H	A + B IgM/IgG
		AA/AO	A		A(H)	B IgM
		BB/BO	B		B(H)	A IgM
		AB	AB		AB(H)	none
hh	—	A/B/O	Oh(Bombay)		—	A B H IgM
				0 10 20 30 40 50 percent		

Fig. 16.4 Although the H antigen is the precursor substance for enzymes encoded by A and B genes, it is genetically independent. In the very rare situation where the H gene is replaced by the allele h, no H antigen is formed and A and B genes cannot be expressed. These individuals have anti-A, anti-B and anti-H antibodies, all active at 37°C, and can be transfused only with blood of the rare 'Bombay' phenotype.

A feature of the ABO system is the reciprocal occurrence of anti-A and anti-B in the absence of the corresponding red cell antigens, but without any obvious immunizing stimulus such as blood transfusion or pregnancy. These so-called 'naturally occurring' antibodies are detectable after the age of about three months. It is thought that exposure, via the gastrointestinal tract, to environmental A and B antigenic material of bacterial or viral origin provides the immunizing stimulus.

The Ig class of anti-A and anti-B, whether naturally occurring or immune, seems to depend on the ABO group of the individual. In group A and B subjects, anti-B and anti-A are predominantly IgM, but in group O subjects there is usually a significant IgG component.

Rh system

This is a very complex system. At its simplest, it is convenient to classify individuals as Rh-positive (85% of the population in the UK) or Rh-negative (15%), depending on the presence of the D antigen. This is largely a preventive measure to avoid transfusing an Rh-negative recipient with the D antigen, which is the most immunogenic red cell antigen after A and B.

At a more comprehensive level, it is convenient to consider the Rh system as a single gene complex on chromosome 1, which gives rise to various combinations of the antigens C or c, D or d and E or e. These antigens are defined by corresponding antisera, with the exception of 'anti-d' which does not exist because d is silent. The gene complex is named either by the component antigens (for example, CDe, cde) or by a single shorthand symbol (for example, R1=CDe; r=cde). Thus, a person may inherit CDe (R1) from one parent and cde (r) from the other, and have the genotype CDe/cde or R1/r.

Rh antigens are restricted to red cells, and Rh antibodies are due to alloimmunization by previous transfusion or pregnancy. They are usually IgG (sometimes with an IgM component), react best at 37°C, and do not fix complement. Therefore when haemolysis occurs, it is extravascular and takes place predominantly in the spleen. Anti-D is the most important clinically: it has caused fatal haemolytic transfusion reactions and, until the recent success of anti-D prophylaxis, was the most common cause of fetal death resulting from haemolytic disease of the newborn (HDN) (see page 16.12). The other Rh antibodies, although less common, may nevertheless cause haemolytic transfusion reactions and HDN.

Other blood group systems

Routine Rh (D) typing before blood transfusion and the success of anti-D prophylaxis for Rh (D)-negative mothers bearing Rh (D)-positive infants have greatly reduced the incidence of alloimmunization to the D antigen. At the same time, the increasing use of blood transfusion has meant that more patients are being immunized by other antigens, especially Rh (c, E), Kell,Duffy and Kidd. These antibodies (predominantly IgG) have all been associated with haemolytic transfusion reactions and HDN.

DEMONSTRATION OF RED CELL ANTIBODIES

The red cell is a convenient marker for antigens, and red cell agglutination or lysis is a visible indication of antigen/antibody reaction. In the laboratory, various manipulations are necessary to promote agglutination of antibody-coated cells, depending on the Ig class of the antibody.

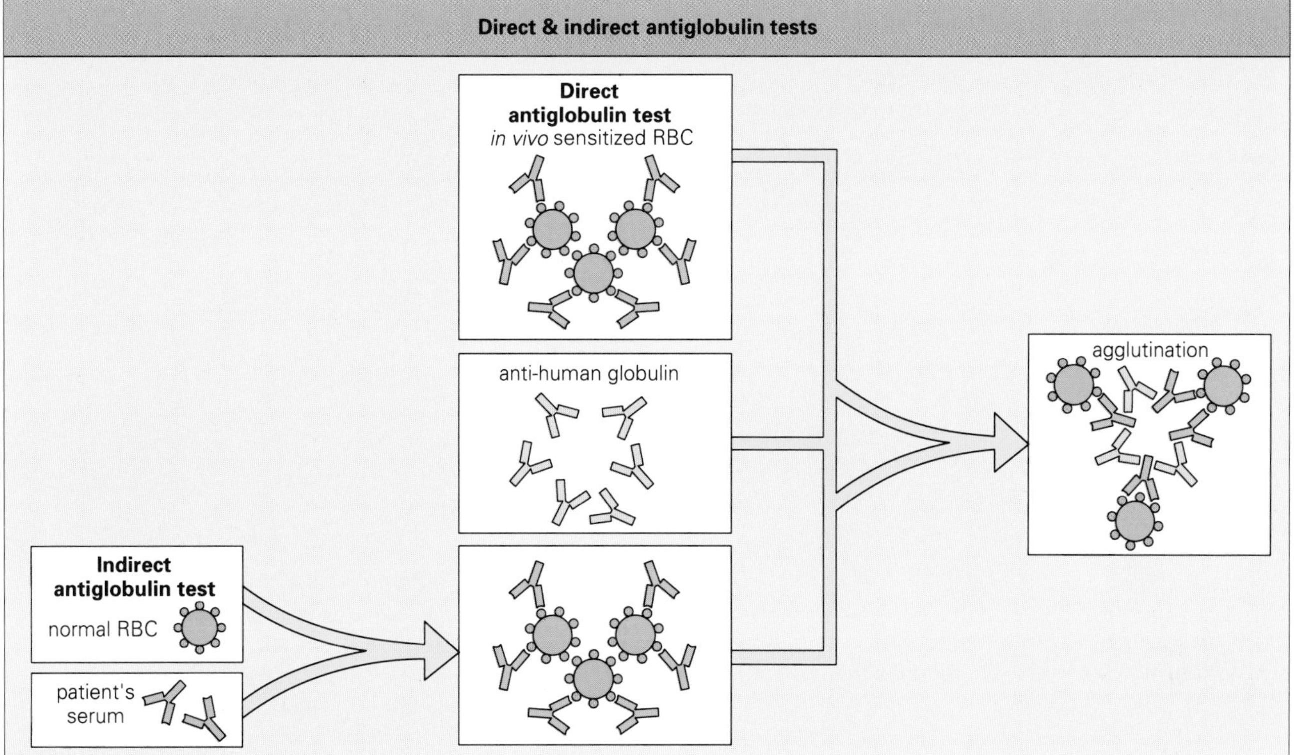

Fig. 16.5 Direct and indirect antiglobulin (Coombs') test. The anti-human globulin forms bridges between the IgG antibody-coated cells, which can be visualized as red cell agglutination. Similar reactions occur between complement components on the red cell and corresponding anti-human complement reagents.

The antibodies involved in immune haemolysis are IgM and IgG. While IgM antibodies can agglutinate red cells suspended in saline, the span length of the Fab arms of IgG antibodies is usually too short to bridge between cells, which are kept apart by a negative surface electrostatic charge. Other techniques are therefore required to promote agglutination of IgG-sensitized cells, such as suspension in albumin or pre-treatment with enzymes (for example, papain), which probably assist agglutination by allowing the cells to come closer together. Furthermore, mild reduction of disulphide bonds in the hinge region of IgG can increase the span length of the Fab arms, thus converting some 'incomplete' IgG antibodies to direct agglutinins.

The antiglobulin (Coombs') test is commonly used to demonstrate IgG antibody on red cells. The cells are thoroughly washed in normal saline to remove Ig not specifically bound to cell-surface antigens and anti-human globulin (AHG) added, which forms bridges between antibody-coated cells to cause visible agglutination (Fig. 16.5). With monospecific antisera, it is possible to determine the Ig class and subclass of the antibody and to detect the presence of complement on the red cells. This provides useful information about the mechanism of haemolysis.

The direct antiglobulin test is used to demonstrate *in vivo* attachment of antibodies to red cells, as in autoimmune haemolytic anemia and alloimmune haemolytic disease of the newborn. In the indirect antiglobulin test, red cells are incubated with serum *in vitro* as the first step, and then tested with the AHG reagent. This has a wide application in blood transfusion serology for red cell antigen typing, antibody identification and cross-matching.

Pre-transfusion compatibility testing

The aim of this procedure is to detect clinically significant antibodies in the patient's serum which would be active against antigens on the donor's red cells. The following procedures are necessary to achieve donor/recipient compatibility:

- ABO and RhD grouping .
- Antibody screening. It is becoming routine procedure to identify irregular antibodies in the recipient's serum before cross-matching.
- Cross-matching. Donor blood of the same ABO and RhD groups as the patient's is selected for cross-matching. This should also lack antigens corresponding to any irregular antibodies in the patient's serum.

A combination of cross-matching tests is used to detect both IgM (saline agglutination test) and IgG antibodies (AHG test). The AHG reagent should contain both anti-IgG and anti-complement. The latter will detect cell-bound C3 which serves as a useful marker of

Platelet specific antigens				
System	**Antigens**	**Phenotype (%)**	**Gene frequency**	**Clinical association**
Pl^{A}(Zw)	Pl^{A1}(Zw^{a}) Pl^{A2}(Zw^{b})	97.6 26.8	0.85 0.15	ANT, PTP ANT, PTP
Ko	Ko^{a} Ko^{b}	14.3 99.4	0.07 0.93	multi-transfused patients
Pl^{E}	Pl^{E1} Pl^{E2}	99+ 5 ±	0.98 0.02	multi-transfused patients ANT
Bak (Lek)	Bak^{a} Bak^{b}	85 63	0.61 0.39	ANT, PTP
Duzo	Duzo	18	0.09	ANT
PEN	PEN	99+	—	ANT, PTP
Yuk	Yuk^{a} Yuk^{b}	1.7 98.3	0.01 0.99	ANT
Br	Br^{a} Br^{b}	20 99		ANT multi-transfused

ANT = alloimmune neonatal thrombocytopenia
PTP = post-transfusion purpura

Fig. 16.6 PEN antigen is the same as Yuk^{b}, which was first identified in the Japanese population.Phenotype and gene frequency refer to the Caucasian population, except Yuk^{a} which was measured in the Japanese population.

Neutrophil specific antigens				
System	**Antigens**	**Phenotype (%)**	**Gene frequency**	**Clinical association**
NA	NA^{1}	53.9	0.32	ANN autoimmune N
	NA^{2}	92.7	0.68	ANN autoimmune N pulmonary TR
NB	NB^{1}	92.1	0.72	ANN autoimmune N
	NB^{2}	31.0	0.17	ANN febrile TR
NC	NC^{1}	96.2	0.80	ANN
ND	ND^{1}	98.5	0.88	autoimmune N
NE	NE^{1}	22.9	0.12	autoimmune N
9	9^{a}	62.6	0.39	febrile TR ANN
HGA-3	a-e	—	—	multi-transfused patients

ANN = alloimmune neonatal neutropenia
TR = transfusion reaction
N = neutropenia

Fig. 16.7 Closely associated (? identical) antigens are linked together by the vertical lines. Gene frequencies were measured in the Dutch population.

antigen-antibody reaction, especially when antibody is present in undetectable amounts or has eluted from the cell in the testing procedure.

LEUCOCYTE AND PLATELET ANTIGENS

Leucocyte and platelet antigens may be exclusive to each cell type (cell-specific) or shared with other cells. There are well defined platelet- and neutrophil-specific antigen
16.6 systems (Figs 16.6 & 16.7), and the corresponding antibodies are associated with significant clinical problems. Of the shared antigens, the most important is the HLA system (see chapter 2). This is best expressed on lymphocytes; only class I antigens (HLA-A, -B, and, to a lesser extent, -C) are expressed on platelets and neutrophils. ABO antigens are also expressed on platelets, but not on neutrophils.

Neutrophil and platelet antibodies

Unlike red cells, neutrophils and platelets are difficult cells to work with serologically, and the many techniques

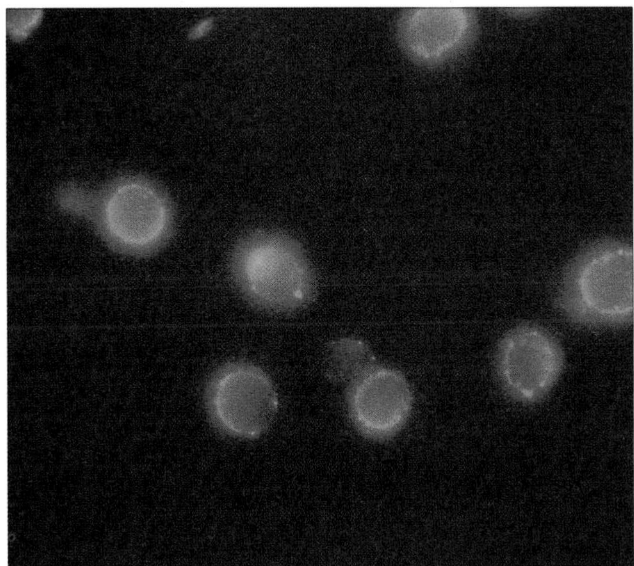

Fig. 16.8 Granulocyte fluorescent antiglobulin test using FITC-labelled $F(ab')_2$ fragment of anti-human IgG and paraformaldehyde-fixed cells. There is a positive reaction between NA_1 positive neutrophils and anti-NA_1, in this case taken from a neonate with alloimmune neonatal neutropenia.

Immunological consequences of blood transfusions
Alloimmunization
red cell, leucocyte & platelet antigens plasma protein antigens
Incompatibility
Red cell incompatibility intravascular haemolysis usually ABO incompatibility extravascular haemolysis immediate delayed **Leucocyte & platelet incompatibility** febrile reaction (granulocytes) pulmonary reaction (granulocytes) post transfusion purpura (platelets) poor survival of transfused platelets & granulocytes graft-versus-host reaction (lymphocytes) **Plasma protein incompatibility** urticarial & anaphylactic reactions

Fig. 16.9 Immunological consequences of blood transfusion.

used to demonstrate antibodies to these cells bear witness to this. The most widely used methods are based on agglutination and antiglobulin techniques. The sensitivity of the latter is improved by using fluorescent (Fig. 16.8), radioactive or enzyme-labelled antiglobulin reagents, and paraformaldehyde-fixed cells to minimize non-specific Ig adsorption.

As platelets and neutrophils have both cell-specific and HLA antigens, the interpretation of a positive reaction requires differentiation between these two antibodies. This can be achieved by stimultaneous tests with lymphocytes (for example, lymphocytotoxicity test) to determine whether HLA antibodies are present. If so, the test can be repeated with chloroquine-treated platelets/neutrophils. This treatment strips off the HLA antigens but leaves the cell-specific antigens intact, so that a persistent positive reaction will indicate that a cell-specific antibody is also present. More recent methods, such as immunoblotting, radio-immunoprecipitation and antigen capture by monoclonal antibodies are also proving useful for the resolution of mixtures of platelet specific antibodies.

IMMUNOLOGICAL CONSEQUENCES OF BLOOD TRANSFUSION

The potential immunological consequences of blood transfusion are classified in Fig. 16.9. These are considered under two broad headings: alloimmunization and incompatibility.

ALLOIMMUNIZATION

All transfusions carry a risk of immunization, as donor and recipient are normally 'matched' only for the A, B and D (Rh) antigens and not for the many other antigens on red cells, leucocytes and platelets. This is usually not a problem in the first transfusion, but it can affect subsequent transfusions. It may also have important delayed consequences for a subsequent pregnancy (for example, resulting in haemolytic disease of the newborn, alloimmune neonatal thrombocytopenia or neutropenia), or tissue transplantation (for example, graft rejection or enhancement).

INCOMPATIBILITY

Alloimmunization may be responsible for cellular and/or protein incompatibility in a subsequent blood transfusion. The clinical effects fall into two main groups:

- shortened cell survival, thereby reducing the effectiveness of the transfusion;
- harmful side-effects of the antigen-antibody reaction, which is often accompanied by complement activation.

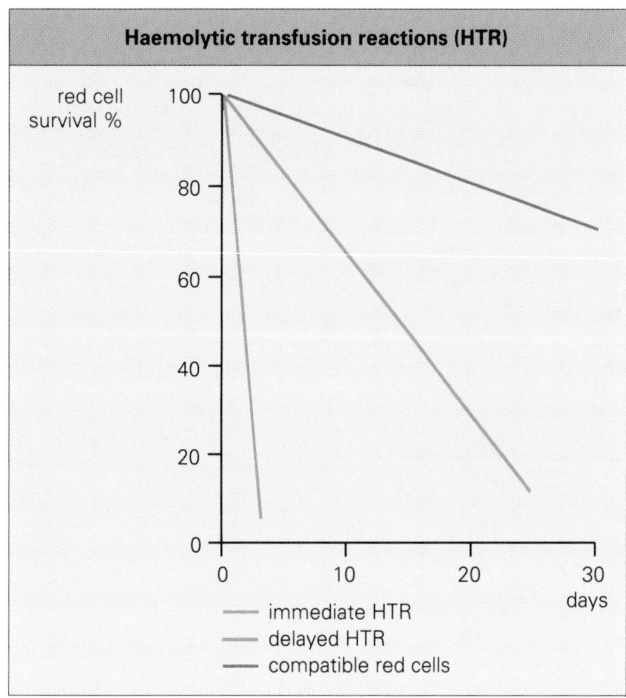

Fig. 16.10 Survival curves of compatible and incompatible transfused red cells. An immediate HTR may be due to rapid intravascular haemolysis (usually due to ABO incompatibility) or slower extravascular haemolysis due to non-complement fixing IgG antibodies. A delayed HTR a few days after the transfusion is due to a secondary (anamnestic) antibody response in a previously sensitized patient.

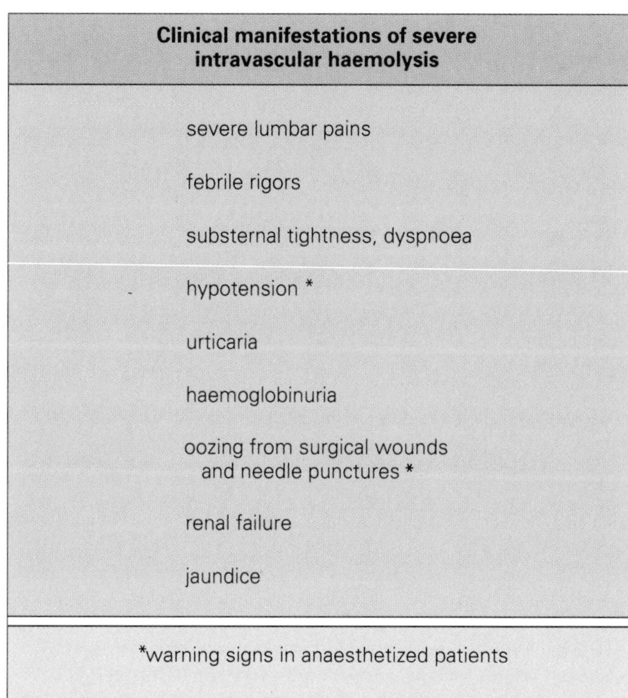

Fig. 16.11 Clinical manifestations of severe intravascular haemolysis.

Red cell incompatibility

There are two main types of haemolytic transfusion reaction (HTR) (Fig. 16.10):

- immediate HTR
- delayed HTR

Immediate HTR may be caused either by rapid intravascular haemolysis due to antibodies (IgM or IgG) that fully activate complement, or by slower extravascular haemolysis due to non-complement fixing IgG antibodies. The most dreaded HTR is acute intravascular haemolysis due to ABO incompatibility, which usually occurs because of patient and/or sample misidentification.

The clinical manifestations (Fig. 16.11) are due to the initial antigen-antibody reaction triggering a series of interactions between the complement and coagulation pathways (Fig. 16.12). Disseminated intravascular coagulation (DIC) is a bad prognostic sign. Fatalities due to ABO-incompatible transfusions are caused either by uncontrolled bleeding due to DIC, or renal failure, which itself may be a consequence of DIC. In some cases, the clinical features are less severe and may even be overlooked, so that the first indication of a possible haemolytic transfusion reaction is the observation of spherocytosis in the blood film (see Fig. 16.3), or a positive direct antiglobulin
16.8 test after transfusion.

Diagnosis depends on demonstrating haemolysis in the patient and incompatibility between donor and recipient (Fig. 16.13). Differential diagnosis from other conditions causing a similar clinical presentation is important, the most serious being the transfusion of infected blood. At the first suspicion of reaction the transfusion should be stopped, as the severity depends partly on the dose of red cell antigen. Emergency treatment should aim to maintain blood pressure and an adequate renal perfusion. If the patient is bleeding, laboratory investigation of DIC should be carried out. Compatible blood should be transfused as required.

Delayed HTR may occur in patients alloimmunized by previous pregnancy or transfusion. The antibody titre is too low to be detected in the pre-transfusion testing,but after re-exposure to the incompatible antigen a secondary (anamnestic) immune response occurs: IgG antibodies develop, and the transfused red cells are destroyed.

Typically, the patient develops anaemia, fever, jaundice and sometimes haemoglobinuria approximately one week after transfusion. The condition may resemble an autoimmune or drug-induced immune haemolytic anaemia with a positive direct antiglobulin test (in this case due to alloantibody on the donor cells), spherocytosis and reticulocytosis. However, the preceding transfusion

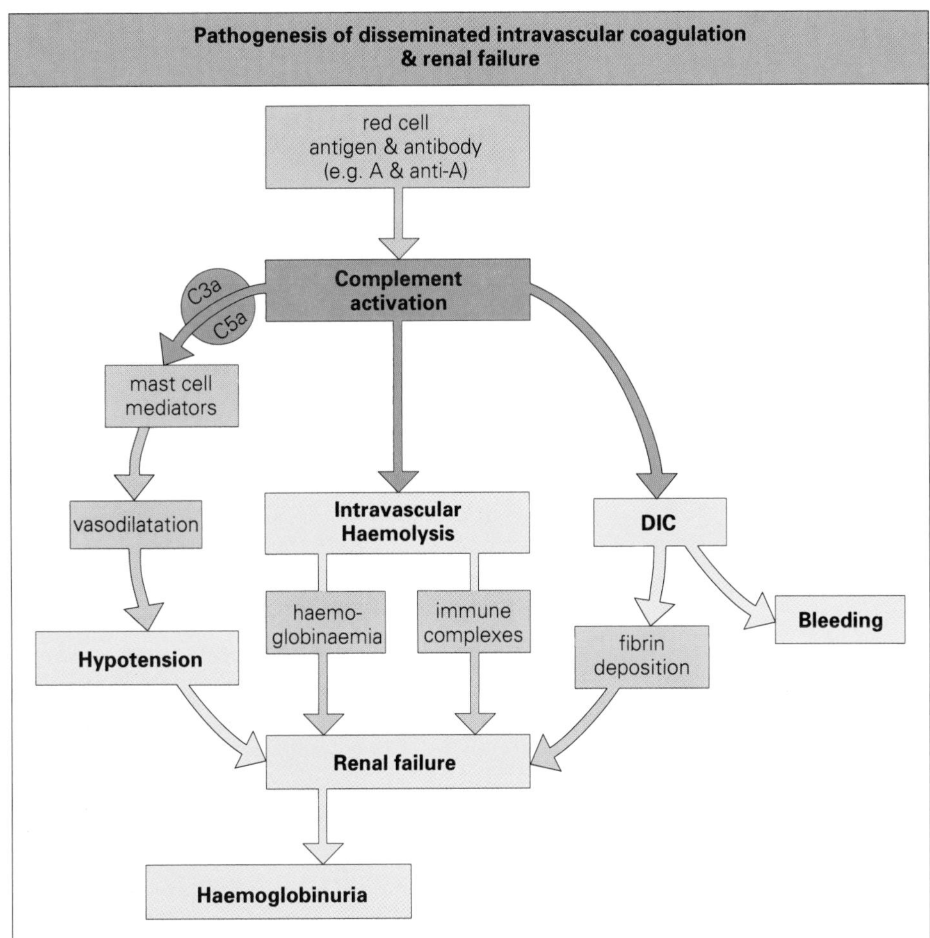

Fig. 16.12 Pathogenesis of disseminated intravascular coagulation (DIC) and renal failure following acute intravascular haemolysis due to red cell incompatibility.

Investigation of haemolytic transfusion reaction

Evidence of haemolysis
examine patient's plasma & urine for haemoglobin
blood film may show spherocytosis

Evidence of incompatibility
clerical check
identification error indicates type of incompatibility

serological check
repeat ABO and Rh(D) group of patient & donor units
screen for red cell antibodies
repeat compatibility test with pre- & post-transfusion serum
direct antiglobulin test (post-transfusion sample)

Evidence of DIC
blood film (red cell fragmentation)
platelet count
coagulation screen

Evidence of bacterial infection
Gram stain
culture donor blood

Fig. 16.13 Investigation of haemolytic transfusion reactions.

should suggest the correct diagnosis. Once confirmed there is usually no need for further action in most cases, as the course is self-limiting. Many delayed haemolytic transfusion reactions of this type almost certainly go undetected.

Leucocyte and platelet incompatibility

Both HLA and cell-specific antibodies may cause transfusion problems. In addition, transfused donor lymphocytes may cause a graft-versus-host reaction in immunocompromized recipients.

Febrile reaction. This is the most common adverse effect of blood transfusion. Anti-leucocyte antibodies in the recipient are the cause, and donor granulocytes are the main target cells. The relative importance of granulocyte-specific and HLA antibodies is not clear.

Febrile reactions occur in patients who have had previous transfusions or pregnancy. Typical signs are flushing and tachycardia, followed by fever (38–40°C) and sometimes rigors, usually about thirty minutes to two hours after starting the transfusion. Although the reaction is usually benign and self-limiting, the transfusion must be stopped to exclude the possibility of a more serious

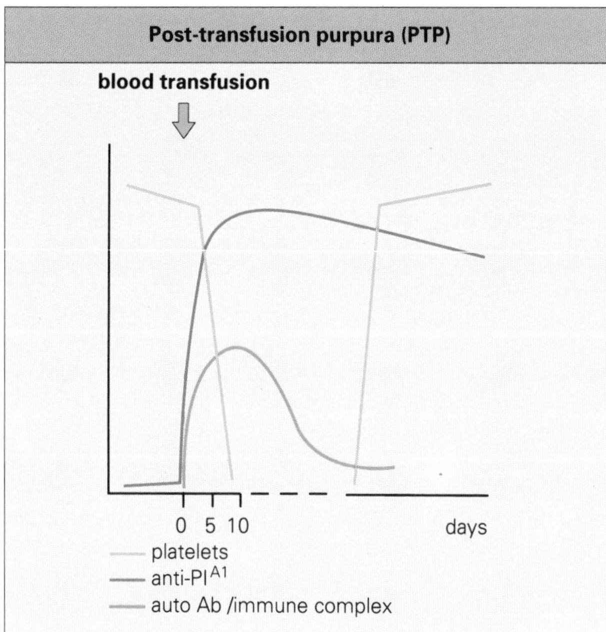

Fig. 16.14 Course of events in post-transfusion purpura showing the onset of severe thrombocytopenia about one week after the precipitating transfusion, and the anamnestic response of anti-Pl ^{A1}. The transient appearance of a platelet autoantibody and /or immune complexes (Pl ^{A1}/anti-Pl ^{A1}) coincides with the nadir of the platelet count.

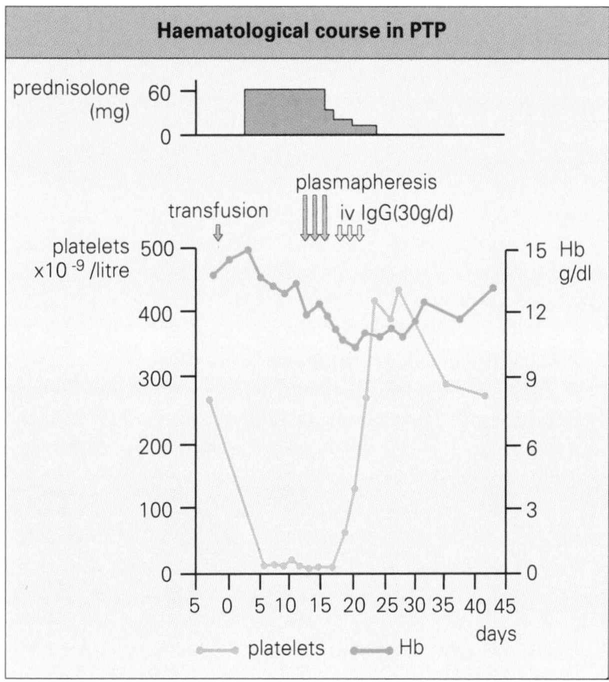

Fig. 16.15 Haematological course of a patient with post-transfusion purpura showing the onset of profound thrombocytopenia (platelets <10 x 10^9/litre) 5 days after a blood transfusion. There was no increase in the platelet count after prednisolone or plasmapheresis, but a prompt remission following high-dose intravenous IgG.

haemolytic reaction. Febrile reactions can be prevented in alloimmunized patients by using leucocyte-poor red cells, which are usually prepared by filtration.

Pulmonary reaction. Some donors (usually multiparous women) may have high titres of leucocyte antibodies that react with the recipient's granulocytes. In the few reported cases, this type of reaction is associated with a complement-fixing granulocyte-specific antibody which causes pulmonary leucostasis and neutropenia. This is accompanied by fever, cough, dyspnoea and a characteristic chest radiograph.

Post-transfusion purpura (PTP). PTP is an acute episode of severe immune thrombocytopenia, occurring about one week after a blood transfusion. It is an uncommon but well-defined syndrome.

Typically, the patient is female and there is always a history of previous pregnancy or blood transfusion. Most PTP patients lack the platelet antigen Pl^{A1}, which is present in about 98% of the population, and anti-Pl^{A1} is usually demonstrated in their serum. The precipitating mechanism appears to be an anamnestic response to Pl^{A1}-positive platelets in a recent blood transfusion, which boosts the level of anti-Pl^{A1}. The unique feature of PTP is the paradoxical destruction of the patient's own platelets (which are Pl^{A1}-negative); the exact mechanism is unknown (Fig. 16.14). One explanation is that the patient's platelets are destroyed either by the adsorption of Pl^{A1}/anti-Pl^{A1} immune complexes or by the adsorption of Pl ^{A1} antigen from the transfused platelets, which subsequently react with anti-Pl^{A1}. Alternatively, the transfusion-induced alloimmunization may stimulate a platelet autoantibody, and there is some evidence for this from animal models of PTP and from recent studies of patients with the condition.

Although PTP is a self-limiting condition, the period of severe thrombocytopenia may exceed two weeks, and intervention is indicated once a definite diagnosis is made. Platelet transfusion is ineffective and may even aggravate the condition. Steroids relieve the bleeding manifestations but usually do not improve the platelet count. Plasmapheresis is beneficial in some cases, and recent experience with high-dose intravenous IgG shows that this can induce a prompt platelet response (Fig. 16.15).

Platelet and granulocyte transfusions. Alloimmunization resulting in an unsatisfactory post-transfusion increase in platelet counts is often a problem in patients receiving repeated platelet transfusions from random donors. This is usually due to HLA antibodies, although platelet-specific antibodies are sometimes responsible. Once refractoriness develops, transfusion of platelets from donors matched for the HLA-A and -B antigens of the recipient usually produces improved platelet increments (Fig. 16.16). Occasionally, however, this is unsuccessful due to the presence of platelet-specific alloantibodies directed against the donor cells, and direct cross-matching of the

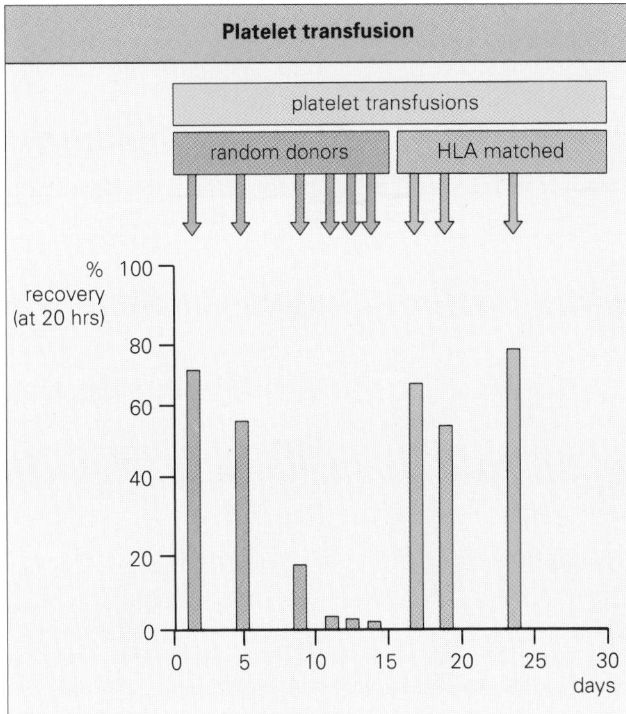

Fig. 16.16 Response of a patient with acute leukaemia during remission induction chemotherapy, showing the development of refractoriness to platelet transfusions from random donors and subsequent improved responses to HLA-matched donor platelets. Recovery % measures the percentage of transfused platelets circulating 20 hours after transfusion.

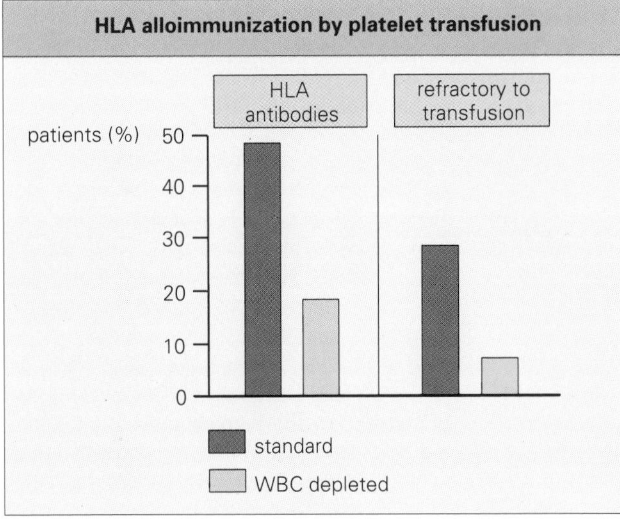

Fig. 16.17 Comparison of the incidence of HLA alloimmunization and refractoriness to platelet transfusion in two groups of multi-transfused patients with acute leukaemia receiving either leucocyte-depleted blood products (19 patients) or standard (non-depleted) blood products (31 patients). Modified from Murphy *et al.* (1986).

donor's platelets against the patient's serum may help to select compatible donors for such patients.

Contaminating lymphocytes in the platelet concentrate appear to be responsible for primary HLA alloimmunization associated with platelet transfusion, and the use of leucocyte-poor red cell and platelet transfusions results in a much lower incidence of HLA alloimmunization and more effective platelet transfusions (Fig. 16.17).

Repeated granulocyte transfusions may immunize the recipient against neutrophil-specific and HLA antigens. Alloantibodies reactive with neutrophil antigens may cause not only a severe febrile transfusion reaction, but also poor survival of the transfused granulocytes and poor localization at sites of infection, thereby reducing the clinical benefit of the transfusion to the patient.

Graft-versus-host reactions

Since viable lymphocytes survive in stored blood, transfusion of immunocompromized recipients may lead to engraftment of donor lymphoid cells. This has caused fatal graft-versus-host disease (GVHD) in some patients. To avoid the risk of GVHD, cellular blood components should be gamma-irradiated if the recipient is receiving immunosuppressive therapy or is immunodeficient from other causes.

Plasma protein incompatibility

After the febrile type, urticarial reactions are the second most common transfusion reaction to occur. These are rarely severe or life-threatening and, although often attributed to plasma protein incompatibility, the cause is unexplained in most cases. However, in some patients, antibodies with only limited allospecificity to IgA can be detected.

Occasionally, severe anaphylactic reactions occur in patients lacking IgA who have made class-specific anti-IgA, which then reacts with IgA in the transfused blood. This is associated with complement activation and severe life-threatening anaphylaxis.

ALLOIMMUNE NEONATAL CYTOPENIAS

Pregnancy is a special transfusion situation in which fetal blood cells cross the placenta and may immunize the mother against antigens inherited from the father. Alloimmunization *per se* has no harmful effect on the mother, but it does predispose to possible immunological complications from a subsequent blood transfusion or tissue transplantation. However, maternal IgG antibodies formed in this way are actively transported across the placenta into the fetal circulation.

The clinical effects depend on the specificity of the antibody. Although HLA antibodies are often formed during pregnancy, they do not appear to cause any harm to the fetus. On the other hand, each cell-specific antibody causes a characteristic disease:

• red cell-specific antibodies cause haemolytic disease;

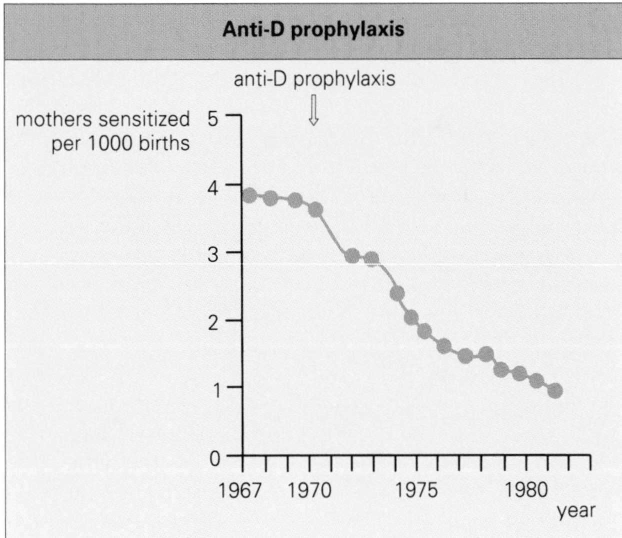

Fig. 16.18 Incidence of new cases of maternal Rh sensitization in the Yorkshire Health Region after 1970, when post-delivery anti-D prophylaxis was introduced for RhD-negative mothers at risk (L A D Tovey, personal communication). New cases occurred for three main reasons: (i) failure to give anti-D to some mothers at risk, especially after abortion; (ii) failure to give enough anti-D to the mother to match the volume of the fetal blood; (iii) intrapregnancy immunization, which could be reduced by antenatal administration of anti-D to mothers at risk.

- platelet-specific antibodies cause alloimmune neonatal thrombocytopenia;
- granulocyte-specific antibodies cause alloimmune neonatal neutropenia.

Although these are designated 'neonatal' conditions, immune cell destruction begins *in utero* during the second trimester and may damage the fetus before birth.

HAEMOLYTIC DISEASE OF THE NEWBORN (HDN)

HDN is a form of haemolytic anaemia affecting the fetus and newborn infant. It occurs when maternal alloantibody to fetal red cell antigens crosses the placenta and causes haemolysis of fetal red cells. As IgG is the only immunoglobulin transferred across the placenta, only red cell antibodies of this class cause HDN.

Rh HDN

Anti-D causes the most severe form of HDN. This may occur when an Rh-negative (dd) mother has an Rh(D)-positive fetus. At the time of delivery, when the placenta separates, fetal red cells enter the maternal circulation. The risk of Rh(D) immunization depends on the maternal dose of fetal red cells and the mother's ability to respond to the antigenic stimulus; approximately 30% of individuals are 'non-responders' in this respect. Furthermore, ABO incompatibility between mother and fetus reduces the risk

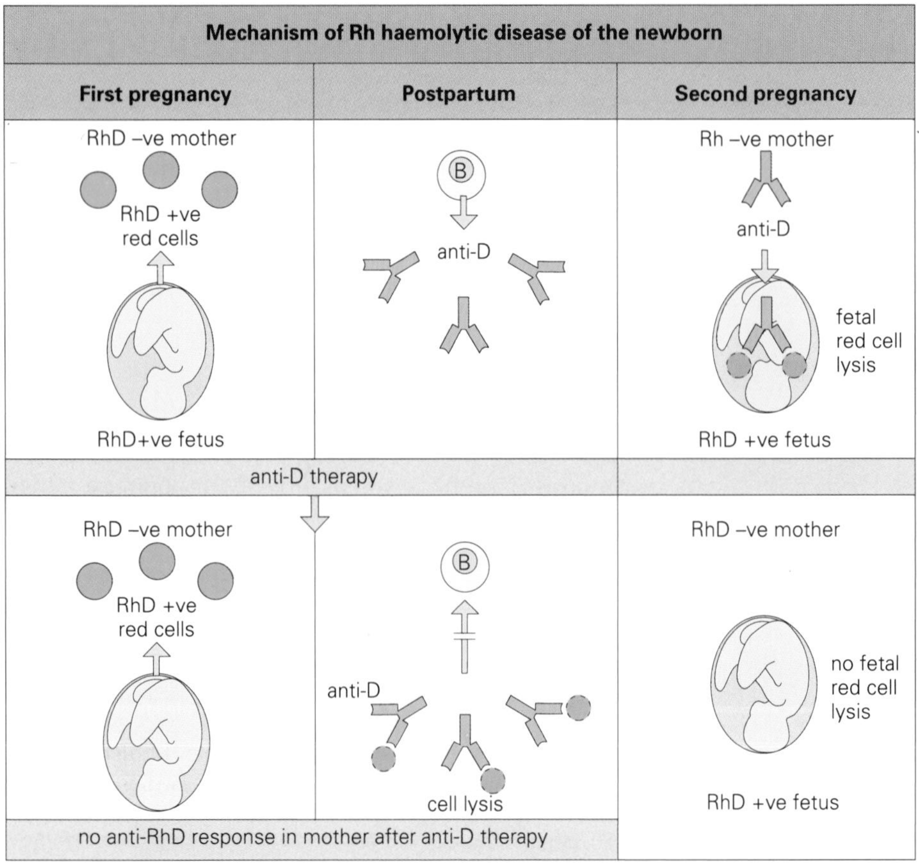

Mechanism of Rh haemolytic disease of the newborn

First pregnancy	Postpartum	Second pregnancy
RhD –ve mother RhD +ve red cells RhD+ve fetus	B anti-D	Rh –ve mother anti-D fetal red cell lysis RhD +ve fetus
anti-D therapy		
RhD –ve mother RhD +ve red cells	B anti-D cell lysis	RhD –ve mother no fetal red cell lysis RhD +ve fetus
no anti-RhD response in mother after anti-D therapy		

Fig. 16.19 Upper: Rh HDN occurs when an RhD-negative woman has an RhD-positive fetus. Parturition is the primary immunizing event, when significant numbers of fetal red cells enter the maternal circulation. The first pregnancy is therefore usually not affected. Once sensitized, the mother will have a secondary response to the small number of fetal red cells that leak across the placenta during the course of the next RhD-positive pregnancy. Maternal anti-D IgG crosses the placenta and destroys fetal RhD-positive red cells by extravascular phagocytosis. Lower: Primary sensitization can be prevented by the administration of anti-D after delivery of every RhD-positive baby.

of maternal Rh immunization by fetal Rh(D)-positive red cells. The precise mechanism of the protection afforded by ABO incompatibility is not clear, but it is thought to be related to rapid clearance of ABO-incompatible fetal red cells, so that the mother is not immunized by the D antigen which is also carried on the red cells. Similarly, the administration of anti-D immunoglobulin to an Rh(D)-negative person, at the same time as a dose of Rh(D)-positive red cells, will suppress primary immunization. The practical application of this could potentially eliminate anti-D HDN, and the prophylactic administration of anti-D is now standard treatment for mothers at risk (Fig. 16.18)

The fetal consequences of maternal anti-D alloimmunization vary in severity. As maternal immunization occurs at the end of the first pregnancy, the first child is spared, but subsequent pregnancies are at risk (Fig. 16.19). The fetus may die *in utero* of severe anaemia ('hydrops fetalis'). However, some severely affected fetuses can be rescued by intra-uterine transfusions until it is safe to interrupt the pregnancy. After delivery, exchange transfusion is used to minimize further haemolysis and reduce the level of bilirubin (a breakdown product of haemoglobin), which may cause toxic brain stem damage (kernicterus). The mildest form of the disease occurs when the mother has very little antibody, which reacts only weakly with the fetal red cells. In these cases the baby's red cells are antibody-coated (positive direct antiglobulin test) at birth, but there is little or no evidence of haemolysis, and no treatment is required.

HDN due to other antibodies

The success of anti-D prophylaxis has reduced the number of cases of HDN due to anti-D, and consequently the relative proportion of cases due to other antibodies has increased. The other most common causes of HDN are anti-c, anti-E and anti-K (Kell), but almost every other red cell IgG antibody has been reported as a cause of HDN.

ABO haemolytic disease of the newborn

This is considered separately, as a number of special factors combine to protect the fetus from the effects of ABO incompatibility. For practical purposes, only group O individuals make IgG anti-A and anti-B. Therefore, only A or B infants of group O mothers are at risk from ABO-HDN. Although 25% are susceptible, only about 1% are affected, and even then the condition is usually mild and very rarely severe enough to need exchange transfusion (approximately 1 case in 3,000). Two mechanisms protect the fetus against anti-A and anti-B: one is the weaker expression of A and B antigens at birth; the other is the widespread distribution of A and B glycoproteins in body fluids and tissues, which diverts much of the IgG antibody that crosses the placenta away from the red cell 'target'.

ABO-HDN may be seen in the first incompatible pregnancy, because the group O primigravida has already made IgG anti-A and anti-B in response to various immunizing stimuli. This is unlike Rh-HDN where immunization usually takes place at the end of the first pregnancy, thus sparing the first child.

At birth, ABO-HDN is suspected if a group O mother has a group A or B child who is jaundiced. The direct antiglobulin test usually demonstrates IgG on cord red cells, which can be eluted and shown to have anti-A or anti-B specificity. Other red cell antibodies must be excluded, as well as other causes of neonatal jaundice.

ALLOIMMUNE NEONATAL THROMBOCYTOPENIA AND NEUTROPENIA

These conditions, which are relatively common, are due to immunization of the mother against fetal platelet- and neutrophil-specific antigens inherited from the father. The high frequency of first pregnancy immunization suggests that neutrophils and platelets invade the maternal circulation at a much earlier stage than red cells.

Diagnosis depends on demonstrating a cell-specific alloantibody in the maternal serum that reacts with the baby's platelets or neutrophils. At the time of diagnosis, the baby's cells are often not available in adequate numbers for testing, and so the father's cells, which carry the relevant antigen, are a more convenient alternative. Neonatal thrombocytopenia may also be due to placental transfer of an IgG platelet autoantibody from a mother with autoimmune thrombocytopenia. Similarly, maternal IgG neutrophil autoantibodies may cross the placenta and cause neonatal neutropenia.

AUTOIMMUNE CYTOPENIAS

Autoimmune haemolytic anaemia is a convenient model for the study of autoimmune disease. A similar condition may affect platelets (autoimmune thrombocytopenia) and neutrophils (autoimmune neutropenia). Although these cytopenias usually occur separately, they may occasionally be present together (Evans' syndrome).

AUTOIMMUNE HAEMOLYTIC ANAEMIA (AIHA)

Haemolytic anaemia is due to an increased rate of red cell destruction. In immune haemolytic anaemia this is due to antibody and/or complement on the cell surface.

Diagnosis

The laboratory plays a key role in the diagnosis and management of AIHA. The essential diagnostic test is the direct antiglobulin (Coombs') test (DAT). With monospecific AHG reagents, it is possible to determine the Ig class/subclass and complement components on the red cell. This will suggest the possible mechanism of cell destruction and assist the diagnosis. Antibodies in an eluate from the patient's red cells and in the patient's serum should also be identified.

Classification

AIHA is broadly divided into 'warm' and 'cold' types. The aetiology may be primary (idiopathic) or secondary (associated with other conditions which may be causally related) (Fig. 16.20). The clinical course may be acute or chronic.

Clinicopathological effects

The immunochemical properties of the antibody determine, to a very large extent, its clinical effects.

Warm Type AIHA. The autoantibody is active at normal body temperature (37°C) and is usually IgG (subclass IgG1 and/or IgG3). Haemolysis is typically extravascular, occurring in the spleen. Some warm IgG antibodies may fix C3, which is often associated with red cell destruction in both liver and spleen (see Fig. 16.2), leading to more severe haemolysis.

The effects of the antibody are reflected in the peripheral blood as spherocytosis (immune damage) and variable autoagglutination due to red cell antibody coating (Fig. 16.21). The bone marrow may occasionally show erythrophagocytosis of sensitized red cells. Examination of the bone marrow may also reveal an associated lymphoproliferative disorder which may be causally related to the immune dysregulation responsible for the production of red cell autoantibodies. Steroids are the first line of treatment to reduce phagocytosis of sensitized red cells and depress autoantibody production. Splenectomy is the second line of treatment, if steroids fail to control haemolysis; this may be followed by a trial of immunosuppresion with cytotoxic drugs (for example, azathioprine, cyclophosphamide) in refractory patients.

Cold Type AIHA. Naturally occurring IgM cold agglutinins (anti-I) have a low thermal range up to 10–12°C and do not cause clinical problems. However, abnormal IgM cold agglutinins have an extended thermal range and cause clinical problems if this approaches peripheral body temperature (30–32°C), leading to cold haemagglutinin disease (CHAD). This is more likely in cold weather, when peripheral red cell agglutination may cause viscosity problems (Raynaud's phenomenon), and complement activation may proceed to intravascular haemolysis at the higher body core temperature.

Acute CHAD following mycoplasmal pneumonia is a winter problem. The polyclonal IgM antibody has both a high titre and a high thermal range; it is a potent haemolysin, and severe haemolytic anaemia may result. This is a self-limiting condition, and once the diagnosis has been made treatment consists of keeping the patient's peripheral body temperature above the thermal range of the IgM antibody, for example with a 'space blanket' (Fig. 16.22). If transfusion is indicated, the blood should first be warmed.

Chronic CHAD presents a different clinical problem. The monoclonal IgM antibody is less effective in activating complement, and mild haemolytic anaemia is usually present. Red cell agglutination causing viscosity problems is often the main feature; Raynaud's phenomenon affecting the extremities may be severe enough to cause necrosis, and it is essential to keep the extremities warm to prevent this occurring.

In both acute and chronic CHAD the DAT is positive, with C3d on the red cells. Examination of the blood film at room temperature shows occasional spherocytes and marked autoagglutination, which can be dispersed by

Classification of autoimmune haemolytic anaemia	
Warm type (IgG ± complement)	**Cold type**
primary (idiopathic) secondary other autoimmune diseases e.g. SLE lymphoproliferative conditions e.g. CLL, lymphoma	CHAD (IgM + complement) acute post-infectious e.g. mycoplasma chronic primary (idiopathic) secondary e.g. lymphoma PCH (IgG+ complement) acute post-infectious chronic idiopathic or secondary

Fig. 16.20 Classification of autoimmune haemolytic anaemia. CHAD = chronic cold haemagglutinin disease. PCH = paroxysmal cold haemoglobinuria.

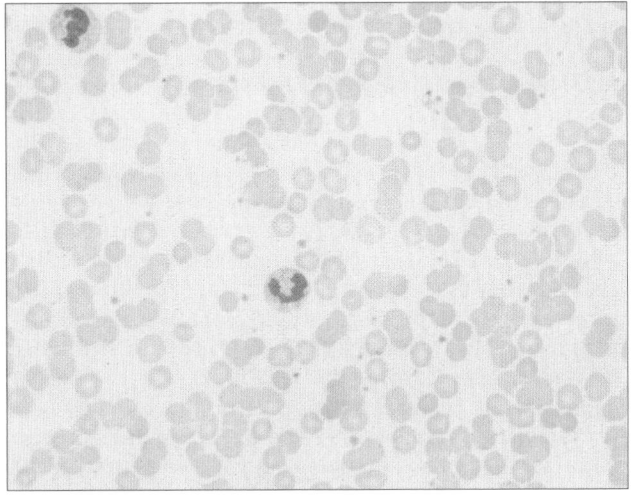

Fig. 16.21 Warm type AIHA. Stained blood film from patient with warm type AIHA (caused by IgG autoantibody) showing autoagglutination (small clumps of red cells) due to IgG antibody coating and a few spherocytes due to immune damage. The DAT was positive with anti-IgG.

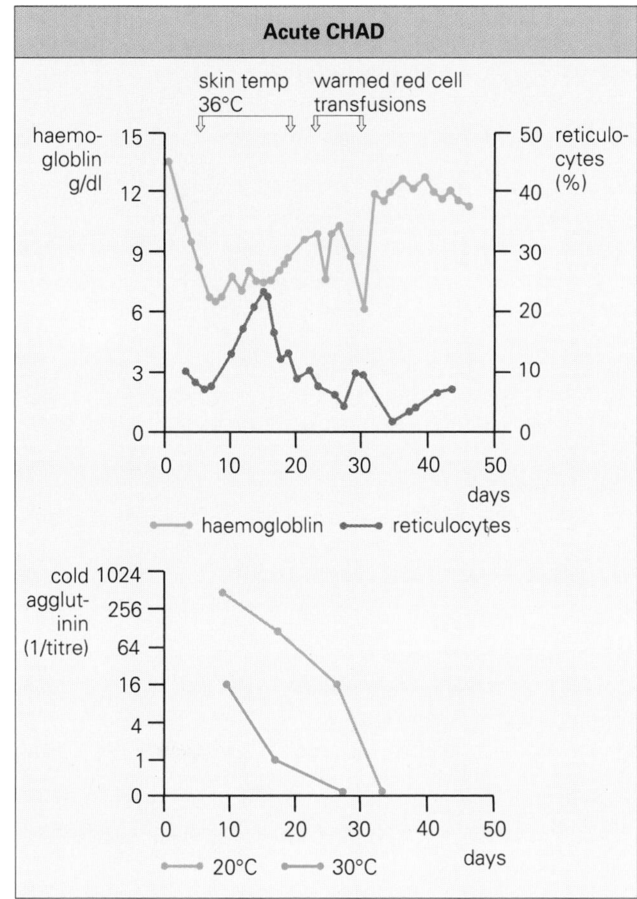

Fig. 16.22 Acute cold haemagglutinin haemolytic anaemia following *M.pneumoniae* infection in a 61-year-old woman. The chart shows a rapid fall in Hb due to haemolysis, followed by a reticulocytosis and slow rise in Hb after warming the patient with a 'space blanket' to raise skin temperature to 36°C. The cold agglutinin titres at 30°C and 20°C show a progressive fall. During recovery the patient had a haematemesis due to peptic ulceration which required gastric surgery. This was managed by transfusion of warmed blood.

Autoimmune thrombocytopenia

Primary (idiopathic - ITP)

Secondary
- acute post infectious
- other autoimmune diseases
  - e.g. SLE, Evans' syndrome
- lymphoproliferative conditions
- other malignancy
- immune system imbalance
  - e.g. AIDS
    - post bone marrow graft

Fig. 16.23 Classification of autoimmune thrombocytopenia.

warming the blood sample. The serum contains a high titre of IgM monoclonal antibody which reacts best at 4°C, but has a variable thermal range depending on the severity of the disease. The antibody usually has specificity for the I antigen, but is sometimes specific for the i antigen, especially in chronic CHAD associated with lymphoma. Treatment consists of keeping the patient warm and treating the underlying cause (for example lymphoma), if present. Alkylating agents (for example chlorambucil) may be helpful in some cases in reducing the production of the monoclonal IgM antibody.

Paroxysmal cold haemoglobinuria (PCH) is a rare form of AIHA which usually occurs as a transient acute condition in children following viral infection. The IgG antibody (Donath-Landsteiner) fixes complement at the low peripheral body temperature that occurs in winter; this causes severe intravascular haemolysis at the higher body core temperature. This can be reproduced *in vitro* by cooling the patient's blood sample to 4°C and then warming it to 37°C, when haemolysis will occur. If supportive blood transfusion is required for severely anaemic patients, washed red cells should be used to avoid the introduction of fresh complement, and the blood should be warmed before transfusion.

AUTOIMMUNE THROMBOCYTOPENIA

Like AIHA, this condition may be classified as primary (idiopathic) or secondary (associated with other conditions) (Fig. 16.23).

Diagnosis

The characteristic haematological features are a low platelet count (<100 x 10^9/litre) and the presence of megakaryocytes in the bone marrow, which excludes poor production of platelets. Diagnosis depends on exclusion of other causes of thrombocytopenia. Demonstration of a platelet autoantibody is not mandatory because, even with a combination of the most suitable techniques now available, platelet autoantibodies remain elusive in a small proportion (10–20%) of patients.

Three other immunological conditions may mimic autoimmune thrombocytopenia, and should always be considered:

- post-transfusion purpura — a recent transfusion will suggest this;
- drug-induced immune thrombocytopenia — a drug history is important;
- pseudothrombocytopenia — the patient has an EDTA-dependent platelet antibody which is active only *in vitro*.

Pseudothrombocytopenia causes platelet agglutination in the standard EDTA blood sample resulting in a false low platelet count; the blood film will, however, show large platelet clumps. The platelet count and blood film will be normal from a blood sample taken into citrate anticoagulant.

Pathogenesis

Platelet autoantibodies are of IgG and IgM classes, and both are often present in the same patient. Platelet destruction by IgG autoantibodies is similar to IgG-mediated red cell destruction. However, the mode of action of IgM autoantibodies is uncertain, as the relative importance of complement is controversial.

The autoantibody in ITP commonly reacts with the platelet membrane glycoprotein IIb/IIIa complex and may cause an acquired thrombasthenia in addition to producing thrombocytopenia.

Management

Patients usually present with cutaneous signs of thrombocytopenia — petechiae, purpura (Fig. 16.24) and mucosal bleeding. The major clinical problem is the risk of spontaneous bleeding into vital organs, especially the brain. The aim of treatment is to restore the platelet count to safe, but not necessarily normal, levels. The approach to treatment is the same as that for AIHA. In addition, high-dose intravenous IgG (iv IgG) has a place in the management of autoimmune thrombocytopenia; it produces an initial transient platelet response, but longer term effects are less predictable.

High-dose iv IgG may have a special place in the management of autoimmune thrombocytopenia during pregnancy, when a prompt platelet response is required towards term. It may also help to reduce placental transfer of the maternal IgG platelet autoantibody by blocking placental Fc receptors, thus sparing the fetus.

The precise mechanism of action of high-dose iv IgG is largely speculative. The initial platelet response is at least partly due to blocking macrophage Fc receptors. However, there also appears to be a direct effect on the immune system, with an absolute increase in T suppressor cells and a decrease in B cells with reduced Ig production. Longer term effects require explanation, but may be due to anti-idiotypic suppression of autoantibody synthesis.

AUTOIMMUNE NEUTROPENIA

Autoimmune neutropenia is the least well studied of the autoimmune cytopenias. This is partly because of the limitations of neutrophil serology, especially in the differentiation of autoantibodies and circulating immune complexes, and partly because the peripheral neutrophil count is an inadequate reflection of total granulocyte kinetics.

Classification

As with other cytopenias, autoimmune neutropenia may be primary (idiopathic) or secondary (Fig. 16.25). Idiopathic autoimmune neutropenia is well documented in infants but uncommon in adults, in whom autoimmune neutropenia is usually associated with other immunological disorders.

Diagnosis and pathogenesis

The relative importance of autoantibodies, immune complexes and cellular mechanisms in the pathogenesis of autoimmune neutropenia has yet to be resolved and the diagnosis is therefore based on the interpretation of a combination of tests (Fig.16.26).

Neutrophil autoantibodies (usually IgG) are unusual in that they may have well defined specificity for neutrophil-specific alloantigens. However, it is not always possible to

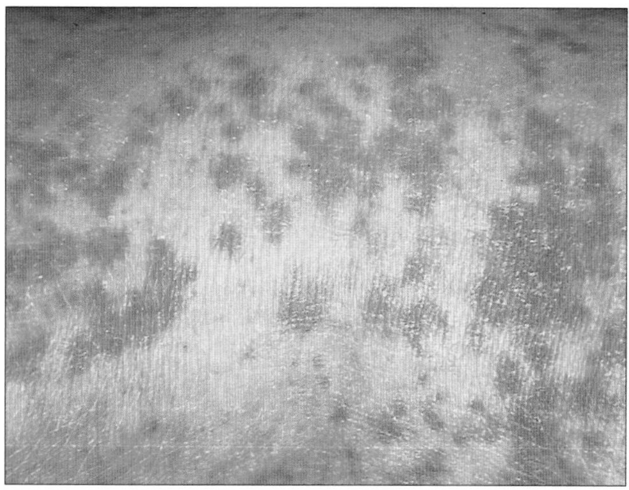

Fig. 16.24 Idiopathic thrombocytopenic purpura showing characteristic petechial spots. Courtesy of Dr Patricia Hewitt.

Autoimmune neutropenia
Primary (idiopathic)
Secondary
autoimmune conditions
SLE
Felty's syndrome
AIHA ± thrombocytopenia (Evans' syndrome)
immune system imbalance
hypogammaglobinaemia
AIDS
post bone marrow graft
lymphoproliferative conditions
± chemo/radiotherapy

Fig. 16.25 Classification of autoimmune neutropenia.

demonstrate antigen specificity, and such autoantibodies may have a wider target specificity than mature neutrophils, and are probably better described as granulocyte autoantibodies. These autoantibodies may suppress granulocyte precursors in the bone marrow and cause more severe neutropenia. The investigation of suspected autoimmune neutropenia should therefore, include tests on bone marrow precursors as target cells, especially when antibodies to mature neutrophils are not found.

When an autoantibody cannot be demonstrated the possible role of cell-mediated mechanisms of neutropenia should also be investigated, as in granulopoietic failure associated with proliferation of large granular lymphocytes with a phenotype (for example $CD3^+$, $CD8^+$, HNK-1^+) suggesting immature NK cells.

Management

Most infants with autoimmune neutropenia undergo a benign, self-limiting course. Steroids are sometimes used to treat severely neutropenic children with severe infections, but this may further prejudice immune function, and it may be preferable to use high-dose iv IgG in this situation.

In adults, secondary autoimmune neutropenia is a feature of the associated disease, which should be treated appropriately. Steroids may be given, but their effect is unpredictable.

AUTOIMMUNE SUPPRESSION OF PROGENITOR CELLS

Immune suppression of progenitor cells may be responsible for pure red cell aplasia, agranulocytosis and aplastic anaemia in some patients. Laboratory confirmation is difficult and depends on carefully controlled bone marrow cell culture assays. The contribution of humoral and cellular mechanisms requires further study.

Investigation of idiopathic neutropenia
neutrophil antibody
cell bound
serum
serum immune complexes
myeloid precursors
CFU-GM assay
antibody assay
ancillary tests
serum lactoferrin (PMN mass)
serum myeloperoxidase (granulopoiesis)
T cell markers

Fig. 16.26 Investigation of idiopathic neutropenia.

AETIOLOGY OF AUTOANTIBODY PRODUCTION

Autoantibody production reflects the loss of ability to recognize antigens as self. This may be an inherited susceptibility or an acquired dysregulation of the immune system as, for example, in some lymphoproliferative disorders or after bone marrow transplantation. If the basic defect is the loss of T cell regulation of B cells, further refinement is required to explain the target cell specificity of autoantibodies in different autoimmune diseases. This could be induced by external triggering factors, such as viruses and drugs, which in the case of AIHA may cause subtle alterations in red cell antigens. The fact that the autoantibody in AIHA often has blood group specificity supports this theory. In warm type AIHA the IgG antibody usually has broad specificity for the Rh complex, and a similar autoantibody may be induced by the drug α-methyldopa (see page 16.19); in CHAD, the IgM antibody is usually anti-I (and sometimes anti-i, especially in chronic CHAD associated with lymphoma); and the IgG Donath-Landsteiner antibody in PCH has blood group P specificity. Similar antigen specificity is also well defined for neutrophil autoantibodies in patients with idiopathic autoimmune neutropenia. Platelet autoantibodies do not have alloantigen specificity, but they commonly react with the platelet membrane glycoprotein IIb/IIIa complex, which carries the major platelet specific antigen systems (Pl^A, Bak).

DRUG-INDUCED IMMUNE CYTOPENIAS

Drug-induced antibodies may cause selective haemolytic anaemia, thrombocytopenia, neutropenia or a combination of these in the same patient. Drugs act as haptens and become immunogenic after binding to a macromolecular carrier, usually protein. They may bind weakly or strongly to the cell surface, the strength of the bond determining to a large extent the mechanism of subsequent immune destruction of the cell by the drug-induced antibody (see chapter 19).

MECHANISM OF CELL DESTRUCTION

Immune-complex mechanism

Shulman proposed this mechanism to explain quinidine-induced thrombocytopenia. It is based on the observation that the drug has only weak affinity for the cell, whereas the drug/antibody complex binds more strongly and activates complement, which destroys the cell. The target cell

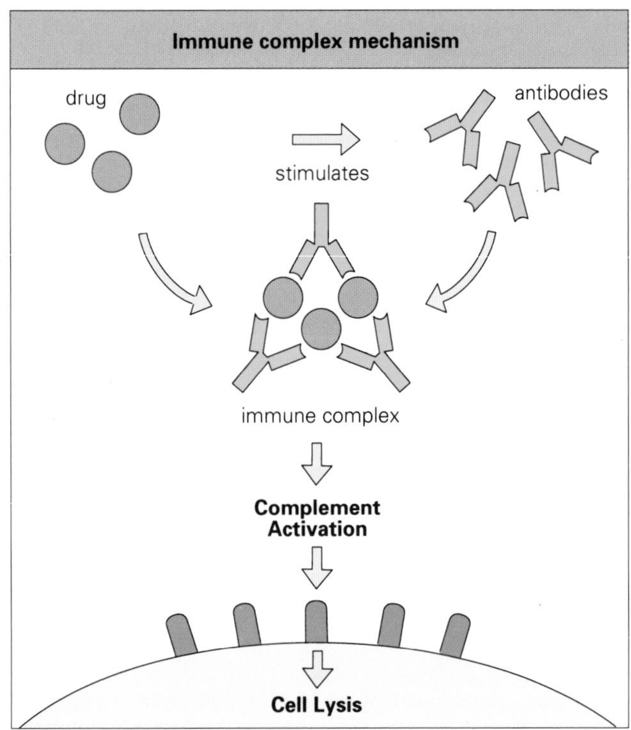

Fig. 16.27 The drug stimulates production of antibody. Subsequent exposure to the drug leads to a drug/antibody interaction, forming immune complexes which may damage the cell (? an innocent bystander) by complement activation.

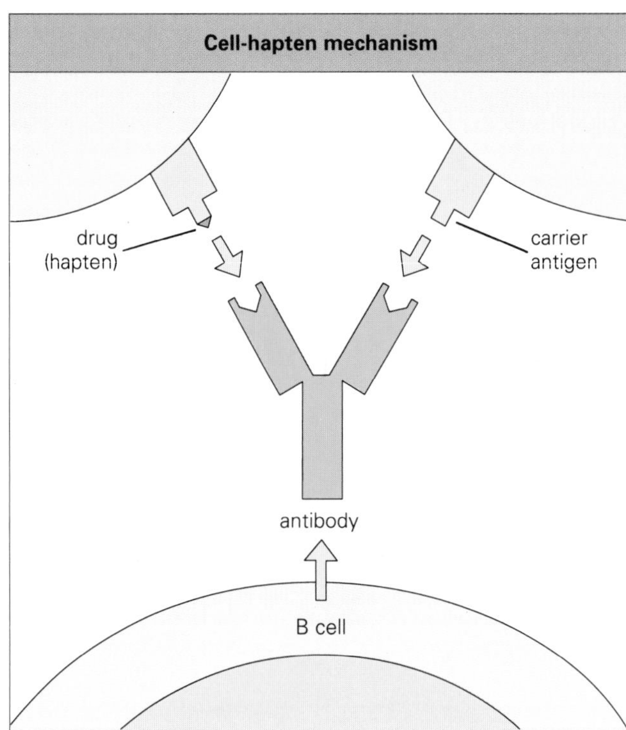

Fig. 16.28 A drug acting as hapten is attached to a larger molecular carrier to stimulate antibody production. The antibody then reacts with the drug as antigen. The antibody may also have specificity for the 'carrier' of the drug, which may be a molecular component of the cell membrane.

appeared to be an 'innocent bystander' (Fig. 16.27), but more recent evidence suggests that specific membrane glycoproteins are required as receptors for particular drug/antibody complexes. In quin(id)ine thrombocytopenia, for example, the drug/antibody complex reacts only weakly or not at all with Bernard-Soulier platelets which have reduced or absent membrane glycoprotein Ib.

As an alternative, Ackroyd proposed the 'cell-hapten' mechanism, which explained the target orientation of the drug /antibody from the outset (Fig. 16.28). He postulated that the antibodies so formed would have specificity for both the drug and a cell-membrane component (carrier). This is consistent with recent observations that a predominant drug-dependent antibody may be accompanied by an apparent autoantibody, usually giving weaker serological reactions.

Drug adsorption

Penicillin is the prototype drug for this mechanism, and immune haemolysis is the most usual clinical effect (Fig. 16.29), although immune thrombocytopenia and neutropenia may also occur. Penicillin binds strongly to the cell membrane. This is not necessary for the immunogenicity of the drug, but it determines the mechanism of
16.18 cell destruction. Preformed IgG penicillin antibody reacts with cell-bound penicillin; cell destruction is characteristically extravascular, occurring in the spleen. In penicillin immune haemolysis, large doses are necessary to deposit enough drug 'antigenic' sites on the red cell membrane to cause significant haemolysis.

Autoantibody induction

This was first described for immune haemolysis due to α-methyldopa. This drug induces red cell autoantibodies similar to the IgG autoantibody in warm type AIHA. The precise mechanism of autoantibody production is not clear, but it is proposed that the drug may:

- cause T cell imbalance and dysregulation of B cell function, which predisposes to autoantibody production;
- alter the Rh complex to explain the Rh specificity (commonly anti-e, -c) of the autoantibody. This is consistent with the red cell being the main target of the autoantibody, although occasional cases of thrombocytopenia have also been reported.

Although the autoantibody is often present in patients receiving α-methyldopa (15–20%), haemolysis is not common (<1%). Recent studies of mononuclear-phagocyte clearance in patients receiving α-methyldopa suggest

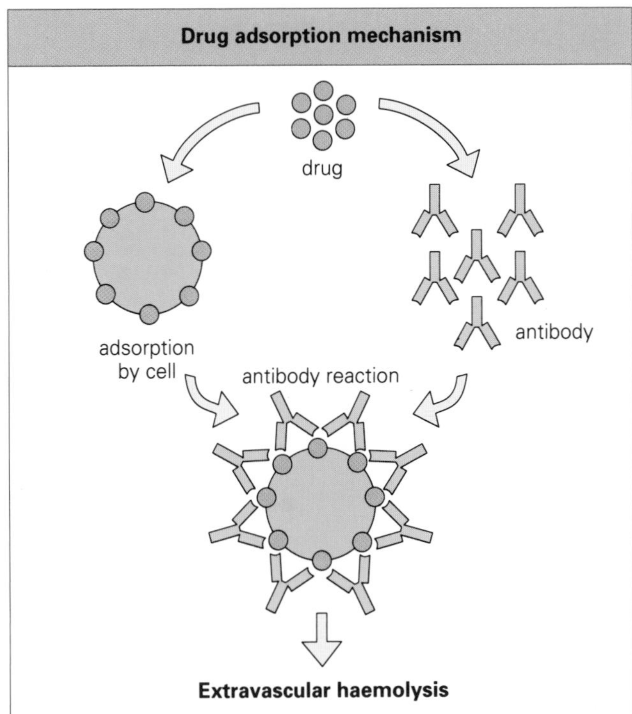

Fig. 16.29 Penicillin stimulates antibody production. On subsequent exposure, the adverse effect of the drug depends on the dose given, which determines the amount of drug (antigen) adsorbed onto the cell surface. The antibody is usually IgG and the cell is destroyed by extravascular phagocytosis.

Failure to demonstrate drug-induced antibody
insensitivity of method used
drug metabolite as antigen
test cells lack specific receptor
drug-antibody acting at precursor cell stage
cell mediated mechanism involved

Fig. 16.30 Failure to demonstrate drug-induced antibody.

that the drug itself may blockade the MP system in most patients, effectively blocking the autoantibody.

Action of Drug Antibody on Precursor Cells. The above mechanisms refer to the immune destruction of mature circulating cells, but the drug-induced antibody may also affect bone marrow precursor cells, which may contribute significantly to the peripheral cytopenia in some cases. This aspect of the pathogenesis of drug-induced immune cytopenias has not been well studied, but improvements in bone marrow clonal assays should make this more feasible.

Idiosyncrasy of Drug-Induced Cytopenias. As previously mentioned, the antibody may recognize not only the drug, but also a specific cell membrane component. Antibodies from patients with drug-induced thrombocytopenia or neutropenia show restriction in that they react with variable proportions of normal donor cells exposed to the drug. This is not related to HLA or known cell-specific antigens, and family studies suggest that another polymorphic membrane determinant is involved.

Failure to Demonstrate the Antibody. It should be pointed out that it is not always possible to demonstrate the antibody in cases of suspected drug-induced immune cytopenia. Fig. 16.30 lists some possible explanations for this.

FURTHER READING

Chaplin H, ed. *Methods in hematology 12: Immune hemolytic anaemias.* New York: Churchill Livingstone, 1985.

Dacie J V. *The haemolytic anaemias: Part II: The autoimmune anaemias* (2E) London: Churchill, 1962.

Engelfriet CP, Van Loghem JJ & Von dem Bornes, AEGKr, eds. *Research monographs in immunology 5: Immunohaematology.* Amsterdam: Elsevier Science Publishers BV, 1984.

Kelton JG. The interaction of IgG with reticuloendothelial cells: biological and therapeutic implications. In: Garratty G, ed. *Current conceps in transfusion therapy.* Arlington VA: American Association of Blood Banks, 1985:51–107.

McCullogh J. The clinical significance of granulocyte antibodies and *in vitro* studies of the fate of granulocytes. In: Garratty G, ed. *Current concepts in transfusion therapy.* Arlington VA: American Association of Blood Banks, 1985:125–181.

McMillan R, ed. *Methods in hematology 9: Immune cytopenias.* New York: Churchill Livingstone, 1983.

Mollison PL. *Blood transfusion in clinical medicine* (7E). Oxford: Blackwell Scientific, 1983.

Murphy MF, Waters AH. Immunological aspects of platelet transfusions (annotation). *Br J Haematol* 1985;**60**:409–414.

Petz LD, Garratty G. *Acquired immune hemolytic anemias.* New York: Churchill Livingstone, 1980.

Waters AH, Minchinton RM (1985). Immune thrombocytopenia and neutropenia. In: Hoffbrand AV, ed. *Recent advances in haematology 4.* Edinburgh: Churchill Livingstone, 1985:309–331.

17

Allergic Disorders

Definition

The original definition of allergy (von Pirquet, 1906) was a 'specifically changed reactivity of the host to an agent on a second or subsequent occasion'. This covers a whole spectrum of immune responses, both protective and harmful. However, more recently, the term allergy has become restricted to the latter and is now synonymous with type I hypersensitivity. In fact this rigid definition is too narrow to cover the range of conditions seen by allergists in clinical practice. It is likely that all four types of hypersensitivity are involved in various allergic diseases and indistinguishable reactions can sometimes be produced without immunological involvement: so-called 'pseudo-allergy'.

TYPE I HYPERSENSITIVITY

Immediate hypersensitivity reactions occur following the interaction of antigen (allergen) with specific IgE antibody which is predominantly bound to tissue mast cells and circulating basophils. This leads to mast cell degranulation and the release of pharmacological mediators of inflammation (Fig. 17.1). This scheme is an over simplification, as the IgE mediated reaction often acts as a gatekeeper for further cell influx and a second wave of inflammatory responses (the late phase response).

ATOPY

Coca and Cooke (1923) coined this term (from the Greek 'out of place') to describe the difference between the anaphylactic animal and the allergic human. Atopy is now used to describe the tendency of 10–15% of the population to suffer from allergic diseases such as asthma, eczema, hay fever, urticaria and food allergy. Coca and Cooke noted a family history of such complaints and positive wheal and flare skin reactions to common inhalant allergens. Atopy provides a convenient umbrella term for those diseases which are associated with the production of specific IgE following exposure to low concentrations of allergen.

IMMUNOGLOBULIN E

Sensitization

The IgE response is a local event occurring at the site of allergen entry at mucosal surfaces and at local lymph nodes. This IgE will first sensitize local mast cells, and 'spill-over' IgE enters the circulation and binds to receptors on circulating basophils and tissue mast cells throughout the body.

Structure

As with other immunoglobulins, IgE comprises two heavy

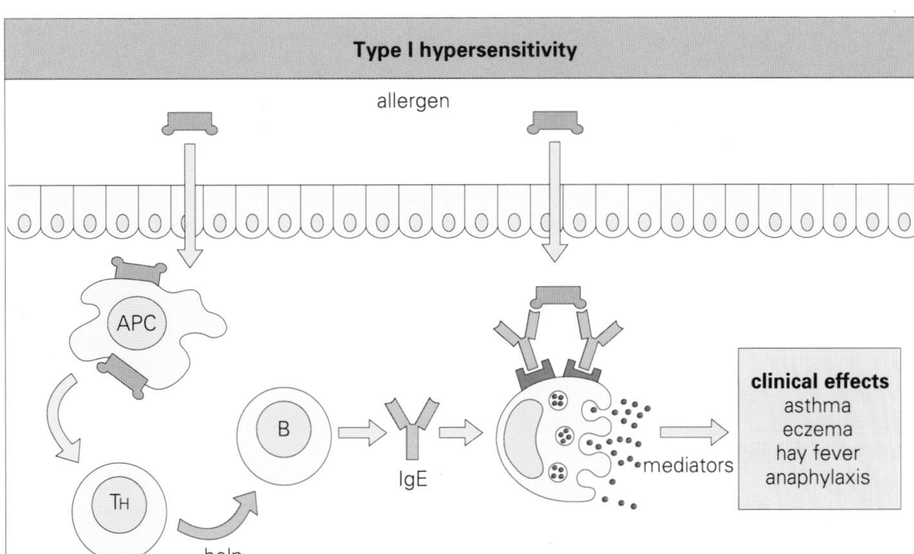

Fig. 17.1 Initial exposure to allergen in atopic individuals results in IgE production by B cells. This sensitizes cells such as mast cells and basophils so that on subsequent exposure to allergen, degranulation occurs, releasing preformed mediators and inducing the synthesis of newly formed mediators to produce the symptoms associated with type I hypersensitivity.

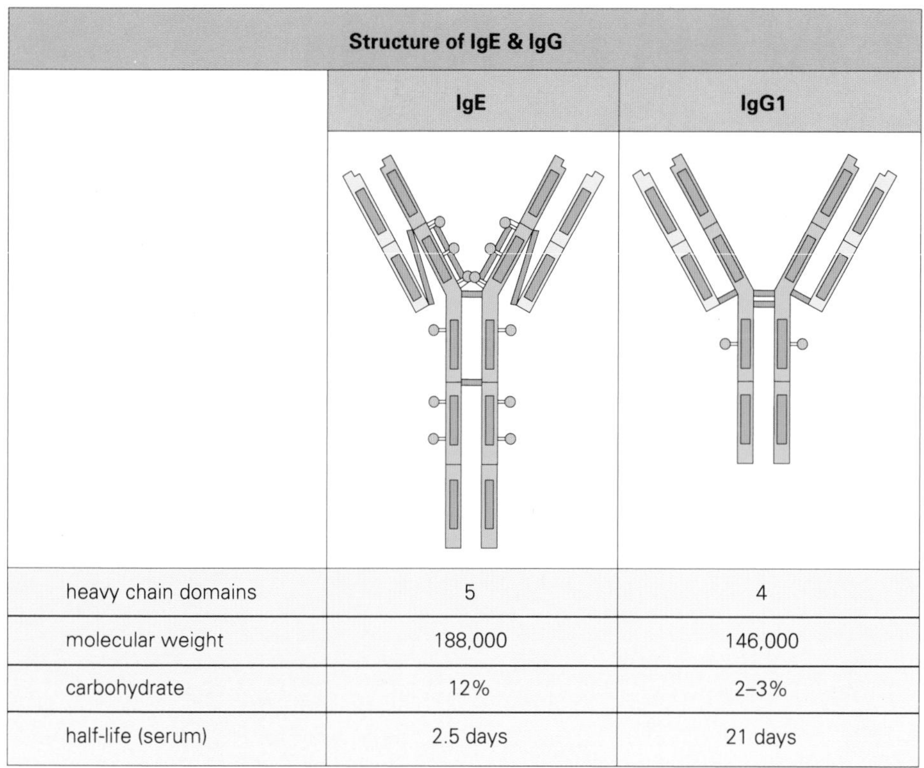

Structure of IgE & IgG		
	IgE	IgG1
heavy chain domains	5	4
molecular weight	188,000	146,000
carbohydrate	12%	2–3%
half-life (serum)	2.5 days	21 days

Fig. 17.2 The heavy chain of IgE has an extra domain compared with IgG and contains a greater percentage of carbohydrate. The CH2–CH3 region binds to $Fc_{\epsilon}R$ and it is the cytophilic capacity, not the antigen binding capability that is destroyed by heating.

and two light chains, the IgE heavy chain having five-domains (Fig. 17.2). The major characteristics of IgE are its heat lability and tight binding to the Fc receptors on mast cells and basophils, which are termed the high affinity receptors or $Fc_{\epsilon}RI$. There are also low affinity IgE receptors on other cell types — $Fc_{\epsilon}RII$. The heat lability reflects alterations in the Fc portion of the molecule following which it no longer sensitizes skin mast cells. The antigen binding capacity which resides in the Fab portion is preserved.

Although the serum half life of IgE is only 2.5 days, mast cells in human skin may remain effectively sensitized for up to 12 weeks following passive sensitization with atopic serum containing IgE.

IgE levels in disease

Serum levels of IgE are minute compared to those of IgG even in highly allergic subjects. Levels of IgE are raised in atopic individuals and even more so in those with parasitic infections. When considering the possibility of atopic disease, a raised level of IgE aids the diagnosis but a normal level does not exclude it (Fig. 17.3 left). A recent survey has shown that up to 30% of a random group of 5000 subjects has a positive wheal and flare reaction on skin testing to one or more common allergens, but only 10–15% of the population is clinically allergic. Thus, these subjects can produce specific IgE but lack some factor which precipitates the actual symptoms of atopy. However, the higher the IgE level, the more likely the presence of atopy (Fig. 17.3 right).

CONTROL OF IgE PRODUCTION

Cellular control: early studies

Tada and colleagues (1970) demonstrated the cellular control of IgE production in rats. In several clinical conditions there is an association between low T suppressor cell numbers and high levels of IgE, thus supporting the hypothesis for T cell control of IgE production in man. The inherent allergic potential of stem cells has been shown recently by bone marrow transplantation between siblings, in which the recipient (previously non-atopic) developed allergic disease similar to that in the sibling donor.

Molecular control: recent studies

Complex interactions which regulate IgE production have been studied at the cellular and molecular levels in experimental animals and man. There are many factors which interact to modulate IgE production by B cells. At the T cell level, two types of IgE binding factor are produced — an IgE potentiating factor (IgE-PF) and IgE suppressor factor (IgE-SF), which differ only in glycosylation. The relative amounts of each are in turn controlled by antigen-specific T cell factors. These either enhance (glycosylation enhancing factor, GEF) or inhibit (GIF) glycosylation of IgE binding factor. GEF is produced by an $Fc_{\epsilon}RII^{+}$ T helper (TH) cell and GIF by a T suppressor cell (Ts).

IgE secretion by B cells. There are also B cell factors that regulate B cell production of IgE (Fig. 17.4). Resting B cells with surface IgM and IgD can differentiate under the

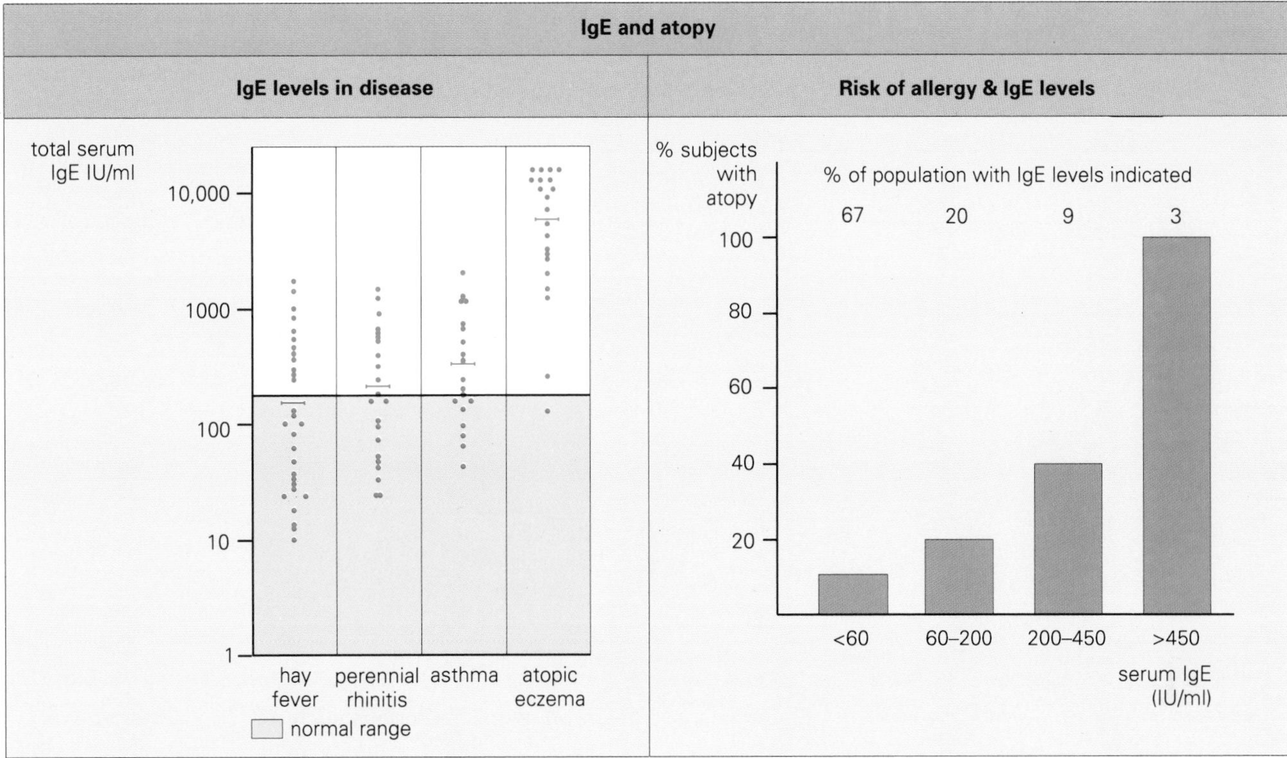

Fig. 17.3 Left: the serum concentration of IgE (around 100 IU/ml) is 10^5 times less than that of IgG (around 10mg/ml) and comprises less than 0.001% of the total immunoglobulin. Levels in atopic patients are usually raised, especially so in atopic eczema (1IU=2ng). Right: the higher the level of IgE the greater the likelihood of atopy.

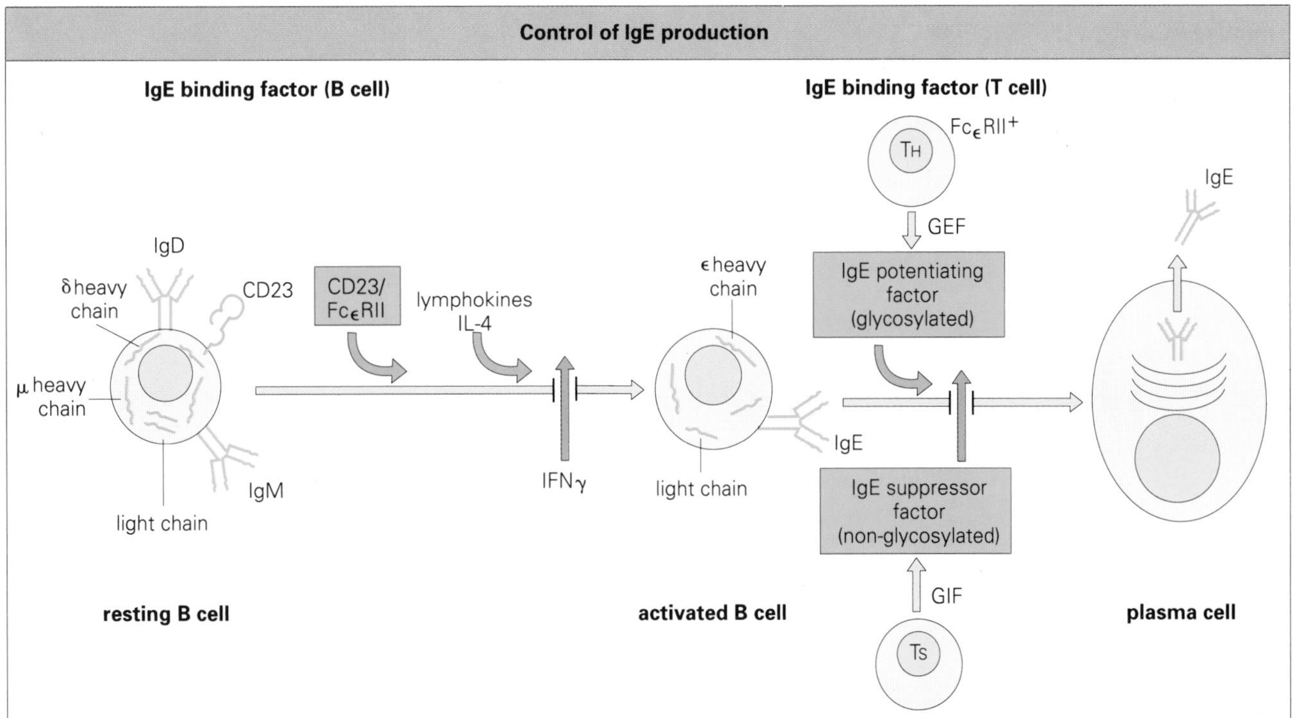

Fig. 17.4 Different T helper cells produce IL-4 and IFNγ; the former promotes IgE synthesis in association with soluble CD23 (the low affinity IgE receptor) and the latter inhibits it. Human lymphocytes also produce IgE binding factors, IgE-PF and IgE-SF.

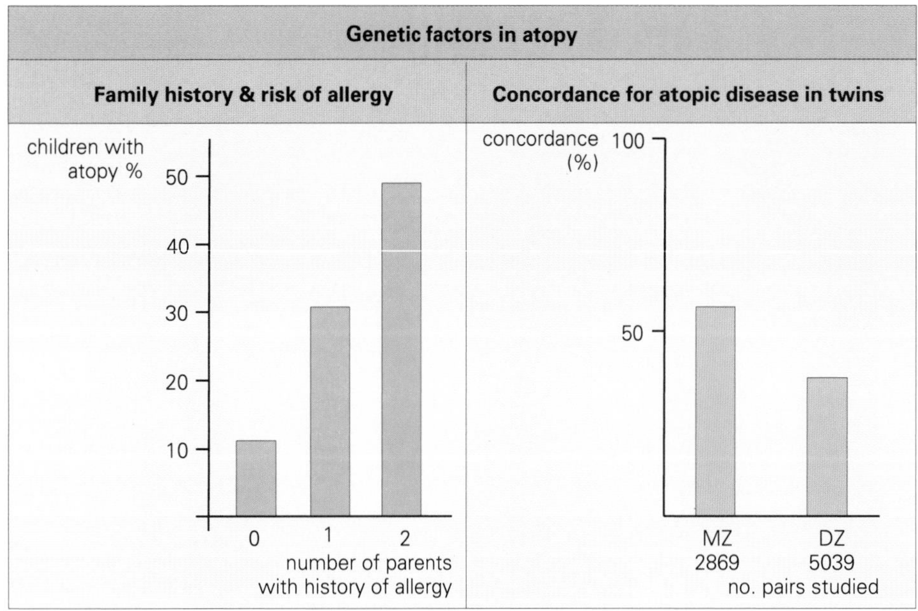

Fig. 17.5 Left: the greater the parental history of allergy, the greater is the risk of atopy in the child. Right: the concordance for atopic disease in dizygotic (DZ) twins is slightly greater than in the general population. However the concordance in monozygotic (MZ) twins is well below the 100% that might be expected if genotype was the sole factor in determining atopic disease.

synergistic influence of B cell factors, such as soluble CD23 (soluble $Fc_{\epsilon}RII$) and IL-4, to a precursor B cell which for the first time expresses surface IgE. Under the influence of T cell factors (IgE-PF), further differentiation occurs to a committed IgE-producing plasma cell. Inhibitory control occurs at both stages, with IFNγ influencing the early stage and IgE-SF the later stages.

THE ALLERGIC RESPONSE IN MAN

There is epidemiological data to show that allergic parents are more likely to have allergic children (Fig. 17.5 left). Thus both genetic background and elevated serum IgE levels are risk factors for allergic disease.

ENVIRONMENTAL FACTORS

The annual challenge of individuals by airborne pollens is about 1 μg and it is surprising that one in six of the population respond to this low level of allergen challenge. The response is influenced by a variety of non-genetic factors, such as quantity of exposure, nutritional status (see chapter 25), and the presence of underlying infections or acute viral illnesses.

Twin studies

That environmental factors are crucial to the expression of atopy is shown by studies of identical (monozygotic) and non-identical (dizygotic) twins (Fig. 17.5 right). There are two major aspects to consider:

- the exposure to allergens with development of specific allergic responses;
- the effect of pollution in the environment, which can act as a non-specific trigger factor.

NON-SPECIFIC FACTORS

Environmental pollutants such as SO_2, nitrogen oxides, diesel fumes and fly ash may increase mucosal permeability and therefore enhance antigen entry and IgE responsiveness. The effect of smoking seems to be biphasic: IgE levels are enhanced with low cigarette consumption and suppressed with high consumption. Smoking also causes a reduction in the immune response to inhaled antigens.

Diesel exhaust particulates (DEP)

DEP can act as a powerful adjuvant for IgE production (Fig. 17.6). They are less than 1 μm in diameter, are buoyant in the atmosphere of polluted districts and are inhaled. Concentrations in urban air of approximately 2–500 $\mu g/m^3$ have been recorded. Their adjuvant effect is seen experimentally with low dose antigen exposure, simulating that which occurs naturally. The increase in allergic rhinitis and asthma in the last three decades parallels an increase in air pollution and diesel exhaust.

SPECIFIC FACTORS

Cedar pollen

In 1934, 3.5% of the Japanese population resident in Southern California experienced allergic rhinitis due to pollen, at a time when the disease was unknown in Japan. In 1986, pollen-induced rhinitis had increased markedly in Japan to involve 30% of children aged 6–17. The incidence was higher in urban districts with high levels of pollution from automobile exhaust, despite the fact that cedar trees are more common in the countryside.

Grass pollen

Between 1960 and 1980, the peak pollen counts over Central London declined, the fall occurring in June, with

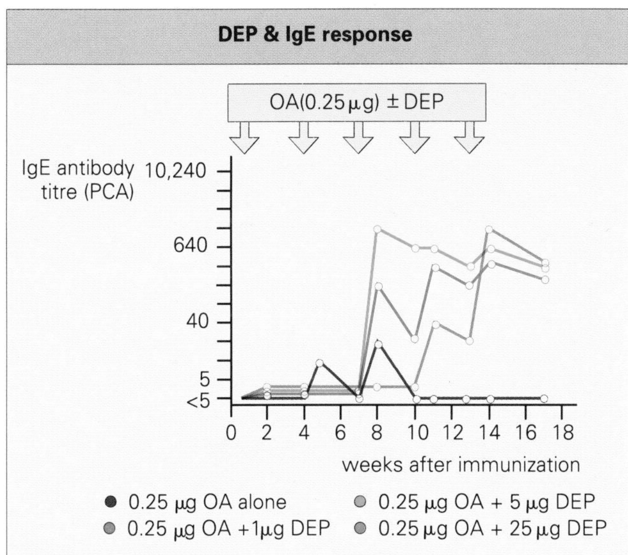

Fig. 17.6 When mice are immunized intranasally with ovalbumin (OA), a small peak of IgE antibody is seen at weeks 5 and 8, and none thereafter. If DEP are added to the OA, there is dose-related increase in IgE persisting after immunization ceases. Modified from Takafuji (1987).

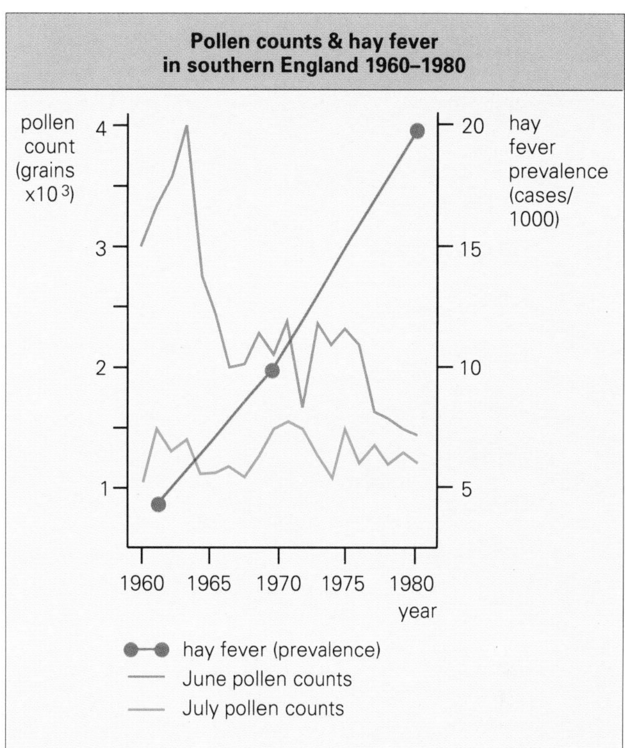

Fig. 17.7 Mean pollen count in London show a steady fall of peak counts in June over a 20 year period. The July levels are much lower and have remained static. This has been associated with a considerable increase in the prevalence of hayfever. Data from Dr R R Davies.

the July counts remaining stable. This was due to the change from hay-making to the production of silage, in which grass is cut before it flowers. However, in the same period there was an increase in the prevalence of hay fever from 3% in 1962 to 19.7% in 1981 (Fig. 17.7). Thus, the decline in pollen concentrations has been accompanied by an increase in the prevalence of hayfever, possibly due to air pollution.

House dust mite

In a prospective study of 92 children, Mitchell and colleagues showed that children exposed to high levels of antigen were more likely to develop clinical sensitivity. With high exposure (>5000 ng/g of DerP1 — the major house dust mite antigen — in dust) the incidence of allergy was greater, with a significant correlation between the amount of mite allergen in the environment and the concentration of serum IgE antibodies. Other important factors for the development of allergic disease in childhood are shown in Fig. 17.8.

GENETIC MECHANISMS

There are three main mechanisms regulating the allergic response; these mechanisms affect the total IgE levels, the antigen specific response and general hyper-responsiveness.

Total IgE levels

In family studies where at least one member has a high serum IgE level, low IgE levels are associated with a dominant gene.

Environmental factors in development of allergic disease in childhood	
Pregnancy	smoking β-blocking drugs month of birth
Perinatal	stress early operations gastroenteritis
Childhood	low IgA levels viral infections inhalant allergens smoke diet position in family

Fig. 17.8 Being born just before or during a major allergen season increases the likelihood of sensitization, as does early exposure to inhaled or ingested allergens. First born children are more likely to suffer from hayfever.

IgE response: genetic association			
	skin test		
HLA	positive (%)	negative (%)	p
A1	28.7	24.1	0.4
B8	22.3	11.5	0.01
Dw3	25.2	11.7	0.002

Fig. 17.9 The IgE response to antigens is clearly genetically linked, both in terms of the ability to respond to a given antigen (ragweed) and the general 'atopic ability' to produce an IgE antibody response to any antigen.

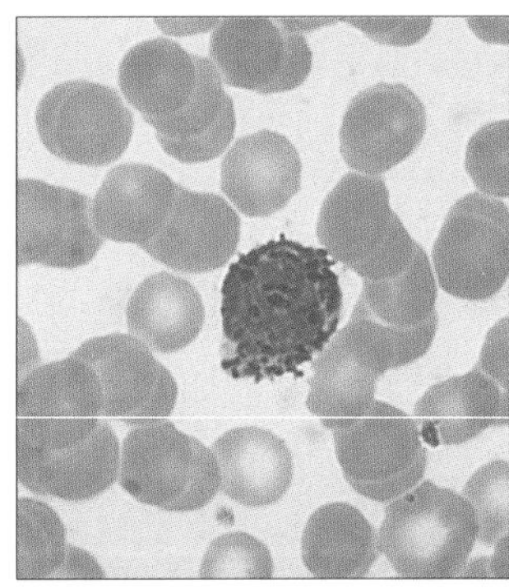
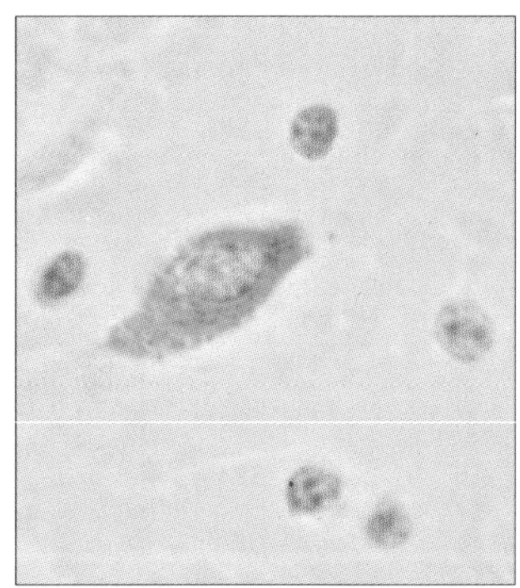

Fig. 17.10 Left: blood smear showing a typical basophil with deep violet granules. Wright's stain, x150. Right: histological appearance of human connective tissue mast cells, which have dark blue cytoplasm with brownish granules. Alcian blue & safranin, x600. Courtesy of Dr T S C Orr.

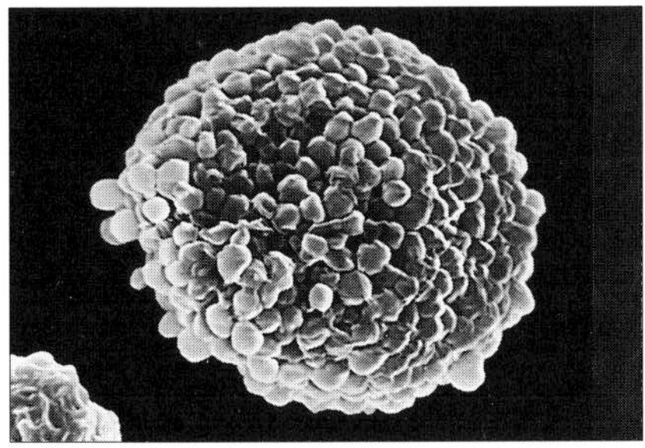
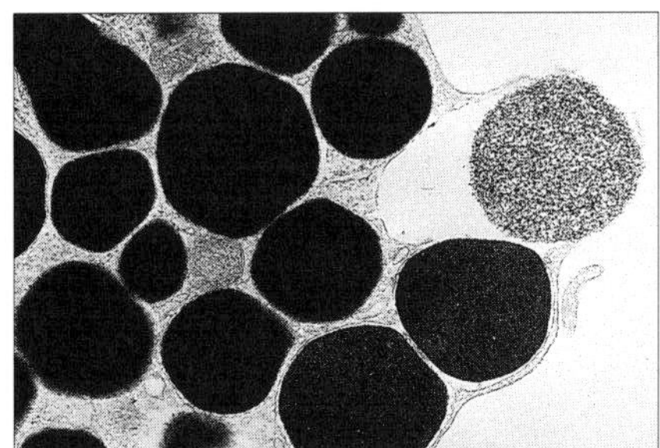
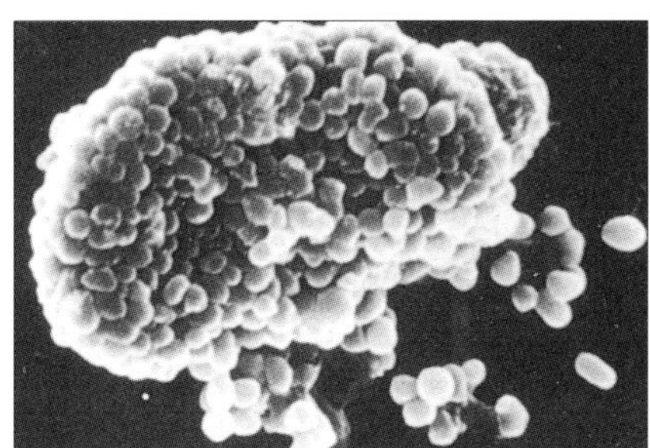

Fig. 17.11 Mast cell degranulation. Left: an intact mast cell on scanning electron microscopy has a typical raspberry-like appearance. Middle & right: following incubation with anti-IgE there is a rapid exocytosis of the granules. x1500. Courtesy of Dr T S C Orr.

HLA-linked allergen specific response

When ultrapure (>99.5% pure) allergens are used there is a good association between HLA and a specific IgE response. This is more impressive for very low dose exposure and low molecular weight minor determinants, such as the ragweed allergen Amb A V (5kDa), than for abundant high molecular weight allergens such as Amb A I (38kDa). With Amb A V over 90% of IgE responders are HLA-Dw2, whereas with Amb A I there is as yet no HLA association.

General hyper-responsiveness

Among patients attending an allergy clinic there was a significantly higher proportion with HLA-B8 and HLA-Dw3 in the skin test positive group than in the negative group (Fig. 17.9). In those already making IgE antibodies to ragweed, those with HLA-B8 have higher titres of antibody and also higher levels of IgE. This HLA profile is also strongly associated with autoimmune disease, raising the possibility of defective T suppressor activity in the development of both autoimmune and IgE responses.

IgE responsiveness (IgER). Recently Hopkin and colleagues have re-examined the inheritance of atopy in more than 500 individuals from a number of extended and nuclear families and have shown that 90% of young atopic asthmatics had at least one parent with demonstrable atopic IgE responsiveness, suggesting a decisive genetic effect. Extended family studies showed clear vertical transmission of IgER, suggesting autosomal dominant inheritance. Supporting this, 61% of children from one responder and one non-responder parent had IgER. This value is higher than in previous studies (see Fig. 17.5 left), probably because extensive testing and questioning were employed. This suggests that there could be one major gene locus largely responsible for IgER, but that this can be modified by other genetic and environmental factors.

CELLS INVOLVED IN THE ALLERGIC RESPONSE

MAST CELLS

The first description of mast cells and basophils as granular cells that stain metachromatically with basic dyes was made more than 100 years ago by Paul Ehrlich. There are similarities between mast cells and basophils but they are distinct cell types (Fig. 17.10). Both synthesize and store histamine, proteogylycan and proteases in their granules and have surface receptors that bind IgE with high affinity ($Fc_{\epsilon}RI$). Cross-linking of the surface IgE leads to a calcium dependent activation with degranulation (Fig. 17.11).

Differences between mast cell populations		
	Mucosal mast cell	**Connective tissue mast cell**
location *in vivo*	gut & lung	ubiquitous
life span	<40 days (?)	>40 days (?)
T cell dependent	+	-
number of Fc_ϵ receptors	2×10^5	3×10^4
histamine content	+	++
cytoplasmic IgE	+	-
major AA metabolite LTC_4:PGD_2 ratio	25:1	1:40
DSCG/theophylline inhibits histamine release	-	+
major proteoglycan	chondroitin sulphate	heparin

Fig. 17.12 Major characteristics of the different mast cell populations.

Mast cell heterogeneity

It was thought that mast cells were homogeneous, with a morphology similar to that which is now recognized as a connective tissue mast cell (CTMC). It is now realized that there are at least two types of mast cell: CTMC and the mucosal mast cell (MMC). Recent evidence suggests that MMCs and CTMCs are derived from the same precursor cell, with the end-cell phenotype depending on factors found in the local micro-environment. The main distinguishing features of mast cell populations are shown in Fig. 17.12).

Neutral proteases have been used to distinguish two populations of human mast cells. The majority found at mucosal surfaces contain tryptase (MCt) whereas those in connective tissue, such as skin, contain both chymase and tryptase (MCct). CTMCs release predominantly PGD_2 on activation, whereas MMCs release mainly LTC4. The development of 'pure' human mast cell lines may be of use in the development of drugs for the management of the allergic patient.

STRUCTURE AND FUNCTION OF Fc RECEPTORS FOR IgE

The high affinity receptor: $Fc_\epsilon RI$

Metzger and colleagues have shown that the receptor is a tetramer of polypeptides (Fig. 17.13 left).

IgE–$Fc_\epsilon RI$ interaction. The receptor interacts with regions of the CH_2 and CH_3 portion of the IgE heavy chain, with

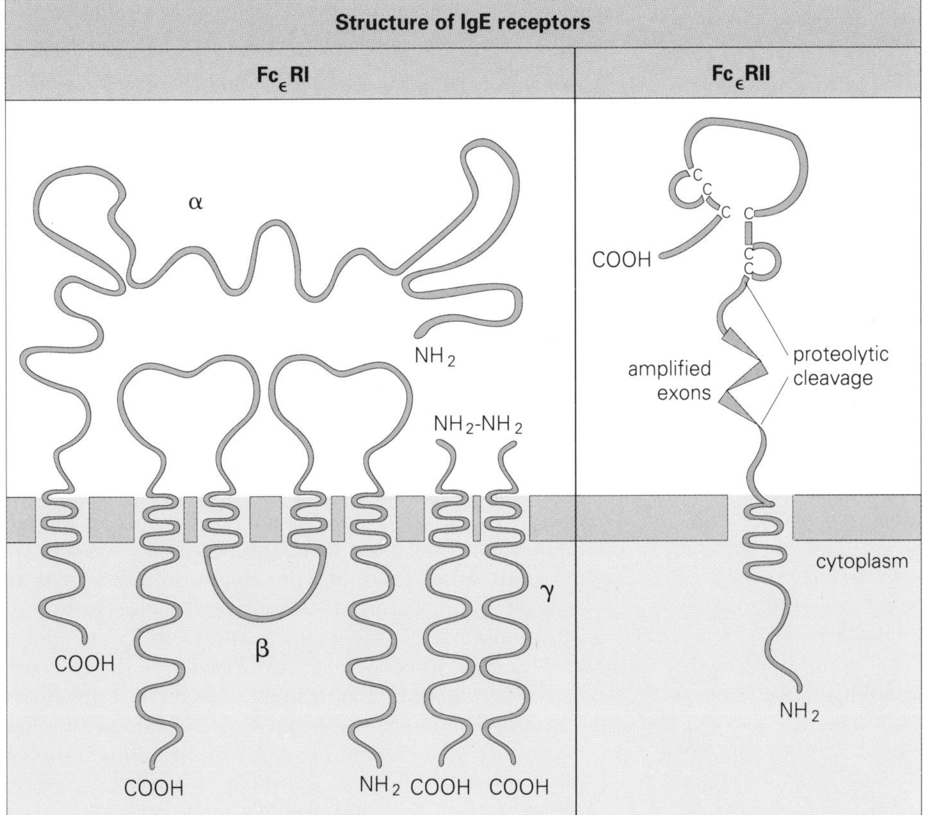

Fig. 17.13 Left: the model for $FC_\epsilon RI$ proposes a tetramer consisting of one α chain with two disulphide-linked immunoglobulin loops. The β chain has two extracellular portions near two γ chains, which are thought to be linked by disulphide bonds. The α chain is crucial for IgE binding. Right: the hypothetical model for the $Fc_\epsilon RII$ is based on sequence data and the homology with animal lectins. Proteolytic cleavage releases IgE-BF. This cleavage is inhibited by IgE, accounting for the apparent increase of $Fc_\epsilon RII$ expression on lymphocytes cultured in the presence of IgE and not influenced by protein synthesis inhibitors.

a high binding constant (approximately $10^{10}M^{-1}$). The interaction of monovalent IgE with the receptor complex does not activate mast cells or basophils since no histamine release occurs. It is the cross-linking of surface bound IgE by antigen and other molecules which stimulates degranulation.

The low affinity receptor: FcεRII

The exact molecular structure of $Fc_{\epsilon}RII$ has not yet been described but a hypothetical model has been made (Fig. 17.13 right). Unlike other Fc receptors, $Fc_{\epsilon}RII$, which is identical to CD23, is not a member of the immunoglobulin superfamily but belongs to a primitive superfamily of animal lectins. A common feature of these molecules is that they lie 'upside-down' in the cell membrane with an intracytoplasmic NH_2 end, and an extracellular COOH end. Cleaving the $Fc_{\epsilon}RII$ produces a soluble CD23 molecule that can bind IgE — IgE binding factor (IgE-BF).

IgE–$Fc_{\epsilon}RII$ interaction. The interaction of IgE with $Fc_{\epsilon}RII$ is independent of any lectin-like activity that the receptor may have. Binding has been mapped to the CH3 region, slightly 'downstream' to the area which binds to the high affinity receptor. Interestingly, IgE-BF (soluble $Fc_{\epsilon}RII$/CD23) can inhibit IgE binding to $Fc_{\epsilon}RII$ and possibly to $Fc_{\epsilon}RI$ by steric hindrance.

Thus, $Fc_{\epsilon}RII$/CD23 can regulate allergic reactions in two ways: by soluble IgE-BF inhibiting IgE binding, and by regulation of IgE biosynthesis through feedback on B cells.

Other $Fc_{\epsilon}R$-bearing cells

The low affinity receptor ($Fc_{\epsilon}RII$) is carried by about a quarter of B cells, and by monocytes which show increased expression during the pollen season. There is a much higher level of receptor on monocytes from patients with atopic eczema, which is suppressed by treatment with corticosteroids. Alveolar macrophages with $Fc_{\epsilon}RII$ can be sensitized with allergen specific IgE to release enzymes after exposure to the relevant allergen, and this could play an important role in allergic lung disease. Eosinophils and platelets can also be activated through IgE dependent mechanisms, leading to substantial damage to parasites such as schistosomes.

MAST CELL TRIGGERING

The cross-linking by allergen of IgE bound to $Fc_{\epsilon}RI$ leads to calcium influx with subsequent release of preformed mediators and the synthesis from arachidonic acid of newly formed inflammatory mediators (Fig. 17.14). Degranulation may also occur when IgE is cross-linked by lectins, such as PHA and Con A which bind to sugar residues on the Fc portion of IgE. This could explain the urticaria seen with some lectin-containing foods such as strawberries.

Direct degranulation

The breakdown products of complement (C3a and C5a)

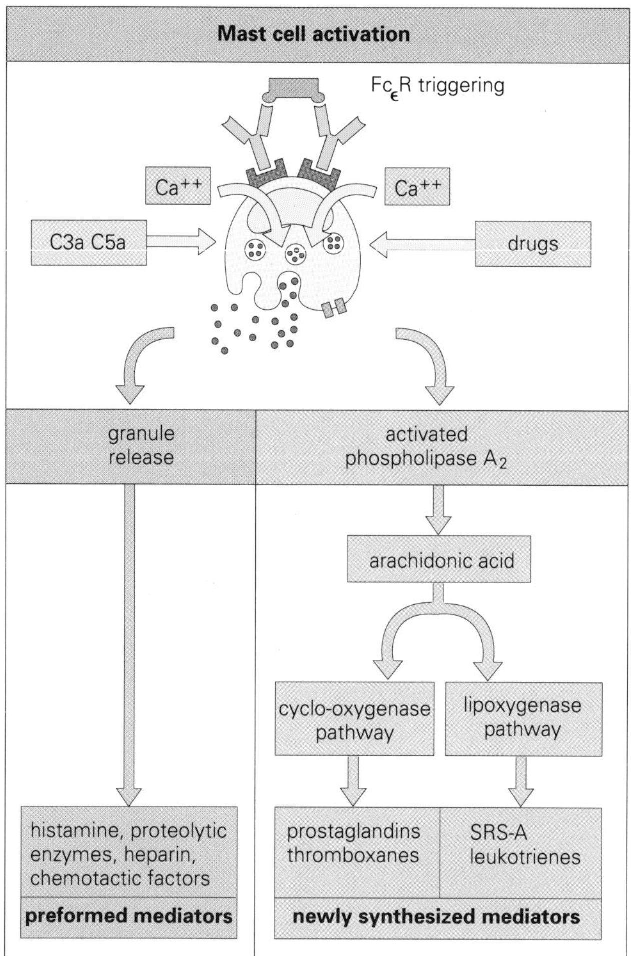

Fig. 17.14 Several stimuli can lead to mast cell degranulation, such as cross-linking $Fc_{\epsilon}RI$ by allergen, drugs such as codeine, morphine, synthetic ACTH, as well as mellitin from bee venom and anaphylatoxins C3a and C5a from complement activation. Calcium ion influx is crucial for degranulation. The changes in the plasma membrane release arachidonic acid leading to the production of newly synthesized inflammatory mediators.

are extremely active in degranulating mast cells directly (not via IgE). Mellitin from bee venom and some drugs such as synthetic ACTH, codeine, and morphine can act in the same way.

Histamine releasing factors (HRFs)

These are poorly characterized factors which can trigger the degranulation of mast cells and basophils. They have been found in lavage fluid from lung and nose, in skin blister fluid and in supernatants from cell culture systems. T and B lymphocytes, alveolar macrophages, neutrophils, platelets and endothelial cells can produce HRFs. Three molecular species of blood mononuclear cell HRF have recently been defined; these have molecular weights of 12, 17 and 41 kDa. An inhibitory factor, histamine release inhibitory factor (HRIF) has also been described recently, and it has been suggested that the normal fine balance

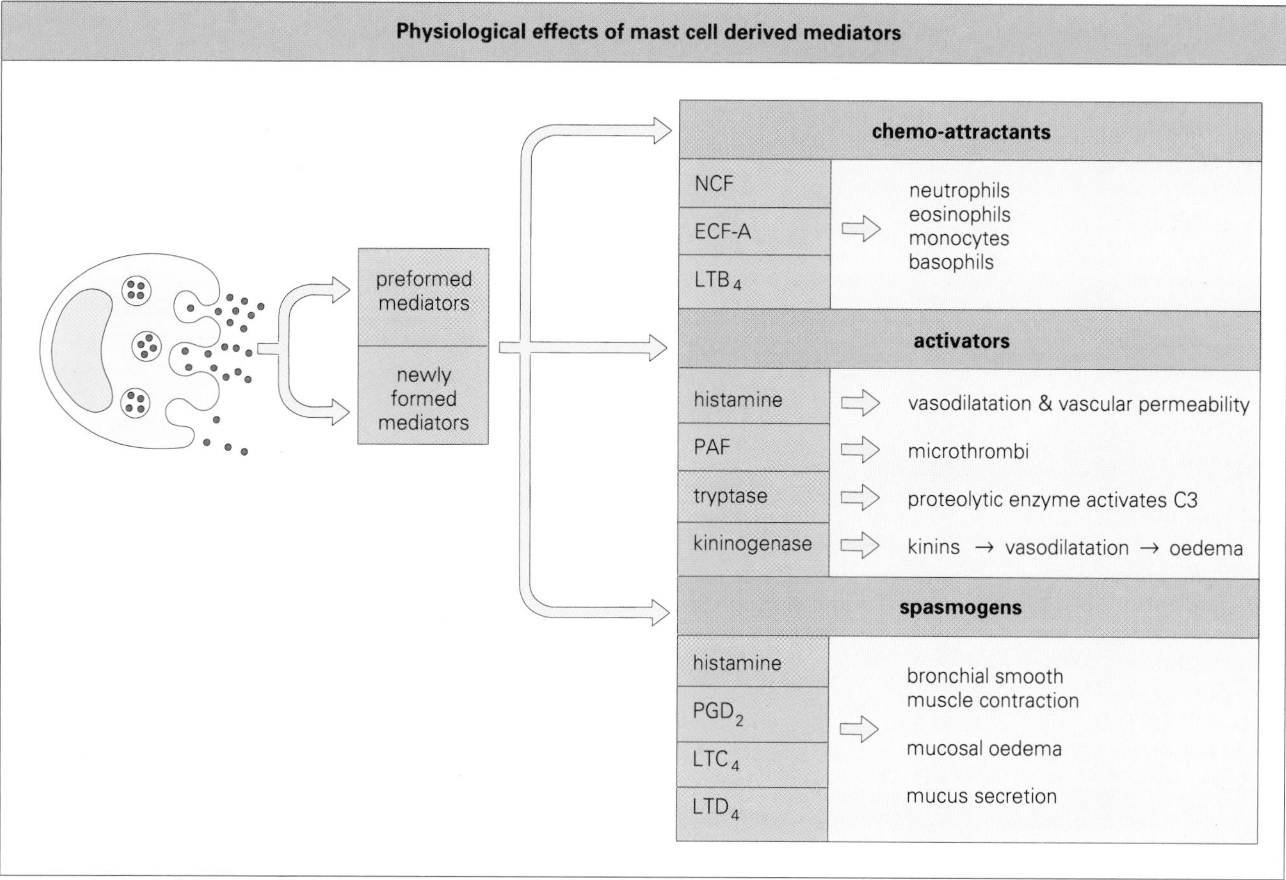

Fig. 17.15 Both type of mast cell mediators act as chemotactic agents (attracting other cells to the site of mast cell activation), inflammatory activators (causing vasodilatation, oedema and tissue damage), and as spasmogens (directly affecting smooth muscle in the bronchi).

between this and HRFs is lost during the development of allergic disease.

MEDIATOR RELEASE

Following receptor triggering, there is calcium influx into mast cells leading to release of preformed and newly formed mediators.

Preformed mediators

Exocytosis of granule contents releases preformed mediators, the major one being histamine. A number of other compounds including β glucuronidase, aryl-sulphatase, superoxide dismutase and peroxidase are present, as are chemotactic factors for eosinophils, neutrophils and monocytes.

Newly formed mediators

There is also synthesis of lipid mediators from arachidonic acid, released from phospholipids by phospholipase enzymes. Arachidonic acid is metabolized either along the cyclo-oxygenase pathway with the formation of prostaglandins (mainly PGD_2) or by the lipoxygenase pathway with the formation of leukotrienes. Platelet activating factor (PAF) is a low molecular weight phospholipid which is generated from alkyl phospholipids in the cell.

More recently, several mast cell lines have been shown to produce lymphokines some hours after stimulation, namely IL-3 to IL-6 as well as TNF and GM-CSF.

Effects of mediators

The release of mediators has a direct effect on local tissues, and in the lung the release from broncho-alveolar mast cells can lead to immediate bronchoconstriction, mucosal oedema and hyper-secretion leading to asthma (Fig. 17.15).

Late phase response. Although IgE-mediated hypersensitivity reactions occur within minutes and decay quickly, there is frequently a second component: the late phase response. This is probably due to slower acting mediators, such as leukotrienes (formerly known as SRS-A, or slow-reacting substance of anaphylaxis), and to further mediator generation from the accumulated inflammatory cells at the reaction site.

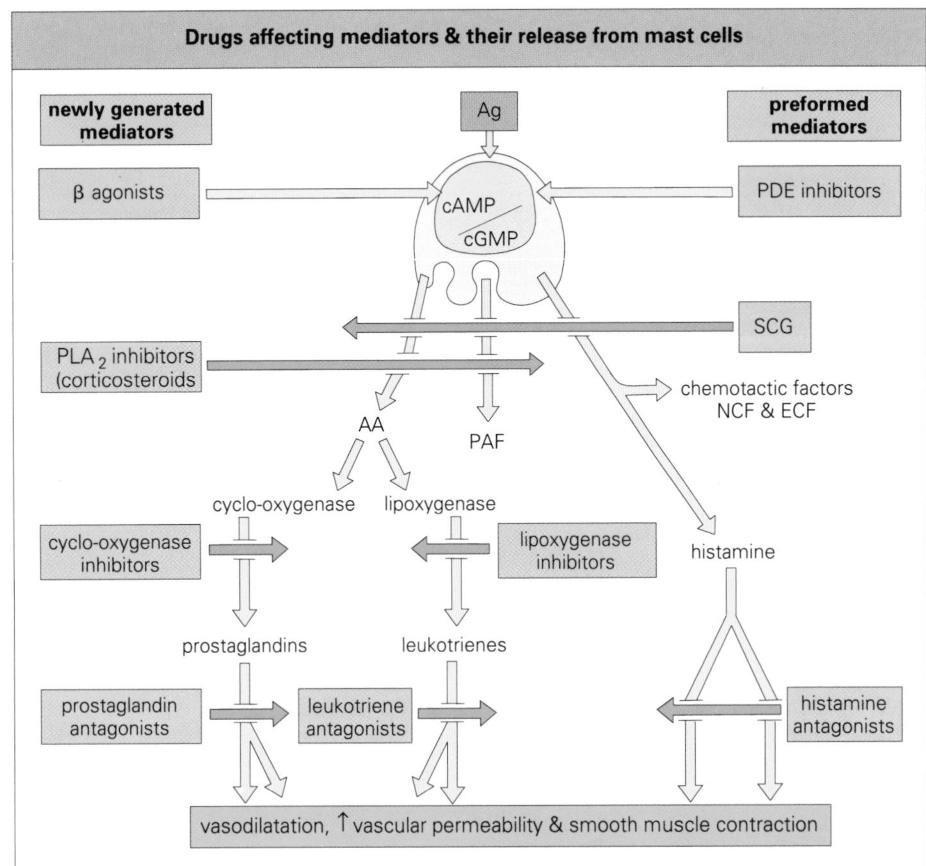

Fig. 17.16 β agonists and phosphodiesterase (PDE) inhibitors raise the intracellular cAMP level and inhibit degranulation, although PDE inhibitors also have other actions, such as increasing adrenalin secretion. β blockers may worsen asthma. Sodium cromoglycate is a mast cell 'stabilizer', blocking mediator release from broncho-alveolar mast cells. Corticosteroids can prevent the release of arachidonic acid (AA) metabolites by inducing synthesis of macrocortin, which inhibits phospholipase A_2 (PLA_2). Cyclo-oxygenase inhibitors can block the late phase response following bronchial provocation but have no role in long term treatment of asthma. Anti-histamines are symptomatically effective in the upper airways and skin but less so in the lower airways.

Drugs affecting mediator release. These are shown in Fig. 17.16. One of the actions of corticosteroids is to inhibit the breakdown of arachidonic acid via macrocortin and lipomodulin. Sodium cromoglycate has many actions, one of which is to inhibit mediator release. However, this does not fully explain its effectiveness in asthma. Aspirin and other cyclo-oxygenase pathway blockers such as non-steroidal anti-inflammatory drugs (NSAIDs) may worsen asthma in some patients, possibly through the formation of extra leukotrienes via the lipoxygenase pathway.

It may be relevant that sodium cromoglycate, methylxanthines, ketotifen and corticosteroids, all of which have prophylactic effects in asthma, inhibit either the release of, or the response to PAF at therapeutic concentrations.

BASOPHILS

Although basophils comprise less than 1% of circulating leucocytes, they contain all the histamine found in human blood and are therefore important subjects for investigation in studies of allergic mechanisms.

There is no evidence that the histamine release mechanism is abnormal in cells from atopic individuals. Peripheral blood basophils from asthmatic patients spontaneously release more histamine when incubated *in vitro,* probably because of *in vivo* activation.

In contrast to mast cells, human basophils release little of the arachidonic acid-derived products such as PGD_2.

Delayed hypersensitivity

Mast cells and basophils are probably involved in delayed hypersensitivity responses. There is evidence from mice that delayed type hypersensitivity depends on the presence of mast cells, is more abundant in mast cell rich sites, and that, at least in animals, delayed responses are inhibited by drugs which block mast cell mediator release.

EOSINOPHILS

These are bone marrow derived granulocytes (Fig. 17.17) which develop under the influence of lymphokines. They are non-dividing granular cells which have a limited life span in the circulation. They have both secretory and phagocytic functions and may play a specific role in defence against parasites.

First identified by Ehrlich in 1879, they were found to be associated with both allergic and parasitic diseases. In these conditions the eosinophils are usually 'activated' in the sense that they have increased expression of membrane receptors for complement and IgG, show increased chemotaxis, an increase in oxidative metabolism, enhanced cytotoxicity and are of lighter density.

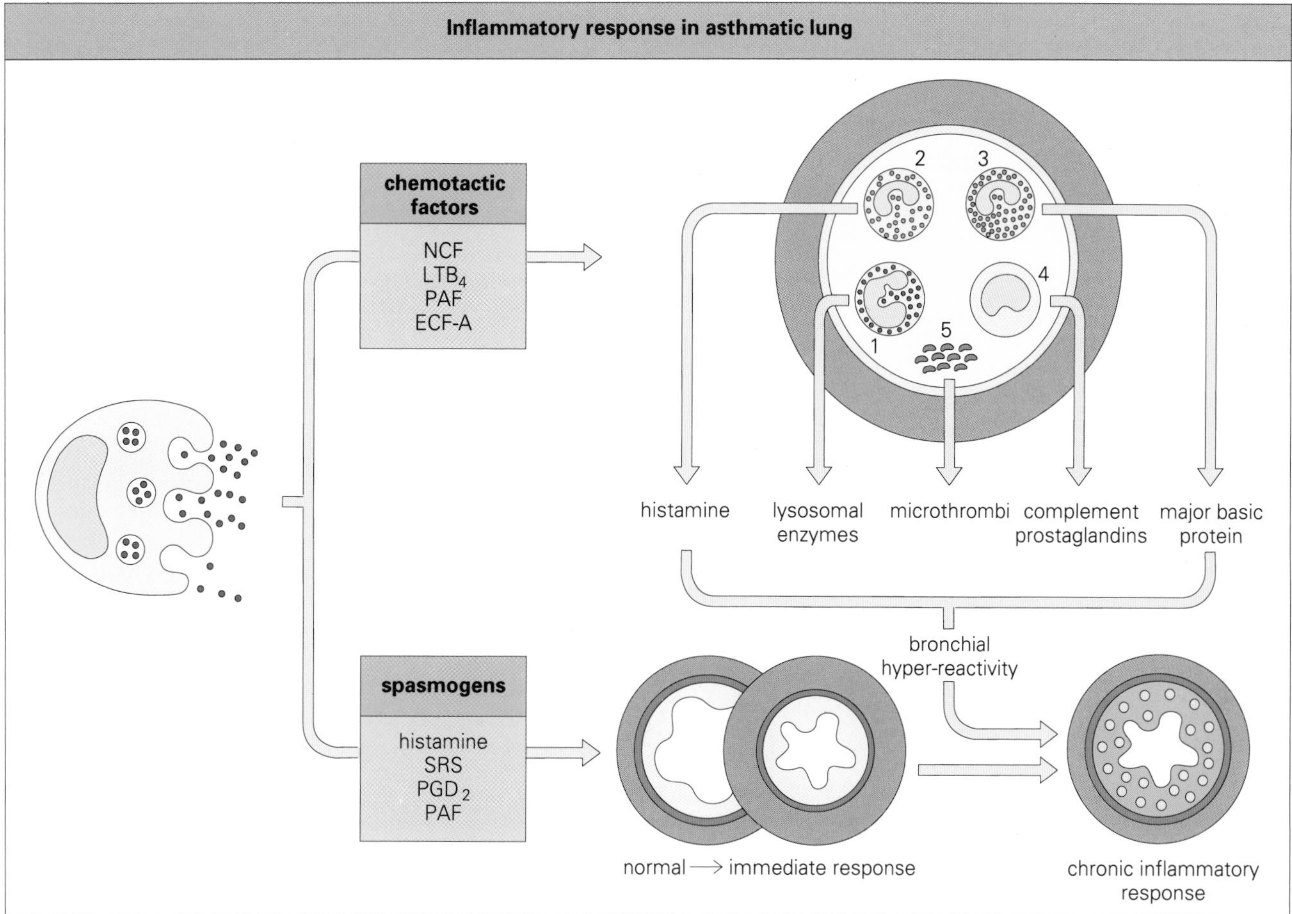

Fig. 17.17 Chemotactic factors lead to active accumulation of granulocytes (1), basophils (2), eosinophils (3), macrophages (4) and platelets (5). Spasmogenic mediators produce the immediate response on bronchial provocation and also lead to increased small vessel permeability, oedema and cell migration.

Eosinophils are probably recruited into allergic reactions via various chemotactic factors including PAF-acether, eosinophil chemotactic factor A (ECF-A) and various tetrapeptides derived from mast cell granules.

Eosinophil mediators.
The mediators of the eosinophil can be divided into granule-associated (for example major basic protein, eosinophil cationic protein) and membrane-derived (for example LTC_4 and PAF). The role of the eosinophil in allergic reactions has been debated. It was initially thought to dampen down such reactions via the possible inactivation of mediators and phagocytosis of mast cell granules and IgE–allergen complexes. However, the capability of this cell to cause tissue damage via its basic proteins, its ability to generate mediators and to cause degranulation of mast cells and basophils has led to the idea that it may be pathogenetic in asthma, especially in the late phase response. Eosinophils are found in mucus plugs, in epithelia and beneath the basement membrane of bronchi in patients dying with asthma. Eosinophil cationic protein is also increased following bronchial challenge with allergen.

It may be that some of the protective action of corticosteroids in asthma is related to their ability to decrease circulating eosinophils by tissue sequestration, decreased egress from the bone marrow and decreased migration into the tissues.

PLATELETS

Large numbers of megakaryocytes have also been observed in the lungs of patients dying in status asthmaticus. Circulating platelet counts fall during and after positive bronchial challenge. Platelet supernatants cause delayed skin responses in atopics and similar responses have been shown following intradermal injection of PAF. This potent inflammatory mediator can activate granulocytes and platelets *in vitro* and causes profound bronchoconstriction after inhalation, with the induction of prolonged bronchial hyper-reactivity. PAF is generated by several cell types including neutrophils, macrophages, eosinophils and mast cells, as well as platelets.

As noted earlier, many of the effective anti-asthma

drugs inhibit the release or activity of PAF. Platelet abnormalities have also been noted in aspirin-sensitive asthmatics. The role of this cell in asthma is still unclear.

CLINICAL ASPECTS OF ALLERGIC DISEASE

Conditions in which allergy is a major underlying factor include extrinsic asthma, rhinitis, conjunctivitis, atopic eczema, urticaria/angioedema, food/drug allergy and anaphylaxis. Several of these are dealt with elsewhere (see urticaria and eczema in chapter 14 and occupational asthma in chapter 18). Asthma, rhinitis, anaphylaxis, venom and food sensitivity will be discussed here.

Precipitating factors in asthma	
Specific antigens	
seasonal (UK)	**perennial**
birch pollen (April)	house dust mite
plane pollen (May)	feathers
grass pollen (June/July)	animal dander
moulds (autumn)	moulds (e.g. *Aspergillus*)
	occupational agents
	food (e.g. milk, wheat, citrus fruits)
Non-specific factors	
exercise	cold
smoke	emotional stress
infection	some drugs (e.g. propanolol)

Fig. 17.18 Specific and non-specific precipitating factors in asthma.

ASTHMA

Intrinsic/extrinsic

Asthmatics are conventionally divided into extrinsic and intrinsic groups, with no obvious causative external allergies in the intrinsic group. However, both types frequently have a family history of asthma and atopy, have eosinophils and mediators in the sputum, raised serum IgE, increased basophil IgE, and lymphocyte sensitivity to histamine suppression. Provocation testing may reveal allergic sensitivity which is not evidenced by skin prick tests; other individuals may be food-sensitive or respond to bacterial allergens. Other causes of intrinsic asthma are carcinoid tumours or aspirin sensitivity.

Clinical characteristics

Asthma is characterized by reversible airways obstruction. Patients present with wheezy dyspnoea which is at first intermittent, but can become constant. The wheeze can be absent, especially in children who may simply have a chronic non-productive cough with shortness of breath on exercise. Asthma is common, affecting 4–10% of the UK population; it is also dangerous and is responsible for about 2,000 deaths per year.

Over 50% of asthmatics are allergic and a careful history may reveal certain precipitating factors such as allergens which could be seasonal or perennial and other non-antigenic factors such as exercise or irritating fumes (Fig. 17.18).

Bronchial response to allergen Bronchial reaction to allergen can show an immediate and late phase response (LPR), with sodium cromoglycate (SCG) being effective in preventing both phases of the response (Fig. 17.19). Most asthmatics with reversible airways obstruction benefit from treatment with corticosteroids which preferentially block the LPR and the cellular infiltration. This suggests that the LPR is of major clinical importance in chronic asthma.

Bronchial hyper-reactivity. Hyper-reactivity of the bronchi to histamine and non-specific stimuli such as cold air,

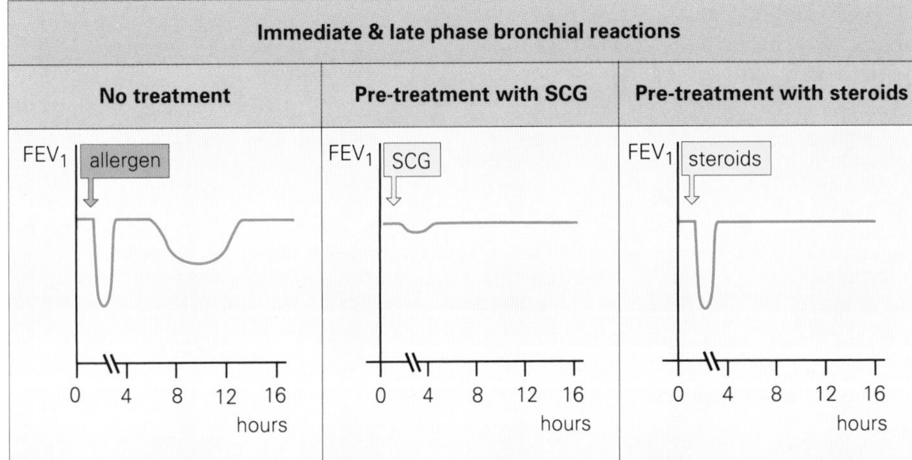

Fig. 17.19 Left: after bronchial provocation with allergen there is an immediate drop in lung function followed by the late phase reaction 4–12 hours later. Middle: pre-treatment with sodium cromoglycate (SCG) inhibits mast cell degranulation and blocks both early and late reactions. Right: pre-treatment with NSAIDs or cortisteroids, which block arachidonic acid metabolic pathways, blocks the LPR but not the immediate response. FEV_1 = forced expiratory volume.

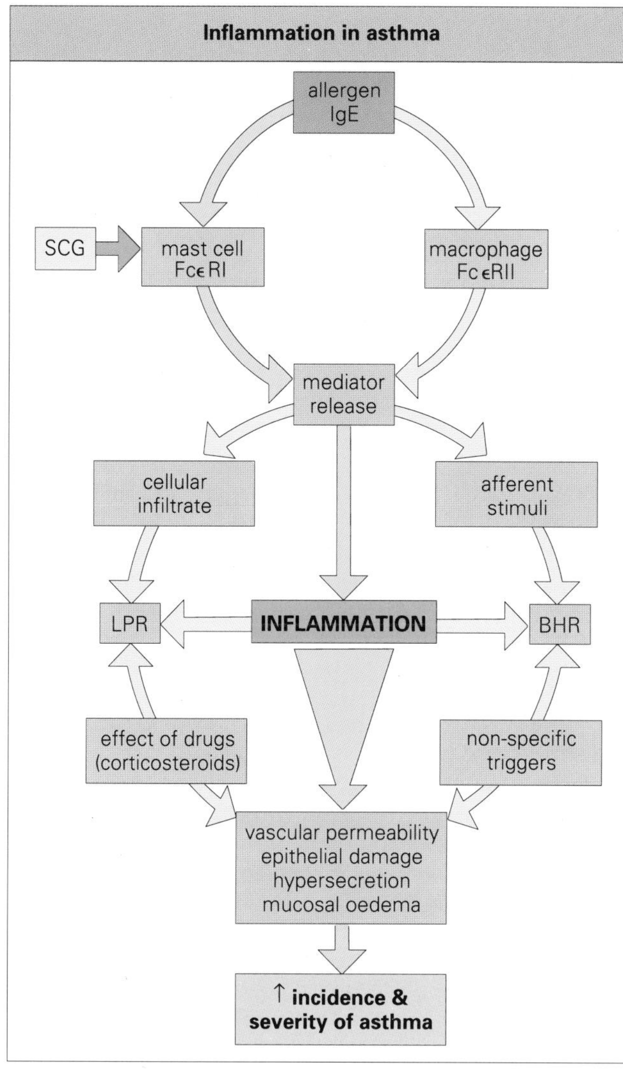

Fig. 17.20 Inflammation in asthma. LPR=late phase response; BHR=bronchial hyper-reactivity.

water vapour and smoke is associated with asthma, especially the LPR. Normal subjects become asthmatic following inhalation of 10ng of histamine whereas asthmatics respond to 100 times less this amount. It is probable that this hyper-reactivity is due to inflammation from chronic allergen exposure, although hyper-reactivity is not confined to allergic asthma. It is also possible that neurogenic mechanisms play a part, because after respiratory epithelial damage, vagal nerve endings can be stimulated to cause further reflex bronchoconstriction. This would be responsive to cholinergic antagonists such as atropine, which are known to be effective in some asthmatics (Fig. 17.20).

VIRUS INFECTION AND ASTHMA

Virus infections are associated not only with asthma (Fig. 17.21) and bronchial hyper-reactivity, but also with the onset of allergies. This has been confirmed in both retrospective and prospective studies, and is more striking in children than adults.

Mechanisms of virus induced changes

Airways inflammation. Even subjects with a simple cold have increased bronchial sensitivity to histamine challenge which can persist for weeks. The cause is probably increased vagus mediated reflex bronchospasm as pretreatment with atropine reduces this sensitivity. Viral infection of the airway mucosa can also lead to increased permeability to environmental allergens and an increased likelihood of sensitization.

IgE antibody production. Some viruses such as respiratory syncytial and parainfluenza virus can elicit a local IgE response in the bronchial mucosa. The persistence or recurrence of viral antigen could therefore lead to increased local mast cell degranulation.

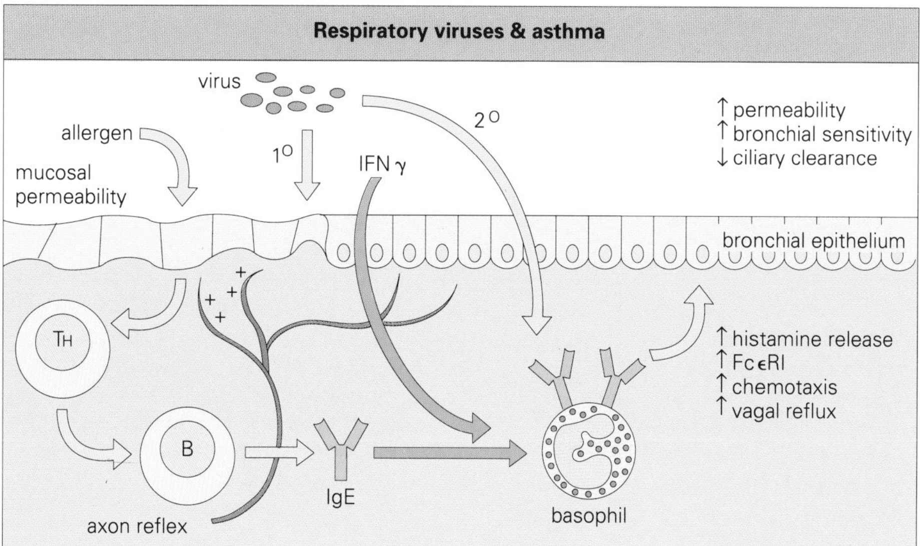

Fig. 17.21 Viruses in the respiratory tract can damage the mucosa and interact with the immune system to produce virus-specific IgE. This can sensitize local mast cells and basophils to release mediators on subsequent exposure to virus, thus exacerbating the local inflammation. This response can be compounded by the release of interferon and local reflex broncho-constriction.

Enhanced mediator release. Following virus infections, lymphocytes release interferon-γ (IFNγ) which enhances basophil histamine release, and increases its Fc receptors for IgE. Blood and sputum basophils increase during an asthma attack and the basophils become more 'sticky' when passing through a sensitized lung. This would fit in with observations that viruses and IFNγ can increase basophil chemotaxis.

ALLERGIC RHINITIS

This is the most common form of allergic disease, affecting about 15% of the population.

Pathophysiology

Inhaled allergens are deposited on the mucosal surface of the anterior nasal cavity where they release water-soluble allergenic components into the mucus layer. These react with cells sensitized with IgE which is produced locally in lymphoid tissues and mucosa. The relevant cells are probably basophils in the mucus and mucosal-type mast cells in the epithelium.

Mediator release occurs with subsequent dilatation of blood vessels and oedema, together with nerve irritation; this leads to symptoms of congestion, sneezing, pruritus, rhinorrhoea and lacrimation.

Late phase response

Some subjects experience a late response during which there is an influx of inflammatory cells into the nasal mucosa over 4–12 hours after initial allergen contact. Nasal lavage studies show that these consist of 50% neutrophils, 30% eosinophils, 20% mononuclear cells and 1% basophils. The absence of PGD2 amongst mediators found at this time supports the role of the basophil rather than the mast cell in the late phase response.

Augmentation of response

Increased antigen sensitivity in the nose after repeated antigen exposure ('priming') has been known since 1967. Increased numbers of mast cells in the nasal mucosa have been demonstrated at the end of the grass pollen season compared to the beginning. Basophil mediator release due to histamine releasing factors (HRFs) can be regulated by allergen exposure. As in the antigen-induced late asthmatic reaction, the nasal response to antigen is accompanied by increased histamine sensitivity lasting up to 10 days after antigen exposure.

Clinical features

Rhinitis may be seasonal when pollens are involved or perennial when house dust mite or animal dander is responsible, or it may be caused by a combination of the two. Occupational allergens such as flour in bakers' yeast or ricin from castor beans can also cause rhinitis. Inhalant allergens are responsible for rhinitis in over 90% of cases; food allergy is a less common cause. However, a proportion of birch pollen sensitive patients also show sensitivity to various foods including apple, celery and nuts. These cross-react on the RAST.

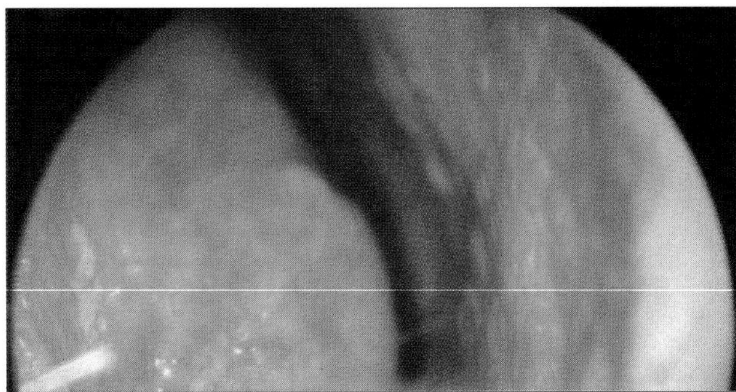

Fig. 17.22 Typical appearance of the allergic nose with pale, bluish, swollen inferior turbinates and clear rhinorrhoea.

Clinically, the allergic nose often shows swelling of the mucosa (Fig. 17.22) which is usually pale and bluish. Nasal polyps may form in severe chronic cases, although the cause of the majority of nasal polyps is unknown. Chronic rhinitis is the cause, co-existing disorder or predisposing factor in many cases of serous otitis media and chronic rhinosinusitis.

Diagnosis

The more useful differentiating symptoms from other causes of rhinitis (see chapter 12) are itch and conjunctival symptoms, which are usually confined to allergic subjects. Nasal smears may reveal eosinophils, which appear in allergic rhinitis and also in the so-called eosinophilic form of vasomotor rhinitis, which may well be the late phase response of an undiagnosed allergic reaction. IgE levels are unhelpful, being normal in about 50% of patients. Skin prick tests may reveal the relevant allergen, but it is possible to have a positive nasal challenge and a negative skin prick test, so nasal challenge with the postulated allergen is the final arbiter.

ANAPHYLAXIS

This is a generalized systemic type I hypersensitivity reaction to an allergen, which is usually introduced parenterally (for example penicillin, wasp and bee venom), but can occur with oral exposure. The widespread use of penicillin in the 1940s provided a new cause of anaphylaxis. Because of its extensive use and appearance in unexpected places (for example milk) it causes around 100–500 deaths annually in the USA.

A common agent used to be horse serum when it was given as passive protection in diphtheria and tetanus. Although this reaction is immediate, the underlying mechanism involves complement fixation with anaphylatoxin release.

Symptoms

In general, symptoms such as skin erythema, itching and

Delayed reactions to food	
skin	eczema
joints	arthralgia
CNS	poor concentration headaches, depression
GI tract	irritable bowel syndrome ? Crohn's disease
UG system	urinary frequency
respiratory system	asthma, rhinitis

Fig. 17.23 Delayed reactions to food sensitivity.

urticaria begin within minutes. Abdominal cramps, vomiting, diarrhoea, faintness and a sense of impending doom are often reported. In a large series of anaphylactic deaths, 70% died of respiratory complications and 20% from cardiovascular dysfunction.

Anaphylactoid reactions

These are similar, and are caused by the same mediators which are released directly from mast cells by a non-immunological mechanism. Thus, previous exposure and IgE production are not necessary. Intravenous contrast agents and anaesthetics can produce reactions in this category. Densensitization is not helpful.

BEE AND WASP VENOM ALLERGY

Death from insect stings occurs in about 40 people per year in the USA, but this is probably an underestimate. The location of the sting may be important; those occurring in the head and neck are more likely to produce symptoms. The types of reaction may be:

- anaphylaxis
- local reactions
- toxic reactions
- unusual reactions

Anaphylaxis is the most serious reaction and may occur in an individual with no previous history of insect sting problems, although a proportion may have had local reactions previously. The local reaction in a non-allergic subject is mild erythema and swelling. In a sensitive person the swelling can be considerable and can last for many days. Multiple stings can cause a toxic reaction, possibly because venom components can degranulate mast cells directly or activate the alternative pathway of complement. Some subjects develop a serum sickness reaction following a sting. Immunotherapy should not be given to such patients for fear of exacerbating the immune complex pathology.

Diagnosis

The clinical reaction to a stinging insect is clear, although the identification of the exact insect can be problem. Skin tests with pure venom usually distinguish allergic from non-allergic subjects. RAST is normally positive, although one in five subjects give a positive skin test and do not show specific IgE in the serum.

Treatment

Acute. Acute reactions should be treated the same way as anaphylaxis from any cause:

- tourniquet above site of sting/injection if relevant;
- adrenalin subcutaneously or intramuscularly around site of sting/injection;
- i.v. hydrocortisone or i.m. promethazine (both take several hours to act);
- cardiopulmonary resuscitation as necessary.

Patients can be taught to give their own adrenalin injections and should also wear an identification bracelet describing their allergy.

Immunotherapy

Using venom (and not whole body extract) immunotherapy, more than 95% of patients with a history of anaphylaxis can be protected. Treatment should be given to patients with a history of sting anaphylaxis and not to those with skin reactions only. A suitable maintenance dose is 100μg of venom at 3–4 week intervals for about 3 years.

FOOD ALLERGY

Immediate reactions

The occurrence of type I hypersensitivity reactions to food antigens is undisputed. They usually occur within minutes to an hour after ingestion and involve symptoms such as perioral erythema, lip swelling, oral irritation, swelling of tongue and pharynx, nausea and vomiting, and may lead to anaphylaxis. The diagnosis can usually be made on the history, but skin prick tests and RAST are usually positive if confirmation is needed. The types of food involved are frequently eggs, cows' milk, fish and nuts in younger children, with the later addition of shellfish and other foods in adults. Avoidance of the food for many years may be necessary, as the sensitivity usually persists.

Delayed reactions

These are more controversial although some, for example those in coeliac disease and dermatitis herpetiformis, are generally accepted. In contrast to type I reactions to foods, delayed reactions need large quantities of food and may take hours, days or even weeks to become manifest. There is no accepted diagnostic test and the diagnosis of food sensitivity rests upon food withdrawal followed by food challenge. The latter is preferably done double-bind on more than one occasion.

The spectrum of clinical symptoms resulting from delayed reactions to food sensitivity is shown in Fig. 17.23. 17.15

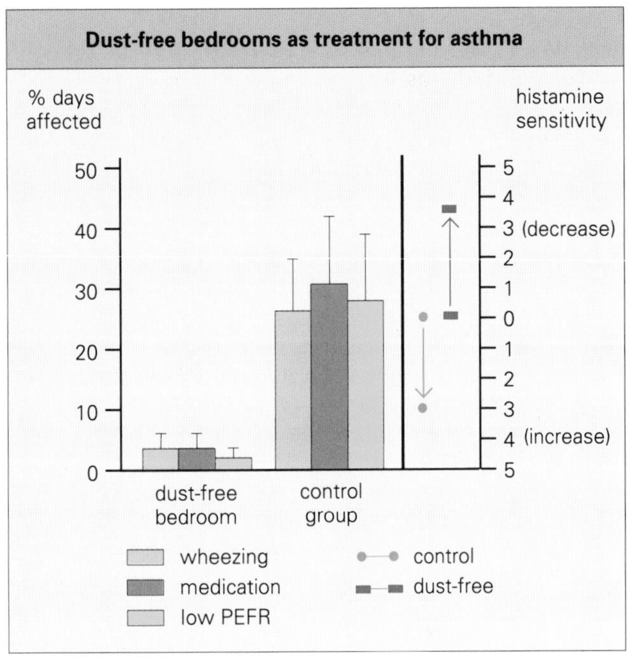

Fig. 17.24 Dust-free bedrooms as treatment for asthma. In a group of children sensitized to house dust mite with a dust-free bedroom, there was a clear reduction in the number of wheezy days, drugs taken and occasions when a low peak expiratory flow rate (PEFR) was recorded. Bronchial hyper-reactivity was reduced, as shown by an increase in the dose of histamine needed to produce a fall of 20% in the FEV_1, as compared with the control group. This attests to the value of reducing the allergen load in the environment. Modified from Murray & Ferguson (1983).

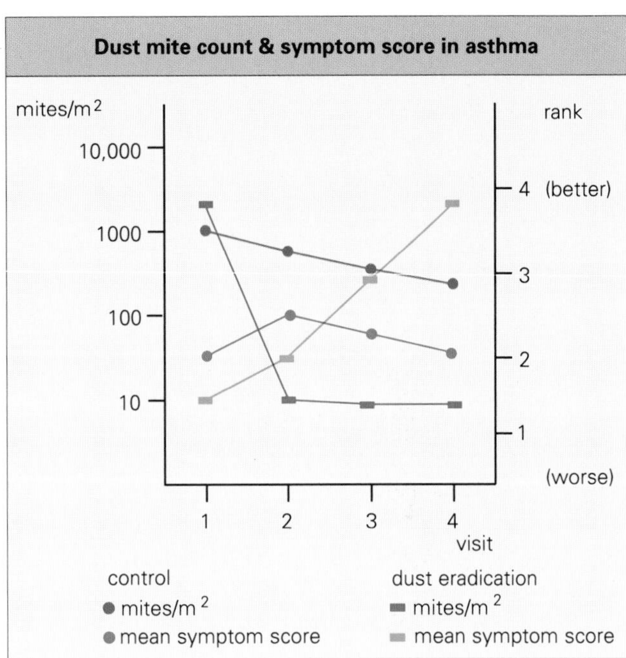

Fig. 17.25 A prospective study of 50 HDM-sensitive adult asthmatics showed that HDM eradication procedures produced a significant drop in house dust mite levels and a considerable clinical improvement which was not seen in the control group. Modified from Walshaw & Evans (1986).

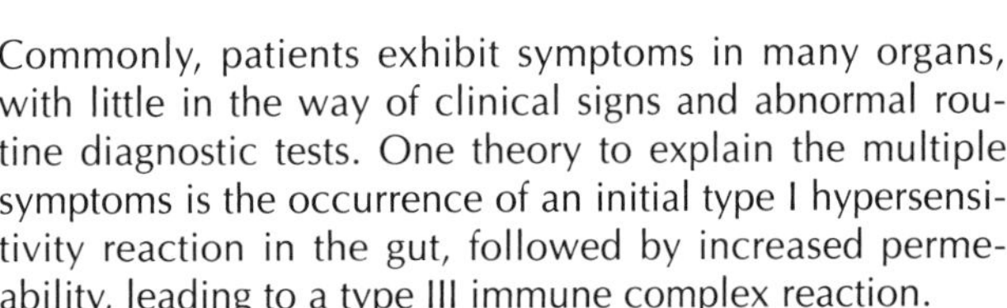

Commonly, patients exhibit symptoms in many organs, with little in the way of clinical signs and abnormal routine diagnostic tests. One theory to explain the multiple symptoms is the occurrence of an initial type I hypersensitivity reaction in the gut, followed by increased permeability, leading to a type III immune complex reaction.

Many delayed reactions to food are probably not immunological, for example idiosyncratic reactions due to enzyme deficiencies and toxic reactions due to microbial contamination. It is possible that defects in the metabolic handling of certain foodstuffs relate to food sensitivity. Recently, a group of food sensitive individuals has been shown to contain a much higher proportion of poor sulphoxidisers than occur normally in the population.

TREATMENT OF ALLERGIC DISEASES

There are three main principles:

- allergen avoidance — inhaled & ingested
- pharmacotherapy
- immunotherapy

Allergen avoidance

Dust free bedrooms as treatment of asthma. A number of studies have addressed house dust mite (HDM) allergen avoidance, with conflicting results. The key to a clinical response is meticulous elimination of the HDM allergen. In a group of asthmatic children, where half had house dust mite reduced as much as possible, there was a significant reduction in wheezing and need for medication, and a rise in peak expiratory flow rate with a marked increase in tolerance to histamine provocation (Fig. 17.24). A further study in adults showed how effective house dust mite eradication regimes could be, with a greater than 100-fold reduction in mite content of the bedroom dust with concomitant improvement in the symptom score (Fig. 17.25). Removal or reduction of the allergen load, where applicable, must go hand in hand with clinical management of the patient.

Pharmacotherapy

The drugs used are shown in Figs. 17.16 and 17.26.

Immunotherapy

Immunotherapy is the art of adminstering sufficient aller-

Major immunological changes during immunotherapy
↑ specific IgG (blocking antibody)
↑ IgE over several months; then slow ↓ IgE over years abrogation of usual seasonal ↑ IgE
↑ specific IgG & IgA in nasal secretions
↓ mediator release from sensitized cells in some patients
↓ lymphocyte proliferation & lymphokine production to immunizing antigen; development of antigen–specific suppressor cells

Fig. 17.26 Major immunological changes during immunotherapy.

gen by injection to atopic subjects to reduce or abolish their allergic response following natural exposure.

The process has been successfully employed since 1911, when it was first described in London by Noon and Freeman. There is no doubt that it is successful in reducing the symptom–medication scores in 60–90% of patients with rhinitis or asthma, although few patients are 'cured'. However the occurrence of anaphylactic reactions, and even death in a few patients, means that this form of treatment should be used only in severely affected individuals who do not respond to other measures. In the UK it must be undertaken only where cardiorespiratory resuscitation facilities are available, with the patient being observed for two hours following each injection.

Immunological changes. The mechanism of action of high dose therapy is not understood, although there are numerous immunological changes (Fig. 17.26). There is often a reduction in sensitivity to the allergen shown by decrease in IgE (frequently preceded by a rise), basophil histamine release, mediator production and nasal provocation test sensitivity. However, clinical benefit can often occur before any of these changes appear and before a significant rise in specific IgG. This suggests that there may be a number of points of interaction of the immunotherapy with the immune system, but with the possibility that reduced T cell responsiveness may play a key part.

FURTHER READING

Brostoff J, Challacombe SJ, eds. *Food allergy and intolerance*. London: Baillière-Tindall, 1987: 1032.

Burney PGJ, Chinn S, Rona RJ. Has the prevalence of asthma increased in children? Evidence from the national study of health and growth 1973–86. *Br Med J*. 1990; **300**: 1306–1310.

Cookson WOCM, Sharp PA, Faux JA, Hopkin JM. Linkage between immunoglobulin E responses underlying asthma and rhinitis and chromosome 11q. *Lancet*. 1989; **i**: 1292–1294.

Ishizaka K. Regulation of IgE biosynthesis. *Hospital Practice*. 1989; **Sept 15**: 51–60.

Pollart S, Chapman MD, Fiocco GP, Rose G, Platts-Mills TAE. Epidemiology of acute asthma: IgE antibodies to common inhalant allergens as a risk factor for emergency room visits. *J Allergy Clin Immunol*. 1989; **83**: 875–882.

Salvaggio JE. The impact of allergy and immunology on our expanding industrial environment. *J Allergy Clin Immunol*. 1990; **85**: 689–699.

Sporik R, Holgate ST, Platts-Mills TAE, Cogswell JJ. Exposure to house dust mite allergen (Der pl) and the development of asthma in childhood — A prospective study. N *Engl J Med*. 1990; **323**: 502–507.

Takafuji S, Suzuki S, Koizumi K, *et al*. Diesel exhaust particulates inoculated by the intranasal route have an adjuvant activity for IgE production in mice. *J Allergy Clin Immunol*. 1987; **79**: 639–645.

Wide L, Bennich H, Johansson SGO. Diagnosis of allergy by an in vitro test for allergen antibodies. *Lancet*. 1967; **ii**: 1105.

18

Occupational Lung Disorders

INTRODUCTION

Agents inhaled at work can cause a variety of inflammatory reactions in the lungs, the nature of which depends on the site and pattern of reaction. The site of reaction is determined by the physical characteristics of the inhaled agent; the pattern is determined by whether the reaction is the consequence of direct cell injury or the outcome of a specific immunological (allergic) reaction.

Site of particle deposition

The site of deposition of inhaled particles is determined primarily by their aerodynamic diameter (Fig. 18.1). Particles deposited in the airways are cleared within hours by the muco-ciliary escalator. Those settling within the acini are cleared more slowly; after ingestion by alveolar macrophages they are transported proximally within the acinus to the terminal bronchioles and muco-ciliary escalator, or to the centri-acinar lymphatics. The acinar clearance mechanisms may be overwhelmed by high concentrations of particle deposition and particles within alveolar macrophages are retained in alveoli in the proximal respiratory bronchioles (Fig. 18.2). Respirable dust particles which absorb X-rays (for example tin and iron) cause nodular opacities on the chest radiograph (Fig. 18.3) when retained in sufficient concentration.

Retained respirable inorganic dusts such as asbestos and silica, which are toxic to alveolar macrophages, provoke inflammation and fibrosis of alveolar walls. Organic dusts, such as thermophilic actinomycetes, avian serum proteins and beryllium stimulate a T cell dependent granulomatous response within alveoli which may progress to fibrosis. Inhaled organic dusts and some reactive chemicals may also cause asthma, usually as the outcome of an immunological response which frequently involves specific IgE antibody.

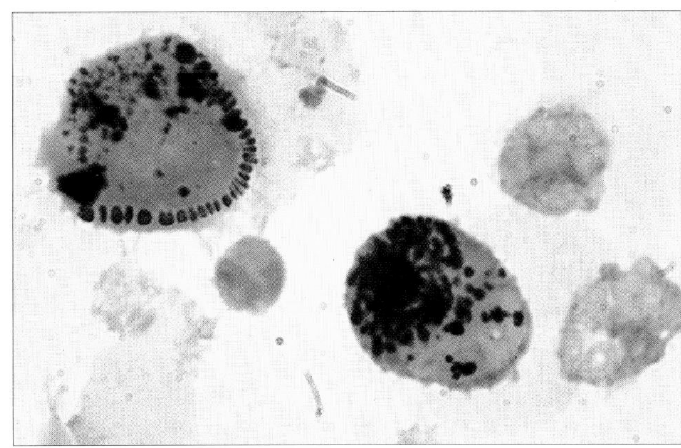

Fig. 18.2 Alveolar macrophage with ingested particles of tungsten carbide in a hard metal worker.

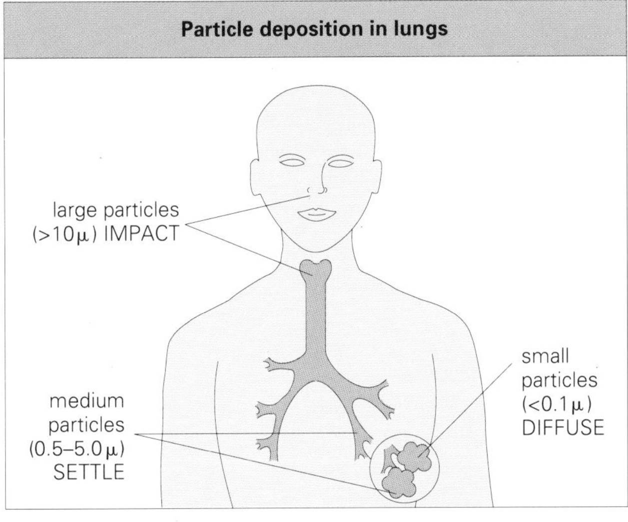

Fig. 18.1 The size of the inhaled particle governs the site of deposition in the lungs.

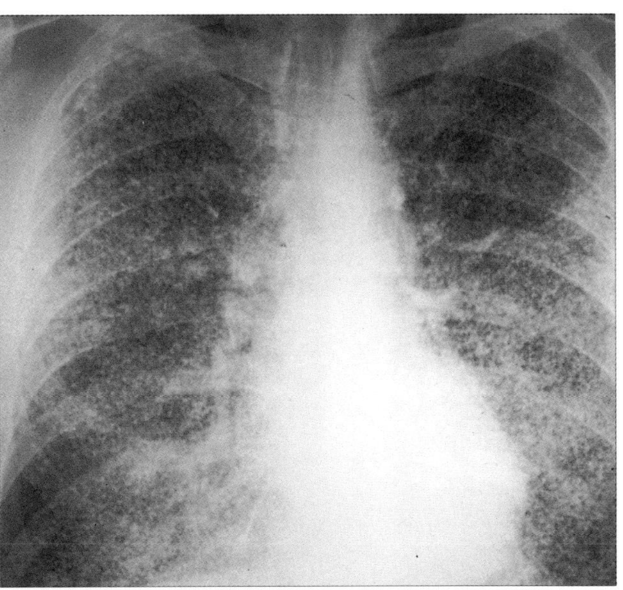

Fig. 18.3 Stannosis. Widespread nodules on chest radiograph due to retained tin oxide in a tin smelter.

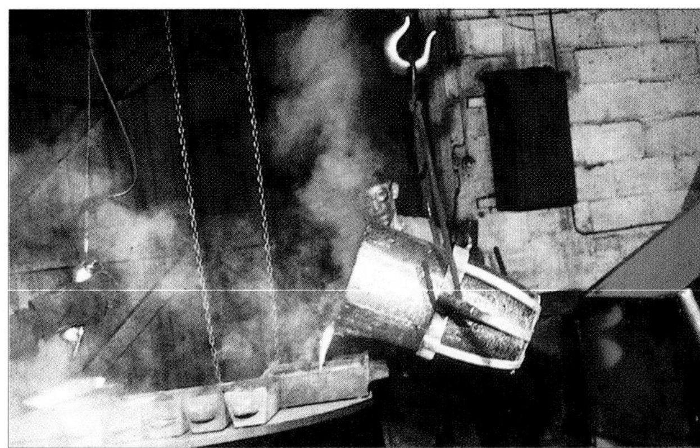

Fig. 18.4 Brown cadmium fumes released during pouring of liquid copper cadmium alloy.

Site of vapour deposition

The site of deposition of gases and vapours is determined primarily by their solubility in the waterline epithelial surface of the respiratory tract — the more soluble the gas, the more proximal their effect. Water soluble toxic gases such as sulphur dioxide and ammonia provide an inflammatory reaction in the moist mucosal surfaces of the upper respiratory tract; only if the exposure is overwhelming does the inflammatory reaction extend into the alveoli.

Insoluble gases, such as oxides of nitrogen and cadmium fumes (Fig. 18.4), are not dissolved in the upper respiratory tract and airways when the dose inhaled is small, but penetrate into alveoli when the inhaled dose is high. In addition to their direct toxic effect on respiratory epithelial cells, there is some evidence that these toxic chemicals may increase the risk of sensitization by proteins inhaled at the same time.

Pattern of allergic reactions

Allergic reactions to agents inhaled at work may be manifested as one of two major patterns of tissue response:

- asthma and airway hyper-responsiveness as an expression of inflammation of the conducting airways;
- granulomatous inflammation of the peripheral gas-exchanging parts of the lungs caused by organic dusts (extrinsic allergic alveolitis or hypersensitivity pneumonitis) or by beryllium salts (beryllium disease).

These diseases are important for several reasons. In individual cases, identification and avoidance of exposure at an early stage can halt the progression to irreversible damage. Prevention is also potentially possible by appropriate environmental control. These diseases provide a model for the investigation of the relationship between environmental stimuli and immunological and tissue responses, and
18.2 the factors influencing these.

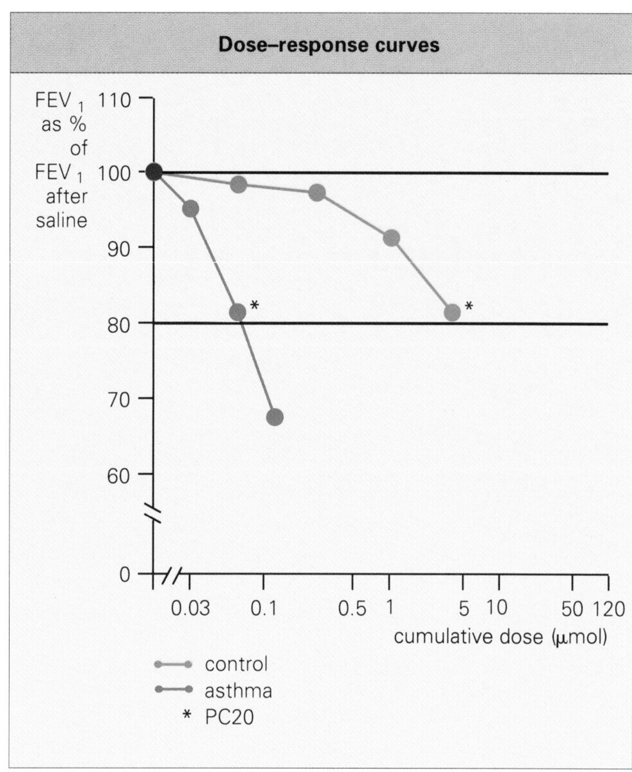

Fig. 18.5 Asthmatics with hyper-responsive airways respond to a much lower concentration of histamine or methacholine than normal subjects. * PC_{20} is the dose of agonist required to provoke a 20% fall in the FEV_1.

DEFINITION OF ASTHMA

Asthma is usually defined as airway narrowing which is reversible over short periods of time, either spontaneously or as the result of treatment. A further characteristic is airway hyper-responsiveness — an increased bronchoconstrictor response to non-specific provocative stimuli. Such stimuli include inhaled cold dry air, exercise, pollutant gases such as sulphur dioxide, and chemical mediators and their analogues such as histamine and methacholine.

Airway responsiveness may be measured by determining the concentration or dose of a stimulus which provokes a specified change in lung function. Most commonly this is the concentration of histamine or methacholine which provokes a 20% fall in FEV_1 (so-called histamine or methacholine PC_{20}). The lower the PC_{20}, the more responsive the airways (Fig. 18.5). The degree of airway responsiveness is related to the severity of asthma and is believed to reflect the desquamative eosinophilic bronchitis characteristic of asthma.

Types of stimuli

Two groups of stimuli which cause asthmatic responses can be distinguished: non-specific factors which provoke

Some causes of occupational asthma		
	Proteins	**Low molecular weight chemicals**
animal	excreta of rats, mice, locusts, grain mites	
vegetable	grain/flour castor bean soya bean green coffee beans Ispaghula	plicatic acid (western red cedar) colophony (pinewood resin)
microbial	harvest moulds *Bacillus subtilis* enzymes	antibiotics, e.g. penicillin
mineral		acid anhydrides isocyanates complex platinum salts polyamines reactive dyes

Fig. 18.6 The causes of occupational asthma are very varied and agents range from complex protein to low molecular weight chemicals.

short-lived airway narrowing in individuals with hyper-responsive airways, and specific agents which induce asthma and increase airway responsiveness to non-specific stimuli. Factors in the first group include exercise and SO_2, which can incite asthmatic attacks and increase their frequency; the second group of factors can initiate asthma and, with continuing exposure, increase its severity.

OCCUPATIONAL ASTHMA

Occupational asthma may be defined as asthma initiated by an agent inhaled at work. The inhaled agent has 'switched on' asthma, and this is an example of a response induced by an identifiable environmental agent:

- Toxic chemicals, such as chlorine gas inhaled in high concentration, can cause direct damage to the epithelial cells of the airways. Persistent asthma which follows such exposure has been given the inelegant name of RADS (reactive airways dysfunction syndrome). Respiratory epithelial damage by toxic chemicals is not a common cause of occupational asthma.
- Proteins and reactive chemicals. Asthma caused by these agents is the result of an acquired hypersensitivity response, thus in many patients occupational asthma can be regarded as the manifestation of an allergic response.

The more important causes of occupational asthma are listed in Fig. 18.6.

INHALED AGENT

Biological materials

Exposure to materials of biological origin occurs in a wide variety of occupations. These include farming, the handling, storage, transport and processing of agricultural products such as grains and beans, food production, the use of laboratory animals in research, forestry and carpentry, and the commercial exploitation of microbes for antibiotics, enzymes and as food sources. The majority of these hazards are dusts, but exposure to some complex biological molecules, such as colophony (pine wood resin used as a soft solder flux) is in the form of fumes.

Synthetic chemicals

Exposure to the synthetic chemicals which cause occupational asthma occur in many different settings.

Isocyanates. These are widely used and are probably the most important causes of occupational asthma. They are bi-functional molecules used commercially to polymerize polyhydroxyl and polyglycol compounds to produce polyurethanes. The polyurethane reaction is exothermic and the heat generated during the reaction is sufficient to vaporize isocyanates with a high vapour pressure, such as toluene (TDI), and hexamethylene (HDI). Significant evaporation of isocyanates with lower vapour pressures, such as diphenylmethane (MDI) and naphthalene (NDI), generally requires the application of heat. Exposure to isocyanates occurs during their manufacture and in the production of polyurethanes. This includes the production of

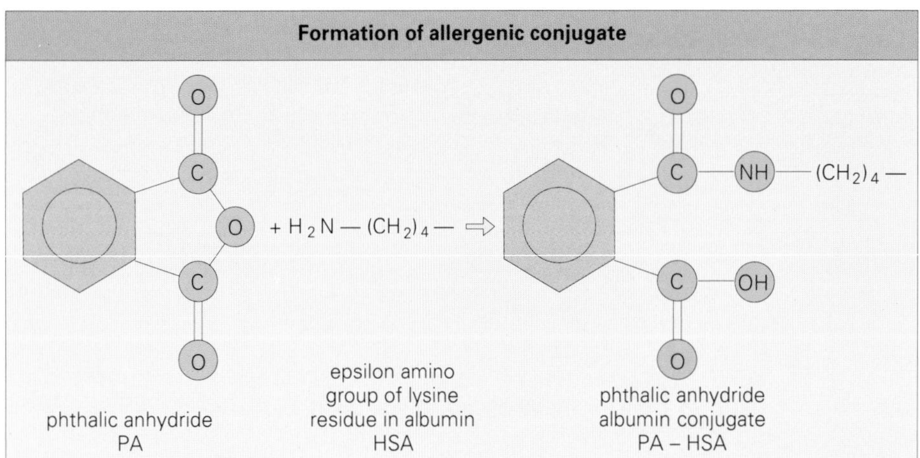

Fig. 18.7 Covalent binding of phthalic anhydride with human serum albumin to form an allergenic conjugate.

rigid and polyurethane foams, and in the application of two part polyurethane paints, particularly when sprayed.

Acid anhydrides. Phthalic (PA) and trimellitic (TMA) acid anhydrides (Fig. 18.7) are used as curing agents in the manufacture of epoxy and alkyl resins; PA is also used in the manufacture of plasticizers.

IMPORTANCE OF OCCUPATIONAL ASTHMA

Occupational asthma is probably the most common type of occupational lung disease. Some 500 new cases are believed to be seen by chest physicians in the UK each year, and at least an equal number probably occur without being so referred.

The most common causes of occupational asthma are isocyanates, laboratory animals and flour. About 5% of those exposed to TDI in its manufacture develop asthma, usually within the first year of exposure, and between one-quarter and one-third of those working with laboratory animals develop allergy to one or more of them, with 5% having asthma. It is estimated that in the USA about 100,000 persons are exposed to TDI in their work and in the UK some 32,000 are in contact with laboratory animals, making these important hazards.

Disease mechanisms

Asthma caused by inhaled proteins, other complex biological molecules and synthetic low molecular weight chemicals fulfils the criteria of an acquired specific hypersensitivity response:

- it develops in only a proportion, usually a minority, of those exposed to the specific cause;
- it develops after an initial disease-free interval, usually of weeks or months from the onset of exposure;
- once initiated, asthma is provoked by exposure to atmospheric concentrations which do not provoke reactions in others and which previously did not provoke a response in the now hypersensitive individual.

18.4 These points fulfil von Pirquet's criteria for an allergic response. Evidence of a specific immunological reaction, in particular of specific IgE antibody, has been demonstrated for many, but not all, of the causes of occupational asthma. These include the majority of the inhaled proteins, such as flour, laboratory animal urine proteins, enzymes, and some of the reactive chemicals dyes which act as haptens, binding covalently to tissue protein. The biological materials possess certain properties; they are water soluble proteins of restricted molecular weight (10–60kDa) which, when inhaled as particles, are rapidly eluted from their carriers. Reactive chemicals capable of stimulating an IgE response seem able to bind covalently to tissue proteins to form stable conjugates.

No consistent evidence of a specific immunological reaction has been found for some occupational asthmas, including those caused by isocyanates and colophony. One possible explanation is that inhaled chemicals may be transformed in the respiratory tract and the relevant *in vivo* conjugate is not used for the *in vitro* test.

CHARACTERISTICS OF RESPONSE

The specific immunological response (most commonly identified as IgE) to inhaled proteins and reactive chemicals is the 'bridge' between inhalation and the development of asthma which, in some cases, becomes chronic:

- inhalation of allergen or hapten induces specific immunological response (commonly IgE);
- subsequent inhalation provokes immunologically dependent inflammation in airways (usually a desquamative eosinophilic bronchitis) which causes both airway narrowing and an increase in non-specific airway responsiveness;
- repeated re-exposure to the specific agent during the working week causes increasing severity of asthmatic symptoms and airway responsiveness;
- with continuing exposure to the initiating cause after the development of asthma, the condition becomes chronic in a proportion of cases, persisting indefinitely despite avoidance of exposure to the original cause.

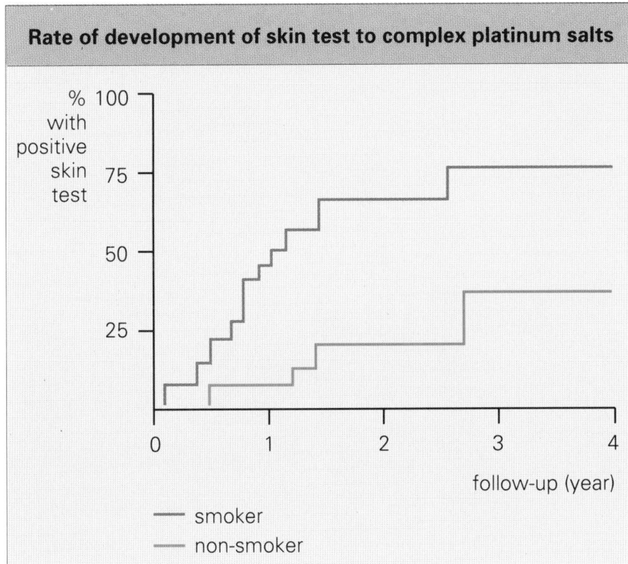

Fig. 18.8 Rate of development of positive skin prick test to complex platinum salts in platinum refinery workers. There is a markedly increased sensitization rate in smokers compared to non-smokers.

Predisposing factors

The development of specific immunological responses and asthma usually occurs within a short period (1–2 years) from initial exposure to an occupational allergen. For those who 'survive' this period, the risk of subsequently becoming sensitized is low. There is limited evidence that the amount of exposure experienced during this period is important. Workers exposed to the enzymes of *B. subtilis* in the manufacture of enzyme detergents showed a relationship between the intensity of exposure and the frequency of development of skin test reaction, those with the highest intensity of exposure experiencing the highest rate of skin test conversion. Exposure to reactive chemicals (such as isocyanates) in high concentration for short periods during 'spills' has also been suggested as particularly likely to sensitize and cause asthma.

Atopy. This is the development of IgE antibody to common environmental allergens such as grass pollens, house dust mite and cat fur, and is usually identified by skin prick test. It is associated with an increased risk of developing IgE antibody and asthma to some, but by no means all causes of occupational asthma. The frequency of asthma caused by laboratory animal secreta and excreta and *B. subtilis* enzymes is increased in atopics, whereas there is no increase in risk among atopics exposed to isocyanates or acid anhydrides.

Cigarette smoking exerts an important influence on the risk of developing occupational asthma, probably through an adjuvant effect on IgE production. IgE antibody production and asthma develop considerably more frequently in tobacco smokers compared to non-smokers exposed at work to many proteins and reactive chemicals including *B. subtilis* enzymes, green coffee beans, acid anhydrides and complex platinum salts (Fig. 18.8). This effect may be the consequence of tobacco smoke damage to the integrity of the bronchial epithelium, increasing its permeability to protein molecules and allowing them access to submucosal immunocompetent cells. A similar enhancing effect on IgE antibody production has been found in experimental animals exposed concurrently to an allergen (for example ovalbumin or platinum salts) and a respiratory irritant (for example ozone or SO_2), suggesting that it is a non-specific consequence of damage to the airways.

DIAGNOSIS OF OCCUPATIONAL ASTHMA

Accurate and early diagnosis of occupational asthma is important so that patients can avoid further exposure to the cause of their asthma and minimize the risk of development of chronic asthma. Misdiagnosis can lead to inappropriate decisions about changes in occupation and is as undesirable as failure to identify the occupational causes of asthma. The diagnosis of occupational asthma is based on the history, changes in lung function in relation to periods exposed and unexposed to the putative causes, and tests of specific immunological responsiveness.

History

The characteristic history is of the development of asthmatic symptoms (which may occur after the end of the working day, in the evening or night time) after an initial symptom-free interval. These improve when away from work (at weekends or on holidays) and recur on return to work, often deteriorating during the working week. The patient may also be aware of others with similar symptoms at the place of work.

Serial peak expiratory flow (PEF) measurements

Asthma can be confidently attributed to an agent inhaled at work when measurements of lung function reproducibly deteriorate during periods at work and improve during absences. Determination of airway calibre for this purpose is most conveniently made by serial self-recording of PEF during a period of several weeks, which ideally includes a long weekend or holiday period. To be useful, such records require honesty and compliance.

A summary of the result as maximum, minimum and average values for each day during the recording period (Fig. 18.9) allows visual assessment of the changes. In general:

- absence of asthma (as screening exposure to its cause during the period of measurement) excludes occupational asthma;
- a pattern of work-related asthma makes the diagnosis of occupational asthma very likely;
- asthma without work relationship does not exclude occupational asthma. This commonly occurs in cases of occupational asthma because of insufficient time of absence from work during the time of the record to allow demonstrable recovery of lung function.

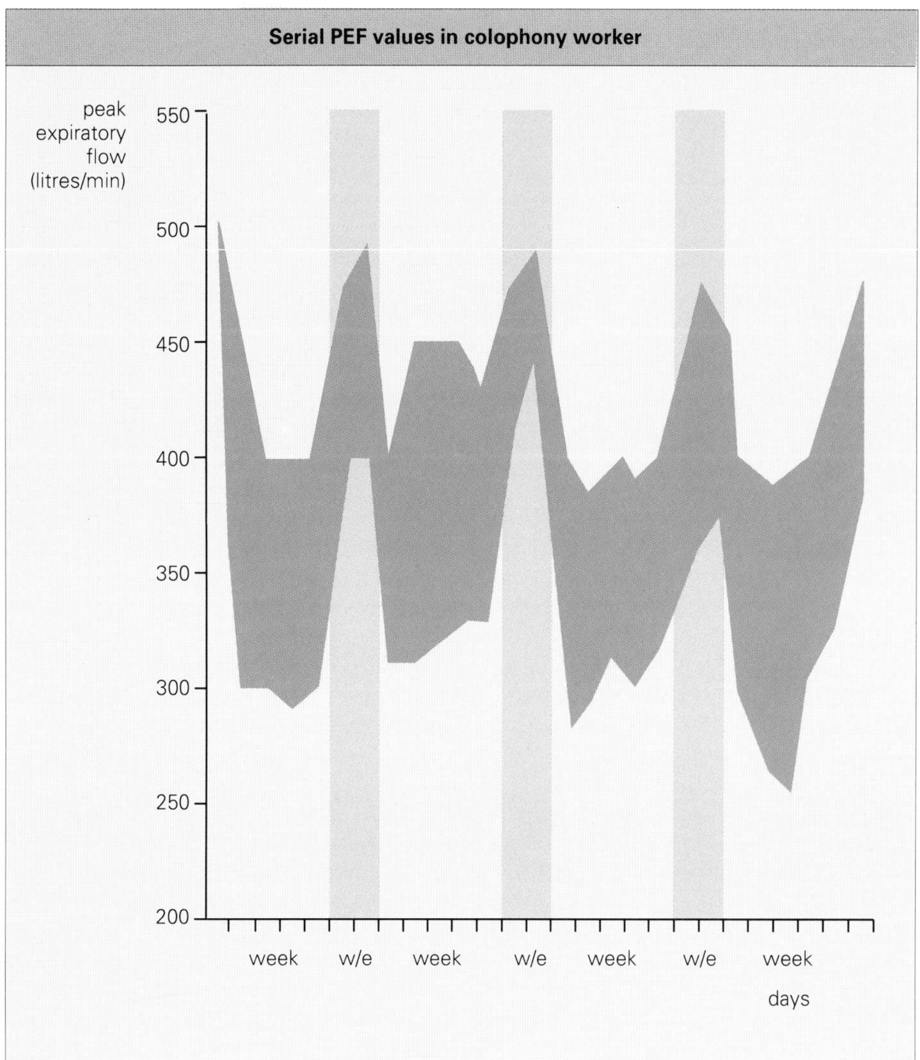

Fig. 18.9 Serial PEF measurements in a solderer exposed to colophony, plotted as best, and worst for each day. This patient showed consistent deterioration at work and improvement during the weekends (w/e).

Immunological investigations

Evidence of IgE-mediated responses to proteins and low molecular weight chemicals (usually conjugated to human serum albumin) can be obtained from skin prick and serological test (most commonly the radioallergosorbent test or RAST). Such tests are diagnostically important where the development of IgE antibody bears a close relationship to the development of asthma and is not simply an unrelated consequence of exposure, or due to cross-reacting antigens binding to IgE antibody stimulated by other environmental allergens. These criteria have not been demonstrated for many occupational agents, but have been shown for asthma caused by laboratory animals, locusts (Fig. 18.10), acid anhydrides and complex platinum salts. This is not the case for isocyanates, where IgE to isocyanate–HSA conjugates can be identified in the serum of only a minority of cases (around 15%) of isocyanate induced asthma, and the relationship of a positive test to
18.6 exposure is unclear.

Inhalation tests

The provocation of an asthmatic reaction by the specific occupational agent in a controlled inhalation test remains, for many, the gold standard against which other diagnositic tests for occupational asthma should be judged. It remains an essential part of the investigation and demonstration of new causes of occupational asthma, and an important tool where other methods of investigation have proved inadequate to provide a confident basis for future management advice.

The aim in an inhalation test is to reproduce the exposure in the work place to a single agent and to provoke reproducibly an asymptomatic but significant asthmatic response. Where possible, the atmospheric concentration of the particular agent should be measured, and exposure in the challenge test based on knowledge of levels of exposures in the work place. The particular method used in an inhalation test will depend on the physical state of the test substance.

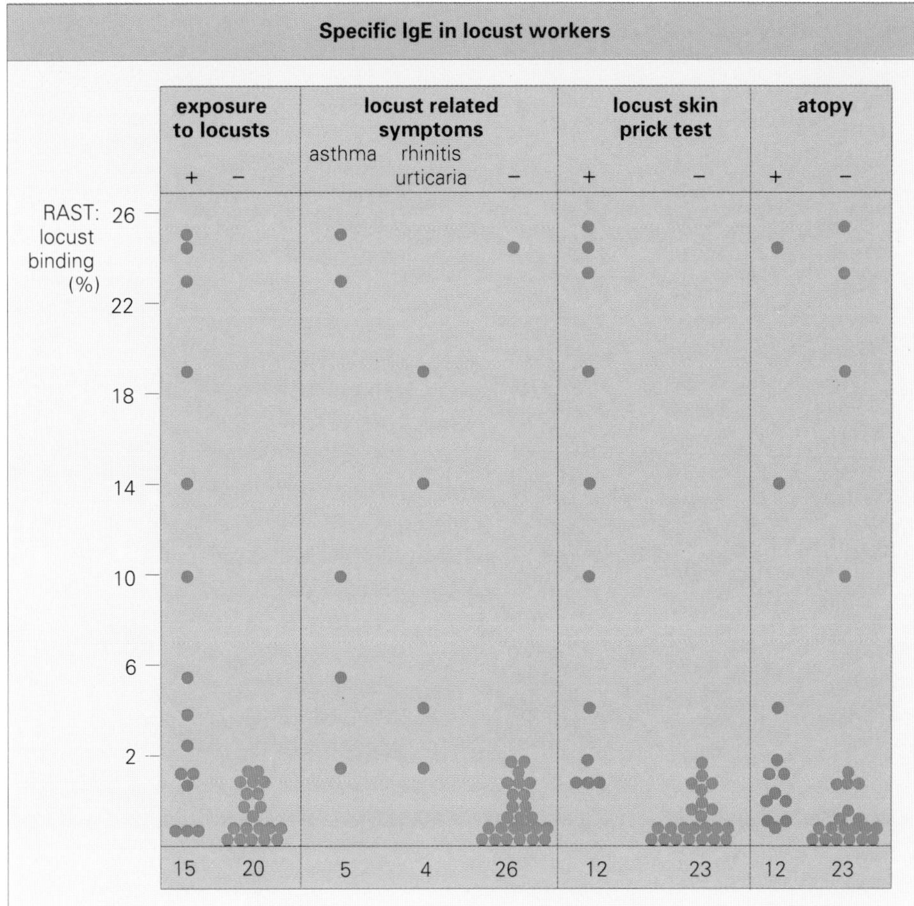

Fig. 18.10 Specific IgE in locust workers. Specific IgE to this antigen is related to exposure, symptoms and skin test reaction, but not to atopic status.

Challenge compounds. Water-soluble proteins, such as rat urine or flour proteins, can be dissolved in saline and inhaled as a nebulized extract. Dusts such as drugs and complex platinum salts can be generated by tipping. Volatile organic liquids such as isocyanate can be generated by evaporation. Colophony fumes can be generated by soldering, and paint aerosols by spraying. The atmospheric concentrations (which can be measured by personal samplers) achieved in these tests can be very reproducible.

The provoked narrowing in airway calibre can be demonstrated by changes in forced expiratory volume in one second (FEV_1) or PEF. In addition, changes in airway responsiveness can be examined by serial tests of histamine (or methacholine) PC_{20}.

Patterns of induced asthma. Three different patterns of asthmatic response to inhalation test, differentiated by their time of onset and duration, have been distinguished (Fig. 18.11):

- the immediate asthmatic response develops within minutes of the test exposure and resolves spontaneously within 1–2 hours;
- the late asthmatic reponse develops one or more hours after the test exposure, and may persist for 24–36 hours. Isolated late responses are almost uniquely caused by occupational chemical sensitizers;
- a dual asthmatic response is a late asthmatic response preceded by an immediate response. The late, but not immediate, response is associated with an increase in non-specific airway responsiveness which can persist for several days.

Recurrent nocturnal asthmatic reactions can follow a single test exposure of short duration; this probably reflects an induced increase in non-specific airway responsiveness.

MANAGEMENT OF OCCUPATIONAL ASTHMA

Established cases should be encouraged to avoid further exposure to the cause of their asthma as far as possible, to prevent the development of chronic asthma.

Ideally, avoidance of exposure can be achieved by relocation. Alternatively, particularly with dusts such as pharmaceutical agents, flour dust and laboratory animal excreta, asthma can be prevented by a combination of improved dust control, reducing dust contact to a minimum and using effective respiratory control when exposed. The effectiveness of these measures must be

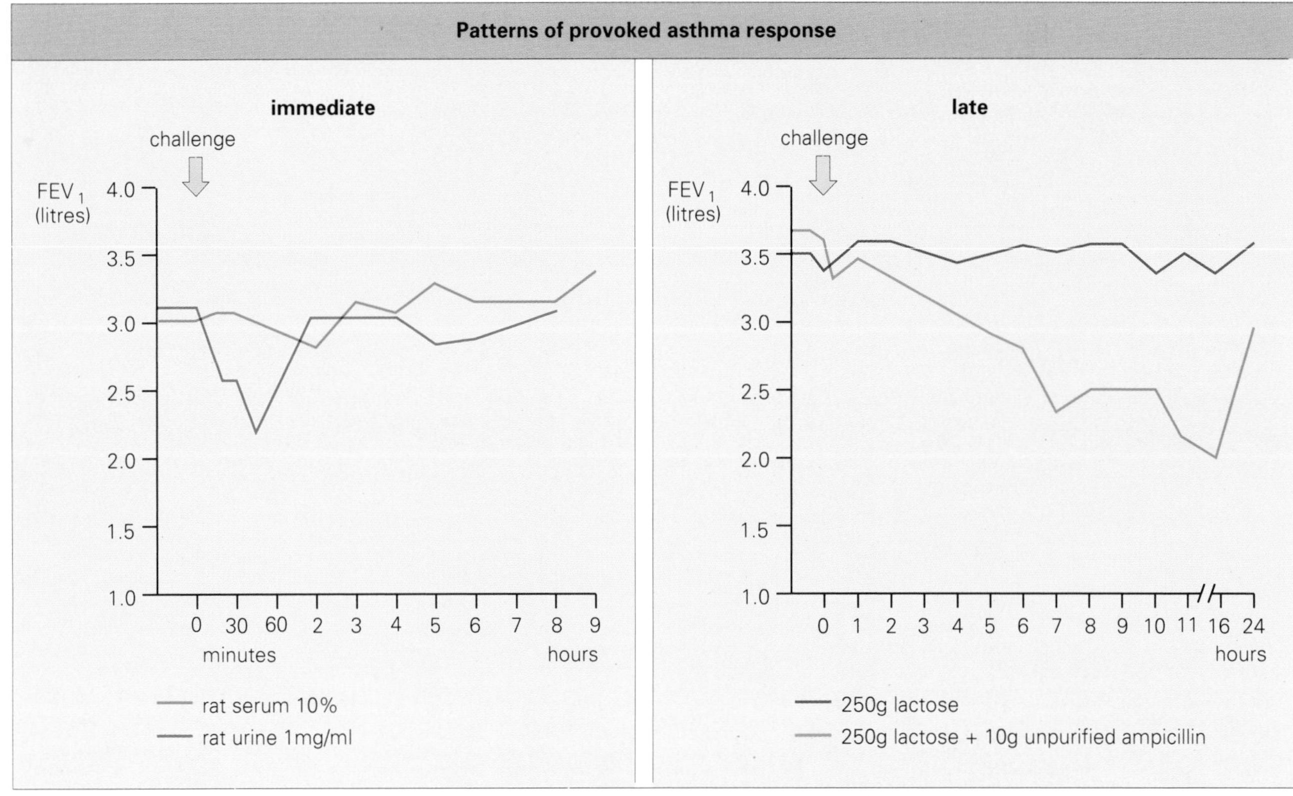

Fig. 18.11 Left: immediate asthmatic response provoked by rat urine extract in laboratory animal workers. Right: late asthmatic response provoked by ampicillin in an individual involved in antibiotic manufacture.

monitored by serial tests of lung function, such as self-recorded PEF measurements. It should be appreciated that, even if direct contact can be adequately controlled, the risk of indirect contact, for example with dust on colleagues' clothing or exhaust from a ventilation system, remains. Thus, if asthma control is to be effective these sources of indirect exposure must also be considered.

GRANULOMATOUS INFLAMMATION

Granulomata are focal accumulations of macrophages and the cells derived from them (epithelioid and giant cells). Material which persists in tissues, such as talc, may stimulate formation of foreign body granulomata; material which is persistent and immunogenic, such as beryllium salts and organic dusts, may stimulate formation of so-called 'immune' granulomata. In these, macrophages are recruited and activated by cytokines (such as interferon) released from T lymphocytes which are responsive to specific inducing antigens (Fig. 18.12). Immune granulomata are distinguishable from foreign body granulomata by the presence of lymphocytes (predominantly $CD4^+$ T lymphocytes) (Fig. 18.13).

Bronchoalveolar lavage (BAL)

18.8 The T lymphocytes participating in extrinsic allergic alveolitis (EAA) and beryllium disease can be studied directly by examining the cells obtained from bronchoalveolar lavage (see chapter 12). Patients with diseases characterized by granuloma formation in the lungs (not only EAA and beryllium disease but also tuberculosis and sarcoidosis) have an increased proportion of lymphocytes in the cells recovered (Fig. 18.14).

T suppressor cells in EAA. Studies of farmers and pigeon fanciers have shown that, in addition to cases of EAA, several exposed but asymptomatic individuals may also have an increased proportion of T lymphocytes with altered CD4:CD8 ratios in the cells recovered at BAL. Those who develop disease are distinguished by a defect in antigen-specific T suppressor (Ts) lymphocyte control. Translation of the specific T lymphocyte response into granulomatous inflammation is prevented in asymptomatic farmers by antigen specific Ts lymphocytes (Fig. 18.15).

CHRONIC BERYLLIUM DISEASE

Chronic beryllium disease is a T lymphocyte dependent granulomatous inflammatory reaction in the lungs and other parts of the body to beryllium inhaled as fumes or dust. Beryllium disease is similar to sarcoidosis in many of its clinical manifestations, although there are some differences: bilateral hilar lymphadenopathy does not occur in

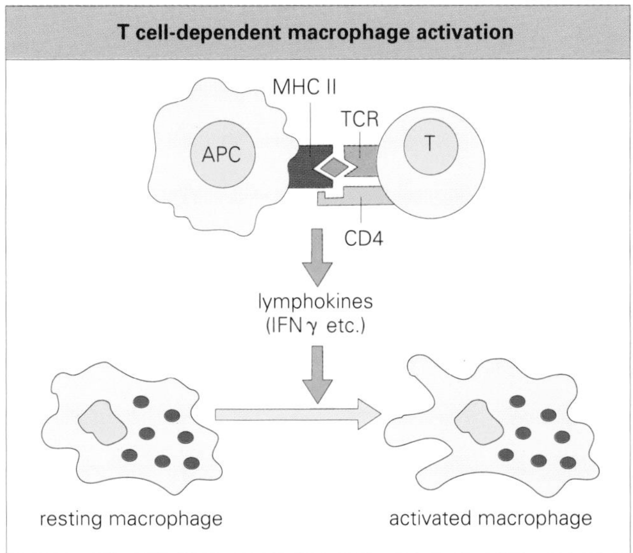

Fig. 18.12 T lymphocyte dependent macrophage activation by cytokines such as interferon-γ (IFNγ).

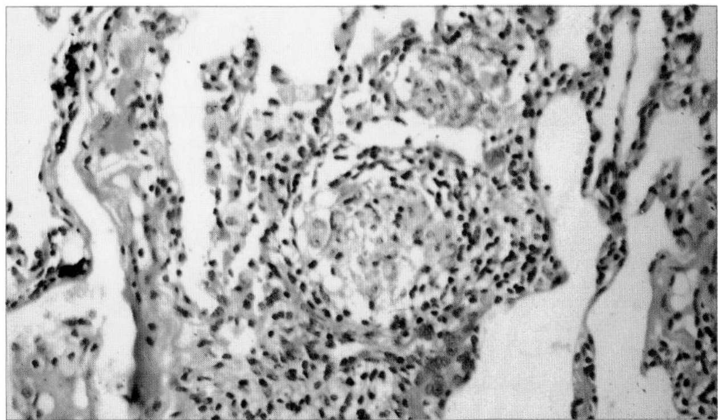

Fig. 18.13 Granuloma in the alveolar wall in a section of biopsy material taken from a patient with extrinsic allergic alveolitis.

Bronchoalveolar lavage cells in granulomatous lung diseases

Group	% lymphocytes	CD4:CD8 ratio
Normals	10	1.5:2
Sarcoidosis	50	5:1
Beryllium disease	50*	5:1
EAA (even some asymptomatic individuals)	60–70+	<1

*lymphocytes show proliferative response to beryllium salts
+lymphocytes show proliferative response to pigeon serum in pigeon fancier's lung

Fig. 18.14 Proportion of lymphocytes recovered at BAL from cases of granulomatous lung diseases.

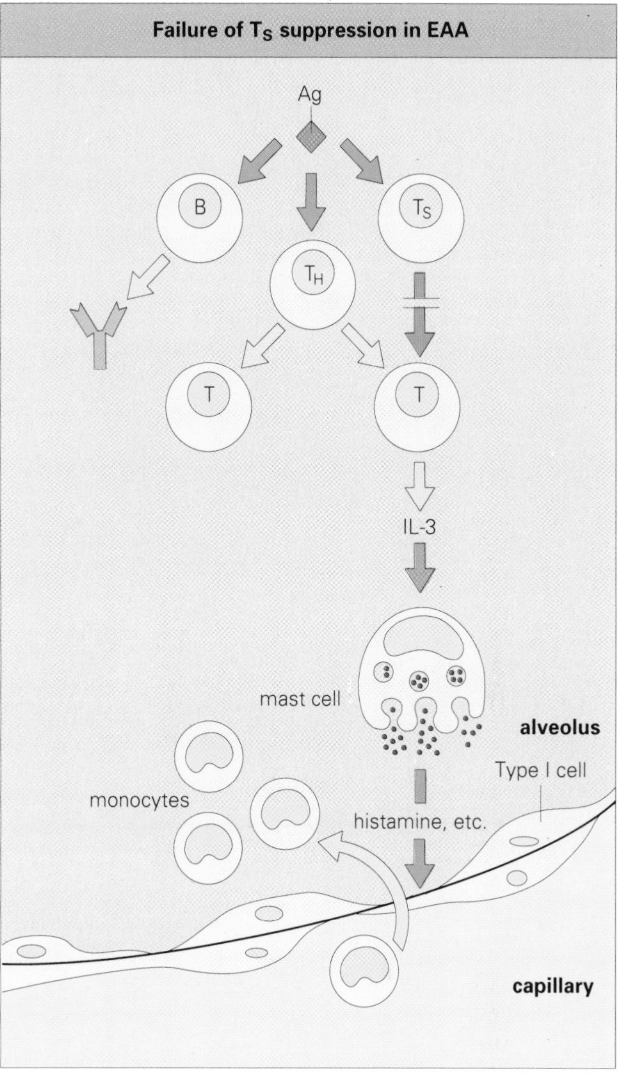

Fig. 18.15 In extrinsic allergic alveolitis (EAA), antigen specific T suppressor (Ts) lymphocytes fail to inhibit the T helper (TH) lymphocyte dependent response to inhaled antigen, and permit the subsequent inflammatory response, which includes IL-3-driven mast cell recruitment.

beryllium disease without pulmonary shadowing, which does not resolve spontaneously. The diagnosis of beryllium disease is made and distinguished from sarcoidosis by:

- history of exposure to beryllium;
- identification of beryllium in elevated concentration in the lungs or mediastinal glands;
- positive beryllium transformation test in blood or BAL lymphocytes;
- negative Kveim test.

Control of exposure to beryllium in the UK has now made this condition uncommon.

Some causes of extrinsic allergic alveolitis		
Disease	**Antigen source**	**Antigen**
Farmer's lung	mouldy hay, straw or grain	*Micropolyspora faeni* *Thermoactinomyces vulgaris*
Pigeon fancier's lung Budgerigar fancier's lung	avian excreta	avian serum proteins
Bagassosis	mouldy bagasse (sugar cane)	*Thermoactinomyces sacchari*
Malt worker's lung	mouldy maltings	*Aspergillus clavatus*
Mushroom worker's lung	spores generated during mushroom spawning	thermophilic actinomycetes
Maple bark stripper's lung	removing bark from stored maple, sycamore, etc	*Cryptostroma corticale*
Ventilation pneumonitis	contaminated air conditioning systems	thermophilic actinomycetes

Fig. 18.16 Some of the causes of extrinsic allergic alveolitis.

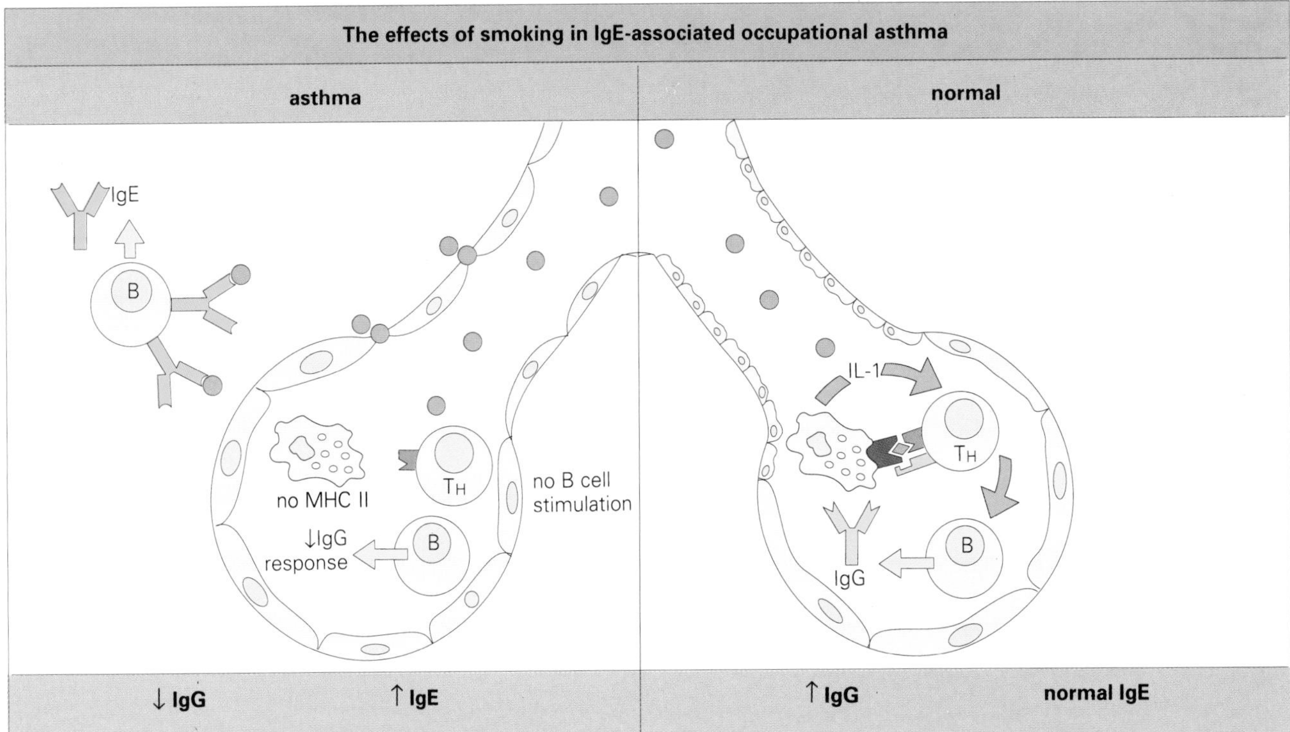

Fig. 18.17 Different effects of smoking in IgE associated occupational asthma. Smoking enhances IgE production, possibly by increasing bronchial mucosal permeability but inhibits the IgG response, possibly by down-regulating MHC class II expression by alveolar macrophages and thus inhibiting antigen presentation.

EXTRINSIC ALLERGIC ALVEOLITIS

Extrinsic allergic alveolitis (or hypersensitivity pneumonitis) is a T lymphocyte dependent granulomatous inflam-
18.10 matory reaction in the lungs to inhaled organic dusts. The disease involves both peripheral bronchioles and the gas exchanging parts of the lungs. The disease may be caused by:

- microbial spores from moulds which grow on vegetable material such as hay, straw, grains and mushroom compost;

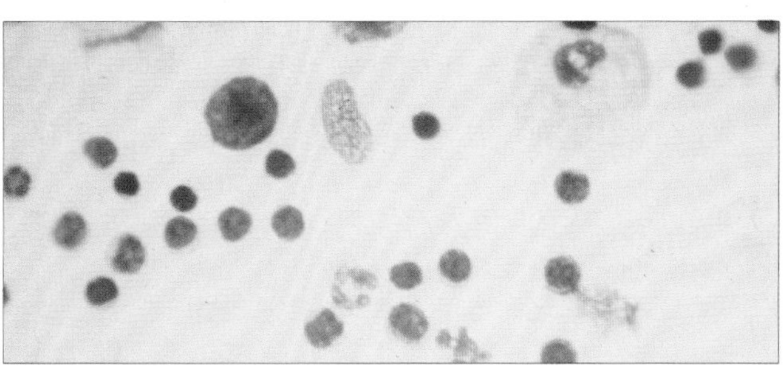

Fig. 18.18 Farmer's lung. There is an increased proportion of lymphocytes in the cells recovered at BAL.

Diagnosis of extrinsic allergic alveolitis (EAA)
history of exposure to potential source, usually at home or in work place
symptomatic, functional & radiographic changes consistent with disease
precipitating antibodies in serum to relevant antigen
BAL ↑ lymphocytes with reversed $CD4^{+}$: $CD8^{+}$ ratio mast cells
lung biopsy granulomatous inflammation centred in bronchioles
inhalation testing with antigen late ↓FEV_1 ↓ CO transfer factors (Kco & DLco)

Fig. 18.19 The last three investigations listed are not essential, but may aid diagnosis.

• foreign animal proteins, particularly from birds, and most commonly pigeons and budgerigars.

Some of the more important causes of EAA are shown in Fig. 18.16. Of these, farmer's lung and bird fancier's lung are the most prevalent causes in the UK and USA.

Farmer's lung

Farmer's lung is the outcome of an allergic response to inhaled thermophilic actinomycetes, most commonly *Micropolyspora faeni* and *Thermoactinomyces vulgaris*. Crops harvested wet and stored with a high water content encourage the growth of moulds, with the generation of heat. Thermophilic actinomycetes such as *M. faeni* and *T. vulgaris* grow and sporulate at temperatures in excess of 50°C. Inhalation of spores and mycelial fragments occur when bales of mouldy hay are opened in enclosed and poorly ventilated barns.

Farmer's lung can be prevented by substitution of silage for hay and by ensuring hay, straw and grain is stored in dry and well-ventilated conditions. It remains a problem on small under-capitalized farms in areas of high rainfall.

In farmer's lung and bird fancier's lung the relevant precipitating antibodies are also both more common in non-smokers than smokers. The reason for this is unclear but may reflect a generalized impairment of alveolar macrophage phagocytosis and antigen presentation in tobacco smokers (Fig. 18.17).

Pathology. The T lymphocytes participating in EAA and beryllium disease can be studied directly by examining the cells recovered at BAL. Patients with disease characterized by granuloma formation (not only EAA and beryllium disease but also TB and sarcoidosis) have an increased proportion of T lymphocytes (Fig. 18.18).

Clinical features

The pattern of disease in EAA depends primarily on the nature and intensity of exposure to the cause (see chapter 12).

Acute recurrent alveolitis. This occurs in those intermittently exposed to high concentrations of antigen, for example farmers going into their barns once a week. Typically, breathlessness with flu-like symptoms develops 4–8 hours after exposure. These episodes are associated with widespread nodular shadowing on the chest radiograph associated with a restrictive ventilatory defect of lung function and impaired gas transfer measurements. In the absence of further exposure, symptoms, radiographic and lung function abnormalities may resolve spontaneously.

Acute progressive alveolitis. Those exposed continuously to high antigen levels develop increasingly severe breathlessness and flu-like symptoms with fever and weight loss. This is associated with progressive shadowing on the chest X-ray and severe abnormalities of lung function.

Chronic alveolitis. Upper lobe fibrosis and volume loss occur either as a consequence of recurrent exposure to high concentration of antigen or as the outcome of continuous exposure to antigen in concentrations insufficient to cause acute systemic and respiratory symptoms but sufficient to cause progressive insidious pulmonary damage. The chest radiograph shows bilateral upper lobe contractions with fibrosis and cystic changes. The abnormalities in lung function tests reflect the small stiff lungs with impaired gas transfer. The changes in the lungs at this stage of the disease are usually irreversible.

Diagnosis and management

The diagnosis of EAA is outlined in Fig. 18.19. The management of established cases is based upon avoidance of exposure so that future damage to the lungs does not occur. Many patients with farmer's lung and bird fancier's lung are able to continue in employment or to enjoy their hobby, provided they minimize exposure to antigen sources and wear adequate respiratory protection when exposure is unavoidable. The effectiveness of these measures should be regularly monitored with serial testing of lung function in conjunction with careful pharmacological management.

FURTHER READING

Chan Yeung M, Lam S. Occupational asthma. *Am Rev Respir Dis.* 1986; **133**: 686–703.

Churg A, Green FY. *Pathology of occupational lung disease.* New York: Igaku Shoin, 1988.

Newman Taylor AJ. Allergy, occupation and the lung. *Postgrad Med J.* 1988; **64 (suppl 4)**: 41–47.

Newman Taylor AJ, Tee R. Occupational lung disease. *Curr Opin Immunol.* 1989; **1**: 684–689.

Parkes R. *Occupational lung disease.* Sevenoaks: Butterworths, 1982.

Saltini C, Winestock K, Kirby M, *et al.* Maintenance of alveolitis in patients with chronic beryllium disease by beryllium specific helper T cells. *New Engl J Med.* 1989; **320**: 1103–1109.

18.12 Salvaggio JE. Hypersensitivity pneumonitis. *J Allergy Clin Immunol.* 1987: **79**: 558–571.

19

Drug Hypersensitivity

INTRODUCTION

This chapter concentrates on the clinical manifestations of drug reactions for which there is some evidence of an underlying immunological mechanism. Many patterns of response affecting various organs have been reported and some are briefly mentioned. However, it must be remembered that the symptoms and signs are not unique to drug-induced immune reactions; many can be associated with the underlying disease, whilst others may be idiosyncratic responses or rare toxic phenomena of the drug. Occasionally, drugs can cause release of intracellular mediators by activation of complement through the alternative pathway, or they may act directly without involvement of the immune system (anaphylactoid reaction). The criteria for induction and elicitation of immune-based responses are described, as well as the mechanisms leading to tissue damage. Often, the antigen has not been identified and reasons for this are given. Conversely, the antigenic basis of penicillin allergy is clearer than for most other drugs and this is used as an instructive model. Finally, suggestions towards making a more definitive diagnosis and some important aspects of management are highlighted.

MANIFESTATIONS OF DRUG HYPERSENSITIVITY

Immune reactions associated with drug therapy can affect virtually every organ (Fig. 19.1):

- Dermatological manifestations. Rash may be one of a variety of types, from localized contact dermatitis or angio-oedema to diffuse urticaria or widespread macular/papular rash. When secondary to bone marrow effects, purpura may be found. The skin is the most commonly affected organ.
- Haematological manifestations may affect the circulating blood (e.g. haemolytic anaemia) or any of the cellular components in the bone marrow (e.g. eosinophilia, thrombocytopenia, agranulocytosis or pancytopenia).
- Hepatic manifestations may occur as cholestatic or hepatic jaundice.
- Renal manifestations may occur as oliguria or nephrotic syndrome.
- Pulmonary manifestations may affect the bronchi (e.g. bronchospasm) or the parenchyma (e.g. eosinophilic infiltrates).

In many instances, the reactions are not confined to one organ, although maximum physiological disturbance may be so focused; for example, renal failure from interstitial nephritis requires specific medical treatment but may be associated with rash, pyrexia and possibly eosinophilia.

The severity of the reaction can also vary, ranging from acute, life-threatening anaphylaxis to a mild rash requiring no specific therapy. Even dermatological reactions vary in the degree of incapacitation which they incur and some, such as purpura, can herald a potentially life-threatening situation.

Features suggestive of drug hypersensitivity include:

- prior contact with the same substance or one of similar chemical structure;
- reaction occurring with doses which are small in relation to the therapeutic dose;
- no dose-response effect;
- reaction unrelated to pharmacological effects;
- other manifestations of allergy occurring concurrently;
- the reaction affects only a minority of the exposed population

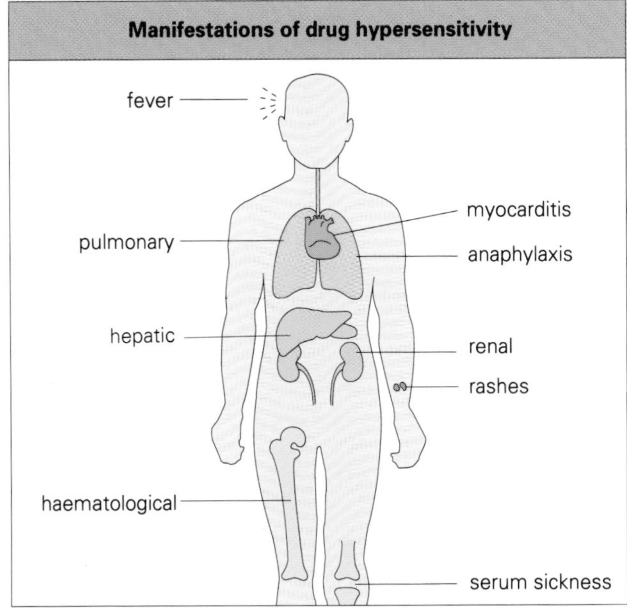

Fig. 19.1 Several organs are often involved, although presentation may be related to one aspect. Thus, a patient may complain of a rash and be found to have eosinophilia and pyrexia. Fever may be low-grade or widely swinging. Serum sickness classically causes swelling and inflammation of the joints, particularly the large joints. Anaphylaxis is a widespread effect due to type I hypersensitivity, whereas myocarditis is probably mediated by a type III mechanism (immune-complex).

These features may be difficult to elucidate and none is specific for a hypersensitive state.

The role of atopy as a predisposing factor is uncertain. Different surveys, even those performed using the same drug and concentrating on the immediate, presumed type I immunological reaction have often produced conflicting conclusions.

Mechanisms of tissue damage

All four hypersensitivity reactions defined by Gell and Coombs are involved in the range of reactions to drugs. These are described in detail in chapter 1.

ORGAN-BASED EFFECTS

DERMATOLOGICAL

Skin lesions not only vary in appearance but can result from any one of the four types of immunological reactions (Fig. 19.2).

Possible mechanisms of skin reactions	
Type I	urticaria angio-oedema
Type II	purpura
Type III	vasculitis ±necrosis
Type IV	fixed drug eruption contact dermatitis exfoliative dermatitis erythema multiforme bullous reactions morbilliform, maculopapular rash

Fig. 19.2 Possible mechanisms of drug-induced skin reactions.

Urticaria

Urticaria and angio-oedema are mediated by type I mechanisms and have been associated with the administration of penicillins (Fig. 19.3).

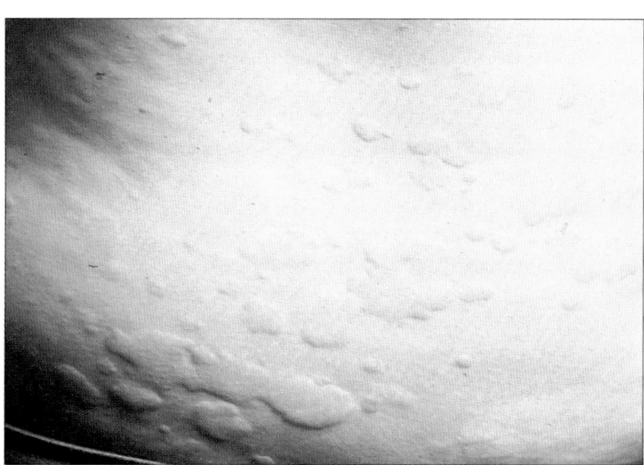

Fig. 19.3 Urticaria, showing typically raised, irregularly-shaped weals, the centre of which will blanch if lightly covered with a transparent rule or microscope slide. Lesions tend to be transient. Courtesy of St Mary's Hospital Medical School.

Purpura

Purpura (Fig. 19.4) is a dermatological manifestation of a type II cytotoxic reaction against circulating platelets, causing thrombocytopenia. The mechanism was elucidated using the hypnotic drug Sedormid, and other studies using quinidine. Antibody and complement are both essential for platelet lysis.

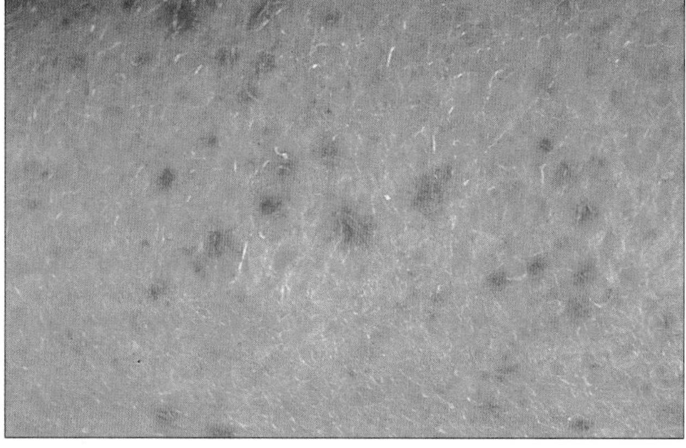

Fig. 19.4 Purpura, showing pinpoint haemorrhagic lesions which do not blanch and remain fixed for days, while fading. Courtesy of The Institute of Dermatology, UMDS Guy's & St Thomas' Hospitals.

Vasculitis

Vasculitis (Fig. 19.5), which is due to the immune-complex (type III) mechanism, is a dermatological manifestation of a generalized condition. Antibody-containing deposits can be detected in histological samples of the lesions using immunofluorescent techniques. An immune complex reaction, seen as erythema nodosum, can occur with the administration of dapsone for lepromatous leprosy. This is not a drug hypersensitivity reaction but is caused by the intravascular interaction of antibodies to *Mycobacterium lepri,* with bacterial antigens released from organisms killed by dapsone.

Erythema multiforme

Erythema multiforme is often associated with administration of barbiturates, co-trimoxazole, penicillins and sulphonamides. Deposits of IgM and C3 have been found around blood vessels in skin biopsies. Circulating immune complexes occur in some patients with erythema multiforme and those with concomitant lesions of the mucosal surfaces (Stevens-Johnson syndrome) (Fig. 19.6).

It is likely that these conditions are a less severe form of toxic epidermal necrolysis (Lyell's syndrome) (Fig. 19.7) and that the mucocutaneous lymph node syndrome (Kawasaki disease) is part of the same spectrum. There are many overlapping features and it is possible that the clinical picture is determined by an interaction of many factors including age, gender, primary infection or disease, and genotype. Whether hypersensitivity to the drug is the direct cause of the reaction remains uncertain.

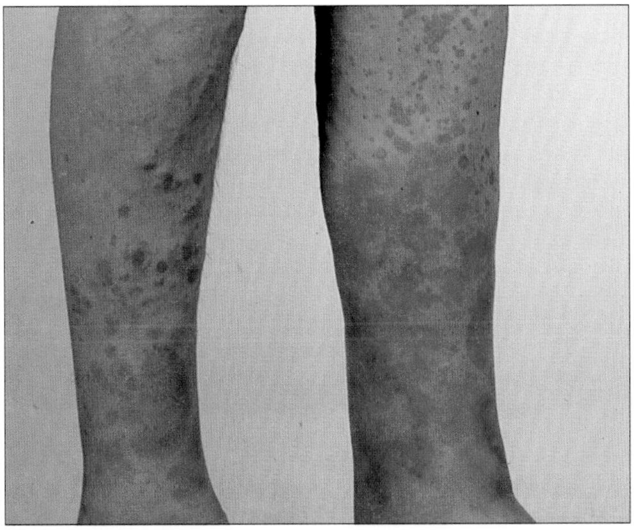

Contact dermatitis

Contact dermatitis (Fig. 19.8) due to drugs occurs either as an industrial disease among production or medical staff, or in patients being treated with topical medicaments. Some drugs which have been implicated include:

- penicillins
- cephalosporins
- streptomycin
- and neomycin.

Fig. 19.5 Vasculitis, showing reddened areas coinciding with inflammatory lesions around superficial blood vessels. Lesions remain fixed for some days. Courtesy of Dr A du Vivier & King's College Hospital.

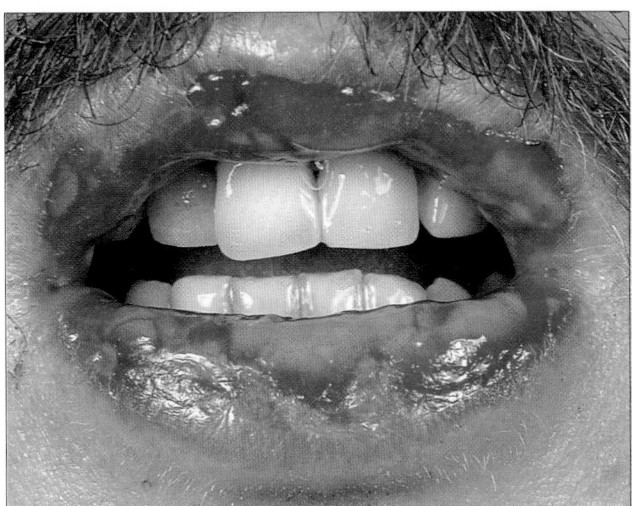

Fig. 19.6 Stevens-Johnson syndrome. This is a severe type of erythema multiforme and is associated with a significant mortality rate. The skin and mucous membranes are involved, as well as the lungs, gut, kidneys, and joints; there is profound systemic upset with fever. Blisters can be confused with bullous pemphigoid but immunofluorescence is negative. Courtesy of Dr A du Vivier & King's College Hospital.

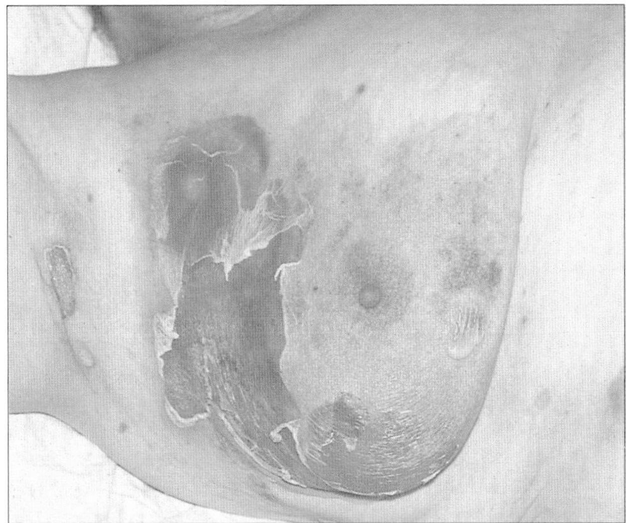

Fig. 19.7 Lyell's ('scalded skin') syndrome. This can be a hypersensitivity reaction to drugs such as sulphonamides, barbiturates, or phenylbutazone. The skin begins to shed all over the body, leaving a raw oozing surface. Even if the drug is identified and stopped, the prognosis is poor. Treatment is with systemic steroids and antibiotics, where indicated, to combat secondary infection. Courtesy of Dr R Staughton.

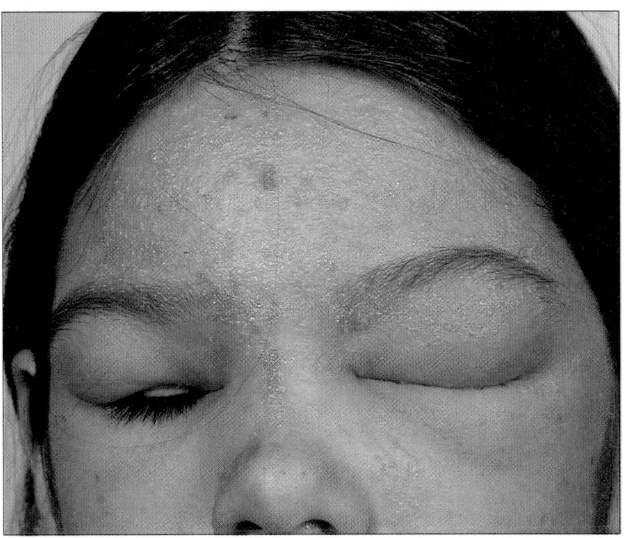

Fig 19.8 Contact dermatitis. Severe eczematous reaction around the eyes caused by mepyramine maleate cream. Courtesy of Dr A du Vivier & King's College Hospital.

Additives in topical medicaments are also likely to cause this problem.

There are many other dermal reactions which may have a type IV reaction as their basis, including fixed drug eruptions (Fig. 19.9), exfoliative dermatitis, and morbilliform or maculopapular exanthemata. Evidence positively linking these manifestations to immune drug reactions is inconclusive.

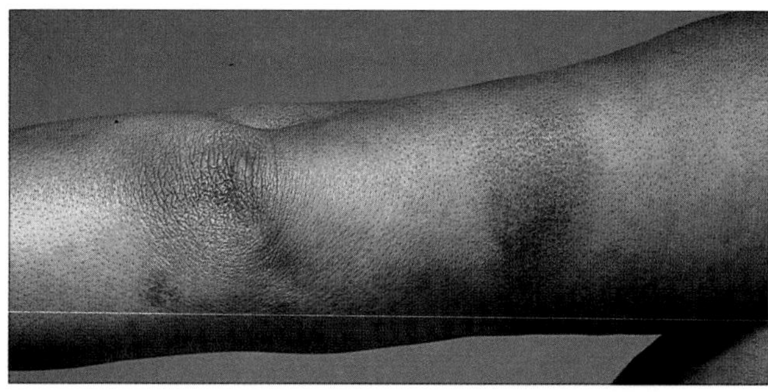

Fig. 19.9 Fixed drug eruption. Single or multiple lesions appear, affecting identical sites each time the drug is taken; they subside quickly once the drug is stopped. Laxatives containing phenolphthalein are the most common cause, but antibiotics such as griseofulvin, tetracycline and sulphonamides, as well as phenacetin and barbiturates, have also been implicated. Courtesy of Dr A du Vivier & King's College Hospital.

HAEMATOLOGICAL

Haemolytic anaemia

Haemolytic anaemia is associated with a number of drugs as a result of at least four distinct mechanisms (Fig. 19.10):

- Penicillin molecules attach to the red blood cell (RBC) membrane and induce the formation of IgG antibodies with penicillin specificity. These antibodies react with the membrane-fixed penicillin (Fig. 19.11 left) in a type II immunological reaction. The phenomenon can be recognized by a positive direct antiglobulin test (see chapter 16). Intravascular haemolysis may occur, but is not invariable.
- Cephalosporin antibiotics have some structural similarities to penicillins. They can also give rise to a positive direct antiglobulin test but haemolysis does not result. The mechanism, although broadly similar, differs because the serum proteins attached to the RBC do not have cephalosporin specificity (Fig.19.11 right). The drug causes a modification of the RBC membrane which facilitates non-immunological adsorption of serum proteins. Thus, the direct antiglobulin test becomes positive. A similar mechanism occurs with clavulanic acid, an inhibitor of bacterial β-lactamase, which is used in combination with certain penicillins, such as amoxycillin and ticarcillin.

Mechanisms of drug-induced anaemia
drug adsorption to erythrocytes → antibodies to drug
drug adsorption → non-specific antibody binding
induction of type III reaction → bystander lysis of RBC
drug → RBCs as autoantigens

Fig. 19.10 Mechanisms of drug-induced anaemia.

Effect of drugs on circulating RBCs

Penicillin	Cephalosporin
induce antibody	non-immune γ-globulin
direct anti-globulin test +ve haemolysis	**direct anti-globulin test +ve no haemolysis**

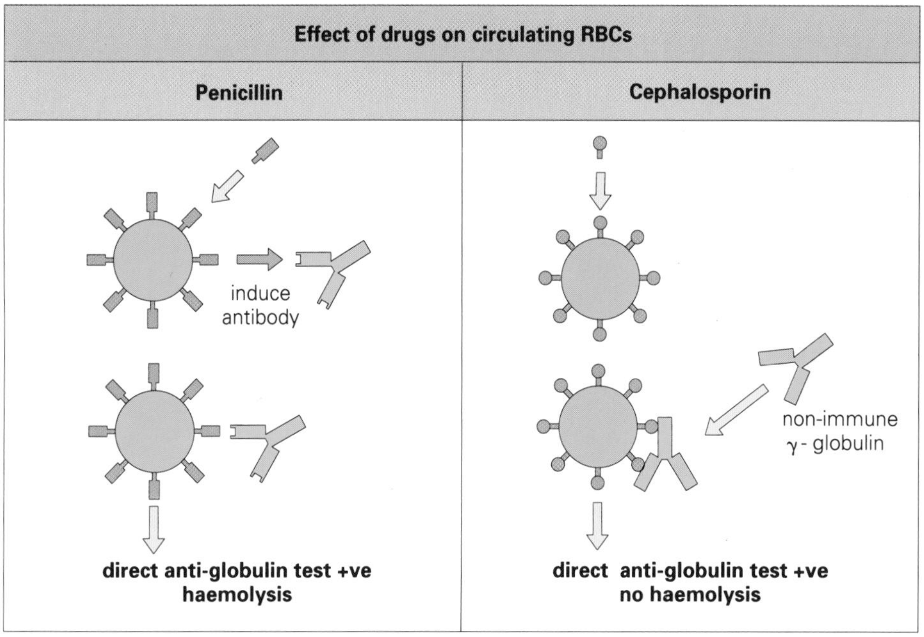

Fig. 19.11 Left: penicillins attach to the RBC membrane and induce specific antibodies, to give a positive direct antiglobulin test. Right: cephalosporins induce a positive direct antiglobulin test by adsorption of cephalosporins and non-specific γ-globulin onto the RBC. Haemolysis occurs in a proportion of patients receiving penicillins but is rare with cephalosporins.

- A third type of haemolytic anaemia, caused by the 'innocent bystander' mechanism, involves a drug-antibody complex fixing complement to the RBC membrane (Fig. 19.12), and is an example of a type III immunological reaction. In some instances, it is the drug metabolite which induces antibody formation after interacting with a carrier protein. The antibodies are usually IgM but may be IgG or IgA, as in the case of nomifensine. Other drugs include antazoline, para-amino salicylic acid (PAS), and phenacetin.
- The fourth mechanism appears to be of an autoimmune type (Fig. 19.13). The drug modifies the developing RBC which then induces T cell sensitization. It is not known whether the new drug–self protein complex formed by processing acts as a T cell epitope. Through cooperation between T and B lymphocytes, antibody

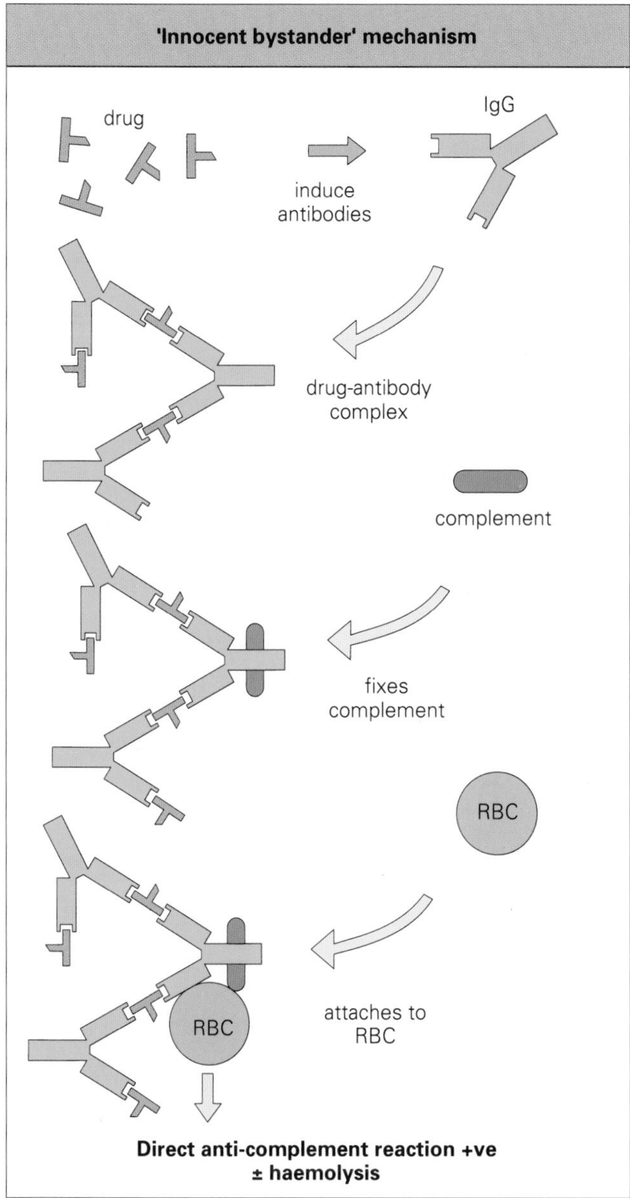

Fig. 19.12 The drug induces formation of antibodies, with which it complexes, and these then fix complement. The tripartite complex attaches to the RBC, probably by way of complement (immune adherence); this gives a positive direct anti-complement reaction. Haemolysis may occur and/or there is faster mononuclear phagocyte (MP) clearance because of the complex attached to the RBC.

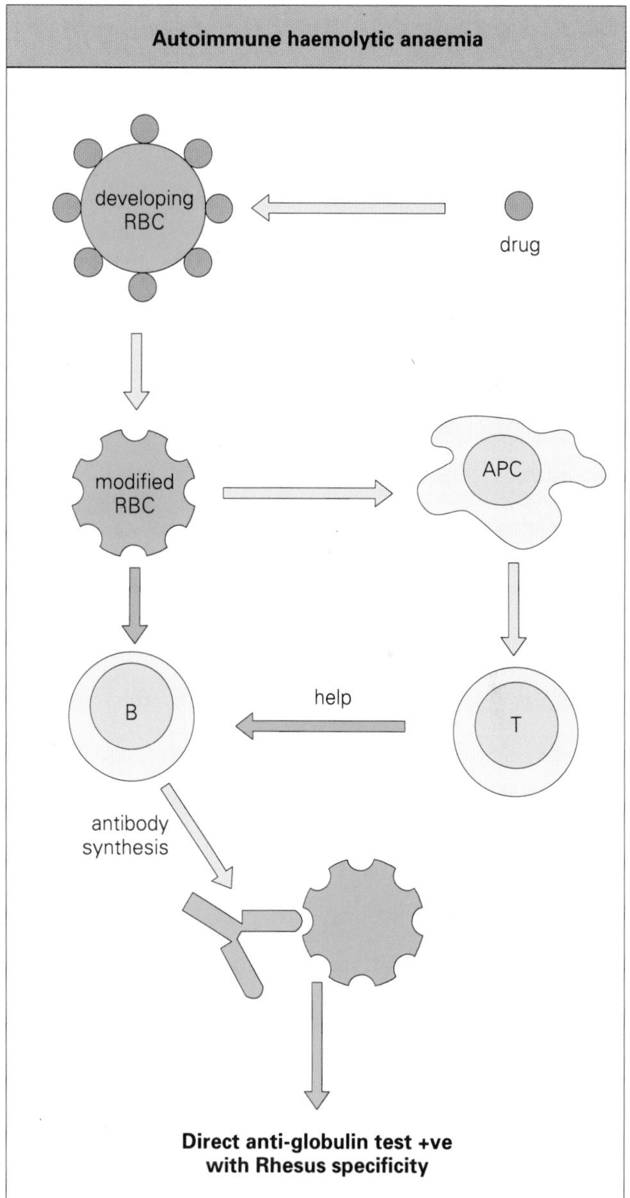

Fig. 19.13 Drug-induced autoimmune haemolytic anaemia has its pathogenesis during the development of the RBC when the drug causes a modification, which manifests itself in the structure of the mature RBC. The altered specificity is commonly within the Rhesus system. Antibodies directed against the altered specificity develop and attach to the RBCs, sometimes leading to haemolysis.

(usually of the warm IgG type and with Rhesus specificity) is produced against the RBC. The direct antiglobulin test is positive but only after several weeks or months of treatment. It remains positive for several months after drug withdrawal until all red cells containing the altered specificity have disappeared. Methyldopa, levodopa, procainamide and mefenamic acid can cause this effect.

Immune-induced thrombocytopenia

Immune-induced thrombocytopenia associated with drug therapy usually results from the 'innocent bystander' mechanism in which a drug–antibody complex fixes complement to the platelet membrane. Chlorothiazide, digitoxin, quinidine and quinine are well recognized aetiological agents.

Agranulocytosis and neutropenia

Agranulocytosis and neutropenia are rarely caused by an immunological mechanism, but rather by toxic effects. However, agglutinating antibodies to WBCs have been found in association with amidopyrine, quinidine, phenytoin, semi-synthetic penicillins, sulphonamides (including sulphasalazine), and thiouracils.

Lupus syndrome

The lupus syndrome can be induced by a number of drugs (Fig. 19.14). The mechanism is unclear but the resulting LE cells, anti-nuclear factor (ANF), and positive direct antiglobulin test (DAT) are probably a result of the drug forming complexes with cell proteins. These altered proteins sensitize leucocytes, which then destroy the cell with release of DNA.

The mechanisms may vary with different drugs. For instance, hydralazine-induced lupus, which appears predominantly in slow acetylators (as does that associated with procainamide), is associated with antibodies to histones H3 and H4 and to both double- and single-stranded DNA. With procainamide the antibodies are directed against histones H2A, H2B and only single-stranded DNA. Furthermore, there seems to be immunological cross-reactivity between procainamide and pyrimidine.

IgG anti-guanosine antibodies, and other autoantibodies against IgG and RBCs are also found in lupus induced by procainamide. Lymphocytotoxic antibodies appear and disappear in parallel with the development and resolution of procainamide-induced lupus, unlike the anti-nuclear antibodies which predate symptoms and persist after clinical resolution. Procainamide alters the normal lymphocyte response to phytohaemagglutinins (PHA or mitogens) in a dose-dependent biphasic manner, and may cause lupus syndrome via lymphocyte membrane alteration. The end result is a form of autosensitization (Fig. 19.15) which will regress after withdrawal of the drug. There seems to be enhancement of T-helper cells in procainamide-induced lupus, in contrast to impaired T-suppressor cell function in spontaneous SLE, although there are conflicting data.

There is some evidence to indicate that inhibition of the covalent binding of activated C3 and C4 occurs with

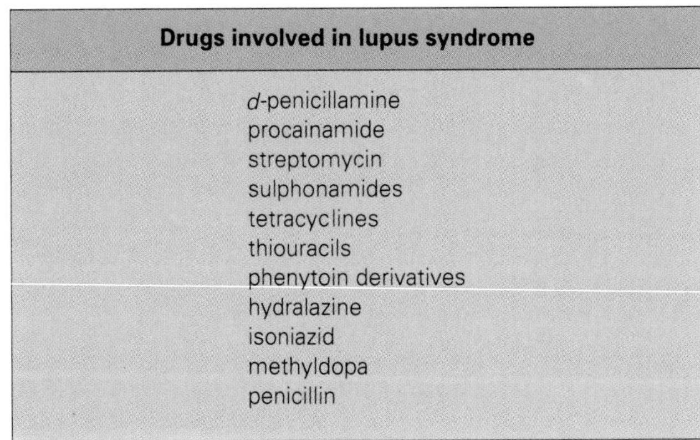

Drugs involved in lupus syndrome
d-penicillamine
procainamide
streptomycin
sulphonamides
tetracyclines
thiouracils
phenytoin derivatives
hydralazine
isoniazid
methyldopa
penicillin

Fig. 19.14 Drugs involved in the lupus syndrome.

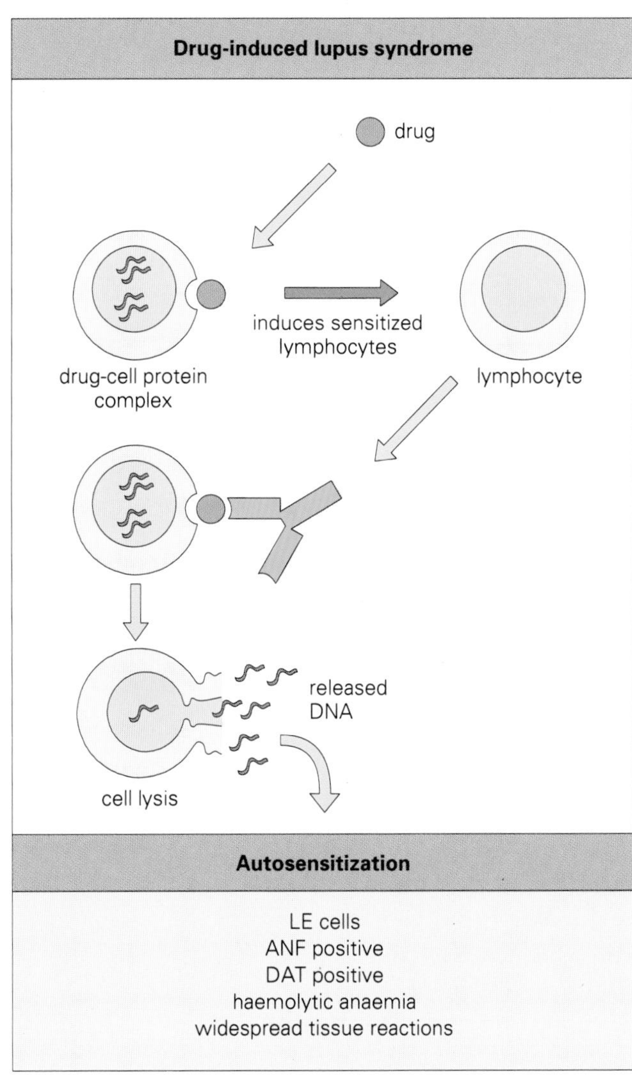

Fig. 19.15 The mechanism of drug-induced lupus syndrome is complicated. The drug forms complexes with proteins of many cells, causing lymphocyte sensitization. Widespread tissue damage results, with cell lysis releasing DNA and other nuclear components. Antibodies occur to some of these components, leading to generalized autosensitization .

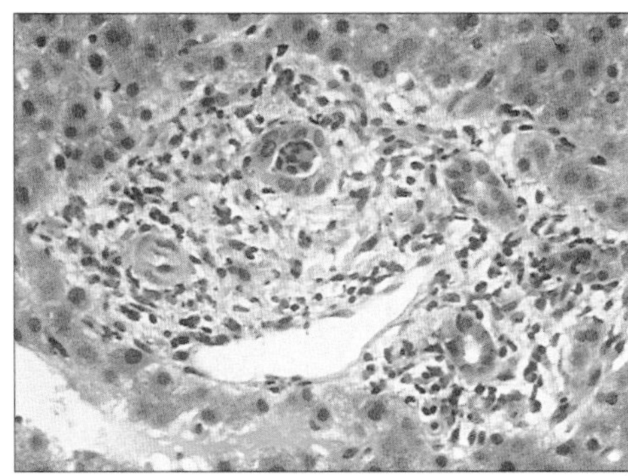

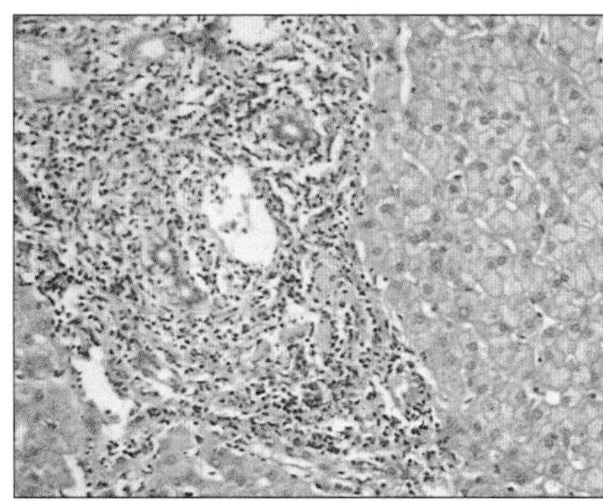

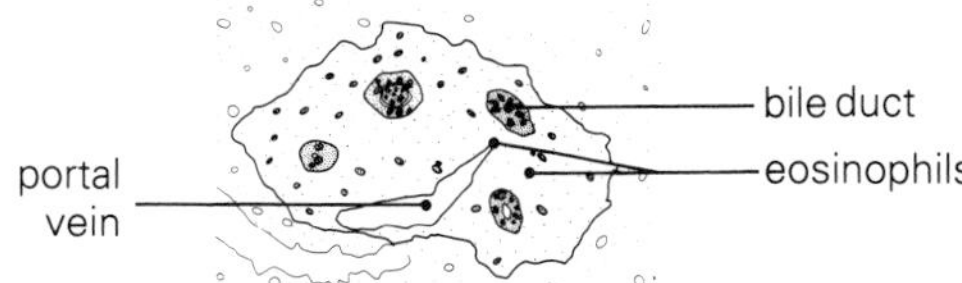

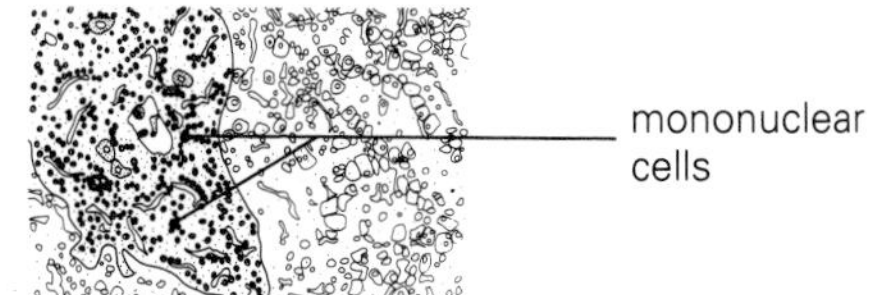

Fig. 19.16 Drugs may cause cholestatic or hepatic jaundice, usually with other manifestations of allergy. Left: chlorpromazine-induced cholestatic jaundice showing eosinophilic infiltrate in the portal tract. Courtesy of Dr I Talbot. Right: hepatic jaundice showing periportal mononuclear infiltrate. Courtesy of Dr A Price.

hydralazine and isoniazid, and can be induced by nucleophilic metabolites of procainamide and practolol. Such inhibition would reduce clearance of immune complexes, increasing the likelihood of developing lupus syndrome.

HEPATIC

Jaundice or other evidence of liver damage can occur during drug treatment but many of these effects are probably toxic rather than allergic in origin. However, there is suggestive evidence that immunological mechanisms are involved in some situations. Chlorpromazine can give rise to cholestatic jaundice accompanied by fever and eosinophilic infiltrates (Fig. 19.16). Hepatic jaundice, characterized by portal and periportal inflammation with mononuclear cell infiltration, has been reported with methyldopa, isoniazid and oxyphenisatin. Anti-smooth muscle and anti-nuclear antibodies are often found in these cases, sometimes with anti-mitochondrial antibodies (see chapter 4) and LE cells. Halothane hepatitis is associated with antibodies, detectable by ELISA, which react with halothane-induced liver antigens.

RENAL

Nephrotic syndrome and oliguric renal failure have been associated with immune reactions to drugs, particularly by a type II mechanism or as a component of serum sickness syndrome. For example, renal biopsies have shown deposits of immunoglobulin and complement on the glomerular basement membrane in the presence of circulating antibodies to *d*-penicillamine (Fig. 19.17). A similar membranous nephropathy also occurs with gold and allopurinol; some patients develop nephrotic syndrome.

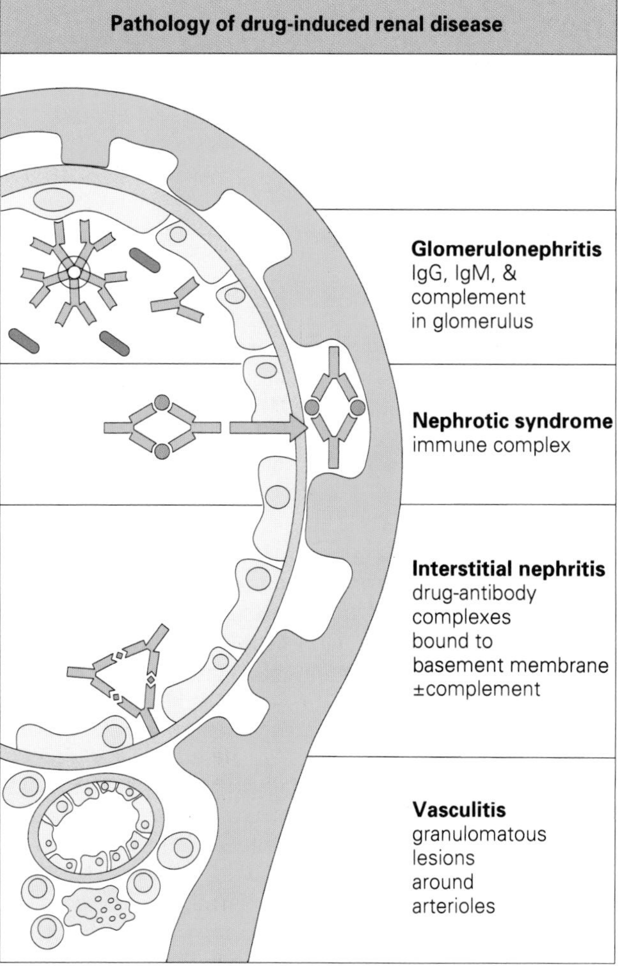

Fig. 19.17 Examination of renal biopsies may reveal deposition of immunoglobulin or complement in the region of the glomerular basement membrane.

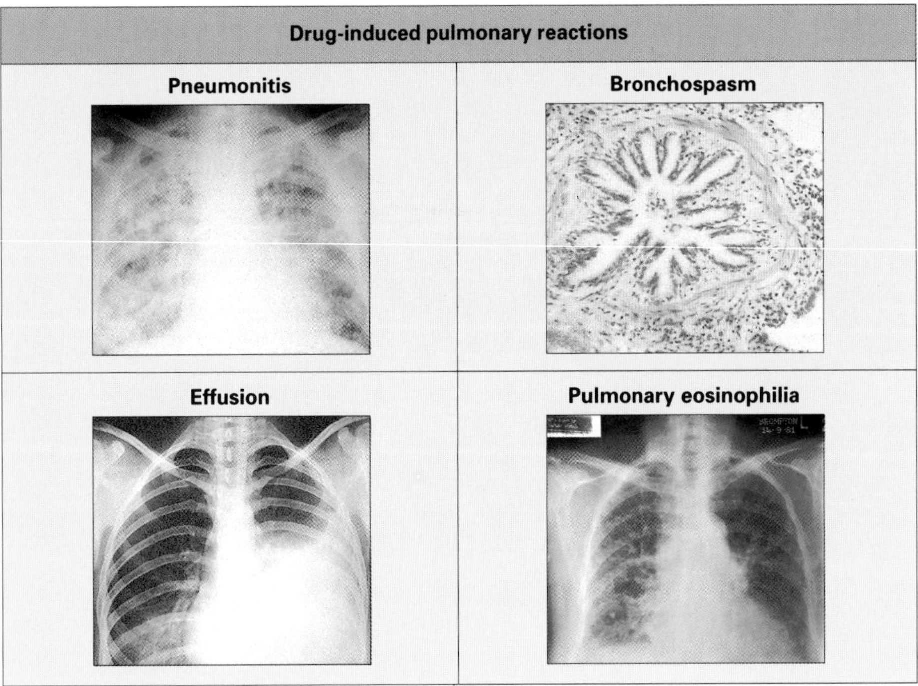

Fig. 19.18 Pulmonary reactions range from widespread pneumonitis (Courtesy of Dr M E Hodson), through diffuse eosinophilic infiltrates (Courtesy of Professor M Turner-Warwick) to bronchospasm (Courtesy of Professor M Turner-Warwick). Pleural effusion (Courtesy of Dr M E Hodson) can also occur as a result of an allergic reaction.

Methicillin has been associated with antibodies to the tubular basement membrane which have been found both fixed locally and circulating in the blood.

PULMONARY

Acute asthma

Acute asthma often occurs as part of general anaphylaxis following massive histamine release in allergies to penicillin and muscle relaxants. It also occurred during reactions, mediated via the alternative pathway of complement activation, induced by the anaesthetic agent Althesin (now withdrawn) .

Pulmonary eosinophilia

Pulmonary eosinophilia (Fig. 19.18) has been reported following treatment with several drugs including aminosalicylic acid, carbamazepine, procarbazine and chlorpropamide. An interstitial pneumonitis can occur during treatment with nitrofurantoin, cytostatics (melphalan, methotrexate) and gold, in the latter instance associated with granulomata.

Methotrexate-induced alveolitis, which can be accompanied by eosinophilic infiltrates and granulomata, is associated with the presence of $CD4^+$ (helper) cells in bronchoalveolar lavage specimens. In alveolitis following amiodarone therapy, however, $CD8^+$ (cytotoxic) T cells usually predominate, suggesting a different pathogenesis.

Nitrofurantoin. This drug induces lymphoblastic transformation in cells from patients with acute pulmonary symptoms; autoantibodies to albumin and IgG–albumin complexes have also been found.

Bleomycin. This drug induces pulmonary interstitial pneumonitis and fibrosis, which is generally regarded as a toxic phenomenon. However, there is evidence that inhibition of T-suppressor cell activity occurs. In addition, laboratory studies have suggested that autoantibodies to collagen are produced. It is possible that the pulmonary fibrosis is, at least in part, an autoimmune reaction.

THE IMMUNE RESPONSE TO DRUGS

Induction phase

Drug molecules are generally too small to act as complete antigens and can only act as haptens (Fig. 19.19). The critical size seems to be around 1000 daltons, therefore combination with a macromolecule, or possibly polymerization, is a prerequisite. The chemical linkage, in most instances at least, is covalent. With the first exposure to the drug a delay of 5–10 days is required to allow formation of specific antibodies.

Drugs with larger molecular weights, particularly polypeptides or proteins, such as insulin, do not require prior combination to become antigenic.

Elicitation phase

Most drugs are monomeric and are therefore incapable of eliciting an allergic response (Fig. 19.20). They must become at least dimeric before they are capable of triggering reactions around the mast cell (and probably other cells) or of forming large complexes. They become divalent or multivalent either by attachment to macromolecules or by polymerization.

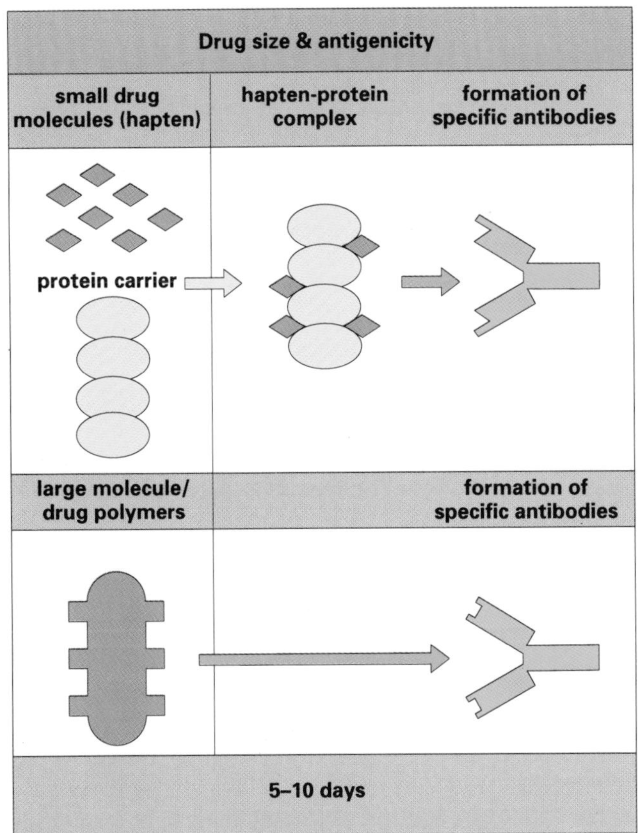

Fig. 19.19 Induction of allergy by drugs depends upon the molecular weight of the drug, which in most cases is too small to be antigenic; the drug can only become antigenic if it attaches to a large molecular carrier. The complex can then induce antibodies or sensitize lymphocytes with specificity directed towards the drug (hapten). For large molecules, combination with a carrier is unnecessary and such drugs can induce allergy directly.

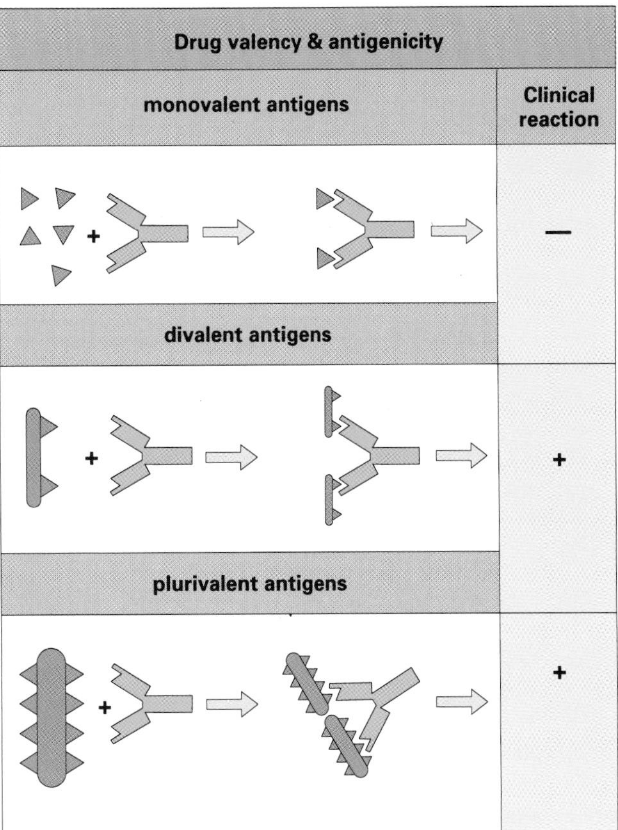

Fig. 19.20 Elicitation of an allergic response requires cross-linking of the antigen binding sites on the Fab sections of the antibody molecules. Monovalent antigens (most drugs) are unable to cross-link and cannot elicit a reaction. Divalent or multivalent antigens, such as haptens attached to a carrier, can readily cross-link and trigger a reaction.

Possible sources of antigens/haptens in drug preparations

From the pure drug
- pure drug substance
- degradation products
  - physical breakdown, polymerization

From added components
- contaminants
  - reactive chemicals, biological products
- pharmaceutical additives

After administration
- metabolites
  - of drugs, of additives/contaminants

Fig. 19.21 A hapten or antigen in a medicinal preparation may arise from several sources. These include those compounds purposely incorporated into the product by the manufacturer (i.e. the stated active component and pharmaceutical additives).

SOURCES OF ANTIGENS IN DRUGS

A clinical reaction associated with drug administration, even if mediated by immunological mechanisms, may not be due to hypersensitivity to the pure drug substance (Fig. 19.21) since the drugs used in clinical practice are often complex formulations.

Pure drug

The pure drug substance may be the specific antigen or act as the important hapten. However, the product used is rarely 100% pure, although the final specification is closely controlled. With storage between manufacture and use, there may be a small degree of degradation, or possibly polymerization, of the original substance or its degradation products. Although the quantity of any such change will be minute provided recommended storage conditions and times are observed, only a small amount of a highly antigenic substance might be necessary to induce sensitization.

Intermediate substances, additives and contaminants

During the manufacturing process of the active ingredient(s), small amounts of intermediate substances, or contaminants within the starting materials, may be retained. These contaminants may be small molecular weight chemicals, which would act as haptens, or they may be large molecules which could behave as complete antigens. The latter circumstance is most likely to occur in products of biological origin. Improvements in the control of manufacturing processes, greater precision and accuracy in analytical methods, and hence tighter specifications, have helped to reduce the potential risk from degradation and contamination.

There are often a number of manufacturing steps between the purification of the drug substance and its final packaging as a product for administration to patients. Some of these steps may consist of blending or mixing the active drug with 'inert' substances, to improve the stability of the active moiety, or to modify the bioavailability of the active substance for pharmacokinetic or therapeutic reasons, or to disguise an unpleasant taste. In addition, the product may be presented in tablets or capsules which contain dyes or other colouring agents of organic or inorganic origin.

Drug metabolites

Once the product has been administered to the patient, the various constituents may be metabolized. Metabolites of the drug substance will normally be identified in the blood, urine and faeces. However, it is always possible that an intermediate metabolite may be produced at the metabolic site and could act as an efficient hapten before further metabolism.

The multiplicity of potential antigens in drugs makes investigation of the mechanism of possible drug hypersensitivity extremely difficult. In addition, more than one hapten may be involved.

PENICILLIN AS A MODEL FOR DRUG HYPERSENSITIVITY

The immunological basis of penicillin allergy is clearer than for most other drugs and provides a useful model for the understanding of drug hypersensitivity.

BENZYLPENICILLIN

Hypersensitivity to benzylpenicillin presents in a variety of ways and through any one of the types of immune reaction. Anaphylaxis, although rare, is life-threatening and is determined by IgE antibodies (type I hypersensitivity). Haemolytic anaemia has a type II mechanism, interstitial nephritis is caused by type III, and contact dermatitis amongst medical staff is classically type IV.

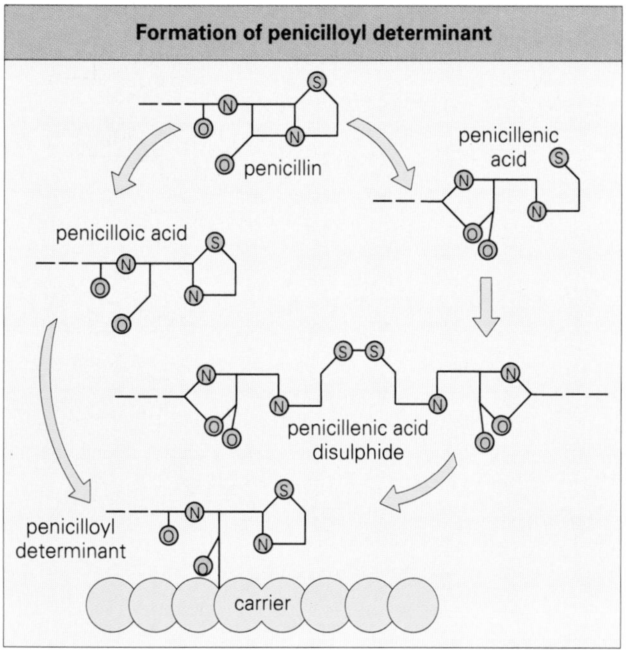

Formation of penicilloyl determinant

Fig. 19.22 Formation of the penicilloyl (major) determinant of penicillin allergy. For simplicity, only the carbon backbone of the penicillin 'nucleus' is shown. The hatched line indicates the portion of the molecule which varies with the type of penicillin. The hapten attaches to the carrier molecule through the β-lactam ring, hydrolysed at the C-N bond.

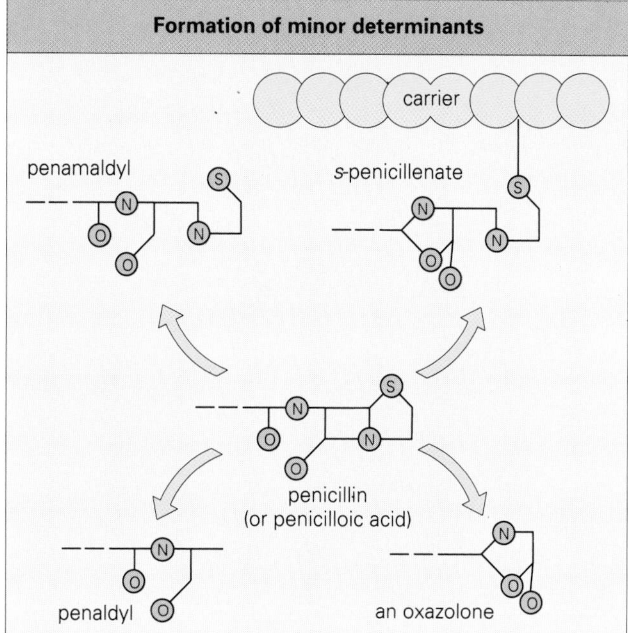

Fig. 19.23 Formation of some minor determinants of penicillin allergy, showing an example of combination with a carrier after hydrolysis of the C-S bond in the 5-membered thiazolidine ring of the 'nucleus'. Again for simplicity, only the carbon backbone of the penicillin 'nucleus' is shown. The hatched line indicates the portion of the molecule which varies with the type of penicillin.

Benzylpenicillin (penicillin G) is produced by fermentation of a *Penicillium* mould and it has been suggested that proteinaceous contaminants from the manufacture are responsible for at least some of the reactions. Manufacture of the semi-synthetic penicillins requires cleavage of the side-chain from penicillin G, originally achieved through a biological process using *E.coli*. It was thought that some of the reactions to ampicillin could be due to large molecular by-products from that process.

Benzylpenicillin has a molecular weight of 334 daltons and is, therefore, unable to act as a complete antigen. It has been shown that several haptens are formed *in vitro* and *in vivo*. The penicilloyl hapten is called the major determinant, as it seems to be the most frequently sensitizing moiety. It is generated either through penicillenic acid, which is formed in penicillin solutions, particularly when unbuffered, or through penicilloic acid (Fig.19.22).

Penicillenic acid can dimerize through disulphide bonds. The penicilloyl derivative reacts with a larger carrier *in vivo* to form a multivalent antigen.

MINOR DETERMINANTS

Various other haptens have been described which are collectively referred to as the minor determinants (Fig. 19.23). These haptens also attach to large carriers *in vivo*. Products of penicillin degradation or metabolism can form dimers by means other than through the disulphide bonds of penicillenic acid (Fig. 19.24). Polymerization can occur with a resulting linear polymer, or a mixture of various products can lead to formation of a complex polymer. All these polymers are of sufficient size to act as complete antigens and are multivalent.

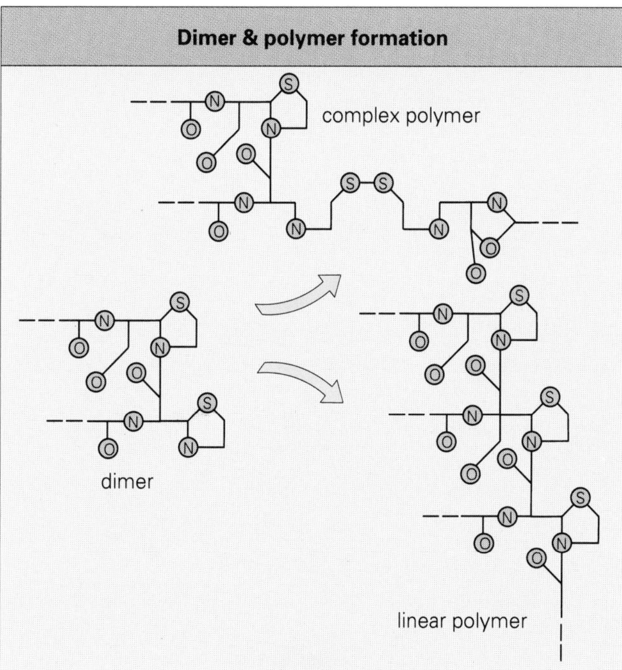

Fig. 19.24 Possible ways in which penicillins may form dimers, complex polymers and linear ploymers. The hatched line indicates the portion of the penicillin molecule which varies with the type of penicillin.

OTHER PENICILLINS

There are now many other penicillin derivatives in clinical use. They all retain the bicyclic 'nucleus' but differ with regard to the side-chain. These differences do not seem to be sufficient to prevent cross-reactivity of the newer analogues with antibodies generated by another penicillin. Thus, the specificity of the side-chain is of minor importance compared to that of the 'nucleus'.

CEPHALOSPORINS

Cephalosporin antibiotics have a similar mode of antibacterial activity to penicillin. Chemically, they have a bicyclic 'nucleus' but one of the rings differs in structure from that in penicillins (Fig. 19.25); in addition, there are two

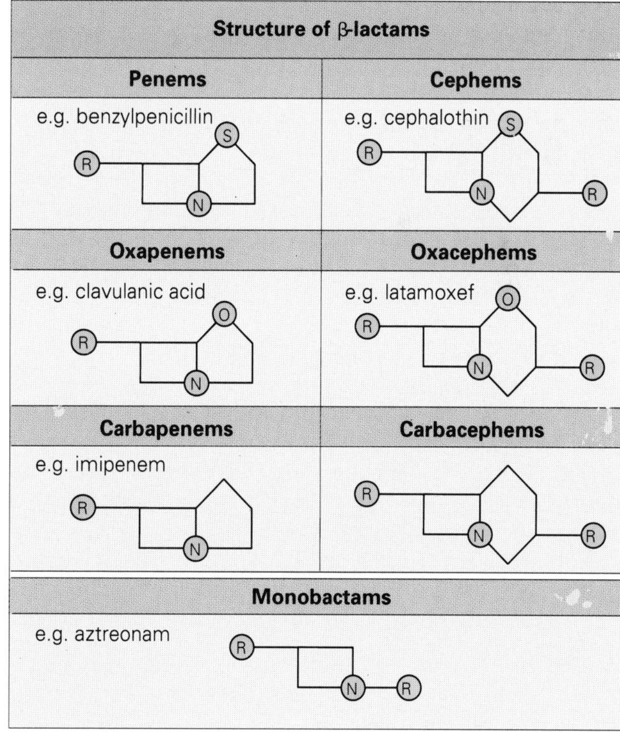

Fig. 19.25 Two differences exist between penems and cephems. Penems have a five-membered ring attached to the β-lactam ring, whereas cephems have a six-membered ring; one side chain is attached to the penem ring (at R), whereas two side chains are present in cephems (at R and R'). Monobactams consist of the four-membered, β-lactam ring to which two side-chains may be attached (at R and R'). Carbacephems are experimental compounds.

side chains (rather than one) attached to the ring structure. Cephalosporins can produce a cephalosporyl derivative, but this seems to be less stable than the penicilloyl equivalent. These differences may account for the better tolerance of cephalosporins than penicillins by hypersensitive patients.

OTHER β-LACTAMS

Both penicillins and cephalosporins contain the β-lactam ring in their 'nucleus'. There are now several other groups of β-lactam antibiotics. Latamoxef is similar to cephalosporins but has an oxygen atom instead of sulphur in the 'nucleus' (see Fig 19.25). Thus, disulphide bonding is not possible. Clavulanic acid has the basic penicillin nucleus but with the sulphur replaced by oxygen; it can cause a positive direct antiglobulin test but through a non-immune mechanism. Imipenem differs from penicillin in having a carbon atom instead of sulphur in the 'nucleus'. All these variations affect the ring attached to the β-lactam unit. Another recent derivative, aztreonam, does not possess this second ring; its 'nucleus' consists solely of the monocyclic β-lactam unit, hence the new family name of 'monobactam'. This difference in structure seems, significantly, to modify the immunological characteristics of these monocylic antibiotics. Aztreonam, for instance, seems to be less immunogenic than other β-lactam antibiotics, despite a small amount of the drug being metabolized to the open ring derivative (that is, breaking of the C-N bond in the ring). However, this derivative is very stable and has a low reactivity, unlike the penicillin or cephalosporin equivalents. In addition, aztreonam shows no significant cross-reactivity with penicillin and cephalosporins in *in vitro* tests, animal models or in patients.

Ampicillin and infectious mononucleosis

The use of ampicillin in patients with infectious mononucleosis is almost invariably followed by a maculopapular rash. The mechanism is unknown, but it is possible that T cell malfunction induced by the acute infection is the critical factor. Cephalexin, a cephalosporin with an identical side chain to ampicillin, does not induce this rash.

Some patients with chronic lymphocytic leukaemia seem to exhibit a similar rash following ampicillin treatment, and patients with AIDS receiving cotrimoxazole can develop rash and fever.

FACTORS PREDISPOSING TO DRUG HYPERSENSITIVITY

Defective or slow metabolism by certain routes is largely genetically determined and is associated with an increased incidence of hypersensitivity and toxic reactions to drugs metabolized predominantly by that route (Fig. 19.26).

The HLA type is also important in some drug reactions:

Factors predisposing to drug hypersensitivity
Metabolic defects
acetylation e.g. procainamide-induced lupus hydralazine-induced lupus
sulphoxidation e.g. *d*-penicillamine-induced myasthenia gravis gold toxicity carbon oxidation e.g. perhexilene-induced liver damage
HLA status
DR3 e.g. *d*-penicillamine side-effects (except myasthenia gravis)

Fig. 19.26 Factors predisposing to drug hypersensitivity.

Tests for diagnosis of drug allergy		
Mechanism	***In vitro* tests**	***In vivo* tests**
type I IgE	basophil degranulation histamine release RAST	Prausnitz-Kustner (PK) prick/intradermal skin tests
type III immune complex	haemagglutination precipitin	Arthus reaction bronchial provocation
type IV delayed hypersensitivity	lymphocyte transformation migration inhibition	patch tests
autoimmunization	LE cells ANF titre	
various	complement fractions biopsy	direct challenge

Fig. 19.27 *In vitro* and *in vivo* tests which may be used to determine drug allergy. The test should be selected on the basis of the likely underlying mechanism for the clinical manifestation. Some of these tests are non-specific, such as LE cells, ANF titre, complement fractions and biopsy. The other tests are specific.

the side-effects of *d*-penicillamine, such as thrombocytopenia and nephritis, are more common in patients possessing the DR3 haplotype.

DIAGNOSIS OF DRUG HYPERSENSITIVITY

It is often difficult to assert that a clinical reaction is due to drug hypersensitivity because of the factors mentioned previously. A good clinical history, including details of temporal relationships and associated allergic pointers, is fundamental. The clinical details may suggest the most likely immunological mechanism and lead to an apt choice of diagnostic tests. Some tests and their immunological basis are listed in Fig. 19.27.

Skin prick tests

Skin prick tests are probably safer than intradermal tests. It is essential that suitable concentrations and appropriate controls are used. They have been successfully used in identifying allergy to penicillins and muscle relaxants. The development of a positive weal and flare reaction, however, may not be due to immunologically-mediated histamine release, but rather to a direct effect of the drug on the mast cell, causing degranulation. It is probable that clinical reactions to radiological contrast media are of this type. Passive cutaneous anaphylaxis (PCA or P-K test) is seldom used because of the potential dangers involved in the injection of human serum into another subject. Many of the *in vitro* tests of IgE-mediated reactions are drug-specific. The RAST test is available only for penicillin allergy caused by the penicilloyl (major) determinant.

Patch tests

Patch testing must be carefully controlled to help distinguish irritant from immunological effects. The various *in vitro* tests can be specific if the correct antigen is chosen.

Rechallenge with the drug, using a small test dose, can be very useful in selected circumstances. Together with measurements of the various markers of an immune reaction, specific information is obtainable. Ethical considerations are of paramount importance in this procedure.

Sequential approach

A sequential approach to investigating whether a drug reaction is immunological in origin involves:

- taking a careful history;
- screening for non-specific evidence of an immunological reaction;
- studying with appropriate specific tests;
- performing a controlled rechallenge with monitoring of immunological markers.

A drug reaction must be fully investigated only if the same (or a similar) drug is likely to be used again in the same individual, for example, reactions to anaesthetics, where the drug should be identified and avoided in future operations. Similarly, children with leukaemia who react to antibiotic therapy should be investigated and, if necessary, desensitized to penicillin. For the majority of individuals, complete avoidance of the suspect drug without full investigation is the simplest and cheapest course.

MANAGEMENT OF DRUG HYPERSENSITIVITY

Details of management depend upon the type of reaction, the drug and the condition being treated. Life-threatening reactions need emergency treatment with adrenaline, corticosteroids and life-support systems as indicated. Other supportive measures may be necessary in some instances, such as severe thrombocytopenia or haemolytic anaemia, and appropriate organ functions should be monitored until they return to normal.

Withdrawal of the drug is logical, even in mild reactions. The patient must be informed and instructed to inform other clinicians in future, before any therapy is prescribed. Carrying or wearing an alerting message is desirable for patients who have experienced severe immediate reactions, particularly to common or emergency drugs.

In difficult clinical situations when the drug in question is by far the most appropriate, a process of desensitization may be necessary. In highly selected cases, this procedure often produced very satisfactory results, but if considered desirable it must be performed in hospitalized patients with full resuscitation facilities readily available.

FURTHER READING

Amos HE, Youlten LJH. Drug allergies. In: Lessof MH, ed. *Allergy: immunological and clinical aspects.* Chichester: John Wiley & Sons, 1984: 397–424.

Cooper JAD, White DA, Matthay RA. Drug-induced pulmonary disease. Part 1: Cytotoxic drugs. *Am Rev Respir Disease.* 1986; **133**: 321–340.

Cooper JAD, White DA, Matthay RA. Part 2: Non-cytotoxic drugs. *Am Rev Respir Disease.* 1986; **133**: 488–505.

Editorial. Myocarditis related to drug hypersensitivity. *Lancet.* 1985; **2**: 1165–1166.

Goldstein RA, Patterson R, eds. Drug allergy. Prevention, diagnosis, treatment (symposium proceedings). *J Allergy Clin Immunol.* 1984; **74**: 4, part 2, suppl.

Hess E. Drug-related lupus. *N Engl J Med.* 1988; **318**: 1460–1462.

Hughes CRV. Recent developments in drug-associated systemic lupus erythematosus. *Adverse Drug React Bull.* 1987; **123**: 460–463.

Kale SA. Drug-induced systemic lupus erythematosus: differentiating it from the real thing. *Postgrad Med.* 1985; **77**: 231–242.

Petz LD. Drug-induced immune haemolysis. *N Engl J Med.* 1985; **313**: 510–511.

Salama A, Mueller-Eckhardt C. The role of metabolite-specific antibodies in nomifensine-dependent immune haemolytic anaemia. *N Engl J Med.* 1985; **313**: 469–474.

Sim E, Stanley L, Gill EW, Jones A. Metabolites of procainamide and practolol inhibit complement components C3 and C4. *Biochem J.* 1988; **251**: 323–326.

Stratton MA. Drug-induced systemic lupus erythematosus. *Clin Pharm.* 1985; **4**: 657–663.

Vervolet D. Allergy to muscle relaxants and related compounds. *Clin Allergy.* 1985; **15**: 510–508.

Wintroub BU, Shiffman NJ, Arndt KA. Adverse cutaneous reactions to drugs. In: Fitzpatrick TB, Eisen AZ, Wolff K, Freedberg IM, Austen KF, eds. *Dermatology in general medicine (2E).*New York: McGraw-Hill Book Company, 1979; 555–567.

20

Cancer

CLINICAL RELEVANCE OF EXPERIMENTAL TUMOURS

A central issue in tumour immunology is the extent to which human neoplasms resemble certain experimental tumours in that they express antigens that are capable, under appropriate conditions, of inducing *in vivo* tumour rejection. Given the multifarious nature of cancer in man, there is, unfortunately, no immunological paradigm in experimental systems.

The argument that the immunological status of human cancers is most closely reflected by spontaneous experimental tumours possessing little or no immunogenicity probably represents an extreme. However, as immunological models of the human disease, experimental tumours induced by high doses of chemical carcinogens, virus-induced tumours and leukaemias in animals other than man, show shortcomings which are all too apparent. Nevertheless, an estimated 75% of human cancer worldwide is attributed to induction by chemical carcinogens, and about 20% of female cancers and just under 10% of male cancers are linked to virus infections.

Increased tumour incidence in immunosuppressed patients	
Patient group	**Tumour type**
organ transplant patients: azathioprine & steroids	non-Hodgkin's lymphoma, liver cancer, Kaposi's sarcoma, cervical cancer
organ transplant patients: cyclosporin A	lymphoma, skin cancer, Kaposi's sarcoma
patients with inflammatory diseases, e.g. rheumatoid arthritis	non-Hodgkin's lymphoma
malaria patients	Burkitt's lymphoma
AIDS patients	non-Hodgkin's lymphoma, Kaposi's sarcoma

Fig. 20.1 Several of these tumour types are thought to be virally associated. The possibility that the drug treatments or infections are carcinogenic *per se* has not been excluded.

IMMUNITY AND TUMOUR PREVENTION

The main function of the immune system is the recognition and elimination of potentially infective agents. This requires an exquisitely specific mechanism of recognition to distinguish normal self antigens from foreign ones. Malignant cells should therefore be antigenically distinguishable from their normal counterparts. This concept led to Burnet's theory of an 'immune surveillance' mechanism by which the majority of potentially malignant cells are recognized and eliminated by the immune system before they can develop into clinically detectable tumours.

A corollary of the surveillance hypothesis is that a defective immune system leads to an increased incidence of cancer. Such immunodepression may be a result of immunosuppressive therapy (drugs, irradiation) and diseases affecting the immune system (Fig. 20.1), or inherited deficiencies in immune responsiveness which lead to lymphoreticular malignancy (Fig. 20.2; see also chapter 21). While there are examples of increased tumour incidence in all of these categories, it should be borne in mind that immunosuppressive treatment may also be carcinogenic, and that genetic defects in, or viral infection of, the immune system may be associated with an increased risk of induction of malignancy which is independent of the concomitant immunosuppression.

Effect of inherited immunodeficiency diseases on tumour incidence			
Immunodeficiency disease	**Defect**	**↑ incidence of malignancy**	
		lymphoreticular	**epithelial & other**
Di George syndrome	↓ T cells	+	–
Wiskott-Aldridge syndrome	↓ T cells	+	–
ataxia telangiectasia	↓ T cells	+	–
severe combined immunodeficiency	↓ B & T cells	+	–
Chediak-Higashi syndrome	↓ granulocytes, monocytes, NK cells	+	–

Fig. 20.2 Chediak-Higashi syndrome is a rare disease in which intracellular granule function is compromised, affecting several cell types.

Immunosuppression and pattern of tumour incidence

Organ transplant patients on conventional therapy with immunosuppressive drugs such as azathioprine and corticosteroids, or the fungal metabolite cyclosporin A, do show an increased incidence of certain types of tumour. Although drug-induced tumours show variations depending on the drug treatment used, a pattern has emerged which differs markedly from that found in the population as a whole. Immunosuppressed patients have an increased incidence of tumours of the haemopoietic system and of those associated with viral infection (carcinomas of skin and cervix), while frequencies of other types of tumour are not markedly increased. Patients receiving immunosuppressive treatment for inflammatory diseases such as rheumatoid arthritis show a similar increase in the incidence of lymphoreticular malignancy.

Immunosuppressive diseases also show a pattern of tumour incidence which differs from that found in the general population. Acquired immune deficiency syndrome (AIDS) patients have an increased incidence of non-Hodgkin's lymphoma and Kaposi's sarcoma (see chapter 24), a malignancy arising from endothelial cells, which is uncommon in developed countries. As both of these tumours may be associated with viral infection (EBV and CMV respectively), it is likely that a deficiency in responsiveness to virally infected or transformed cells is reponsible for tumour emergence in AIDS patients. HIV may infect endothelial cells, but whether this directly influences the development of Kaposi's sarcoma is unclear.

Burkitt's lymphoma

Immunosuppression is also thought to be important in Burkitt's lymphoma. Normally, EBV infection in childhood is asymptomatic, but when it occurs in conjunction with malarial infection there is a greatly increased incidence of this otherwise uncommon tumour (Fig. 20.3). The immunosuppression brought about by malarial infection is believed to diminish the response against EBV-transformed B cells, allowing the development of a B cell lymphoma.

In normal individuals, B cells transformed by EBV are killed by specific cytotoxic T cells. Latent virus infection persists throughout life, but potentially malignant B cells are lysed efficiently before they can develop into a B cell lymphoma. However, in adolescents mild immunosuppression during malarial infection may allow a single clone of transformed B cells to escape elimination and develop into a lymphoma.

IMMUNE RESPONSE AGAINST ESTABLISHED TUMOURS

If an effective immune surveillance mechanism operates against potentially malignant cells it is evident that those tumours which do develop in immunocompetent hosts have successfully evaded elimination. However, there is circumstantial evidence that such tumours do evoke a response, although it may be insufficient to prevent tumour growth. Established tumours frequently show extensive infiltration by cells of the immune system (lymphocytes, plasma cells, macrophages) (Fig. 20.4) and these cells often show phenotypic or functional signs of activation. Only in rare situations (for example medullary carcinoma of the breast) does leucocyte infiltration appear to correlate positively with favourable prognosis.

Concomitant immunity

Progressive tumour growth can occur in the face of demonstrable anti-tumour reactivity. Effective immunity can be compromised by an overwhelming tumour burden or local immunosuppression, as suggested by the phenomenon of 'concomitant immunity' (Fig. 20.5). This illustrates that tumour growth is not invariably the result of a systemic failure of the host immune system to recognize and/or eliminate tumour cells.

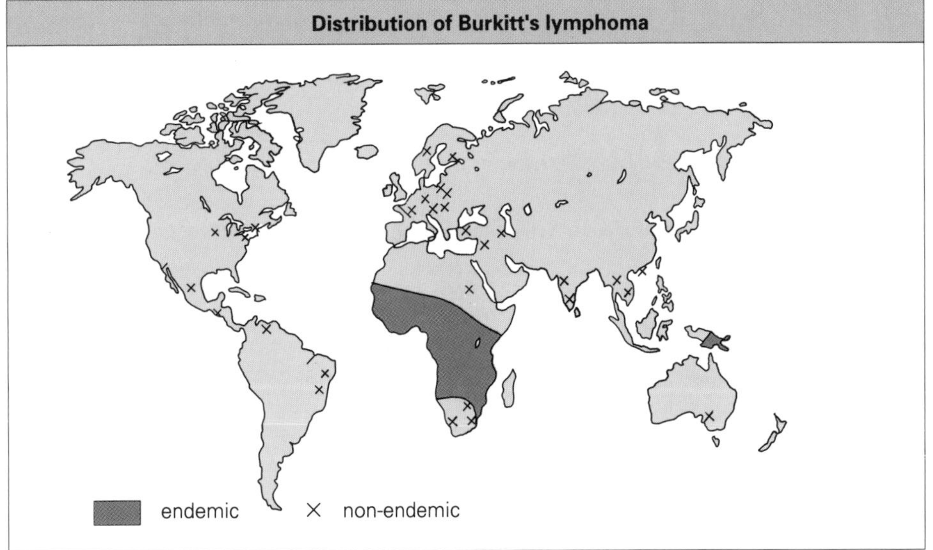

Fig. 20.3 Areas in which Burkitt's lymphoma (BL) is endemic also have a high incidence of malarial infection. Crosses indicate places where non-endemic lymphomas with BL histopathology were described. Modified from Burkitt (1970).

Metastatic insufficiency

The observation that the frequency of metastasis reflects only a fraction of the cells released or shed from a primary tumour into the blood or lymph, also suggests that a tumour-bearing host is able to deal successfully with small, but not large, numbers of tumour cells. However, it is important to realize that other, non-immunological factors also contribute to this phenomenon of 'metastatic insufficiency'. Only a small fraction (around 1%) of most tumour populations may be tumour 'stem' cells (Fig. 20.6), i.e. capable of self-renewal and of repopulating the entire tumour mass, and, as with conventional forms of cancer therapy, it is the ability of the immune system to selectively eliminate these cells which is of primary importance. Further circumstantial observations support the contention that the immune system is at least partially effective at limiting tumour growth (Fig. 20.7).

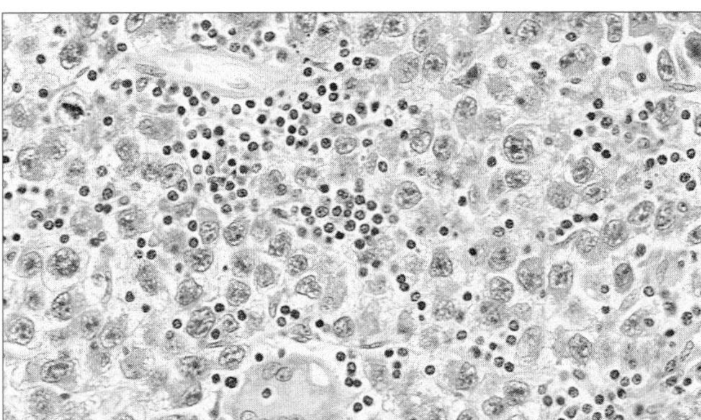

Fig 20.4 Section of seminoma showing dark-staining lymphocytes surrounding the tumour. H & E stain. Courtesy of Professor P G Isaacson.

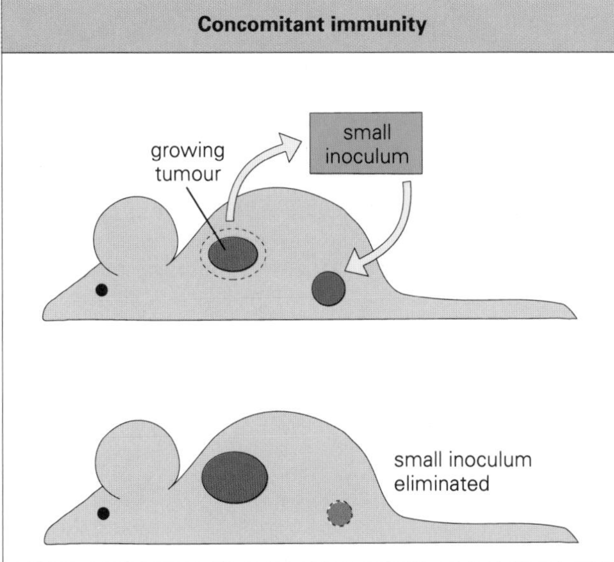

Fig. 20.5 This can be demonstrated by removing a small inoculum of cells from a large, antigenic tumour and injecting it into a distant site in the same animal, whereupon it is effectively eliminated; the original tumour continues to grow.

TUMOUR ANTIGENICITY

Until recently, most of our knowledge about tumour antigens related to those of experimental tumours and, in particular, to serially transplanted lines. This was a reflection of the emphasis within cancer research on tumours which could be conveniently maintained under laboratory conditions in forms that were widely available and relatively stable in their biological properties, including antigen expression.

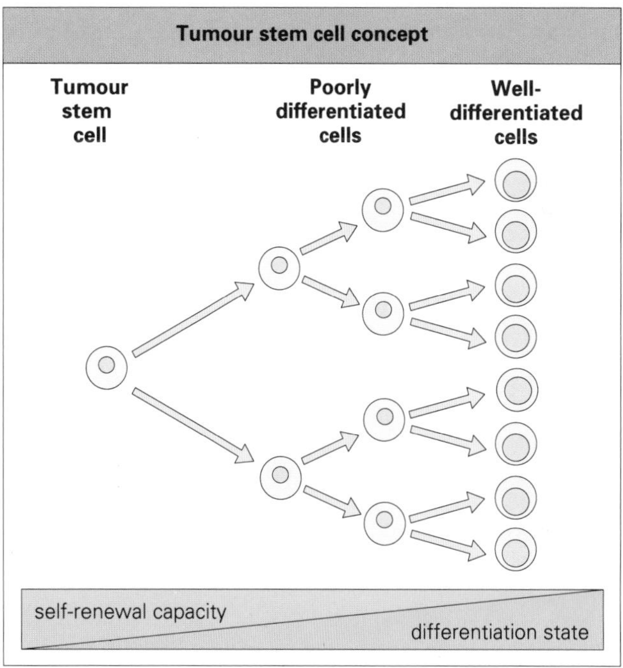

Fig. 20.6 A tumour may consist of a mixture of cells at various stages of differentiation, the more mature types having less proliferative potential.

Evidence for anti-tumour immunity
concomitant immunity
waxing & waning of tumour deposits
latency of secondaries following removal of primary
chemotherapy more effective *in vivo* than *in vitro*

Fig. 20.7 'Waxing' and 'waning' of tumour deposits has been observed in human neoplasms, notably malignant melanoma and non-Hodgkin's lymphoma. This phenomenon has been attributed to fluctuation in anti-tumour immunity. The efficacy of surgical extirpation and chemotherapy/radiotherapy is apparently augmented by an endogenous anti-tumour response, which may be partially, if not wholly, immunological.

Tumour 'antigens'

Several types of experimental neoplasm express antigens which are capable of inducing immunity and evoking resistance to their own transplantation in genetically compatible (syngeneic) hosts, as well as in the primary (autochthonous) host. These antigens are described as tumour-associated transplantation antigens (TATA) or tumour rejection antigens (TRA) because of the *in vivo* tests used to detect them. Animals immunized with transplanted immunogenic tumours are rendered resistant to subsequent challenge with appropriate numbers of live tumour cells of the same neoplasm, whereas non-immunized controls succumb.

The TATA of tumours induced by chemical carcinogens are frequently highly immunogenic, stable, heritable and cellularly homogeneous. It is likely that, depending on the carcinogenic dose, many chemically-induced tumours are multicentric to begin with, in other words they originate in a number of antigenically distinct foci and initially comprise several distinct clones. On serial transplantation this antigenic heterogeneity gives rise to the relative homogeneity which characterizes the most aggressive clone to establish itself as the tumour 'line'. In this respect, artificially-induced cancers differ from human neoplasms, the majority of which are probably clonal in origin.

Antigenic specificity

Operationally, TATA are frequently characterized by a remarkable uniqueness, so that each tumour expresses a distinct antigen, a prototype of which was recently purified to homogeneity, apparently restricted to that tumour. In this respect they are in marked contrast to the TATA of virus induced tumours, which are shared by all those induced by the same virus, but not by those induced by different viruses. These TATA are not necessarily structural components of the virion, but cellular antigens encoded by viral genes integrated in the host cell genome.

It is important to realise that neoplastic transformation is not invariably accompanied by expression of detectable TATA; many experimental tumours evoke little or no immunity. Immunoselection *in vivo* is unlikely to account for this, since cells which transform spontaneously *in vitro* (that is, in the absence of immune surveillance), or which are chemically induced, are not necessarily antigenic in the host from which the cells were originally derived. These observations, which may have important implications for human cancer, indicate that TATA expression is not a universal property of the neoplastic state.

Differentiation antigens

It must also be recognized that tumour cells express many of the antigens which normally characterize the tissues from which they arise, such as differentiation or tissue type-specific antigens. In common with more tumour-specific antigens, some of these 'determinants' evoke humoral responses; they are, however, rarely protective.

Autologous typing. This technique has led to the descrip-
20.4 tion of three major classes of cell surface antigens for malignant melanoma, astrocytoma, renal cancer and acute leukaemia (Fig 20.8). A class I antigen of malignant melanoma was recently partially purified and found to be a glycoprotein of molecular mass 25–40kDa, bearing no relationship to HLA antigens or β_2-microglobulin. Immunoprecipitation analysis with autologous serum showed another such antigen to be a 90kDa glycoprotein.

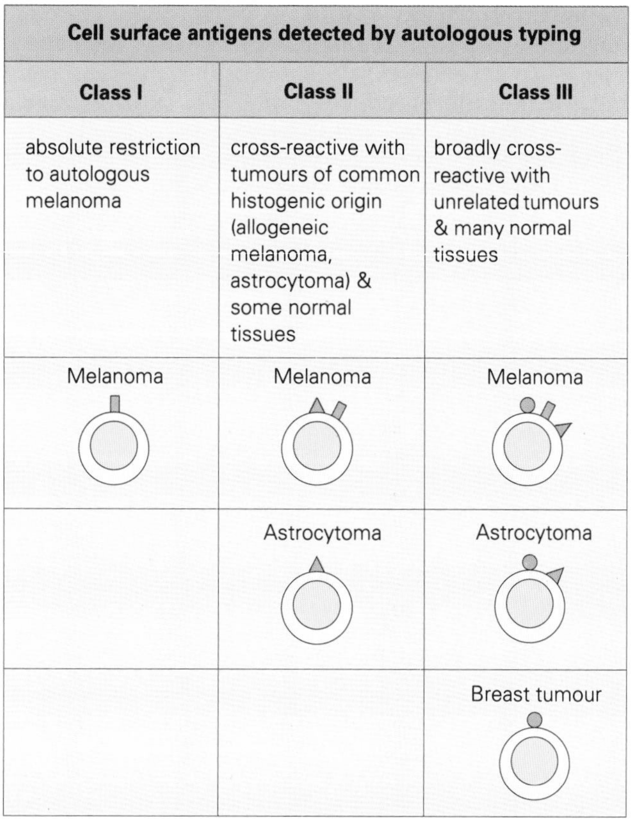

Cell surface antigens detected by autologous typing		
Class I	**Class II**	**Class III**
absolute restriction to autologous melanoma	cross-reactive with tumours of common histogenic origin (allogeneic melanoma, astrocytoma) & some normal tissues	broadly cross-reactive with unrelated tumours & many normal tissues
Melanoma	Melanoma	Melanoma
	Astrocytoma	Astrocytoma
		Breast tumour

Fig. 20.8 Cell surface antigens expressed by malignant melanoma cells and detected by the technique of autologous typing, in which sera from melanoma patients are tested against a panel of tumour cell lines, including the autologous tumour, allogeneic melanomas, histogenically related tumours and unrelated tumours. A tumour may display more than one class of antigen. Note that class I and II tumour antigens should not be confused with MHC class I and II molecules.

B cells: immunoglobulin idiotype. The Ig idiotype of neoplastic B cells can be regarded operationally as a 'tumour-specific' antigen in view of the wide variety of idiotypic structure. These are strictly clonal antigens, rather than markers of transformation.

Cytotoxic T cells recognize antigens on human tumour cells in both an HLA-restricted and non-restricted fashion. Because of the requirements of HLA-compatibility for the demonstration of cytotoxicity (in autologous testing), it is presently difficult to know the extent to which an antigen specifically recognized by T cells might be present on other tumours. 'Determinants' which do not require co-recognition in association with HLA molecules are present on a wide variety of tumours and interact with receptors other than the T cell antigen receptor on both classical T cells and cells of NK lineage.

ESCAPE FROM IMMUNOSURVEILLANCE

If the host immune system is normally capable of preventing tumour growth, the emergence of a clinically apparent tumour must be the result of an alteration either in the efficiency of the immune response, or in the immunogenicity or growth properties of the tumour (Fig. 20.9). These concepts will now be considered in more detail.

Factors influencing escape from immunosurveillance
↓ efficiency of immune response ↓ immunogenicity of tumour ↑ growth of tumour ↑ 'acquired' resistance of tumour

Fig. 20.9 The monoclonality of most tumours could indicate that a potentially malignant cell rarely avoids elimination. It may also reflect the capacity for selective outgrowth of a clone which has acquired resistance to recognition or elimination by the immune system, or which has increased proliferative potential. Note, however, that tumour monoclonality does not necessarily support the existence of immune surveillance, but may merely indicate the rarity of a genetic event(s) leading to malignant transformation.

Lack of tumour antigen and MHC class I

Tumours may fail to stimulate an immune response for various reasons (Fig. 20.10). For example loss or alteration of MHC class I antigens by the tumour cell would prevent lysis by cytotoxic T cells even in the presence of an immunogenic tumour antigen. This assumes that the recognition of putative novel tumour antigens is governed by the same rules as those for recognition of virus-infected targets in that they are subject to restriction by antigens of the major histocompatibility complex. Possible loss of non-antigen-specific adhesion molecules on tumours may also contribute to tumour escape (for example LFA-1 on non-Hodgkin's lymphoma and ICAM-1 on some melanomas).

Lack of T cell response

The host may be genetically incapable of mounting a response against a particular tumour antigen due to failure of the inherited MHC class II molecules to form an effective association with tumour antigen fragments. Evidence for this mechanism is difficult to obtain in man, but there are parallel examples of immune response gene defects in experimental animals. In addition, a particular tumour antigen specificity may not be represented in the T cell pool ('hole in the repertoire'), thereby preventing the tumour from being recognized.

'Sneaking through'

A potentially malignant cell may avoid detection by the immune system, in spite of being antigenic, by a process known as 'sneaking through'. By the time the tumour has attracted recognition, it may have grown beyond a manageable size. This process may reflect the finite statistical probability that an immunogenic tumour antigen may not be recognized rapidly rather than outgrowth of a resistant clone *per se*. Experimentally, this situation can be reproduced by injecting very small numbers of cells from an immunogenic tumour which are then more likely to result in progressive growth than injection of a larger number of cells.

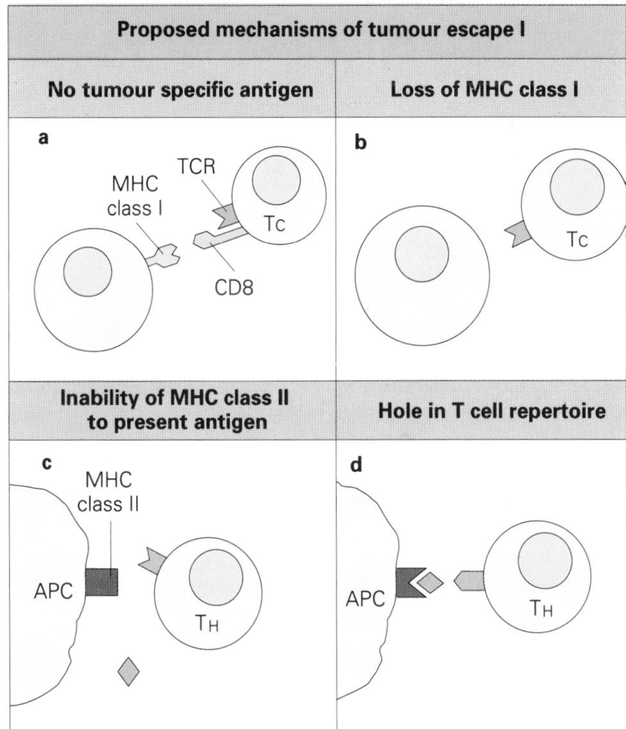

Fig. 20.10 a) lack of tumour specific antigen prevents recognition by T cells. b) lack of MHC class I on tumour cells prevents lysis by specific cytotoxic T cells. c) genetically determined lack of responsiveness due to inability of MHC class II to form adequate complex with processed tumour antigen fragment. d) absence of T cells with specificity for tumour antigen.

Antigenicity of 'stem' cells

On the other hand, a developing tumour may stimulate an immune response immediately, but its rapid growth rate or relative inaccessibility (in immunological 'sanctuaries') may tip the balance between tumour cell growth and killing in favour of net tumour progression. It may be that

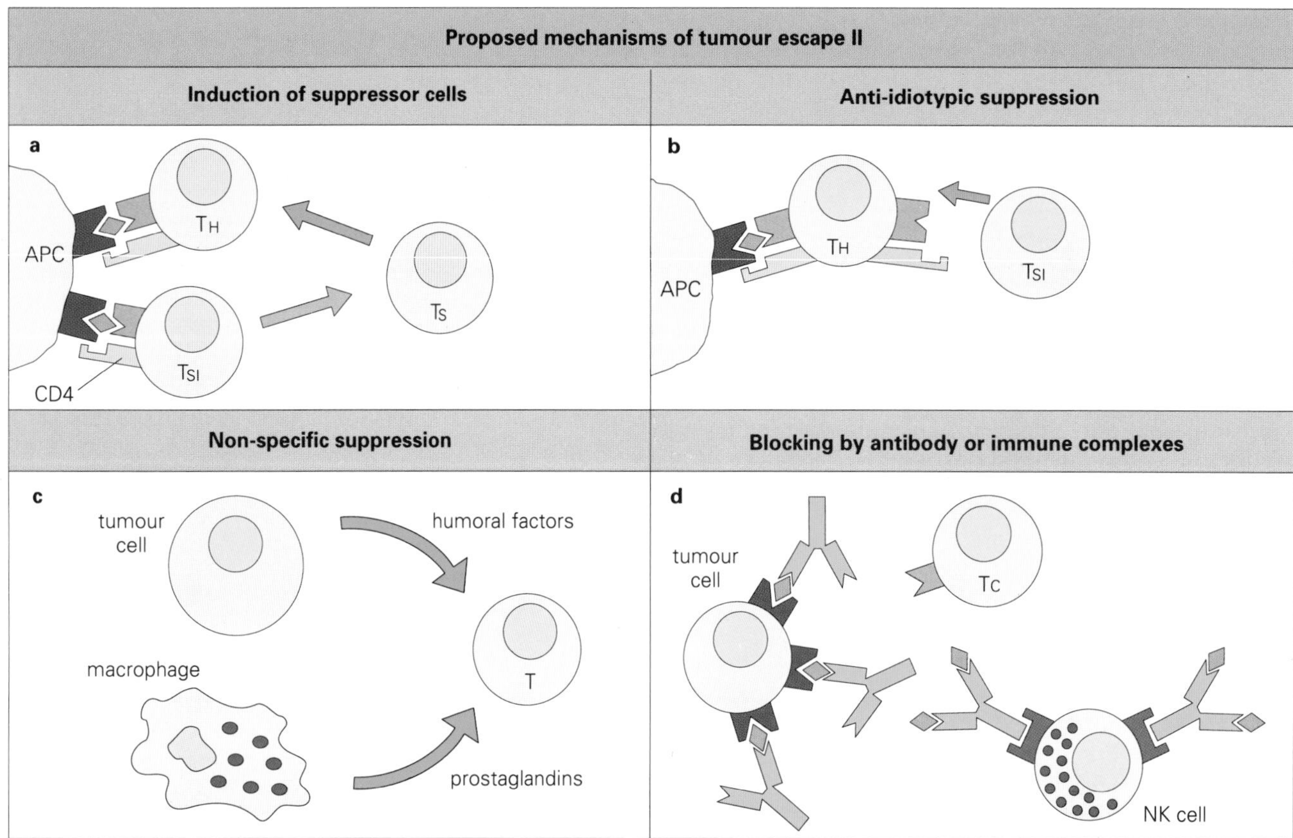

Fig. 20.11 Suppression of immune responses. a) as in certain types of tolerance, specific Ts cells may be induced by $CD4^+$ TSI (suppressor inducer) cells and suppress the immune response. b) TSI cells may act on TH cells by specific anti-idiotypic suppression. c) non-specific suppression of effector T cells at the tumour site by humoral factors produced by tumour cells or via prostaglandins produced by activated macrophages. d) blocking of anti-tumour cytotoxic T cells by tumour specific antibody and blocking of NK cell or macrophage ADCC by immune complexes.

in certain situations the tumour 'stem' cells are relatively resistant to lysis in spite of active elimination of more differentiated cells which are less capable of division.

Suppression of immune response

Tumour growth may occur in the face of an active immune response by the induction of a variety of suppression or blocking mechanisms (Fig. 20.11). Antigens shed by the tumour may block the effector function of specifically tumour-reactive T cells. These antigens may also combine with specific anti-tumour antibody to form complexes which may then be able to block the action of tumour-reactive T cells or K cells. Products of tumour cells other than specific antigen may also be able to block immunoreactivity locally. Certain tumours can release anti-inflammatory and anti-chemotactic substances which may decrease the response in a non-specific manner.

ANTI-TUMOUR EFFECTOR MECHANISMS

20.6 Although the classical view of immunosurveillance envisaged that tumour cells would be primarily the targets of antigen-specific cytotoxic T cells, it is evident that there are a variety of mechanisms which could be involved in the detection of, or response to established tumours. In many cases, the relative importance of these is uncertain and may change with tumour progression.

Cytotoxic T lymphocytes (CTL)

Cytotoxic T lymphocytes, important in the adaptive immune response to viral infections, are found in many tumour-bearing patients. These cells recognize integral cell surface antigen(s) or degradative products (peptides) of antigens expressed elsewhere in the cell (for example in the nucleus) in association with host MHC molecules (normally class I).

Activation of CTL depends on TH cells which recognize tumour antigen in association with MHC class II molecules on host antigen presenting cells (APCs). Certain tumour cell types, notably melanomas, may express MHC class II molecules *in vivo* but the functional significance of this is not clear and may be more a reflection of the differentiation status of the melanoma cells, or a 'transformation trait'. While classical CTL are of $CD8^+$ phenotype and recognize processed antigen in association with MHC class I molecules on target cells, it has recently been

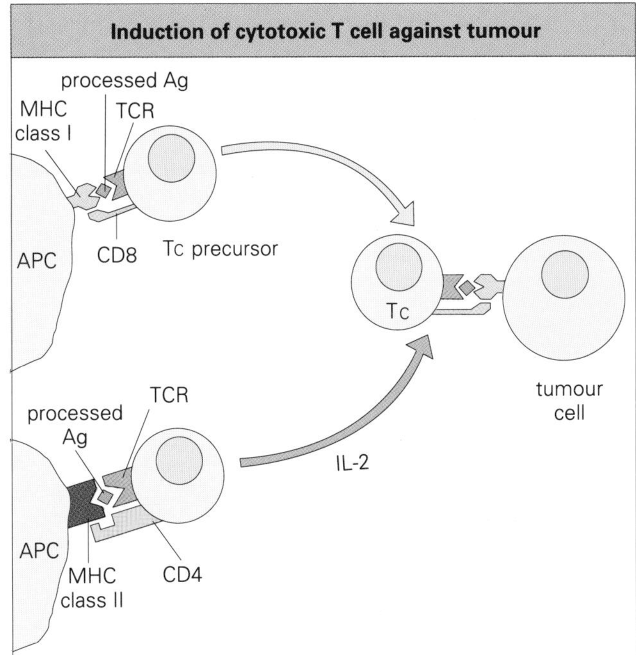

Fig. 20.12 Mechanism of induction of Tc cells against idealized tumour cell expressing tumour specific antigen in association with MHC class I. CD4+ cytotoxic-inducer cells recognize tumour antigen in association with MHC class II on host antigen presenting cells (APC). CD8+ CTL pecursors recognize antigen in association with MHC class I and become responsive to IL-2 produced by the CD4+ cells.

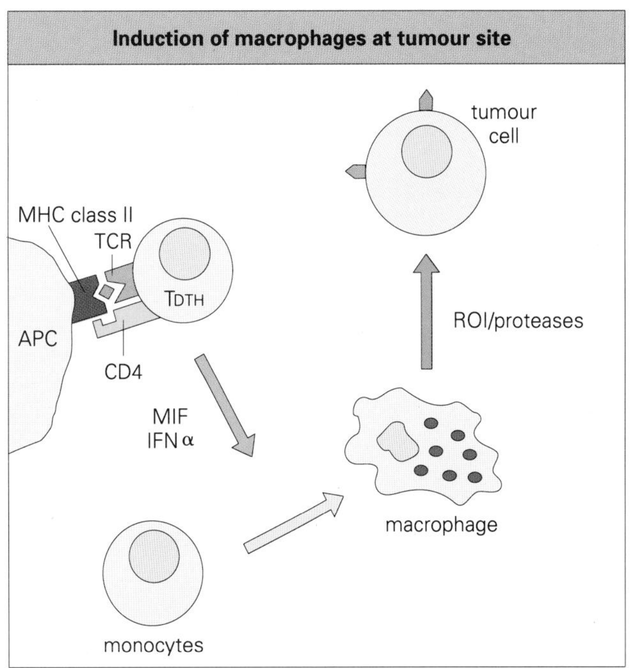

Fig. 20.13 Lymphokines secreted by T cells attract monocytes to the tumour site and bring about their activation, leading to non-specific killing of tumour cells in a mechanism analogous to a delayed hypersensitivity reaction.

found that CD4+ CTL exist which recognize antigen plus MHC class II molecules on target cells. Whether class II expression on tumour cells permits them to be recognized by CD4+ CTL is uncertain (Fig. 20.12).

Activated CD4+ lymphocytes

Activation of TH cells by tumour antigen on host APCs can result in the recruitment and activation of macrophages at the tumour site (Fig. 20.13). In this type of mechanism, lymphokine secretion by TH cells is responsible for macrophage activation and tumour cell killing is brought about by the secretion of cytotoxic proteases and/or reactive oxygen intermediates (ROIs) by activated macrophages. In this instance, although induced by specifically reactive T cells, tumour cell killing is via a non-specific mechanism. Recent evidence has implicated cells of the CD4+ sub-population in direct killing of target cells via secretion of cytotoxins, possibly tumour necrosis factor (TNF).

Anti-tumour antibody

Some tumours stimulate the production of anti-tumour antibodies. These are rarely tumour-specific but are directed against cytoskeletal proteins or nuclear antigens. As with CTL induction, B cell activation depends on CD4+ TH cells, although it is now thought that distinct CD4+ sub-populations are involved. Antibody bound to tumour cells may lead to complement activation and subsequent complement-mediated lysis. It may also lead to tumour cell killing via antibody-dependent cellular cytotoxicity (ADCC) (Fig. 20.14). Such target cell lysis is an extracellular process, but under certain circumstances phagocytic cells such as macrophages or polymorphs may be able to phagocytose opsonized tumour cells via Fc or C3b receptors. Target cell killing by activated macrophages can be enhanced by C3b, even in the absence of antibody.

Natural killer cells

Natural killer (NK) cells are part of the non-adaptive immune system and are capable of spontaneously lysing certain tumour cell types (mainly lymphoreticular tumours) in the absence of antibody. However, they are predominantly confined to the blood and spleen and so their activity against solid tumours may be restricted to an anti-metastatic role. Unlike T cells, neither the NK cell receptor(s) nor the target cell molecule(s) recognized have been identified.

Lymphokines: IFNγ and TNF

A variety of lymphokines produced by cells of the immune system may participate, either alone or in concert, in anti-tumour responses. Interferon (IFNγ), primarily a product of activated T cells, is inducible with IL-2 and can influence the activity of other leucocytes as well as having direct effects on tumour cells. Both NK cells and macrophages can be activated by IFNγ (although IFNα is more effective for NK activation), resulting in more efficient lysis of tumour cells. IFNγ can inhibit the proliferation of certain tumour cells and can also increase or

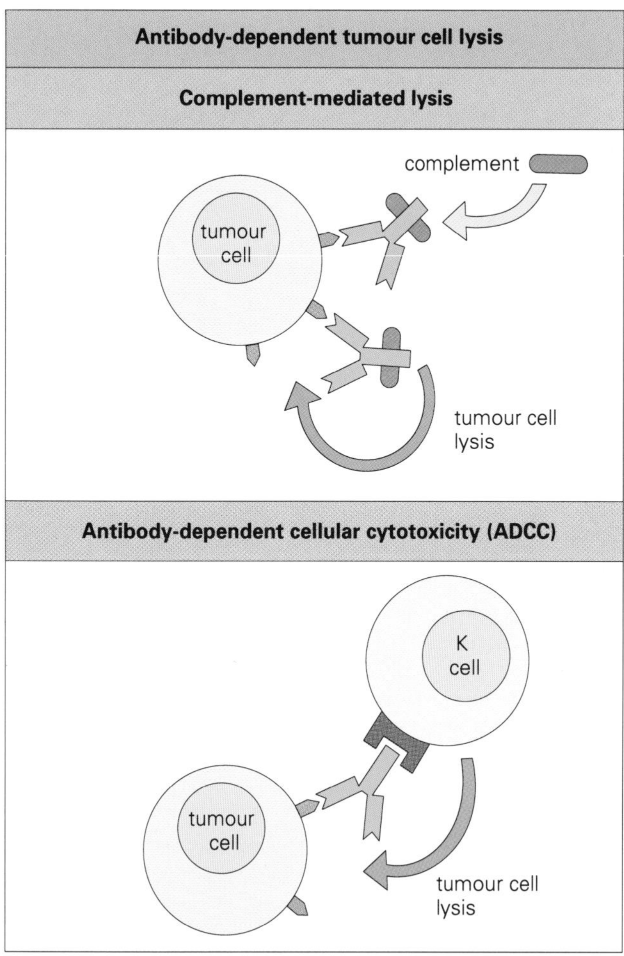

Fig. 20.14 Antibody-dependent lysis of tumour cells. Upper: tumour-specific antibody bound to tumour cells may bring about complement lysis. Lower: in ADCC, cells with surface receptors for the Fc portion of the IgG molecule engage opsonized tumour cells and lyse them. Such cells include macrophages, monocytes and K cells (now thought to be the same population as NK cells).

induce expression of MHC class I and class II antigens, enhancing recognition by T cells.

Tumour necrosis factor (TNFα) and lymphotoxin (now termed TNFβ) have a direct cytotoxic action on some tumour cells. The mechanism of action of TNF is not clear but receptors for it have been described on tumour cells. Recently, it has been reported that IFNγ and TNF can synergize in their anti-tumour activity, possibly via the induction of TNF receptors by IFNγ. The factors governing the secretion of TNF by T cells or macrophages are largely unknown.

Lymphokines: IL-2

Treatment of lymphocytes *in vitro* with interleukin 2 (IL-2), the lymphokine required for T cell proliferation, results in enhanced cytotoxic activity against tumour cells. This is known as the 'lymphokine activated killer' (LAK) phenomenon and the main precursors of LAK cells are probably NK cells, that is, they represent NK cells in a different state of functional activation. Such cells can also be induced *in vivo* by the exogenous administration of IL-2 and this phenomenon has stimulated much interest in their possible therapeutic use. The cytotoxic repertoire of LAK cells is wider than that of NK cells, but for both cell types the determinants governing target cell recognition have remained obscure. Whether LAK cells are generated *in vivo* without administration of exogenous IL-2 is not certain.

IMPORTANCE OF CELLULAR RESPONSES

Cancer is a multifarious disease and tumours of different cell origin and localization are therefore likely to stimulate different arms of the immune response. In addition, the cell type(s) responsible for immunosurveillance (Fig. 20.15) may not be the same as that which is responsive to an established tumour.

Immunosurveillance appears to operate mainly against lymphoreticular and/or virally associated tumours; there is

Characteristics of cytotoxic cells directed against tumour

Cell type	Immune mechanism	Compartment	Induction	Target
T cells	adaptive	recirculating	require priming	differentiated tumour cells
NK cells	non-adaptive	confined to blood & spleen	spontaneously active	tumour stem cells
Macrophages	non-adaptive	fixed in tissues	spontaneously active; stimulated by T cells	? no preference

Fig. 20.15 NK cells tend to react with less mature cell types expressing low amounts of MHC class I antigens (stem cells), while CTL are more likely to recognize targets with higher amounts of MHC class I (differentiated tumour cells).

little evidence that it is effective against the more common epithelial tumours, for example breast, colon and lung.

T cells

Evidence from patients with immunodeficiency diseases strongly implicates T cells as the effector cell type. As CTL are known to be important in resistance to viral infection it is these, presumably in conjunction with $CD4^+$ TCR, which are thought to be responsible. Immunosurveillance against virally associated tumours may be a result of T cell-mediated immunity against virally infected cells rather than virally transformed cells.

T cells are the most likely cell type to be involved in activity by virtue of their recirculatory capacity. In this respect, as well as in the highly specific nature of the response, T cell function may complement that of NK cells and macrophages. The latter would maintain a relatively non-specific response against tumour cells and the former a specific response against those transformed cells expressing abnormal proteins.

Mature macrophages

Mature macrophages are largely compartmentalized in lymphoid organs and other tissues such as liver and lung, where they bind and remove particulate material from the circulation. This function may extend to the clearance of potentially metastatic tumour cells. The high incidence of lung and liver metastases in many tumour types may reflect the ability of macrophages to bind and remove micrometastases from the circulation but not always to destroy them.

NK cells

NK cells are chiefly confined to the blood and spleen, where they regulate the proliferation of haemopoietic stem cells and other immature lymphoid cells. Any anti-tumour reactivity may be thought of as an advantageous secondary function, directed almost exclusively against blood-borne tumour cells. The predominant reactivity of NK cells *in vitro* against lymphoreticular neoplasms indicates that their activity is confined to the vascular compartment.

ANTIBODY RESPONSE TO TUMOURS

A variety of antibodies are detectable in tumour-bearing patients, the majority of which are directed against antigens present on a wide variety of cell types (class III antigens), as well as well-characterized autoantigens (for example anti-nuclear factors). Antibodies to tumour class I and class II antigens are present in patients' sera at a low frequency (about 6% for class I), at least in malignant melanoma, a disease in which they have been intensively sought. There are several possible reasons for this: the antigens might be present on only a small number of melanomas or heterogeneously expressed; they may be of intrinsically low immunogenicity; they may be downregulated upon tissue culture (cultured cells are normally used in antibody assays); or they may evoke cellular rather than humoral immunity. Alternatively, they may be subject to unpredictable cyclical expression.

Enhancing antibody responses

Attempts to induce (or enhance) the serological response to tumour class I and class II antigens with two different types of vaccine have been largely unsuccessful. In the mouse, lysates prepared from tumour cells infected with vesicular stomatitis virus (VSV) or other viruses have been shown to be more effective than lysates of non-infected tumour cells in inducing resistance to tumour engraftment. In man, membrane extracts of VSV-infected melanoma cells elicit delayed hypersensitivity reactions in melanoma patients, under conditions in which extracts of non-infected melanoma cells are virtually inactive.

IN VITRO TESTS FOR TUMOUR IMMUNITY

CELLULAR RESPONSES

Cellular immunity to human tumours can be demonstrated in assays of lymphoproliferation and cytotoxicity.

Lymphoproliferation

Lymphoproliferation (Fig. 20.16 left) is a function of predominantly TH cells upon recognition of tumour antigen in association with MHC class II molecules (that is, the interaction is class II restricted). Antigen released from the dying tumour cells is presumed to be taken up and processed by MHC class II positive dendritic cells and monocytes, present in the PBMC. However, it is also possible that antigenic tumour cells co-expressing MHC class II products 'self present' to TH cells.

Approximately one-third of all 'solid' tumours coming to surgery are capable of inducing significant proliferative responses in autologous lymphocytes, but there is little apparent association with tumour type. Non-transformed cells from corresponding normal tissues lack significant stimulatory potential. There is some evidence that patients with positive responses fare better clinically.

Cytotoxicity

Cytotoxicity is demonstrable against freshly disaggregated tumour cells (and other 'targets' as appropriate) in PBMC following stimulation with autologous tumour (Fig. 20.16 right) or, occasionally, in fresh PBMC in blood taken at surgery. In practice, the target cells separated from contaminating stromal cells, are pre- (or post-) labelled with appropriate radionucleotides and the degree of release (or uptake) measured in the presence and absence of 'effector' lymphocytes with which the targets are co-incubated for several hours at different ratios. The 'specificity' of the cytotoxic reactions is usually determined against a panel of targets comprising the autologous tumour, allogeneic tumour of related and unrelated tissue origin and cell line

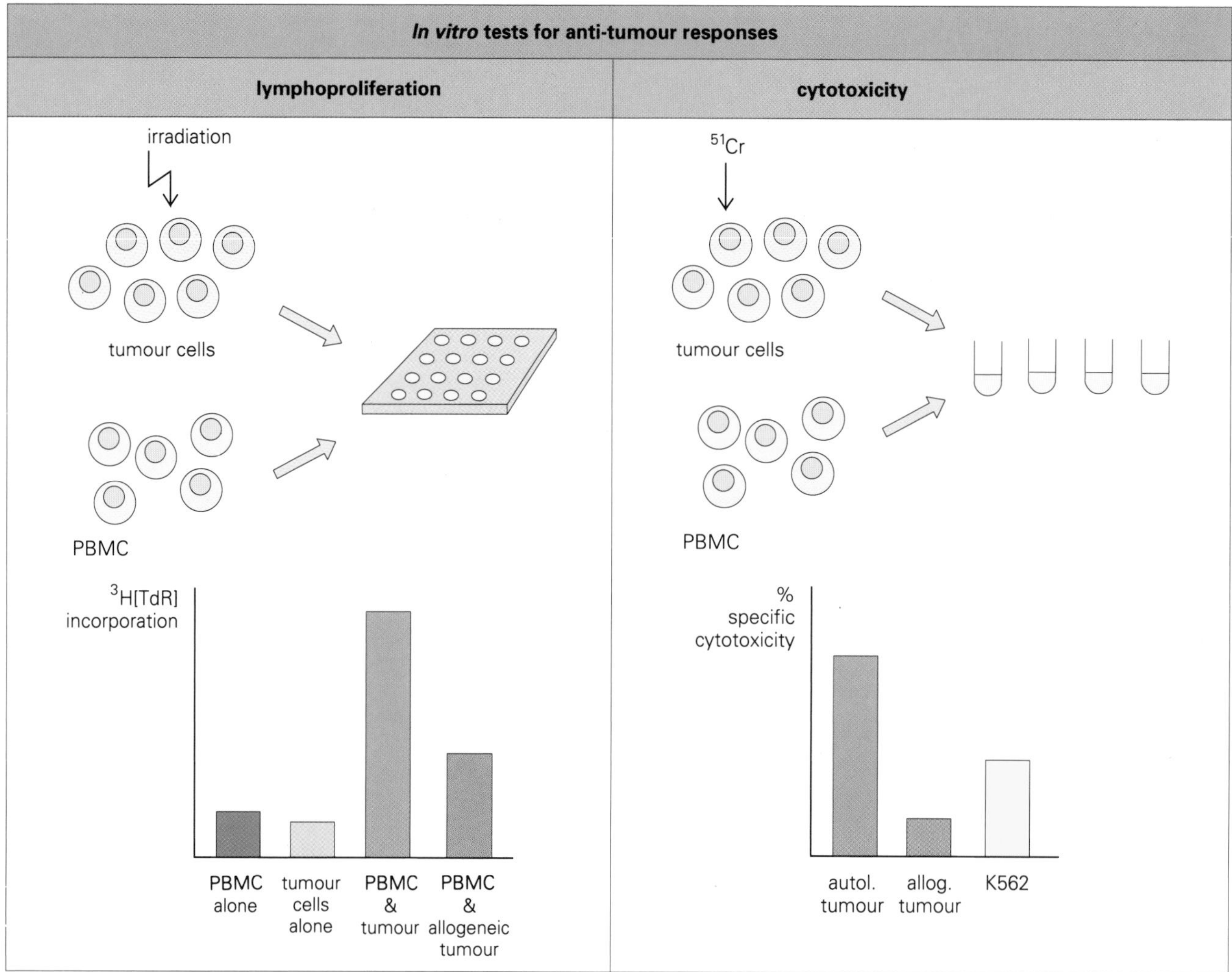

Fig. 20.16 Left: peripheral blood mononuclear cells (PBMC) or tumour infiltrating lymphocytes are co-cultured with irradiated autologous tumour cells and their proliferative response measured by the incorporation of tritiated thymidine. Positive lymphoproliferation relative to unstimulated PBMC controls, provides an index of the secondary immune response to antigen which the lymphocyte population previously encountered *in vivo*. Right: lymphocytes from tumour patients are incubated with a panel of ^{51}Cr-labelled tumour cell targets and the degree of lysis determined by measuring isotope release.

targets (Fig. 20.17). By judicious experimental design, a single experiment can determine the level and specificity of killing against the autologous tumour, the extent of cross-reactivity with other targets, and natural killer (NK) activity.

Approximately two-thirds of all cancer patients coming to surgery have demonstrable cytotoxicity in their PBMC. Much of this is evidently NK activity since it is detectable only against cell line targets, fresh autologous and allogeneic tumours being relatively resistant. By contrast with peripheral blood, lymphocytes recovered from tumours themselves, 'tumour infiltrating lymphocytes' (TIL), are less cytotoxic, possibly on account of suppressor cells *in*
20.10 *situ*, or suppressor substances released from the tumours.

HUMORAL RESPONSES

Autologous tissue typing

This has been one of the most useful approaches to date. It involves identifying patients with surface antigens of cultured autologous tumour cells and analysing the specificity of the reactions by absorption tests with autologous and allogeneic normal and malignant cells.

Other approaches include fluorescence analysis, radioisotope labelling techniques, complement fixation and immune adherence. Although antibody responses provide an indication of which antigens are capable of being recognized by the tumour-bearing patient, it is unlikely that

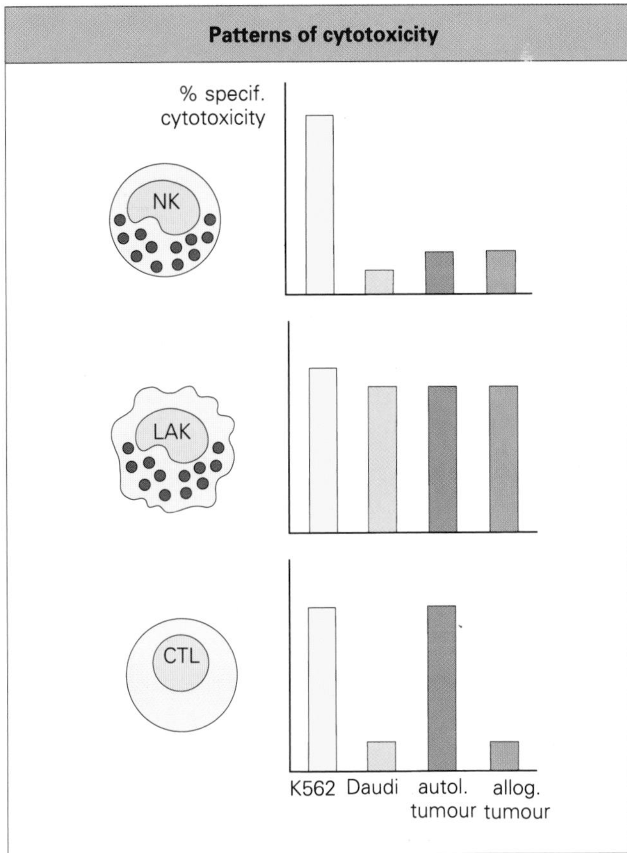

Fig. 20.17 Patterns of cytotoxicity mediated by different effector cell populations. NK cells kill only certain sensitive lymphoid or myeloid tumour cell targets, but LAK cells also kill a range of NK resistant targets in a non-MHC restricted fashion. CTL show restricted specificity for autologous tumour targets but may also show non-MHC restricted killing of NK sensitive and resistant targets.

they play any significant role in protection and the relevant ones are, in any case, too infrequently detectable to be useful as diagnostic or prognostic markers. Immune complexes are found in the sera of many cancer patients but the frequency often does not differ greatly from that seen in inflammatory or degenerative conditions affecting the same tissue. Such complexes could conceivably differ in antigenic moieties, but little work has been done in this area and the idea remains hypothetical.

THERAPEUTIC APPROACHES

The diverse nature of cancer and the multiplicity of potential immune responses have led to a variety of therapeutic approaches. Most have concentrated on augmenting, either actively or passively, the putative existing response: others have attempted to modify the tumour cells themselves in the hope that this will render them more easily recognizable by the immune system.

Prophylatic immunization for EBV-associated tumours

Vaccine	Antigens	Response
vaccinia virus	host epithelial cell & vaccinia antigens	vaccinia immunity
vaccinia virus & EBV gene(s)	vaccinia & EBV antigen(s)	vaccinia & EBV immunity

Fig. 20.18 Vaccinia virus transfected with EBV genes infects host epithelial cells, leading to expression of the EBV gene product(s) and induction of anti-EBV immunity (both humoral and cellular). Although this type of approach is primarily intended for prophylactic immunization of high-risk groups, it could potentially be used to stimulate the immune response of tumour-bearing individuals to virus antigens.

Prophylactic immunization

In view of the undoubted importance of T cells in antiviral immunity, the possibility of protecting against virally-associated cancers by prophylactic immunization is an attractive one. Burkitt's lymphoma and nasopharyngeal carcinoma are two diseases which are associated with EBV infection. Pre-immunization with EBV may therefore be able to protect against the development of these tumours.

Unfortunately, the virus cannot be grown in sufficiently large quantities *in vitro* to facilitate vaccine production and so attempts are being made to transfect EBV genes into vaccinia virus (a good immunogen) to induce EBV immunity (Fig. 20.18). This technique may prove less successful for viruses with a large number of types, such as papilloma virus, unless only a limited number are implicated in tumour causation, or there is considerable antigenic cross-reactivity between the different types; it may also prove less effective for viruses with a high mutation frequency.

Specific immunotherapy

Several kinds of 'specific' immunotherapy have been tested in patients with established tumours (Fig. 20.19). One approach which has been utilized in acute myelogenous

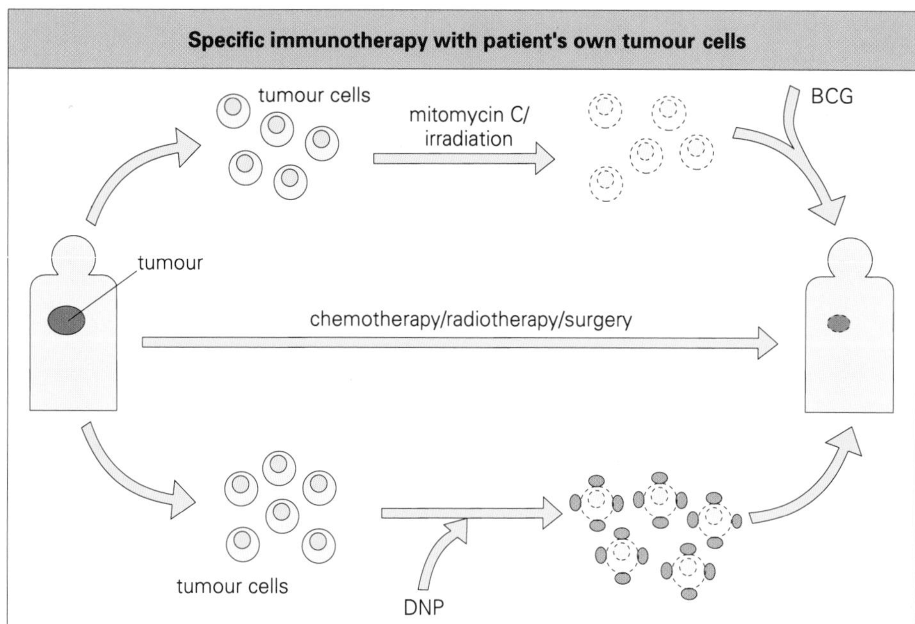

Fig.20.19 Immediately prior to treatment tumour cells are removed and either inactivated or chemically modified and subsequently used to immunize the patient following the induction of remission.

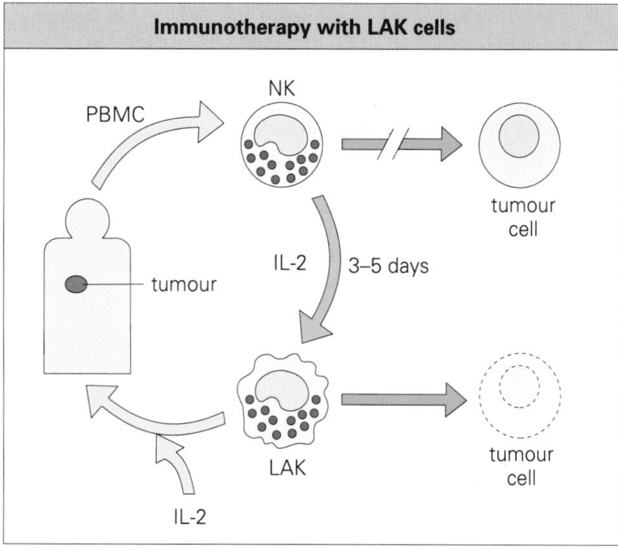

Fig. 20.20 Patient's PBMC obtained by leukapheresis are unable to kill tumour cells but after 3–5 days' culture *in vitro* with IL-2, cytotoxicity is induced against autologous tumour cells. LAK cells are then reinfused into the patient together with IL-2, which is essential for the maintenance of lytic activity.

leukaemia is to remove large numbers of tumour cells immediately prior to intensive chemotherapy or radiotherapy to induce remission. The patient is then immunized with his own inactivated tumour cells, together with an adjuvant such as BCG, in order to stimulate the response against re-emerging leukaemia cells.

Alternatively, tumour cells may be conjugated to a hapten molecule such as DNP and used as immunogens to
20.12 induce an anti-carrier response to tumour antigens. A fundamental problem here, however, is the extent of the response to non-haptenized tumour cells, for example in metastatic sites.

Non-specific immunostimulation

This has been utilized in several different types of skin tumour. BCG injected into the tumour in immune patients results in a delayed hypersensitivity reaction to BCG at the tumour site. This leads to activation of macrophages (and possibly other cell types) which can non-specifically kill neighbouring tumour cells. Although surgery is often superior to this method alone, BCG has had a role in reducing the local tumour burden prior to surgery.

BCG is efficacious in stage I bladder carcinoma, where intravesicular instillation has a profound anti-tumour effect. In a similar way, patients can be immunized with a contact sensitizing agent such as DNP by skin painting followed by challenge with the same agent painted onto the tumour site. The local contact hypersensitivity reaction thus induced can lead to tumour cell lysis by neighbouring activated macrophages.

Passive immunotherapy

Cellular immunotherapy. Some recent progress has been made in the field of adoptive or passive immunotherapy. Cellular approaches involve sensitization of autologous or allogeneic lymphocytes to tumour cells *in vitro* followed by infusion of stimulated cells into the patient. The success of such procedures depends on several factors, including the specificity of the transferred cells for tumour antigens and their ability to gain access to the tumour site *in vivo*. There have been some encouraging results in experiments with LAK cell therapy (Fig. 20.20). The parameters governing LAK cell activity are largely unknown and the success of therapy would also be subject

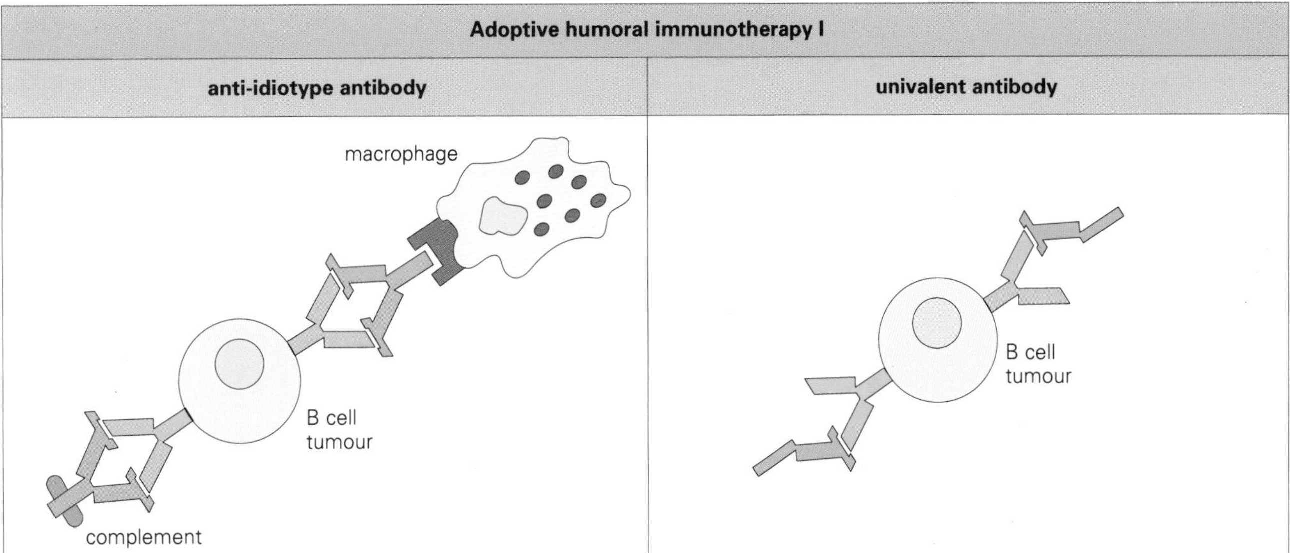

Fig. 20.21 Left: an anti-idiotypic monoclonal antibody is raised against the idiotypic determinant of a B cell tumour. Antibody administration may lead to tumour cell elimination via complement-mediated lysis, macrophage- or NK cell-mediated binding and phagocytosis. Right: univalent antibodies may reduce the likelihood of antigen or antibody modulation.

to the above considerations. Also, systemic IL-2 administration can result in serious side-effects, notably the capillary leak syndrome.

Humoral immunotherapy
With the advent of monoclonal antibodies against tumour antigens, many adoptive humoral immunotherapy regimens have been developed. The rationale governing these methods is that the monoclonal antibody provides the specificity of delivery of a toxic molecule to tumour cells ('magic bullet') and the therapeutic advantage compared to conventional treatment therefore depends on the relative affinity of the antibody for malignant as compared to normal cells. The selection of a highly specific monoclonal antibody is thus of critical importance.

Treatment of B cell lymphomas. This approach has been used in the treatment of some B cell lymphoma patients by developing a unique, highly specific, anti-idiotypic monoclonal antibody against the surface Ig molecules on the tumour cells (Fig. 20.21 left). Whether long-term remission can be induced by this means is not clear. Problems include possible sensitization to mouse Ig with prolonged antibody administration, antigenic modulation and the necessity to produce large amounts of monoclonal antibody specific for the individual tumour. Antigenic modulation can, to some extent, be overcome by the use of univalent antibodies (Fig. 20.21 right). In principle, the anti-idiotypic approach could be extended to certain T cell malignancies.

Drugs coupled to antibodies. Most treatment protocols using monoclonal antibodies have relied on toxic molecules chemically conjugated to the antibody to deliver a lethal signal to tumour cell targets. Cytotoxic drugs such as methotrexate or adriamycin have been successfully coupled to antibody molecules without substantial loss of antibody specificity or drug activity. Similarly, monoclonal antibodies conjugated to highly toxic molecules such as abrin, ricin or tetanus toxoid have also been used (Fig. 20.22 left). However, these methods are generally only able to bring about lysis of tumour cells to which the antibody actually binds. The use of monoclonal antibodies conjugated to radioisotopes such as ^{131}I or ^{90}Y can theoretically serve to increase the range over which the toxic signal is effective provided a sufficient radiation dose can be delivered (Fig. 20.22 right). Similar antibody-isotope conjugates have also been used in the radiological assessment of tumour spread.

Hybrid antibodies. The vast majority of currently available monoclonal antibodies are of mouse origin and prolonged treatment may result in the development of an anti-mouse Ig response, leading to antibody neutralization or more rapid clearance. To some extent, this response may be ameliorated with cyclosporin A, or the use of genetically engineered hybrid antibodies with human Fc and murine Fab portions (Fig. 20.23 left). It is also possible to construct an antibody with one of the Fab arms specific for a tumour antigen and the other for an antigen present on CTL (Fig. 20.23 right) This concept is still at an experimental stage.

Interferons (IFNs)
While IFNα and β are more potent enhancers of NK cell activity than IFNγ, the latter is probably more relevant to cancer immunotherapy by virtue of its direct effects on tumour cells. IFNγ can have anti-proliferative effects on some leukaemia cells by promoting differentiation and thereby diminishing self-renewal capacity. It is also able

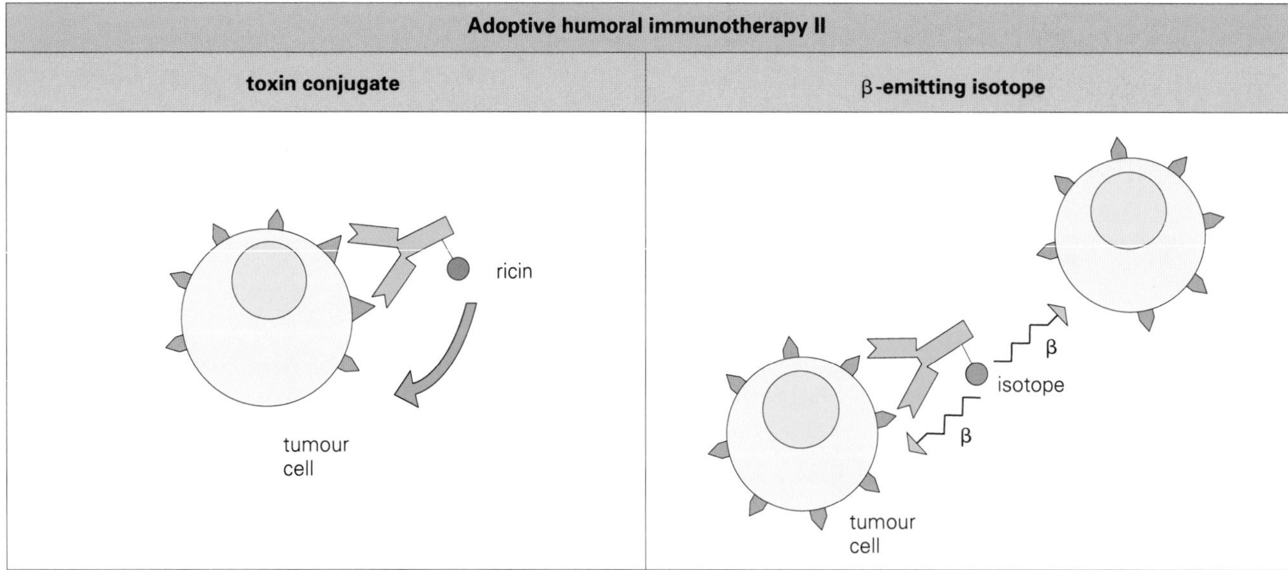

Fig. 20.22 Left: an anti-cancer drug or a toxic molecule such as ricin is conjugated to a tumour specific monoclonal antibody. The therapeutic advantage may be increased by using an unconjugated first antibody followed by a drug- or toxin-conjugated second antibody. Right: conjugation of a monoclonal with a short-range, β-emitting isotope may lead to killing of neighbouring tumour cells which have not bound the antibody in addition to those which have.

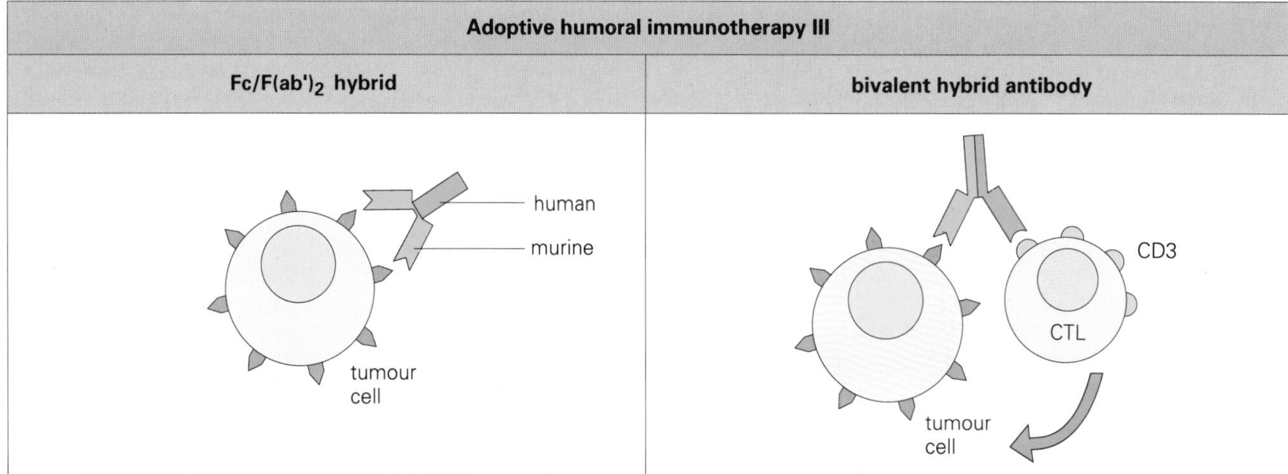

Fig. 20.23 Left: the use of hybrid monoclonals with a human Fc region reduces the risk of inducing immunity to mouse Ig. Right: bivalent hybrid antibodies recognizing tumour specific antigen and a T cell determinant such as CD3 may lead to localization and non-specific activation of CTL at the tumour site.

to induce or increase expression of MHC class I and II molecules on a wide range of tumour cell types, potentially rendering them more easily recognized by T cells.

It has recently been observed that IFNγ can synergize with TNF both in the induction of MHC antigens and in the killing of tumour cells. The precise mechanism of this synergy is not yet clear but the phenomenon has indicated much therapeutic promise. IFNγ is able to induce TNF receptor expression on some tumour cells, although this does not necessarily lead to increased sensitivity to killing by TNF, and TNF can stimulate IFNγ production by lymphoid cells suggesting that a positive feedback mechanism may operate. Therapeutic benefit from IFNα treatment has been limited to a minority of tumour types (for example hairy cell leukaemia). However, with a better understanding of its effects, together with the possibility of combined therapy (for example with TNF) a more rational approach is facilitated.

Bone marrow transplantation

Purged autologous marrow. Although not strictly an immunotherapeutic approach, bone marrow transplantation

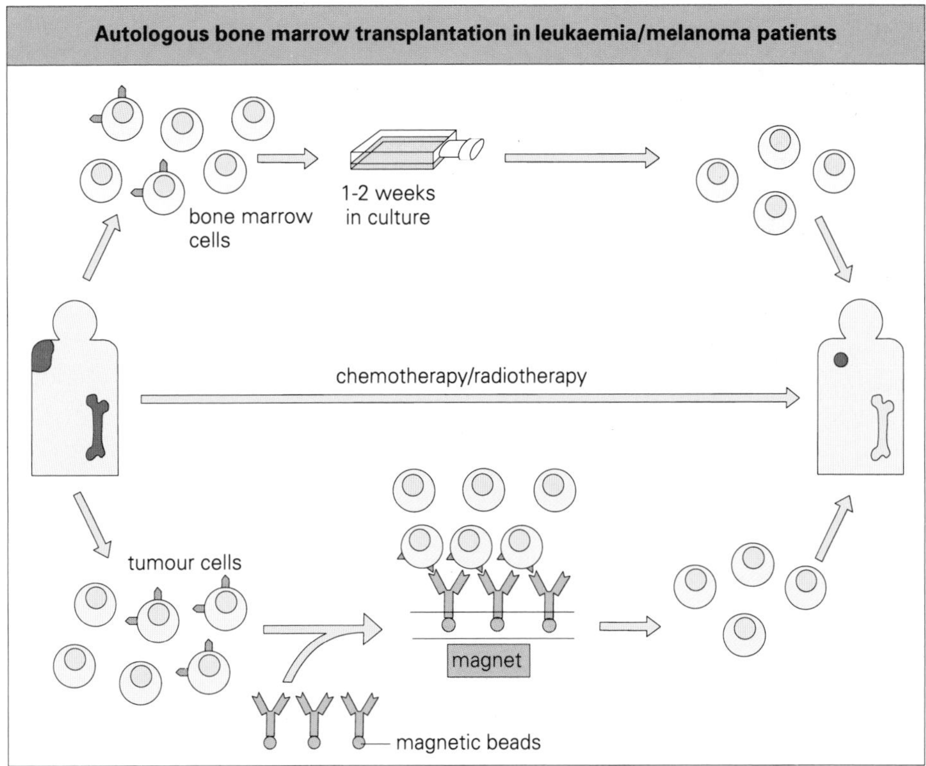

Fig. 20.24 A bone marrow sample taken immediately prior to induction of remission is purged of tumour cells by one of two methods. *In vitro* bone marrow culture permits normal bone marrow cells to survive while many tumour cells die in culture. Alternatively, treatment with monoclonal anti-tumour antibody coupled to magnetic beads allows tumour cells to be removed from bone marrow suspensions by the use of a magnet. The residual normal bone marrow cells are then reinfused into the patient.

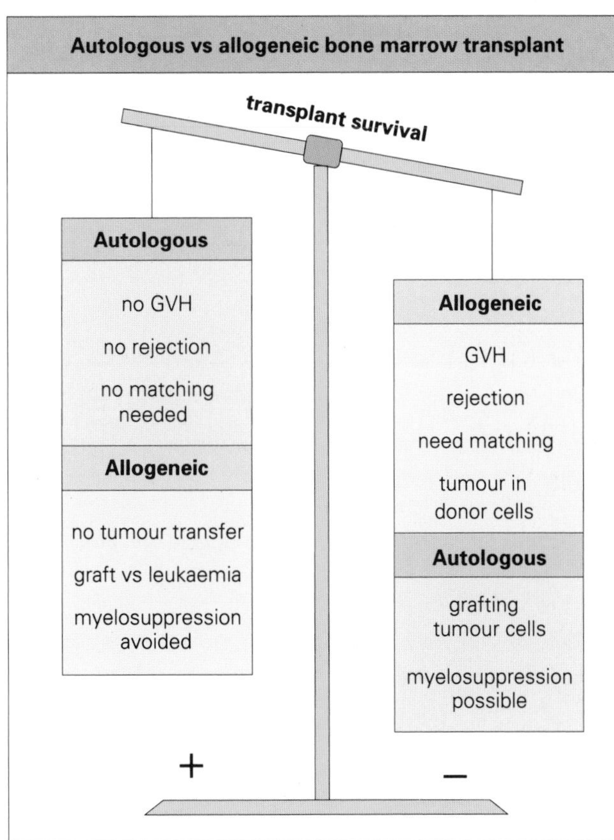

Fig. 20.25 Relative merits of autologous and allogeneic bone marrow transplantation for leukaemia.

(see chapter 3) is being increasingly used as a means of treating leukaemias refractory to conventional therapy as well as other malignancies such as melanoma (Fig. 20.24).

Allogeneic marrow. The alternative approach of transplanting bone marrow from another normal individual removes the need to purge the marrow of malignant cells (Fig. 20.25). The ideal situation of a genetically identical donor (an unaffected monozygotic twin) is only rarely encountered and so in almost all cases allogeneic donors, matched as closely as possible for MHC class I and II antigens, have been used. However, in spite of close matching, problems with graft versus host reactions are frequently noted, presumably due to minor antigen histoincompatibilities. Purging the donor marrow of T cells largely removes these adverse reactions but leads to an increased likelihood of graft failure. It appears that regenerating host alloreactive T cells are often able to bring about rejection of the marrow graft but that these may be inactivated or eliminated by donor alloreactive T cells.

The possibility of inducing specific tolerance to donor marrow by prior blood transfusion is being actively investigated. Also, donor T cells may exert a beneficial anti-leukaemia effect *in vivo* so that removal of donor T cells is not always advantageous. An additional complication which has been reported is the recurrence of leukaemia of donor cells, presumably due to horizontal transmission of an infective agent. In spite of these considerations, bone marrow transplantation is finding an increasing use in the treatment of certain leukaemias and malignant melanomas.

FURTHER READING

Ades EW, Lopez C, eds. *Natural killer cells and host defence.* Basle: Karger, 1989.

Balkwill FR. *Cytokines in cancer therapy.* Oxford: Oxford University Press, 1989.

Fidler IJ, Schroit AJ. Recognition and destruction of neoplastic cells by activated macrophages: discrimination of altered self. *Biochim et Biophys Acta.* 1989; **948**:151–173.

Koprowski H, Rovera G, eds. Cancer. *Curr Opin Immunol.* 1989/1990; **2**:681–722.

Lloyd KO Old LJ. Humoral monoclonal antibodies to glycolipids and other carbohydrate antigens: dissection of the humoral immune response in cancer patients. *Cancer Res.* 1989; **49**:3445–3451.

Parmiani G, Anchini A, Fossati G. Cellular immune response against autologous human malignant melanoma: Are *in vitro* studies providing a framework for a more effective immunotherapy? *J Nat Cancer Inst.* 1990; 82: 361–370.

Thorley-Lawson DA. Immunological responses to Epstein-Barr virus infection and the pathogenesis of EBV-induced diseases. *Biochim et Biophys Acta.* 1989; **948**:263–286.

 Cancer immunotherapy update. *Immunol Today.* 1990; **11**:190–200.

21

Lymphoreticular Disorders

INTRODUCTION

Blood cell malignancies are a diverse group of neoplasms which include the leukaemias, lymphomas and myeloma. They are broadly classified according to histological or morphological criteria and further divided, in the leukaemias, into clinically defined chronic or acute conditions (Fig. 21.1). A set of related conditions recognized as pre-malignant are characterized by benign or smouldering proliferation of lymphoid or myeloid cells with a strong predisposition towards true neoplasia (Fig. 21.2). All of these blood cell malignancies, and at least some of the pre-malignant disorders, have identifiable mutations in DNA which are acquired rather than inherited and are believed to be responsible for the underlying cellular pathophysiology. The aetiological mechanisms by which these mutations arise are, in most cases, unknown.

The emphasis in this chapter is on lymphoid rather than myeloid malignancy and Fig. 21.3 illustrates the variety of morphological and histopathological features that are characteristic of different subtypes of lymphoid malignancies. These features provide important diagnostic clues and are used in conjunction with more recently developed immunological, cytogenetic and molecular tests to arrive at a definitive diagnosis which, in turn, will determine the choice of therapy.

The overwhelming majority of lymphoid malignancies occur in adults, with some disorders such as CLL and myeloma, being exceedingly rare or absent in children (Fig. 21.4). Although lymphoma is predominantly an adult disease, some subtypes do occur in children. Approximately 50% of all childhood cancers are leukaemias or lymphomas, and the majority of these are acute lymphoblastic leukaemia (ALL) with a peak incidence between the ages of 2 and 6 years. Despite the predominance of ALL amongst the paediatric cancers, its overall incidence rate is low (20–40 cases per 10^6 children of under 15 years of age per year). Overall, the childhood lymphoid malignancies are more often curable than those of adults; this holds true even more for a single type of disease such as ALL. The explanation for this difference is not entirely clear, but in part relates to the different subtypes of

General classification of leukaemia/lymphoma & related conditions	
Leukaemias	
acute leukaemias	
acute lymphoblastic leukaemia	**ALL**
acute myeloblastic leukaemia	**AML**
acute mixed-lineage leukaemia	
chronic leukaemias	
chronic myeloid leukaemia	**CML**
(acute blast crisis of CML)	**CML-BC**
chronic lymphocytic leukaemia	**CLL**
prolymphocytic leukaemia	**PLL**
hairy cell leukaemia	**HCL**
adult T cell leukaemia/lymphoma	**ATL**

Hodgkin's disease	Myeloma
lymphocyte predominant †	multiple myeloma
nodular sclerosing	plasma cell leukaemia
mixed cellularity	
lymphocyte depleted	

Non-Hodgkin's lymphoma*	
follicular centre tumours	lymphoblastic lymphoma (cf. ALL)
centrocytic/centroblastic	lymphocytic lymphoma (cf. B-CLL)
immunoblastic (e.g. Burkitt's)	histiocytic lymphoma
lymphoplasmacytoid	T-zone lymphoma
(cf. Waldenström's)•	Sézary syndrome
	mycosis fungoides
	T-CLL

Fig 21.1 *Kiel classification system. Other major systems used includes the Lukes and Collins, and Rappaport schemes. The latter scheme uses the terms nodular versus diffuse and well versus poorly differentiated. Other terms in frequent use include nodal versus extranodal lymphomas and lymphomas of MALT (mucosa-associated lymphoid tissue). • Similar or equivalent leukaemic or pre-leukaemic conditions to lymphomas listed. † Rye classification scheme.

Benign proliferative conditions with pre-malignant clonal dominance	
lymphoproliferative	**myeloproliferative**
Waldenström's macroglobulinaemia	myelodysplastic syndromes (MDS)
α heavy chain disease	polycythaemia vera
angioblastic lymphadenopathy (ALD)	

Fig. 21.2 These proliferations of lymphoid cells (usually B cells but occasionally T in ALD) or myeloid progenitor cells involve only one or a small number of clones and may convert to overt leukaemia or lymphoma with high frequency.

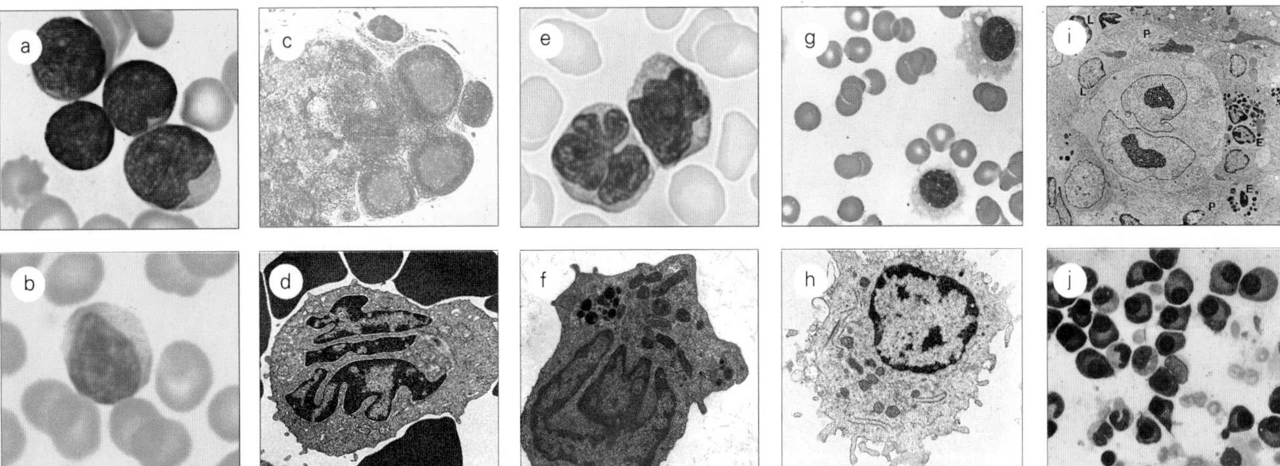

Fig. 21.3 Morphology of predominant cell types in blood cell malignancies. **(a)** ALL. Lymphoblasts with homogeneous chromatin, regular nuclear outline and absent or small nucleoli (L1 in the FAB classification scheme for acute leukaemia). **(b)** CLL. Small homogeneous lymphocyte with relatively condensed heterochromatin and high nuclear/cytoplasmic ratio. Courtesy of Dr B Bain. **(c)** NHL. Section of lymph node showing rounded enlarged follicles with pronounced pale germinal centres and surrounded by a variable mantle zone of small lymphocytes and suppressed (T cell) paracortical areas. **(d)** Sézary cell binding sheep erythrocytes. The nucleus is typically highly convoluted x3,300. **(e & f)** ATL. The nuclei are characteristically cerebriform in shape. **(g & h)** HCL. Large mononuclear cells with very irregular ('hairy') cell surfaces and some cytoplasmic vacuolation. **(i)** Hodgkin's disease ('mixed cellularity' subtype) showing a characteristic bi-nucleated Reed-Sternberg cell. E = eosinophil; P = plasma cell; L= lymphocyte. **(j)** Multiple myeloma. Giemsa stained smear (bone marrow) of tvpical plasma cells.

cells and molecular mechanisms that appear to be involved in childhood versus adult disease.

PHENOTYPIC CHARACTERIZATION OF LEUKAEMIAS AND LYMPHOMAS

Blood cell malignancies have been extensively analysed over the past 15 years with immunological, biochemical, cell kinetic, chromosomal and molecular methods. These studies have helped identify the relationship of different subtypes of disease to the normal cell populations from which they originate and have, in many cases, revealed cytogenetic, molecular and biochemical abnormalities that are unique to the leukaemic cell. As these observations unfolded, there was considerable interest in determining whether the features of leukaemic cells could help identify subsets within the major diagnostic groups that might differ prognostically given the same treatment. Several quantitative and qualitative associations have been found (Fig 21.5), and such correlations have served as a useful guide to further therapeutic developments.

IMMUNOPHENOTYPIC ANALYSIS

Identification of normal lymphocyte subsets has had a major impact on our understanding of the organization, function and pathology of the immune system. Similarly, the identification of subsets of leukaemic cells via their immunophenotype, that is the antigens they express, has provided important insight into the cellular diversity and origins of lymphoid malignancies, as well as diagnostic aids and potential new therapeutic approaches. The value of immunological characterization of leukaemias has been greatly helped by a number of technical innovations, especially the production and standardization of hybridoma derived monoclonal antibodies, and the workshop classification of antibodies and their corresponding cellular antigens into distinct biochemical groups (defined as CD or cluster of differentiation, followed by an arbitrary workshop number). Application of these reagents has been considerably aided by the development of flow cytometry methods, new fluorochromes for labelled antibodies and enzyme labelling methods that can be applied directly to blood smears as well as tissue sections. Figs. 21.6 & 21.7 illustrate some examples of the immunophenotypic analysis of leukaemic cells using these different methods.

Normal lymphoid cell immunophenotypes

Interpretation of leukaemic cell immunophenotype requires detailed information of the normal differentiation-linked programme of antigen expression in lymphocytes. This, in turn, requires careful investigation of lymphoid precursor cells in fetal liver, bone marrow and thymus. Equally important is the examination of lymphocyte subsets in peripheral lymphoid tissue and, particularly in the context of lymphomas, in germinal centres. From these analyses, it has been possible to construct a hypothetical developmental sequence of B and T lymphocytes in

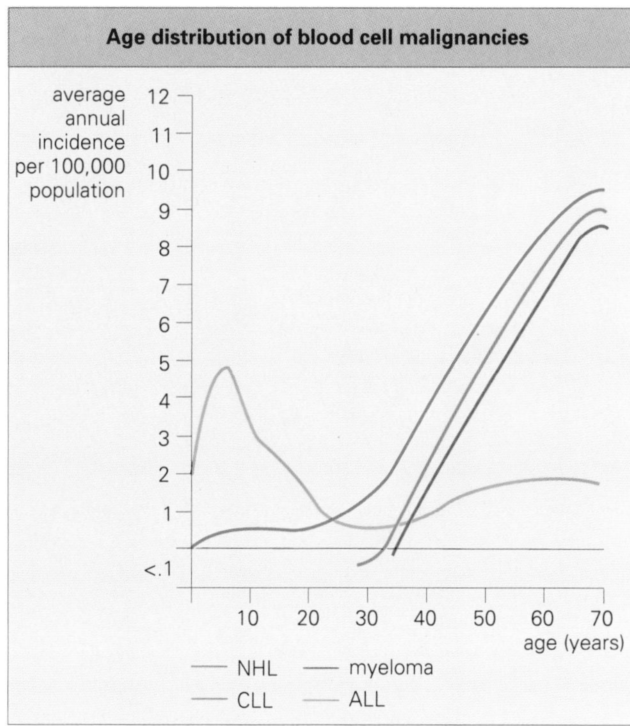

Fig. 21.4 ALL is the major leukaemia in childhood whereas most other blood cell malignancies have an increasing incidence with age, as observed with the common (epithelial) cancers. This incidence profile is typical of western, developed countries. A different pattern is seen in developing countries (e.g. Africa) and in the Far East. In Japan for example, the incidence of CLL, myeloma and follicular NHL is 2–3 times lower than that in the USA or Europe. In contrast, ATL associated with the retrovirus HTLV-1 is common in Japan and the Caribbean.

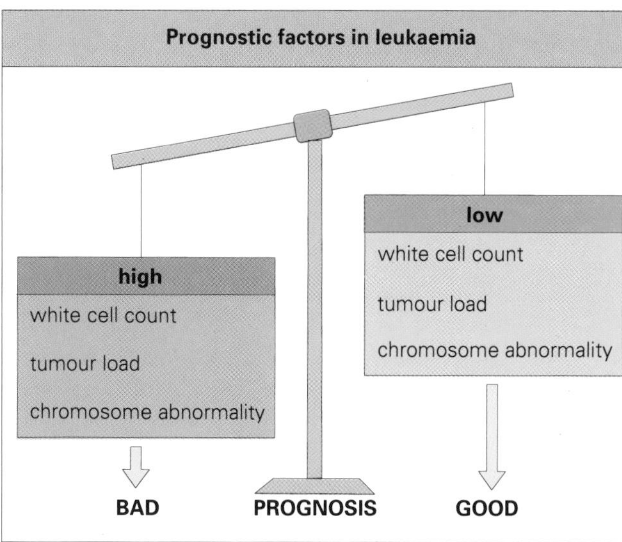

Fig. 21.5 All features listed provide some independent association with prognosis (i.e. remission induction or remission duration) in the context of particular therapeutic regimes.

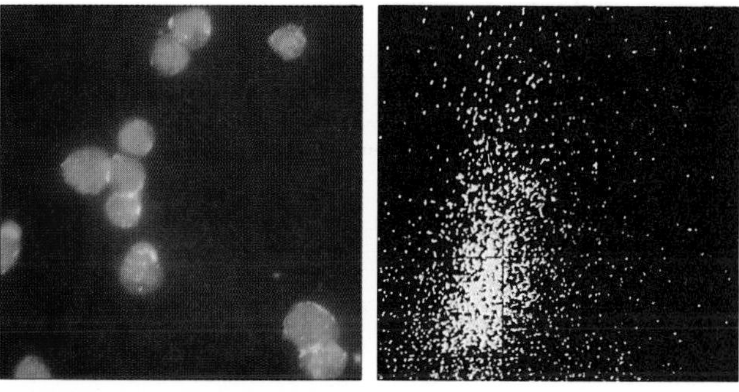

Fig.21.6 Immunophenotypic analysis by immunofluorescence. Left: microscopy. Leukaemic cells (ALL) stained with rhodamine labelled anti-terminal transferase (red nuclear stain) plus fluorescein labelled anti-CD10 (yellow/green cell surface stain) and viewed with incident UV illumination. Right: flow cytometry. Vertical axis = relative fluorescence intensity; horizontal axis/relative cell size. Leukaemic cells (ALL) stained with fluorescein labelled anti-CD10.

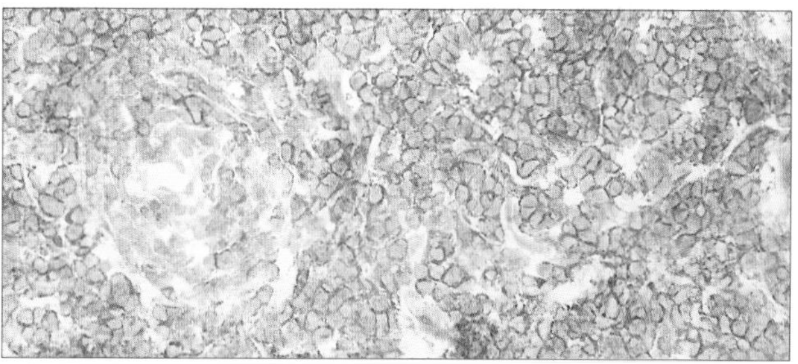

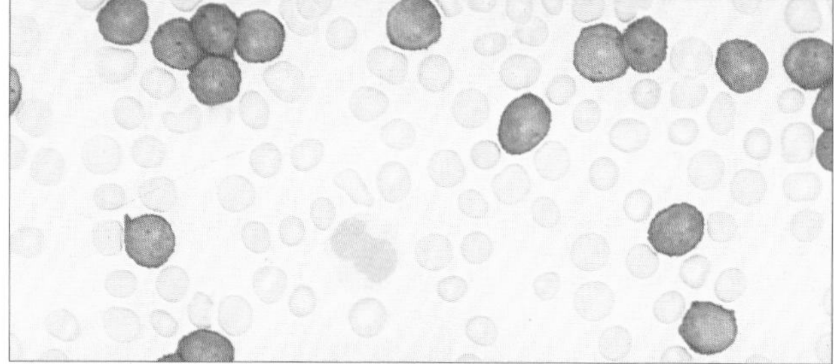

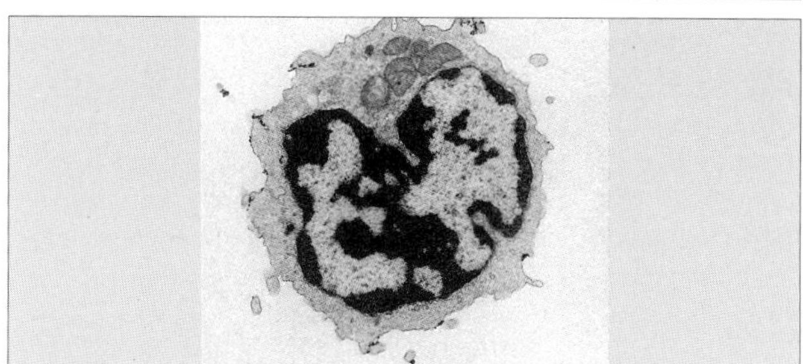

Fig. 21.7 Immunophenotypic analysis by immunocytochemistry.Upper: tissue section of testis infiltrated with leukaemic cells, stained with peroxidase labelled anti-CD10. Middle: blood film. T cell leukaemia stained with alkaline phosphatase labelled anti-CD5. Lower: immunogold EM showing T lymphocyte labelled with anti-CD4 linked to 30nm gold particles.

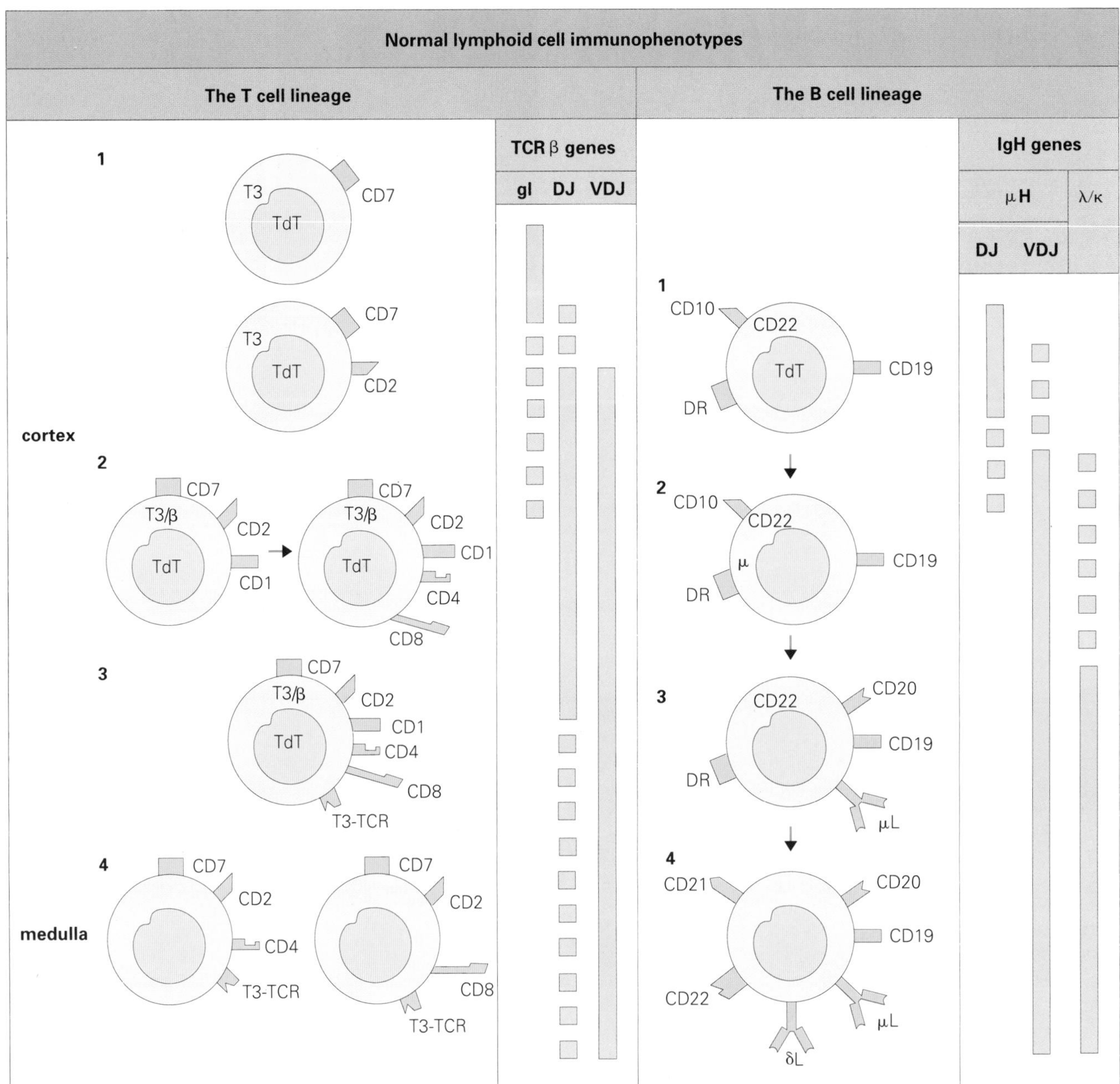

Fig. 21.8 Left: the putative linear sequence of intrathymic development is shown. A CD (cluster of differentiation) number given to each cell surface antigen detected. Note that early immature T cells have intracellular CD3 and T cell receptor (TCR) proteins but not on the cell surface. The rearrangement configuration of the T cell receptor (β) gene is shown. Fragmented lines indicate variable phenotypic features. Right: the putative linear sequence of B cell development is shown. μ = free μ heavy chain; μL = cell surface IgM. The rearrangement pattern of heavy and light chain Ig genes is shown. Cells in 1 and 2 are precursor B cells. Cells in 3 and 4 are mature, immunocompetent B cells. Note that plasma cells lack most B cells markers and are not included here.

which the co-ordinated expression of cell surface antigens, intracellular antigens and immunoglobulin or T cell receptor gene rearrangement can be mapped (Fig. 21.8). Note that some cells' surface antigens (CD22 and μ heavy chains in B cells, CD3 and T cell receptor β chains in T cells) appear in the cytoplasm of precursor lymphoid cells before they are detectable on the cell surface.

Immunophenotypic classification

These developmental maps of antigen expression in lymphopoiesis (in much more detail than can be illustrated here) and similar data on myelopoiesis provide the framework for an immunological classification of blood cell malignancies. In such schemes as these (Fig. 21.9), the common or dominant immunophenotype of the

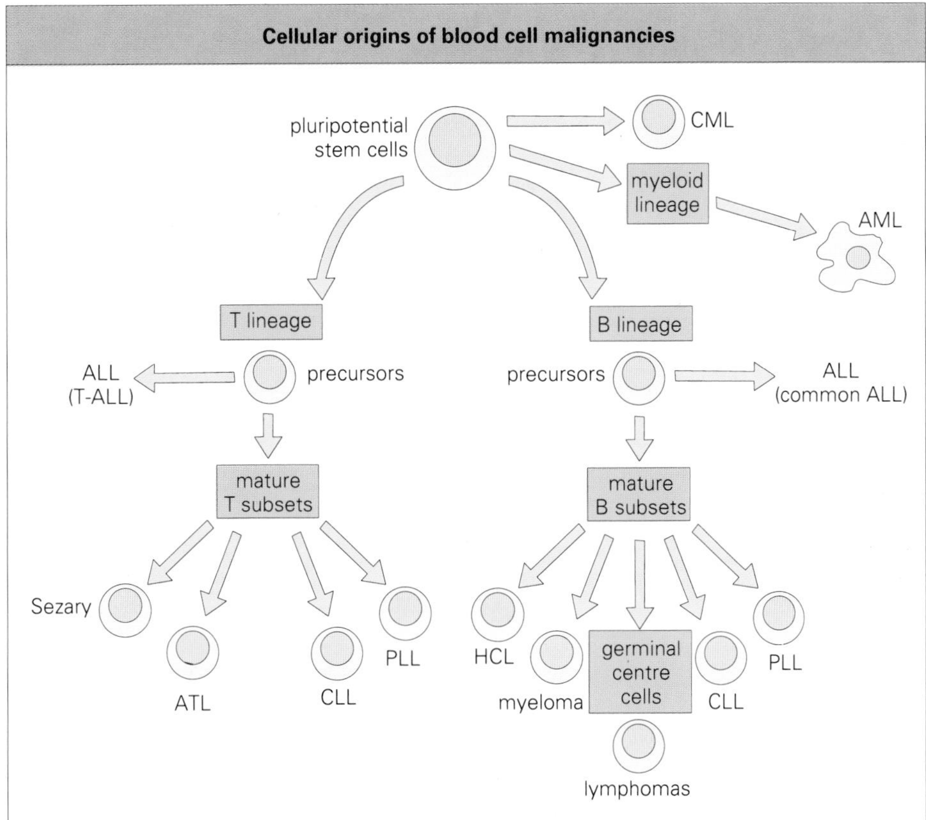

Fig.21.9 Immunophenotypic classification of leukaemias and lymphomas by comparison with normal developmental/functional equivalents. This illustrates the approximate level of maturation arrest of the majority of leukaemia or lymphoma cells in particular subtypes of disease.

leukaemia or lymphoma is affiliated to the nearest normal counterpart. From these comparisons, it emerges that acute lymphoblastic leukaemia (ALL) cells have the overall features of B or T precursor cells, whereas other lymphoid malignancies are equivalent to subsets of mature lymphoid T or B cells. The majority of childhood ALL have the immunophenotypes of B lymphocyte precursor cells. These are often referred to as common ALL and account for the pronounced 2–6 year age peak (Fig. 21.10).

One corollary of these findings is that some leukaemia cells, especially in ALL, have the composite immunophenotypes of normal cells that are numerically quite infrequent, and very careful analysis of bone marrow or thymus is required to detect them. In some non-leukaemia circumstances, for example fetal haemopoietic tissue or regenerating bone marrow (after chemotherapy and/or radiation), the number of these normal precursor cells with 'leukaemic' phenotypes may increase substantially but transiently (Fig. 21.11).

Complications of immunophenotypic analysis

The comparison between leukaemic and normal cells is not quite as simple as implied in summary diagrams such as Fig. 21.9. There are a number of complications of immunophenotypic analysis that are important to appreciate (Fig. 21.12). Perhaps the most important of these is the fact that the dominant phenotype of a leukaemic cell population reflects the degree of maturation achieved by a leukaemic clone and may not, therefore, correspond either precisely to a specific normal equivalent cell or to the initial 'target' cell for the disease, which might be a more primitive cell type than is suggested by immunophenotype.

The latter caveat may have important implications for therapy and curability and is most evident in chronic myeloid leukaemia. In this, the leukaemic cells have the phenotypic properties of immature granulocytes, but the transformed cell is known from clonal analysis (see below) to be a multi-potential lymphomyeloid stem cell. In the chronic (or benign) stage of disease, the progeny of the transformed stem cell are still able to mature relatively normally into all lymphoid and myeloid lineages with additional proliferative advantage in the granulocyte lineage (hence the terminology CML or CGL). Subsequent genetic events (after an average of three years) may block differentiation and produce an acute leukaemia (or 'blast crisis' of CML) with the phenotype of either precursor myeloid or lymphoid cells.

Mixed lymphomyeloid lineage. A proportion of acute leukaemias have a mixed lymphomyeloid lineage immunophenotype. In those that are a mixture of separate or dual populations of lymphoid plus myeloid precursor cells, the interpretation is quite straightforward: a leukaemia originating in a common lymphomyeloid stem cell

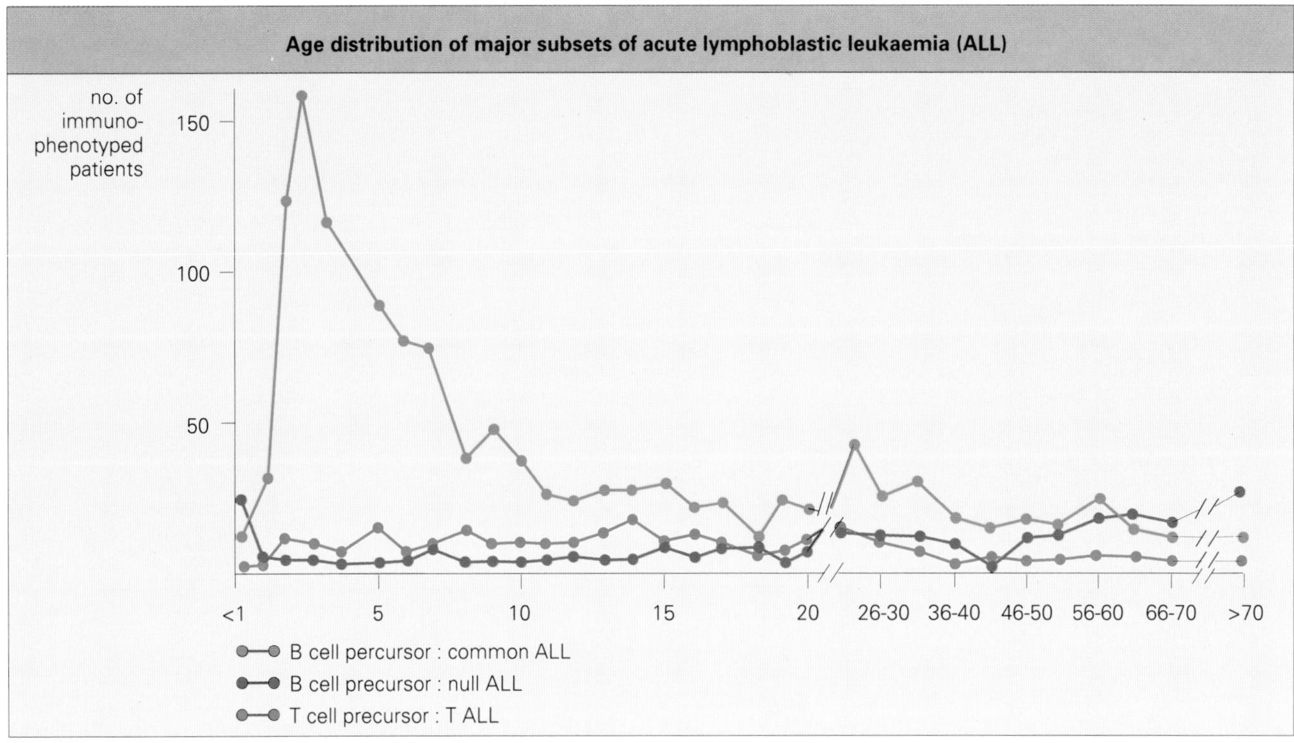

Fig. 21.10 Age distribution in ALL based on a data set of approximately 1,500 patients.

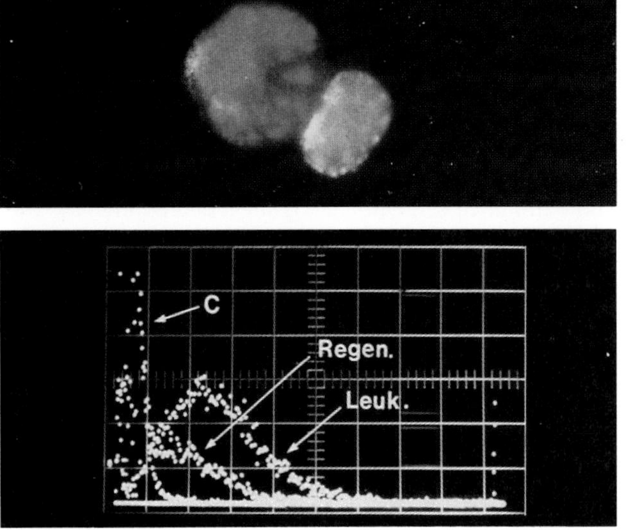

Fig. 21.11 Detecting the rare normal equivalent to leukaemic cells. Upper: cells in non-leukaemic regenerating bone marrow stained simultaneously with rhodamine labelled anti-TdT (red nuclear stain) and fluorescein labelled anti-CD10 (yellow/green cell surface stain). These two cells have the same immunophenotype as common acute lymphoblastic leukaemia cells (see Fig. 21.6 left). Lower: flow cytometry of the same cells. Note that in this non-leukaemic sample, the number of staining cells (19%) is less than in a leukaemic (ALL) bone marrow; the cells also tend to be smaller and stain less intensely. Vertical axis = relative cell number; horizontal axis = relative fluorescence intensity.

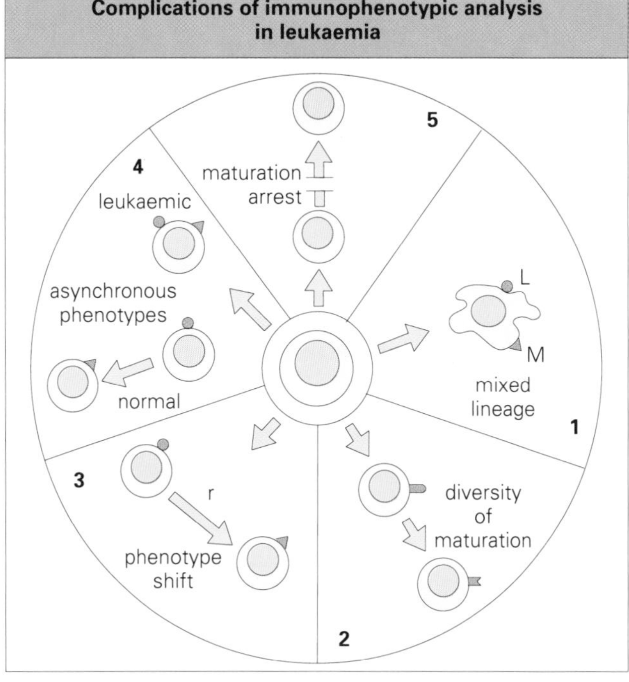

Fig. 21.12 1) phenotypes may be mixed lineage or 'aberrant'. L = lymphoid; M = myeloid. 2) diversity of maturation linked phenotype within clone. 3) shift of phenotype in relapse (r). 4) individual cell phenotypes may be asynchronous compared with normal, e.g. they may express antigens simultaneously that are normally expressed sequentially. 5) major immunophenotype indicates approximate level of maturation arrest, not developmental level of original 'target' cell.

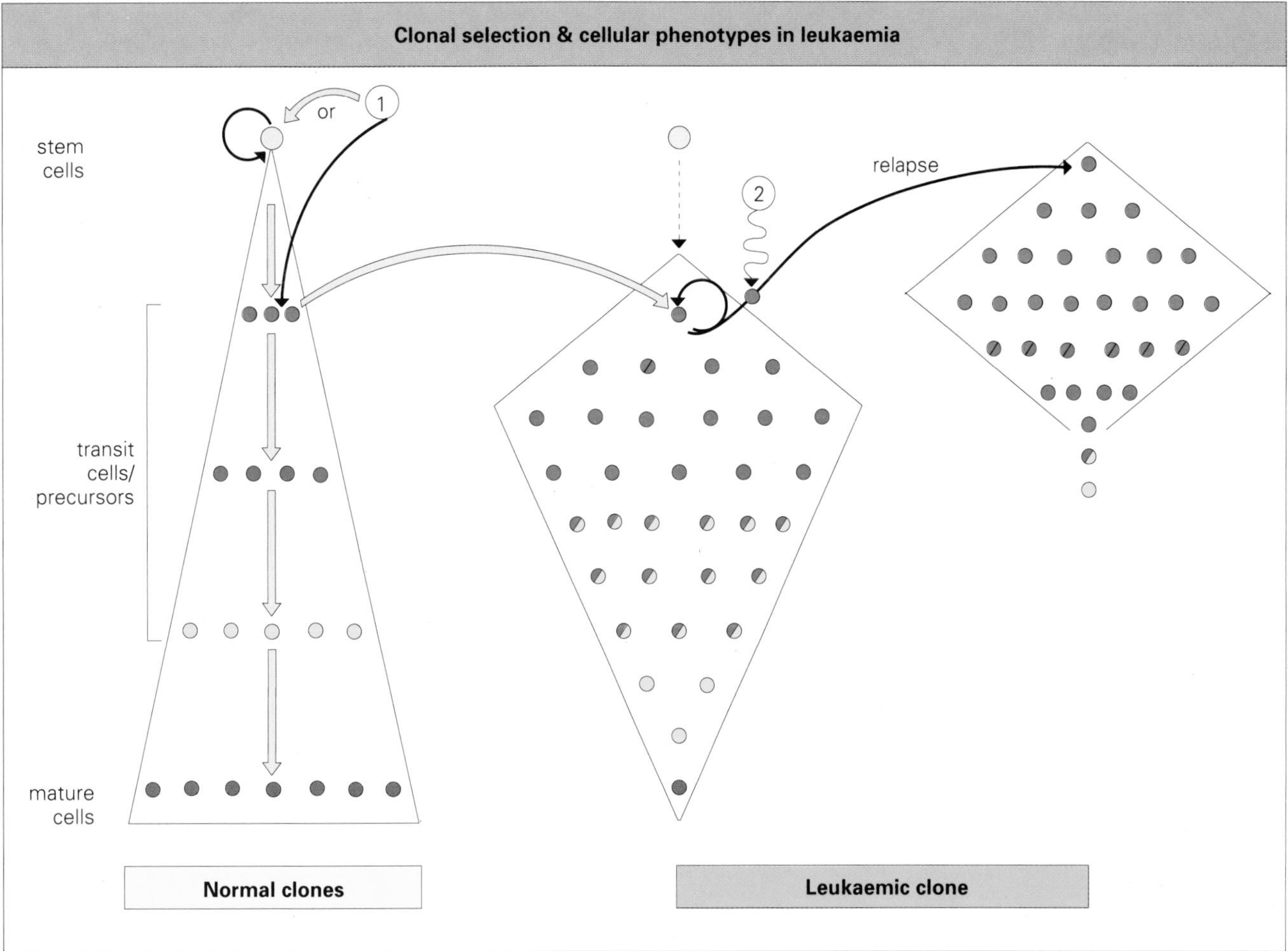

Fig. 21.13 The normal developmental sequence is illustrated on left. The leukaemic clone and its subsequent sub-clone (in relapse) show a dysregulation of uncoupling of proliferation and differentiation resulting in abortive maturation and some asynchrony of phenotypes (mixed colour cells). 1 = first genetic (transforming) event in primitive stem cell or one of its immediate progeny; 2 = second key genetic event occurring in clonogenic, poorly differentiated cell within leukaemic clone which then has further selective growth advantage (and perhaps drug resistance) and produces a dominant (sub) clone in relapse with more pronounced maturation arrest.

with concomitant differentiation of daughter cells into both lineages. In other circumstances, individual leukaemic cells may express both lymphoid and myeloid markers. Here, the biological interpretation is more tricky. These leukaemias probably also originate in common lymphomyeloid stem cells and their mixed lineage features may arise from either or both of the following:

- the leukaemic transformation mechanisms disrupt the normal molecular programme of lineage differentiation, producing a single aberrant phenotype;
- or, if normal lymphomyeloid stem cells are transformed into leukaemic cells and continue to proliferate in the absence of effective differentiation, then they will express multiple lineage genes that are normally available for expression in such stem cells.

Irrespective of the precise biological meaning of these complex phenotypes, it is important to note that leukaemias originating in lymphomyeloid stem cells are only very rarely curable by conventional chemotherapy and radiation. Bone marrow transplantation offers the best prospect for such patients. Adults tend to have a higher proportion of stem cell leukaemias than children, which partly explains the variable success rates of conventional treatment in relation to patient age.

Phenotypic diversity. Phenotypic diversity, phenotypic switch and maturation asynchrony, are other important features of leukaemic cells. Such heterogeneity at the antigenic and molecular level occurs despite the fact that leukaemic cells are monoclonal (note that in rare cases, an apparent leukaemic relapse may be a new cancer induced by therapeutic agents and originate in a separate clone). Fig. 21.13 summarizes the impact that this intrinsic diversity has on the comparison of normal and leukaemic cells.

GENOTYPIC ALTERATIONS IN LEUKAEMIA AND LYMPHOMA

Leukaemia, lymphoma and myeloma, in common with other cancers, arise as a consequence of mutations in DNA. *A priori,* the genes involved are likely to be those critically involved in regulating proliferation and differentiation of cells. Insight into these genes has been possible because of:

- identification of oncogenes (in oncogenic viruses) and their normal cellular counterparts (proto-oncogenes);
- chromosomal localization of both proto-oncogenes and other important genes (e.g. Ig, T cell receptor genes) by *in situ* hybridization;
- the discovery of non-random chromosome alterations, especially translocations, in leukaemia.

The latter observations provided crude geographic clues (to within 10^7 base pairs or 10^3 genes) and allowed candidate genes to be identified and subsequently verified by molecular cloning and sequencing.

There are now many examples of consistent molecular rearrangements in blood cell malignancy (more that 15 in ALL alone) and in this section a few of the best understood examples are described.

INVOLVEMENT OF Ig AND TCR GENES IN LEUKAEMOGENESIS

In the lymphoid malignancies, the most striking molecular discovery has been the high frequency with which chromosomal rearrangements involve the immunoglobulin and T cell receptor (TCR) loci on their respective chromosomes (Fig. 21.14). Fig. 21.15 summarizes most of the

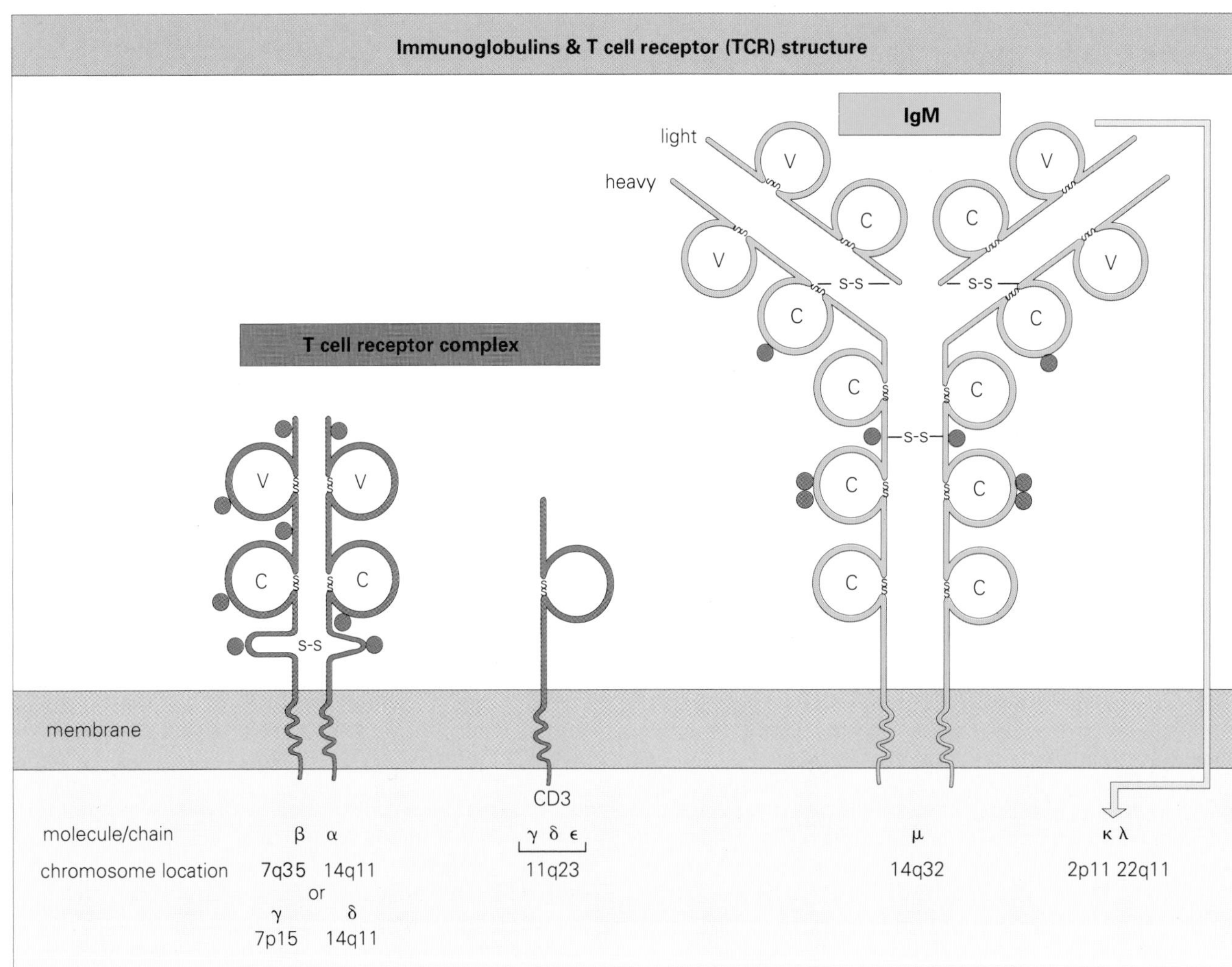

Fig. 21.14 The chromosome location of the various chains is shown. V = variable region domains; C = constant region domains; s-s = disulphide bonds, helping the formation of globular domain structures (shown as loops). Blue circles = carbohydrate side chains.

changes which bring immunoglobulin or TCR genes in juxtaposition to other, normally unlinked, genes in a form of illegitimate recombination. The generally accepted explanation for this remarkable observation has two parts:

- that the Ig and TCR loci are prone to physical disruption and rearrangement in lymphoid cells and, moreover, are constitutively expressed (unlike many other genes) in lymphoid cells;
- and that if another gene, that regulates, say, proliferation, is brought within the physical domain of immunoglobulin or TCR gene control, then it too may be constitutively expressed (i.e cannot easily be turned off) and its product may therefore drive proliferation independently of the normal extracellular regulatory signals.

The c-MYC gene in Burkitt's lymphoma

In no case yet have all the molecular and biochemical details been understood, but in several, the 'partner' genes and their protein products are identified and likely mechanisms have been explored. The first of these to be unravelled was the association of Ig genes with the MYC proto-oncogene in Burkitt's lymphoma (Fig. 21.16) which occurs as a consequence of a reciprocal chromosomal translocation between chromosome 14q32 (where the IgH gene is located) and 8q24 (where the c-MYC gene is located).

Two different types of molecular rearrangement occur, in so-called 'endemic' Burkitt's lymphoma (in tropical Africa) and in 'sporadic' Burkitt's lymphoma (outside of the endemic area). These rearrangements differ in where the IgH gene breaks and joins up to c-MYC. The latter may also lose exon 1 or acquire mutations in this exon (Fig. 21.17). Although the precise function of the c-MYC protein is not known, it is a nuclear protein sharing DNA recognition motives with other transcription factor proteins and is normally expressed in a co-ordinated fashion with the cell cycle. It seems likely, therefore, that constitutive expression of c-MYC, driven by the Ig locus, forces constitutive cell proliferation. Transgenic mice carrying a human c-MYC gene fused to an IgH region have a very high predisposition towards B cell malignancy, providing evidence for the oncogenic effect of this rearrangement. The 'sporadic' Burkitt's lymphoma IgH–c-MYC rearrangement also occurs in non-Burkitt B cell malignancies.

Involvement of immunoglobulin & T cell receptor genes in leukaemogenesis

	Chromosome	Partner chr/gene
Ig		
IgH	14q32	11q13 ('BCL-1'), BCL-2 (18q21), MYC (8q24)
κ	2p12	MYC (8q24)
λ	22q11	MYC (8q24)
TCR		
δ	14q11	11p13 11p15, 10q24, 1p32
γ	7p15	-
α	14q11	MYC, 11p13, 14q32
β	7q35	9q32, 9q34, 19p13, 14q32

Fig. 21.15 Involvement of immunoglobulin and T cell receptor genes in leukaemogenesis.

The BCL-2 gene in follicular lymphoma

In a high proportion (75%) of B cell non-Hodgkin's lymphomas of the nodular or follicular type, there is a consistent translocation between chromosomes 14q32 and 18q21 which brings the IgH gene in juxtaposition to a gene at 18q21, BCL-2 (B cell leukaemia gene 2). Breaks occur in the J region of the IgH gene and either within the second exon (e2) or downstream from it in BCL-2 (Fig 21.18). The fused hybrid gene does not transcribe across the fusion junction and, as in the case of c-MYC, the net result appears to be dysregulated expression of a normal protein, in this case BCL-2. The latter is a 24kDa cytoplasmic protein found predominantly in non-cycling lymphoid cells and has the unusual property of protecting cells from apoptosis or active cell death. Since most cells in the germinal centre die in the absence of antigenic stimulation, BCL-2 appears different from typical proto-oncogenes in exerting its effect via life-span effects. BCL-2 can complement or synergize with more classical

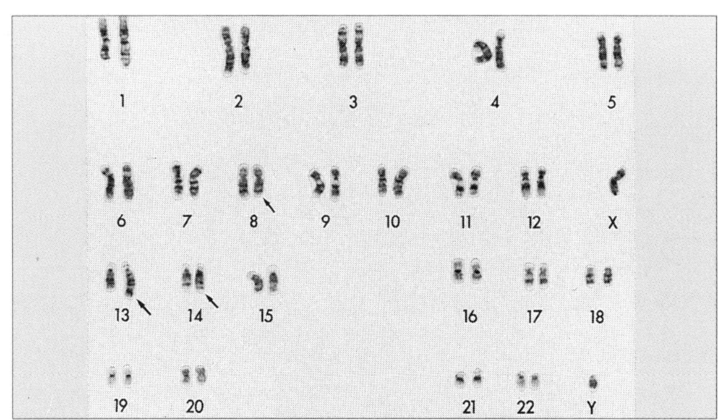

Fig. 21.16 Metaphase from a tumour mass of a male child with non-Hodgkin's lymphoma (diffuse non-Burkitt's) and stained with trypsin-Giemsa. This cell has the typical Burkitt's translocation involving chromosomes 8 and 14 with breaks in band 8q24 and 14q32; this translocation was seen in all cells. There is also an abnormal chromosome 13 with added material of undetermined origin which was observed in 80% of cells.

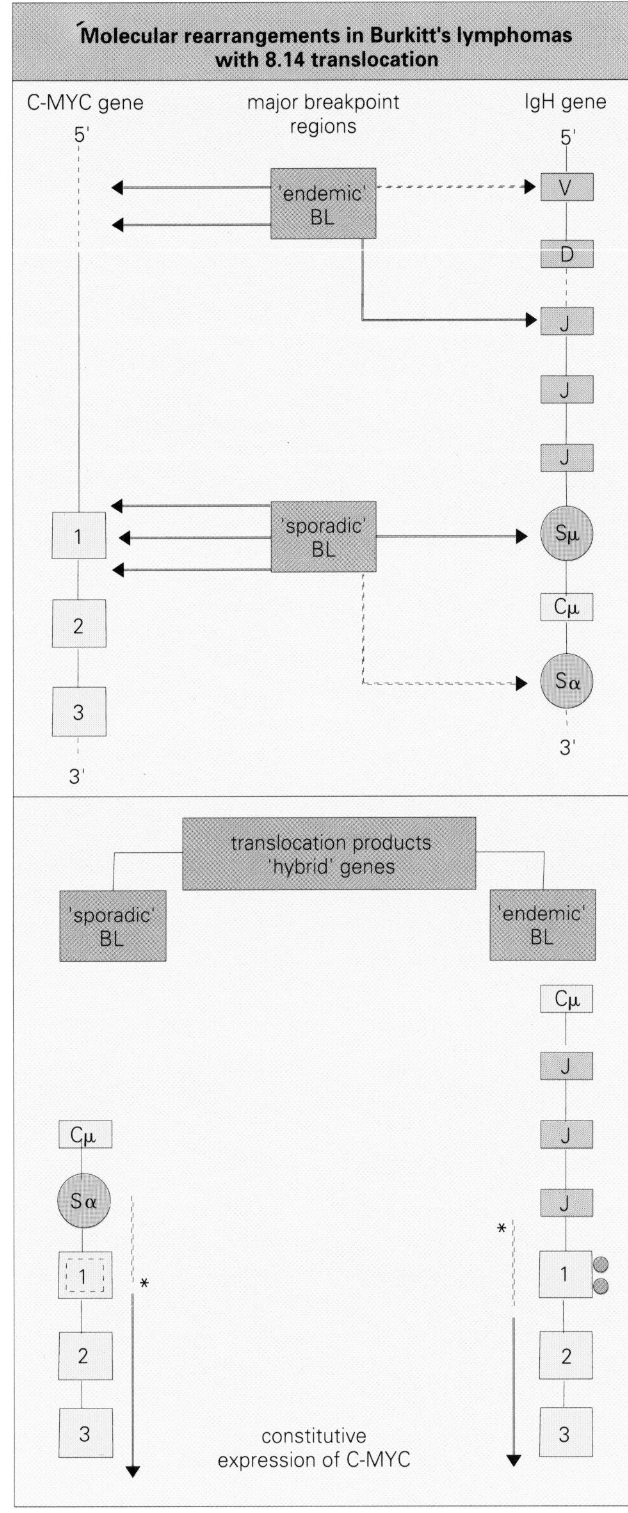

Fig. 21.17 **S** = switch region.*= untranslated first exon of the MYC gene. 1 (in broken box) = first exon of MYC gene may be variably deleted or truncated in the 'sporadic' form of Burkitt's lymphoma. Purple circles indicate mutation commonly found in this region in 'endemic' Burkitt's lymphoma.

oncogenes in experimental *in vitro* systems and it is likely that genetic alterations, in addition to BCL-2 dysregulation, may be required for the development of follicular lymphoma.

Transcription factor genes in acute lymphoblastic leukaemia

Transcription factors are proteins that can bind to particular DNA sequences via distinctive domain-like structures (leucine zippers, zinc fingers, helix-loop-helix structures, homeoboxes or homeodomains) as well as interact with other proteins and in so doing, help form stable DNA transcription complexes with RNA polymerase II. Modulation of transcription factor proteins themselves, by, for example, dimerization or phophorylation, provides a major mechanism for regulating gene expression, differentiation and hence cell phenotype. Defects in transcription factor genes produce profound developmental defects in *Drosophila* and several oncogenes are now known to encode this type of product (for example JUN, ERB-A/thyroid hormone receptor, INT-1). MYC probably belongs to this class of proteins. Recent evidence implicates new transcription factor genes in chromosome translocations observed in ALL. Fig. 21.19 illustrates two such translocations. In B cell precursor ALL, transcription factor gene (E2A), known to regulate the IgH gene is rearranged by fusion to a portion of a novel gene (Pr-1) on chromosome 1 that itself has a DNA recognition element (homeodomain). In this fusion, the DNA binding region of E2A is effectively replaced by the homeodomain of Pr-1 producing a fusion protein that probably functions as a novel transcription factor.

In the second example, occurring in T-ALL, another transcription factor gene (Lyl-1) on chromosome 19p13 is fused, out of frame for transcription, to the J region of the T cell receptor β gene. There is no fusion product in his case and the presumption is, as with MYC translocations, that the Lyl-1 protein is dysregulated by illegitimate association with the T-cell receptor. Whether these types of rearrangements promote cell proliferation or block differentiation, or both, remains to be determined.

The Philadelphia (Ph) chromosome in CML and ALL

The fourth example of a chromosomal rearrangement was in fact the first to be discovered in 1960, although a further 25 years were required to decipher the underlying molecular mechanism. As illustrated in Fig. 21.20, the Ph chromosome is formed by a reciprocal exchange between chromosomes 9 and 22, producing a fusion between the ABL proto-oncogene from 9q32 and a gene at present called the BCR gene (Breakpoint Cluster Region for CML). The two genes are fused in frame for transcription and produce a novel hybrid mRNA and protein in which the N-terminal is encoded by BCR. The biochemical consequence of this fusion is that the otherwise weak or unstable tyrosine kinase activity of c-ABL now becomes stable or greatly enhanced.

Breaks can occur in two distinct regions of the BCR gene (Fig. 21.21). When they occur in the 'major breakpoint region' between exons b2 and b3 or b3 and b4, they

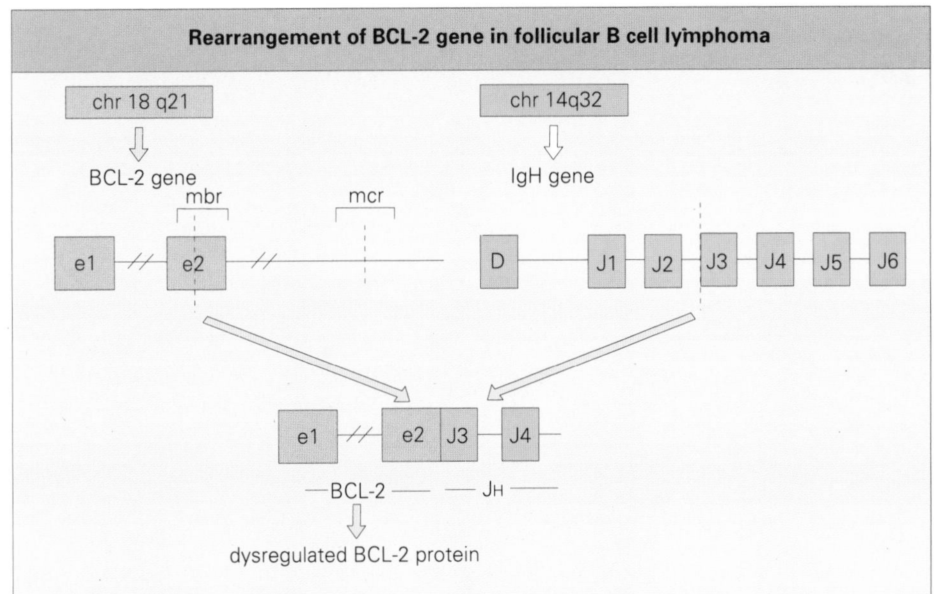

Fig. 21.18 Rearrangement of the BCL-2 gene in follicular B cell lymphoma. e = exon (of BCL-2 gene). mbr = major breakpoint regions. mcr = minor cluster (of breakpoints) region.

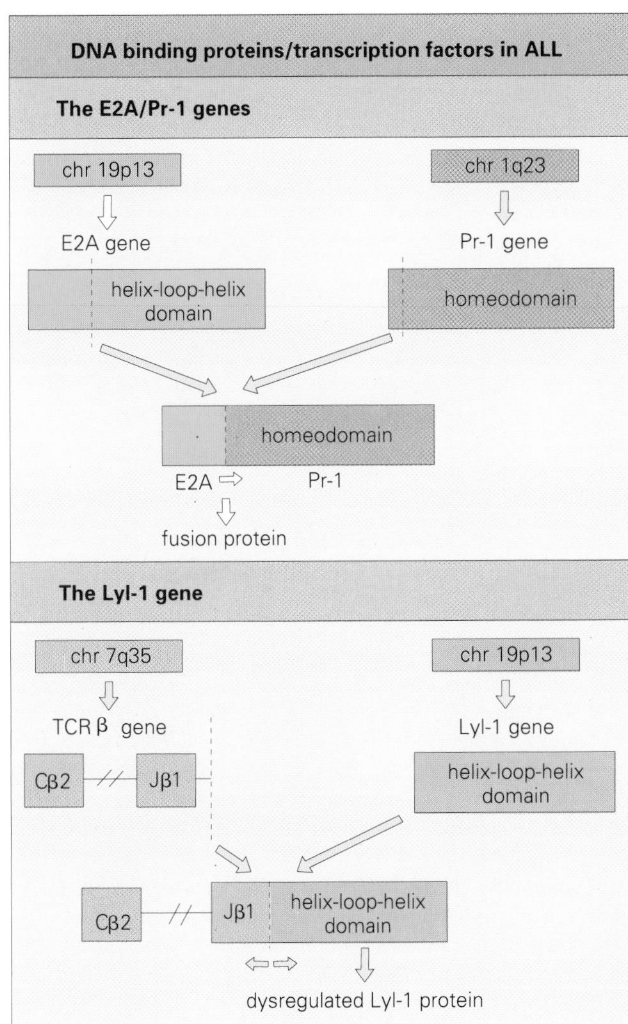

Fig. 21.19 Involvement of DNA binding proteins/transcription factors in acute lymphoblastic leukaemia.

result in a 210kDa BCR-ABL protein and this is the form found in over 99% of CML with the Ph chromosome. In some cases, however, the break occurs in the first intron of BCR (the 'minor breakpoint region'); this fusion then produces a shorter protein of 190kDa. Interestingly this latter breakpoint and p190 protein is often found in acute lymphoblastic leukaemia with the Ph chromosome.

Cloned BCR-ABL p210 or p190 genes, when transfected in fertilized eggs to produce transgenic mice, initiate or cause CML or ALL respectively providing persuasive evidence that this molecular liaison is a critical part of the causal mechanism in CML and some ALL.

Clonality of lymphoid malignancy

The majority of leukaemias and lymphomas so far investigated, in common with other human cancers, are monoclonal, the few exceptions being some multi-focal lymphomas in immunosuppressed transplant or AIDS patients. The rationale of monoclonality is that very rare and specific genetic events are required to transform normal cells to a leukaemic state and the probability of these occurring is so small that only one cell at most in the body is likely to undergo such a change.

Evidence for clonality comes from the use of X-linked polymorphisms (in females), complex chromosome alterations (for example translocations) and, specifically in lymphoid malignancy, the pattern of rearrangement of immunoglobulin or T cell receptor genes. Since normal lymphoid cells develop in a clonal fashion with respect to the rearrangement and expression of these genes, this can be conveniently exploited to demonstrate clonality in leukaemia or lymphoma. Normal lymphocyte populations in blood, in germinal centres of lymphoid tissue or in cell populations transformed *in vitro* with Epstein Barr virus (EBV) will be a mixture of multiple clones in which some cells produce κ light chains and some cells λ light chains (Fig. 21.22). In contrast, in EBV-associated Burkitt's

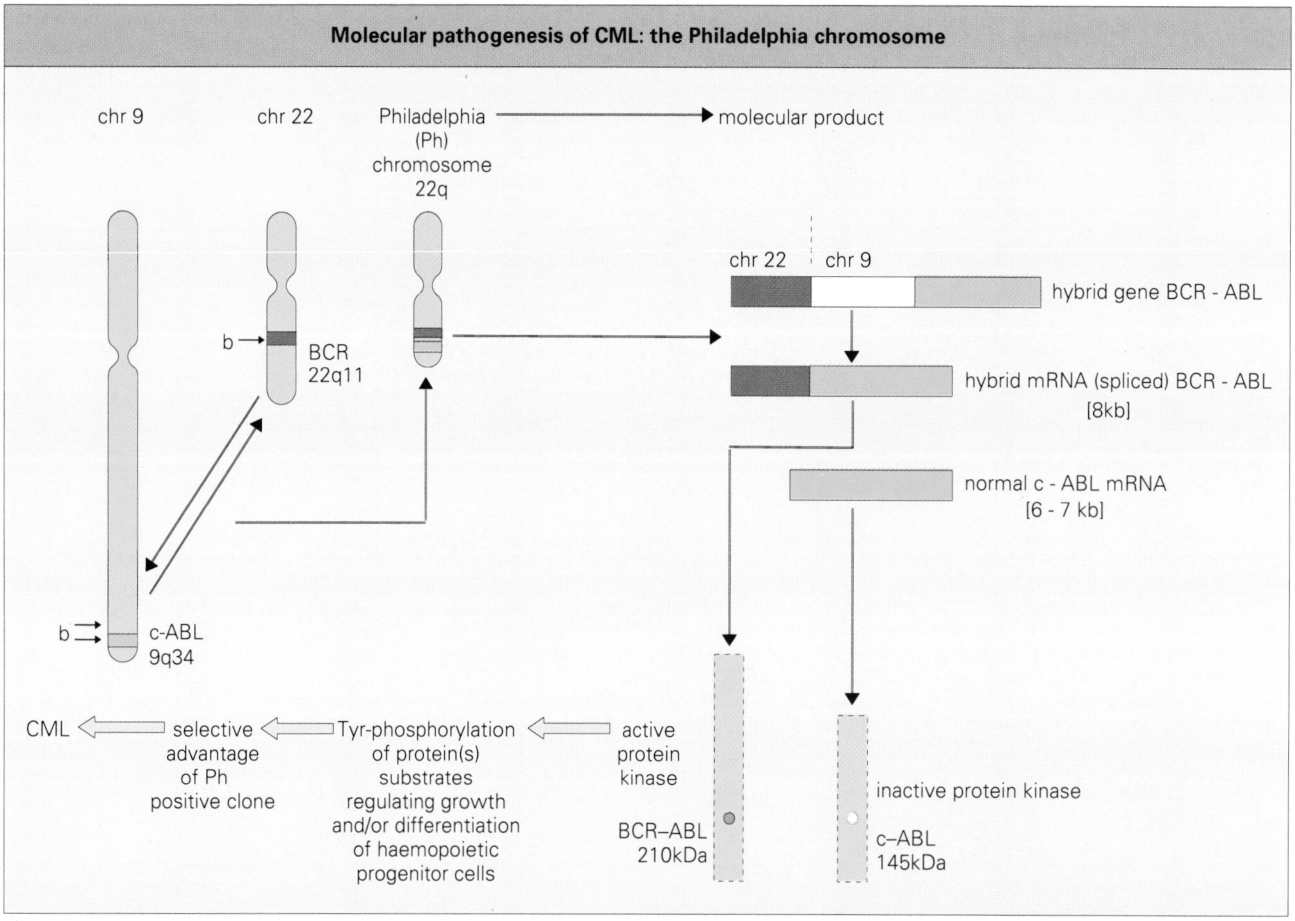

Molecular pathogenesis of CML: the Philadelphia chromosome
chr 9
chr 22
Philadelphia (Ph) chromosome 22q
molecular product
chr 22
chr 9
hybrid gene BCR - ABL
b
BCR
22q11
hybrid mRNA (spliced) BCR - ABL [8kb]
normal c - ABL mRNA [6 - 7 kb]
b
c-ABL
9q34
CML
selective advantage of Ph positive clone
Tyr-phosphorylation of protein(s) substrates regulating growth and/or differentiation of haemopoietic progenitor cells
active protein kinase
BCR–ABL 210kDa
inactive protein kinase
c-ABL 145kDa

1
2
3
4
5
6
7
8
9
10
11
12
X
13
14
15
16
17
18
19
20
21
22
Y

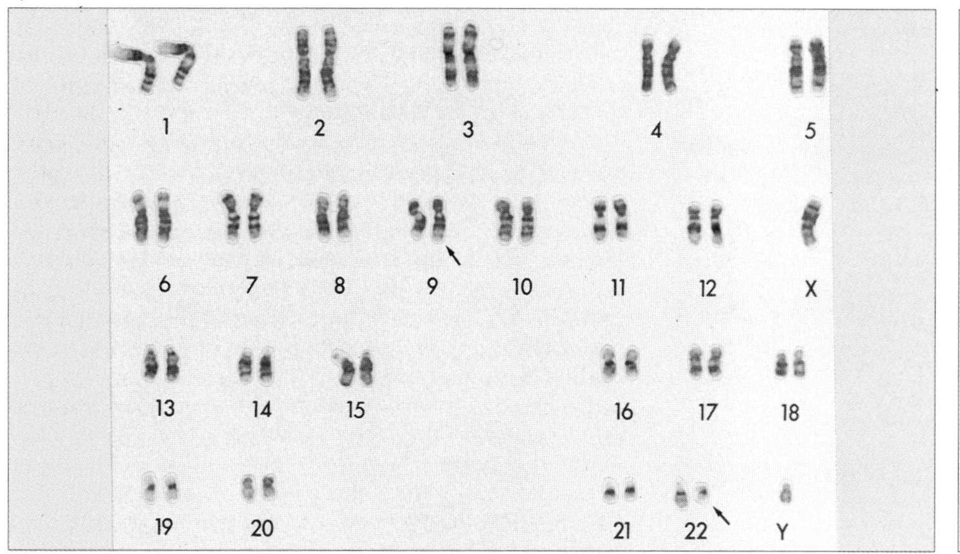

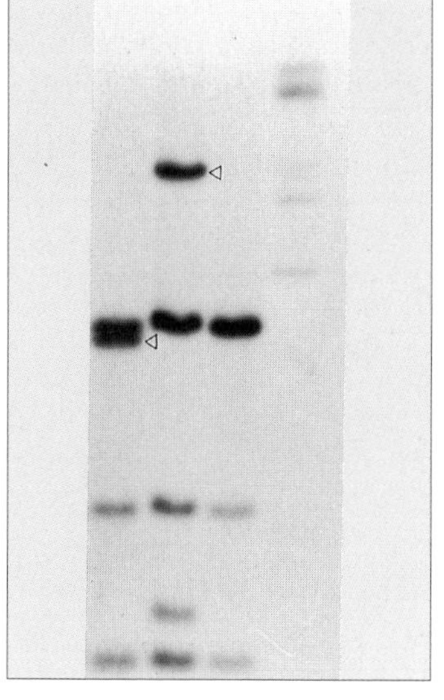

Fig.21.20 Upper: molecular (translocation) events associated with Ph chromosome formation and its functional consequences. The key event is the increased protein tyrosine kinase activity of the c-ABL protein which arises as a consequence of the additional N-terminal protein sequence added onto the c-ABL protein by the BCR gene. Lower left: banded metaphase chromosomes from a Ph-positive CML showing an abbreviated chromosome 22 and an elongated chromosome 9. Lower right: Southern blot analysis of BCR gene rearrangement in Ph-positive CML. DNA from leukaemic cells is digested with restriction endonulcease (Bg/II) and probed with a radioactive BCR DNA probe. Control sample (lane 3) shows the normal three fragments (i.e. unrearranged). Lanes 1 and 2 have DNA from CML patients and have clonal rearrangements (arrowed). Lane 4 has molecular weight standards.

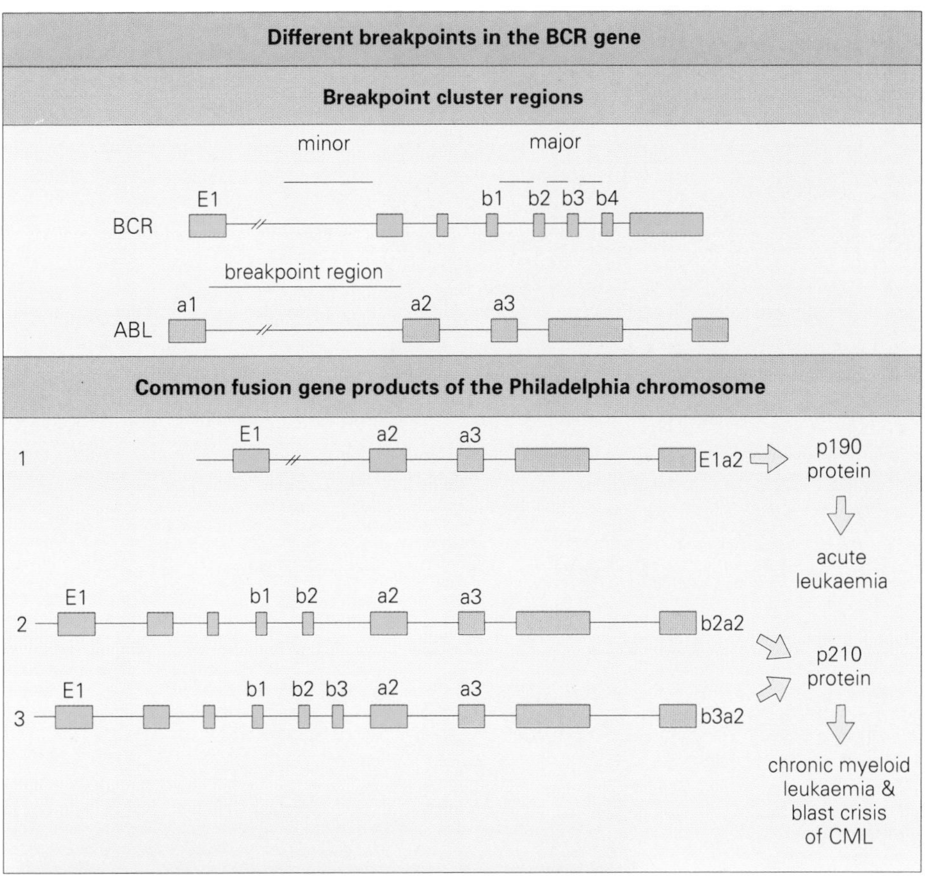

Fig. 21.21 Different breakpoints in the BCR gene. E1, b1 etc = exon numbers. E1a2 = fusion of E1 exon (of BCR) to a2 exon (of ABL). -//- = intron not drawn to scale.

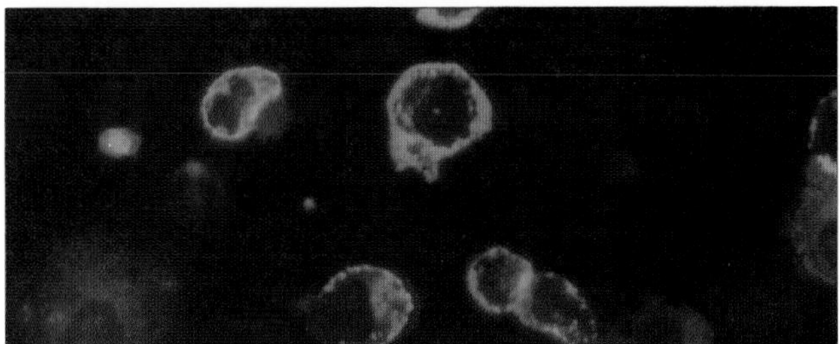

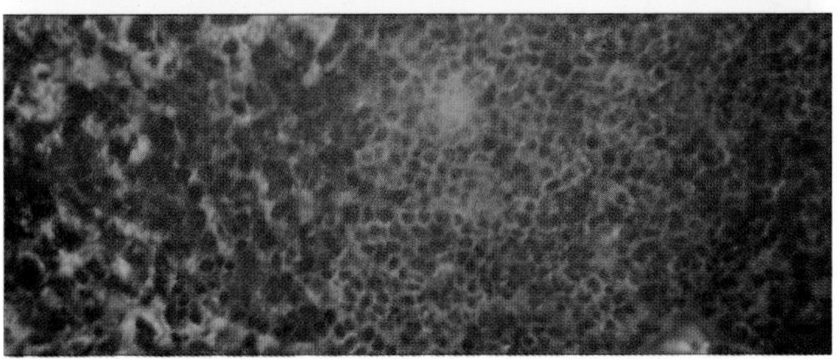

Fig. 21.22 Upper: immunofluorescent staining of EBV transformed normal blood B cells for intracellular kappa light chains (red/rhodamine anti-κ) and lambda (green/fluorescein anti-λ). Both κ and λ producing cells are present in this polyclonal population. Lower: immunofluorescent staining of a normal lymph node germinal centre for kappa (red/rhodamine anti-κ) and lambda (green/fluorescein anti-λ) light chains. As illustrated here, normal germinal centres are poly- or oligoclonal, producing both types of light chains (in separate cells).

lymphoma and in follicular lymphoma the lymphoma cells produce either κ or λ light chain but not both (Fig. 21.23). Clonal restriction can also be demonstrated at the DNA level by Southern blot rearrangement patterns of IgH or T cell receptor DNA (Fig 21.24). In contrast to the multiple restriction fragment sizes (and resultant gel smear) observed with normal lymphoid cell populations, clonal lymphoid malignancies usually show only one or two rearranged fragments. Clonal rearrangements of immunoglobulin or TCR genes will usually distinguish malignant from immunoreactive conditions but it should be borne in mind that in some non-malignant conditions, clonally restricted lymphocyte populations may be present (for example clonal T cells in synovial fluid in patients with rheumatoid arthritis and in the cerebrospinal fluid of patients with multiple sclerosis).

THE NATURAL HISTORY OF LYMPHOID MALIGNANCY

Although specific molecular alterations have been identified in most varieties of lymphoid cancer, we are still some way from having a comprehensive understanding of the aetiological mechanisms involved. This is for several reasons;

- firstly, because the precise function of the altered protein is, in many cases, unknown;

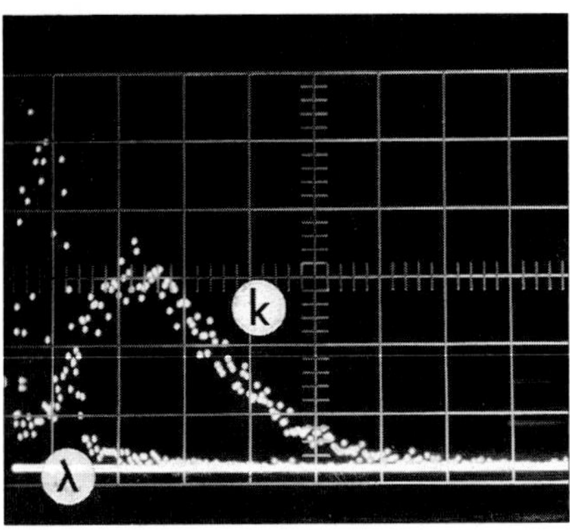

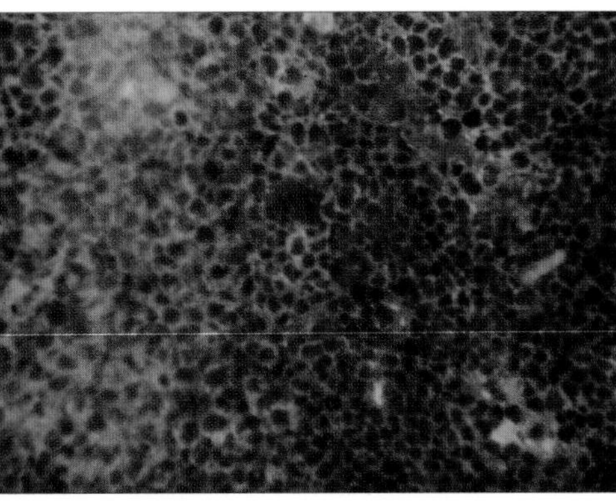

Fig. 21.23 Left: flow cytometry analysis of Burkitt's lymphoma cells for cells surface Ig light chain expression. Vertical axis = relative cell number; horizontal axis = relative fluorescence intensity. All cells stain for κ but not λ light chains. Right: immunofluorescent staining of a lymph node section in follicular lymphoma for κ and λ light chains. Almost all cells in this population are producing κ (red/ rhodamine anti-κ) light chains.

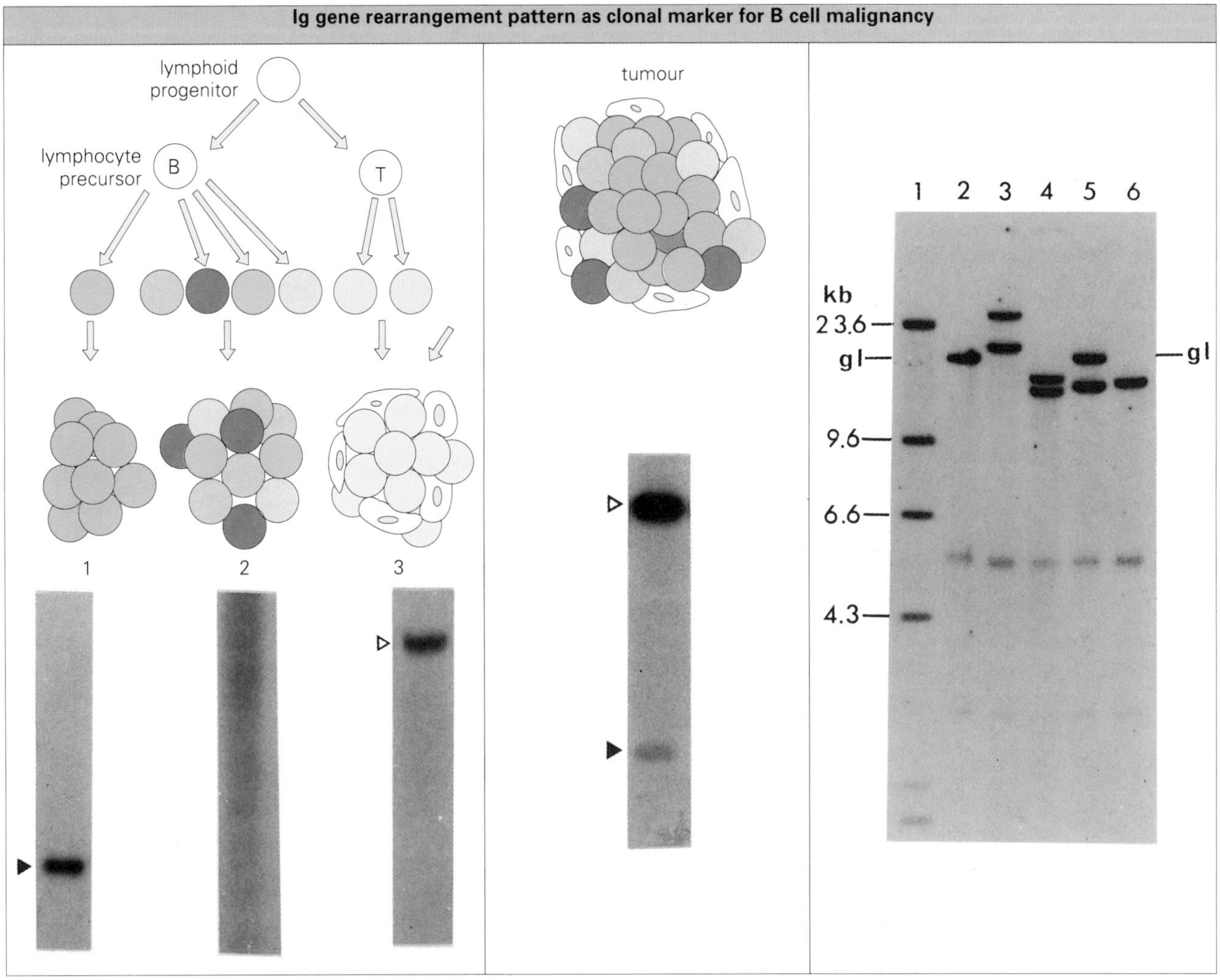

Ig gene rearrangement pattern as clonal marker for B cell malignancy

Fig. 21.24 Left: comparative patterns on Southern blot autoradiographs of DNA restriction fragments probed with a radioactive IgH DNA probe. 1) monoclonal B cell population showing loss of germ line fragment and appearance of single novel rearranged fragment. 2) polyclonal B cells (centre) showing smear of multiple rearranged bands and loss of germ line fragment. 3) non-B cell showing unrearranged (germ line) fragment. Middle: restriction fragment pattern when clonal tumour B cells are present but are in a minority. Right: variable patterns of clonal rearrangements identified in different B cell leukaemias/lymphomas (clinical examples). Track 1 = molecular weight markers (in kilobases); Track 2 = myeloid leukaemia DNA (unrearranged or germ line); Tracks 3–6 = examples of B cell lineage malignancy with monoclonal IgH gene rearrangements. Three patterns are observed: both chromosomal IgH alleles rearranged (tracks 3 and 4), one allele rearranged, one germ line (track 5) and one allele rearranged, the other deleted (track 6).

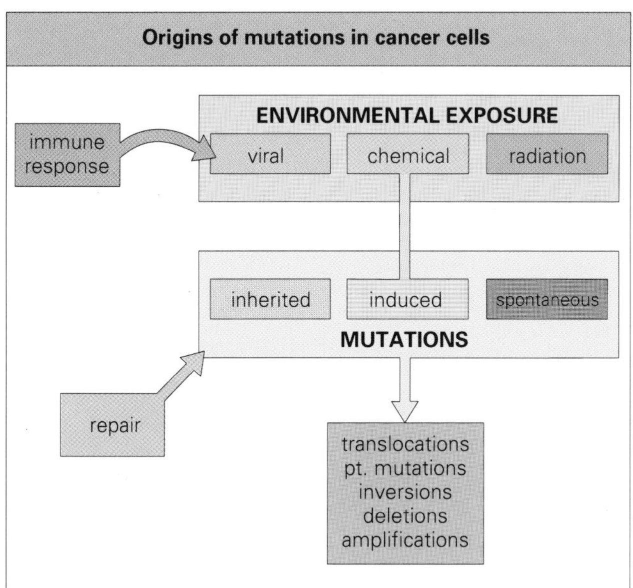

Fig.21.25 Origins of mutations in cancer cells. pt = point mutation, i.e. single base pair change.

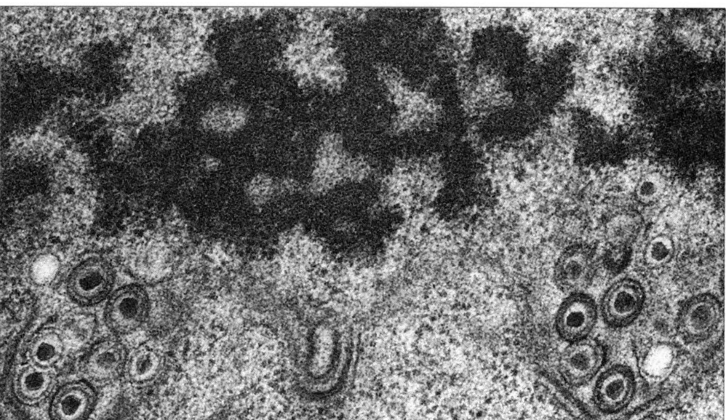

Fig.21.26 Epstein-Barr virus particles.

- secondly, because more than one mutation is probably required to produce leukaemia and some key events are as yet unidentified;
- and thirdly, because the mechanisms producing the observed mutations are largely unknown.

Fig. 21.25 illustrates the complexity of this situation where multiple types of mutations can arise via these separate mechanisms. Those that are environmentally induced could involve (as in animal leukaemias) radiation, viruses or chemical leukaemogenic substances. In addition, the immune response will play some role, at least in cases where infection is relevant. Diet may also be a co-factor since calorie restriction in experimental rodents greatly reduces the frequency of radiation or virally induced lymphoid leukaemias. The intrinsic efficacy of DNA repair mechanisms will also be crucial contributors to risk of leukaemia, as evidenced by individuals with inherited deficiencies in this activity (Bloom's syndrome, Fanconi's anaemia, ataxia teleangiectasia) who have a greatly increased frequency (20–300 times) of leukaemia. Two agents known to be involved in the causation of lymphoid malignancy are Epstein-Barr virus and human T cell leukaemia virus 1 (HTLV-1).

EBV and Burkitt's lymphoma

Burkitt's lymphoma was first described in the 1950s by Denis Burkitt, a British surgeon working in Africa. He noticed that this lymphoma, often presenting with a jaw mass in children, was widely distributed throughout tropical Africa and largely coincident, both in geographic distribution and altitude, with malaria (see chapter 20). EBV, a DNA virus of the herpes family (Fig 21.26) was subsequently isolated from Burkitt's lymphoma biopsy material by Epstein and Barr. The same virus is responsible for infectious mononucleosis in the western world but is only rarely implicated in lymphoma development — and then specifically in the context of immunosuppression. The same virus will also transform normal blood B lymphocytes *in vitro* into continuous cell lines. These have a normal diploid karyotype and are non-tumorigenic in experimental animals (for example immunodeprived mice). Transfection of such cells with an activated c-MYC gene renders them malignant.

Epidemiological evidence strongly implicates EBV in the aetiology of Burkitt's lymphoma in tropical Africa, even though infection is endemic and only a small proportion (<1%) of infected infants will develop lymphoma with a latent period averaging around five years. Other factors are therefore involved. In contrast to the infection and transformation of B cells with EBV *in vitro*, Burkitt's lymphoma cells are monoclonal. These data suggest a likely scenario for the development of Burkitt's lymphoma. In this model, T cell immunosuppression by malaria (and possibly also by malnutrition) permits EBV to proliferate and infect more B cells; these proliferate polyclonally (perhaps promoted by mitogenic products of malarial parasites) and thereby greatly increase the risk that a single cell will, by chance, undergo a chromosomal translocation that activates c-MYC constitutively and thereby precipitate overt lymphoma. Fortunately, a combination of surgery and cyclophosphamide provide an effective treatment for this lymphoma. EBV is also the causative agent (or initiator) of nasopharyngeal carcinoma — one of the most common cancers in South-East Asia.

HTLV-1 and adult T cell leukaemia/lymphoma (ATLL)

Adult T cell leukaemia/lymphoma is a highly malignant lymphoid cancer which was first described in 1976 in

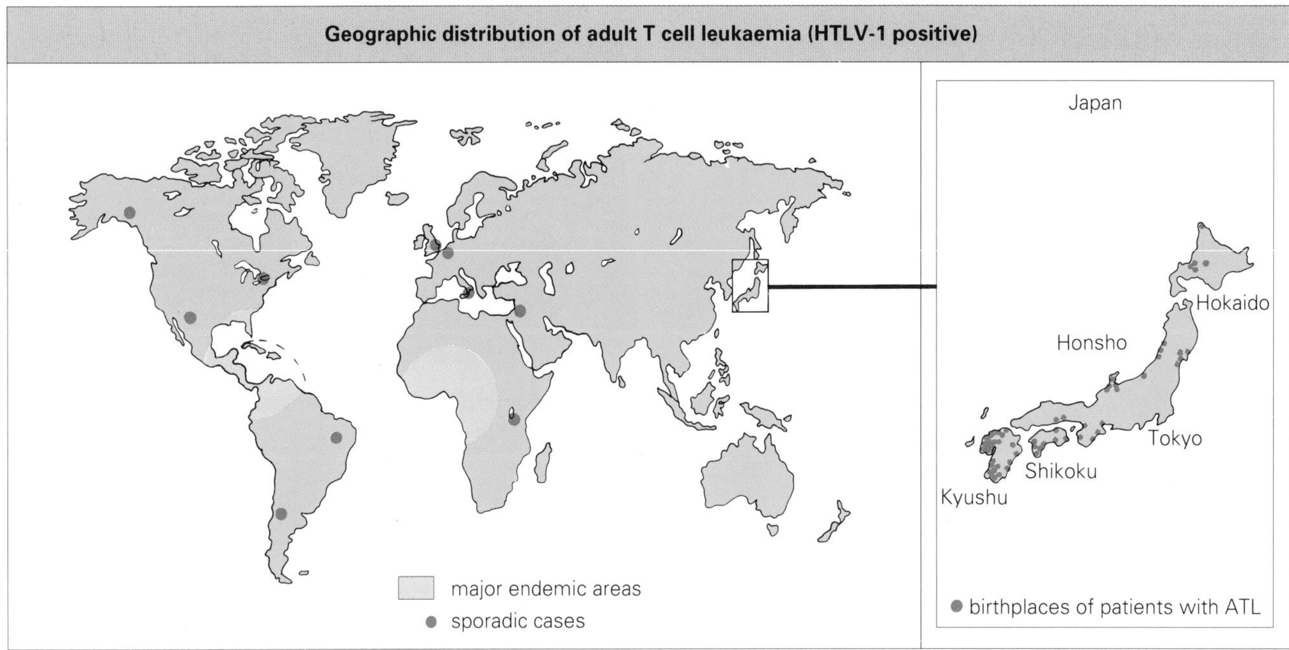

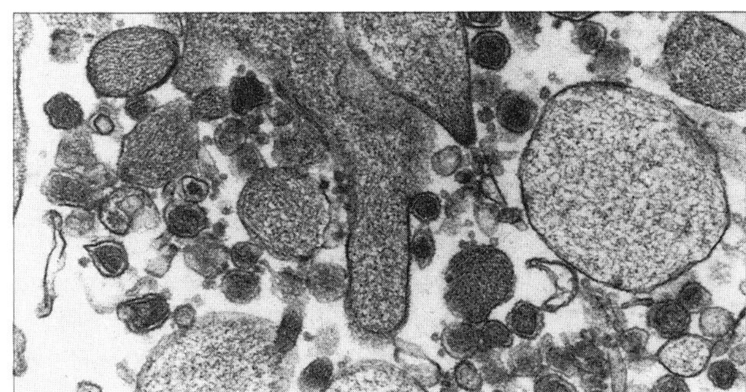

Fig. 21.27 Upper: HTLV-1 associated leukaemias/lymphomas (ATLL), are seen predominantly in southern Japan, the Caribbean basin and West Africa. Other sites include southern Italy (Calabria) and within the Afro-Caribbean immigrant community of the UK and the Netherlands. Left: electron micrograph of HTLV-1 particles.

Japan, the majority of patients being born in the southern island of Kyushu (Fig. 21.27). The leukaemic T cells have a characteristic, highly cerebriform nucleus (see Fig. 21.3e) and the lymphoma histopathology is very diffuse and pleomorphic. Subsequently, a similar disease was recognized in Caribbean immigrants to the UK and, later still, the disease was observed in West Africa, the Caribbean region and other areas. With a few interesting exceptions, the disease is limited to individuals of Afro-Caribbean or Japanese descent. This geographic distribution suggested that an infectious agent was involved and the culprit, a retrovirus termed HTLV-1, was first isolated from a black American patient in 1980. The same virus is now known to be involved in different geographic regions and racial groups. The geography of the disease world-wide parallels the map of endemicity of the virus.

Although HTLV-1 is likely to be causative agent of ATLL, the story is not quite so simple. The life-time risk of developing ATLL in the endemic regions (for example Kyushu) is around 1%. In one respect, this is quite high — the life-time risk of developing any blood cell malignancy (in 'developed' countries) is also around 1%. Nevertheless, this indicates that 99% of individuals infected with HTLV-1 do not develop leukaemia. Furthermore, it is known from studies of immigrants to the UK that the latency of the disease (that is, the period after infection until diagnosis of ATLL) is often 30 years or more and the resultant leukaemia is monoclonal (by T cell receptor, ß gene rearrangement pattern and retroviral gene integration pattern) and can have a variety of clonal chromosomal rearrangements, frequently, though not exclusively, involving the TCRα gene.

It is therefore likely that there are important co-factors in the development of ATLL which increase the risk of further essential mutations or chromosomal rearrangements. These co-factors could be infections of one sort or another. Curiously, neither in Burkitt's lymphoma nor ATLL is there any firm evidence for risk associated with HLA genotype. Indeed, the only human blood cell malignancies where there appears to be such a link are Hodgkin's disease and possibly ALL. HTLV-1 is also the causative agent of a neurological disease — tropical spastic paraparesis. Claims that HTLV-1 is involved in multiple sclerosis have not been confirmed.

Lymphoid malignancy in immunodeficiency conditions

The Burkitt's lymphoma scenario suggests that T cell surveillance against EBV is a critical regulator of risk for

Lymphoid malignancy in immunodeficiency conditions
Wiskott-Aldrich syndrome ataxia telangiectasia common variable immunodeficiency severe combined immunodeficiency (SCID) selective IgA deficiency X-linked hypogammaglobulinaemia
Organ transplant recipients
secondary to infection: malaria HIV/AIDS

Fig. 21.28 Patients with ataxia telangiectasia usually develop T cell leukaemia with no evidence of viral involvement; in this instance, defective DNA repair is more likely to be the crucial underlying mechanism. Not all lymphomas in AIDS patients are EBV-associated and some are T rather than B cell neoplasms.

Clinical application of monoclonal antibodies in lymphoid malignancy
Differential diagnosis
anti-cell/lineage associated (differentiation) antigens proliferation related antigens e.g. transferrin receptor, cyclin, incorporated BrdU
Assessing remission (rare cell/ minimal disease detection)
differentiation antigens thymic phenotype in bone marrow T,B precursor phenotype in extra medullary sites e.g. CNS, testis asynchronous phenotypes in bone marrow Ig/TCR idiotypes altered proto-oncogene encoded proteins
Therapy
in vivo — anti leukaemia cell *in vitro* — pre-transplantation bone marrow purge anti-leukaemia Ab: autologous transplants anti-T cell Ab: allogeneic transplants

Fig. 21.29 Clinical application of monoclonal antibodies in lymphoid malignancy. BrdU = bromodeoxyuridine.

lymphoma. Since EBV is a ubiquitous virus, it is not surprising that immunosuppression, other than via malaria, is associated with a greatly increased risk (up to 200 times) of developing lymphoma (Fig. 21.28). Many immunodeficient patients with lymphoma have an EBV-associated disease but some do not.

CLINICAL APPLICATIONS OF LEUKAEMIA BIOLOGY

Clearly, an understanding of the immunology, cellular and molecular biology of blood cell malignancies has increased dramatically during the past decade. Not surprisingly, there is an inevitable time-lag before this information and associated technology is translated into the practical arena of patient management. Already, however, there are very real, as well as plausible, potential applications that can be of benefit to patients in the context of differential diagnosis, monitoring of treatment and therapy. These developments are to be encouraged, especially in the therapeutic field. Despite very substantial improvements in the treatment of leukaemia and related diseases by chemotherapy, radiation and bone marrow transplantation, these are usually traumatic treatments with substantial morbidity. Furthermore, a considerable proportion of adults remain incurable. There is, therefore, a great need for new or complementary treatment modalities that are efficacious and non-toxic.

Monoclonal antibodies

Monoclonal antibodies have a number of important advantages as diagnostic or therapeutic agents, including well-defined specificity, reproducibility, ease of preparation in bulk, and tagging (for example with dyes or toxins). Some current, as well as potential, applications of these reagents are summarized in Fig. 21.29.

Diagnosis. The routine application of panels of monoclonal antibodies for the differential diagnosis of leukaemia and lymphoma is well established, and plays an important part in choice of therapy. The complexities of cellular immunophenotypes demand that appropriate reagents are used collectively to define the 'composite' phenotype of a leukaemic cell population as a basis for diagnostic classification. Fig. 21.30 illustrates the markers used and major immunophenotypes observed in a fairly typical laboratory screening assay.

None of the monoclonal antibodies currently in routine use are leukaemia- specific but nevertheless, it may be possible to identify individual cells as leukaemic by exploiting normal differentiation antigens, for example finding intrathymic T cell phenotypes on T cells outside the thymus indicates that such cells are likely to be leukaemic. Finding cells with asynchronous phenotypes or combinations of antigens not normally observed together provides another possible marker of leukaemic cells. Also, it may be possible to produce genuinely leukaemia-specific antibodies in those cases where the leukaemia has a consistent molecular alteration which produces a qualitatively unique protein, for example BCR-ABL. Anti-idiotype reagents are operationally

Immunophenotypes as an aid to diagnosis																
	Cell surface												Nuclear	Cytoplasmic		
	T lineage			B lineage				Myeloid			Others					
	early		late	early		late							early lymphoid	early T	early B	
CD no.	2	7	TCR-T3	10	19	22	κ/λ	13	33	14	DR	34	Tdt	3	22	μ
ALL																
T pre	○	○	◕	◕	●	●	●	●	●	●	●	◕	○	○	●	●
B pre																
common	●	●	●	○	○	●	●	●	●	●	○	◕	○	●	○	◕
null	●	●	●	●	○	●	●	●	●	●	○	◑	○	●	○	●
pre-B	●	●	●	○	○	●	●	●	●	●	○	◕	○	●	○	○
B-CLL B-NHL	●	●	●	◕	○	●	●	●	●	●	○	●	●	●	●	●
AML	●	◕	●	●	●	●	●	◔	○	◔	◑	◑	◕	●	●	●

Fig. 21.30 Only the predominant reactivity patterns are shown. Turquoise circles indicate <5% cases positive; Dark blue circles indicate >95% cases positive.

clone-specific for B or T cell leukaemia/lymphoma cells but pose serious logistical as well as other problems in their application (for example modulation of idiotype expression). Some of these immunological approaches to distinguish leukaemic from normal cells are currently being applied to the detection of rare cells or of minimal residual disease in treated patients.

Treatment. Another exciting area of clinical application of monoclonal antibodies is in therapy. Some preliminary studies suggest that particular monoclonal antibodies may be very effective at eliminating leukaemic cells *in vivo* but most applications to date have concerned the use of antibodies to manipulate or 'purge' the cellular composition of bone marrow prior to allogeneic or autologous transplantation (see chapter 20). Strictly speaking, this is not a therapeutic use of antibody, but an application designed to improve the success of haemopoietic reconstitution following intensive *in vivo* therapy with drugs and radiation. Whether removal of residual leukaemic cells from autologous bone marrow makes a real clinical impact remains controversial and unproven. There seems little doubt, however, that removal of T cells from allogeneic marrow (combined in most cases with *in vivo* T cell suppression) can greatly reduce the incidence of life-threatening graft-versus-host disease and hence survival of transplant patients. Unfortunately, and ironically, in several such studies the removal of allogeneic T cells appears to increase the risk of leukaemic relapse via the loss of what is referred to as a graft-versus-leukaemia effect of allogeneic donor bone marrow. Understanding this latter mechanism could have important implications for future treatment strategies.

Manipulation of growth factor response pathways

Since leukaemia cells are proliferating abnormally and failing to differentiate effectively, this may provide another effective and specific channel for targeting therapeutic agents. Some possibilities currently under investigation in both leukaemias and cancers in general include:

- growth factors to induce effective terminal differentiation;
- growth factor receptor antagonists to inhibit aberrent receptor activity and proliferation;
- growth factor–toxin conjugates or anti-receptor conjugates to kill proliferating leukaemic cells;
- competitive inhibitors of growth factor response pathways e.g. IFNα, TNF, TGFβ.

Application of these is currently limited in lymphoid

Clinical application of molecular probes
Differential diagnosis
BCR-ABL rearrangements in CML, Ph^+ALL BCL-2 rearrangements in follicular lymphoma clonal rearrangements of Ig/TCR gene (cf. immunoreactive conditions)
Rare cell/minimal disease detection
southern blot assay for the gene rearrangement (1% sensitivity) polymerase chain reaction for amplifying unique sequences (e.g. BCL-2, BCR-ABL (1 in 10^6 sensitivity)
Therapy (?)
anti-sense mRNA to block altered gene translation antibody to altered gene products inhibitors/antagonists of altered gene product activity (e.g. ABL kinase)

Fig. 21.31 Potential clincial application of molecular probes.

malignancies to the use of anti-IL-2 receptor or IL-2 reagents in ATLL, in which leukaemic cells produce very high levels of IL-2 receptor, and IFNα treatment in hairy (B) cell leukaemia. The latter appears to be particularly effective. As we learn more about the growth factor responses of normal and leukaemic lymphoid cells, more possibilities for beneficial manipulation will become available.

Molecular probes

One of the key issues for the future is whether insight into the molecular biology of leukaemia will provide any practical benefit to patients. As with monoclonal antibodies, three areas of application can be considered — differential diagnosis, monitoring of residual disease and therapy (Fig. 21.31). Some DNA probes are already being used for diagnostic purposes, for example BCR, BCL-2 gene rearrangements, and IgH/TCR rearrangements for distinguishing true lymphoma from immunoreactive conditions or non-lymphoid cancers. A potentially very useful application is for the detection of rare leukaemic cells. Unique DNA or RNA sequences, for example across the fusion junction of BCR-ABL and other fused genes in leukaemia, can be detected using the polymerase chain reaction method (PCR) with a sensitivity of 1 leukaemic cell in 10^5–10^6 normal cells. Unique IgH or TCR gene sequences can be similarly used by the PCR method. Moreover, this no longer requires cloning and sequencing of the unique patient-specific regions, thus overcoming the logistical problems of the idiotype strategy. These methods are already being applied and are clearly able to detect covert disease that is missed by conventional haematological or pathological assessment. It remains to be seen whether modification of available treatment on the basis of these new tests produces any improvement in remission duration and survival.

The major unanswered question is whether there is a future for therapy tailored to attack the specific molecular lesions of leukaemic cells. Several possibilities suggest themselves (Fig 21.31) and some of these can be shown to work at least transiently *in vitro* for example anti-sense mRNA. This is currently an area of great activity and offers considerable promise for the future.

One possible limitation to the potential success of molecular intervention is the fact that, in common with most cancers, individual blood cell malignancies may, by the time of diagnosis, have acquired multiple molecular abnormalities and thus be difficult to 'switch off'. The best strategy, at least initially, would therefore be to focus research efforts on those diseases in which the number of mutations is limited to only one or two, for example. BCR-ABL in CML, and BCL-2 in follicular lymphoma.

FURTHER READING

Boehm T, Rabbitts TH. The human T cell receptor genes are targets for chromosomal abnormalities in T cell tumours. *FASEB J.* 1989; **3**: 2344–2359.

Clark SS, Crist WM, Witte ON. Molecular pathogenesis of Ph-positive leukaemias. *Ann Rev Med.* 1989; **40**: 113–122.

Dow LW, Martin P, Moohr J, Greenberg M, Macdougall LG, Najfeld V, Fialkow PJ. Evidence for clonal development of childhood acute lymphoblastic leukaemia. *Blood.* 1985; **66**; 902–907.

Furley AJ, Mizutani S, Weilbaecher K, *et al.* Developmentally regulated rearrangement and expression of genes encoding the T cell receptor–T3 complex. *Cell.* 1986; **46**: 75–87.

Furth M, Greaves MF, eds. *Cancer cells 7: Molecular diagnostics of human cancer.* New York: Cold Spring Harbor Laboratory Press, 1989.

Greaves MF. Differentiation-linked leukaemogenesis in lymphocytes. *Science.* 1986; **234**: 697–704.

Heim S, Mitelman F. *Cancer cytogenetics.* New York: Alan R Liss Inc, 1987.

Janossy G, Campana D. The pathophysiological basis of immunodiagnosis in acute lymphoblastic leukaemia. *Cancer Rev.* 1988; **8**: 91–122.

Linet MS. *The leukemias: Epidemiologic aspects.* New York: Oxford University Press, 1985.

O'Connor NJT, Gatter KC, Wainscoat JS, *et al.*. Practical values of genotypic analysis for diagnosing lymphoproliferative disorders. *J Clin Pathol* 1987; **40**: 147–150.

Penn I. Lymphoproliferative diseases in disorders of the immune system. *Cancer Detection Prevention.* 1990; **14**: 415–422.

Stamatoyannopoulos G, Nienhaus AW, Leder P, Majerus PW, eds. *The molecular basis of blood diseases.* Philadelphia: WB Saunders Co, 1987.

Waldmann TA. The arrangement of immunoglobulin and T cell receptor genes in human lymphoproliferative disorders. *Adv Immunol.* 1987; **40**: 247–321.

Zucker-Franklin D, Greaves MF, Grossi CE, Marmont AM. *Atlas of blood cells: Function and pathology (2E).* Philadelphia: Lea & Febiger, 1988.

22

Principles of Immunity to Infection

CLASSES OF PARASITIC ORGANISMS

The five classes of parasitic organisms (viruses, bacteria, fungi, protozoa, helminths) constitute the principal raison d'être of the immune system, since defects in the latter generally lead to impaired control of the former, often resulting in increased morbidity and mortality from infectious disease. It is important to appreciate that death of the host is not part of the strategy of successful parasites, most of which have evolved along with their hosts for millions of years to reach a more or less stable balance; this can, however, be disturbed by alterations either in the parasite (for example antigenic change or spread to a new host species) or in the host (for example immunodeficiency or vaccination). This chapter will briefly review the various levels at which the host and parasite interact, with representative examples of the major mechanisms involved but with no attempt to deal individually with every infectious organism.

It is convenient to consider the host-parasite relationship under eight separate headings (Fig. 22.1).

ROUTES OF ENTRY

Surface of the body

The surface of higher animals is bounded by the relatively impermeable epithelial layers of skin and mucous membranes. Some parasites manage to colonize these while remaining outside the body; indeed, certain fungi (for example dermatophytes) and bacteria (for example staphylococci) on the skin and a variety of bacteria in the intestine are so universal and generally harmless that they might well be considered perfectly adapted parasites. These organisms do not normally come to the attention of the immune system unless, like staphylococci, they invade the tissues via broken skin. Under normal circumstances, their numbers are probably controlled by ill-defined products of the various secretory glands in skin and mucous membranes.

Inside the body

On the other hand, many parasites have chosen a habitat inside the body, whether intracellular or free in the interstitial tissues or body fluids, and such organisms must somehow breach the body's outer barriers (Fig. 22.2). A number of ingenious strategies have evolved, including the destruction of epithelium by secreted toxic molecules (employed, for example by amoeba), attachment to specific

Host-parasite relationship
1. entry of the parasite 2. multiplication & spread 3. pathology 4. natural immunity 5. adaptive immunity 6. immunopathology 7. parasite survival mechanisms 8. host-parasite balance

Fig. 22.1 Aspects of the host-parasite relationship.

Routes of microbial entry		
Site of entry	**Method of entry**	**Examples**
skin	wounds, burns	staphylococci streptococci tetanus
	insect bites	malaria trypanosomiasis typhus yellow fever
	dog bite	rabies
	direct penetration	schistosomiasis
nose & throat	attach to cells	adenovirus
	attach to teeth	*Strep. mutans*
respiratory tract	receptor on epithelium	influenza
	mucus/ciliary defects	*B. pertussis*
gut	attach & penetrate	salmonella polio *Entamoeba*
	attach without penetration	cholera *Giardia* hookworm
genito-urinary	attach to epithelium	gonococcus

Fig. 22.2 Routes of microbial entry into the body.

Cell surface receptors for parasites		
Organism	**Receptor**	**Cell infected**
Viruses		
EBV	CR2 (C3d receptor)	B cells
HIV	CD4	T cells, macrophages
Coxsackie A	ICAM-1	respiratory tract
rhinovirus	ICAM-1	
polio	ICAM?	intestine
mycoplasma	neuraminic acid	respiratory tract
rabies	acetylcholine receptor	neurons
adenovirus	MHC I	
Bacteria		
E. coli	CR3 (C3bi receptor)	intestine
V. cholerae	mannose-fucose receptor	intestine
Protozoa		
Entamoeba	asialo-fetuin	colon
Giardia	mannose-D-phosphate	small intestine
malaria	glycophorin	red cell
	sialic acid	
	Duffy blood group	
Leishmania	fibronectin	macrophage
	mannose-fucose receptor	
	CR3	
Fungi		
Histoplasma	CR3	macrophage
	LFA1	

Fig. 22.3 Receptors are used by a wide variety of bacteria and protozoa, and by most viruses.

cell-surface molecules (receptors; Fig. 22.3) via complementary molecules on the parasite, and passive entry with the assistance of biting insects and other vectors.

Method of entry

The method of entry selected may have great significance for the pattern of disease and immunity that results. For instance the protozoa causing malaria, trypanosomiasis and leishmaniasis, and the yellow fever virus are normally spread by insects. This enables them to infect over great distances and therefore thrive in thinly populated areas, but they are restricted to those parts, mainly tropical, where their vectors can survive. By contrast, spread of respiratory viruses by sneezing is effective over only a few feet and is favoured by the crowded living conditions of modern cities.

Vectors. Quite minor differences between vectors can have far-reaching effects. For example malaria transmission is more effective in Africa than in India mainly because the African mosquito species are longer-lived; thus, most people have repeated attacks every year in
22.2 Africa and those who do not die as children develop effective immunity, while in India the pattern is of occasional epidemics and slower-developing immunity, with many deaths in adults.

Beneficial receptor interactions. Specific receptor interactions offer an opportunity for antibody to interfere with entry, and this represents one of the most important ways in which the immune response can prevent infection — specific IgA in the gut being an important example.

Detrimental receptor interactions. In special situations, however, antibody may actually enhance entry by binding to Fc receptors on the target cell, as in the case of dengue virus and the macrophage. The molecule chosen by an organism as a binding site may have profound consequences for the immune system. This is illustrated by HIV which, by selecting the CD4 molecule, invades and leads to the destruction of the vital helper T cells which use this molecule as part of their normal function (see chapter 24).

MULTIPLICATION AND SPREAD

After entry, the strategies adopted by different parasites vary widely. Viruses, fungi and protozoa usually undergo extensive replication, so that even a small infective inoculum can result in a large number of organisms a few days later. Immune elimination of even the majority may be relatively useless since they can quickly be replaced. Multiplication can be very rapid, as in the case of staphylococci (3 divisions per hour) or quite slow, as with mycobacteria (approximately once a week); this clearly affects the rate at which the parasite burden increases and the ability of the immune response to keep pace. In the classical pre-antibiotic situation of (untreated) pneumonia due to *S. pneumoniae*, bacterial multiplication and the development of the primary antibody response were so well matched that the outcome was in the balance for a week, after which time the patient either died or dramatically recovered.

Worms are rather different in that they do not replicate within the human host, so that parasite density is directly related to the number that achieve entry. Therefore even partial success in cutting down the numbers of surviving worms may be of value to the host, whilst on the parasite side quite sophisticated escape mechanisms may be required to avoid total elimination, as will be seen later.

Local spread

Some parasites remain at or near the site of entry, spreading from cell to cell, to produce a localized infection; examples are the vaccinia virus, used to immunize against smallpox, and many of the respiratory viruses. Local tissue spread may be enhanced by the secretion of toxins, especially common in bacteria such as streptococci and staphylococci, which produce a veritable barrage of secretions aimed at establishing superiority over the local defence mechanisms in the skin or other organs.

Blood and lymphatic transmission

More commonly however, organisms enter lymphatics or the bloodstream. This has the virtue for the host that they are rapidly exposed to the lymphocytes (for example in lymph nodes) and the macrophages (for example in the liver) that form a vital part of the immune defence system, but it may also allow the parasite to colonize other parts of the body not otherwise available to it. Usually parasites do not spend more than a few hours in the blood, because there they are susceptible to so many potent anti-microbial mechanisms (complement, antibody, neutrophils, monocytes). Exceptionally, however, an organism manages to evade these and, like the African trypanosome and the liver fluke *Schistosoma*, adopts the blood as its natural habitat.

Other routes of transmission

Spread by the blood is of course rapid, but other slower routes are available; for example herpes simplex and rabies viruses travel along nerves. In the case of rabies, the journey from the bite in the skin to the central nervous system is slow enough for there to be time to immunize the patient after exposure — a most unusual bonus for the vaccinator. Another special situation is the placenta. Few organisms are capable of traversing it, but those that do can cause severe damage by colonizing the still immunologically incompetent fetus: rubella virus and *Toxoplasma* are important examples.

Once again parasitic worms represent the extreme case, often migrating from organ to organ, causing different symptoms and immunological problems in different sites. The lung is commonly affected, for example by the roundworm *Ascaris*, with resulting asthmatic crises.

PATHOLOGY

Most people most of the time consider themselves to be healthy, yet they harbour dozens of species of parasite, particularly viruses and bacteria, so disease is obviously not an inevitable consequence of infection. Nevertheless tissue destruction does often occur, whether as part of the normal replication mechanism (for example of many viruses or of blood-stage malaria), as an aid to colonization (for example amoebae), or in an attempt to overcome host defence mechanisms (for example staphylococcal destruction of neutrophils). Sometimes this tissue damage is carried out by secreted exotoxins, as in cholera, diphtheria, tetanus, and diseases caused by staphylococci, streptococci and clostridia. These molecules offer an excellent target for neutralizing antibody and can be used in vaccines when they can be rendered inactive without losing antigenicity.

In many cases, however, tissue damage is not directly due to the parasite but to elements of the body's defence system produced inappropriately (Fig. 22.4). A striking example is the production by macrophages of the cytokine, tumour necrosis factor (TNF) in response to endotoxin from Gram-negative bacteria. TNF plays a part

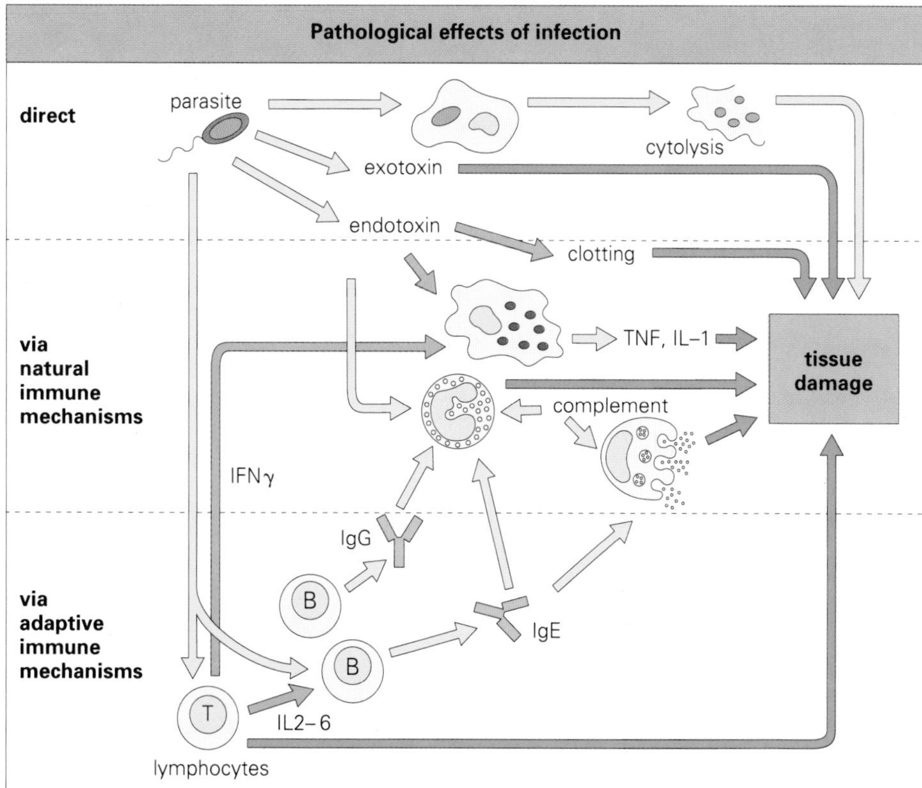

Fig. 22.4 This general scheme shows the major pathways by which microbes or their products can cause tissue damage, either directly (top), or by activating natural (middle) or adaptive (lower) immune mechanisms.

in protection against many viruses and bacteria, but in excess it can damage the vascular endothelium, leading to collapse and shock. Other microbial toxins, and probably other cytokines, may similarly be involved in pathological changes.

Matters may be made worse by the involvement of the adaptive immune system; these immunopathological or 'hypersensitivity' responses will be considered later.

NATURAL IMMUNITY

A great variety of host defence mechanisms have evolved to limit entry, spread or multiplication of parasites selectively — that is, with the minimum damage to the host itself. Most of these are well-developed at birth, are more or less general or 'non-specific' in their effects, and do not alter significantly from one infectious episode to the next, all of which distinguishes them from adaptive immunity (Fig. 22.5).

Natural immune mechanisms that restrict entry of micro-organisms include the secretions of glands in the skin, the acid pH of the stomach, the beating cilia and the layer of mucus overlying most of the respiratory epithelium, and enzymes such as lysozyme in tears and other secretions (Fig. 22.6).

Phagocytes

Organisms that succeed in entering the tissues are rapidly exposed to phagocytic cells, principally polymorphonuclear leucocytes (PMNs) and macrophages. In that they recognize, attach to, endocytose and digest foreign material of all kinds, these cells are remarkably similar to primitive free-living protozoa, and can be regarded as the fundamental units of defence. Indeed the entire adaptive (lymphocyte-based) immune system owes most of its power to its effects on these phagocytic cells. Their function is improved by antibody which enhances recognition and attachment, and by T cells which 'activate' various intracellular functions. Deficiencies of phagocytic cells tell us where their real value lies; PMN defects predispose particularly to bacterial and fungal infection, and defects in macrophage activation lead to chronic intracellular infections of all kinds (see chapters 23 & 24).

Killing mechanisms of phagocytes are usually classified as oxidative (that is, requiring a supply of oxygen) or non-oxidative. The oxidative pathway, in which a variety of transient but highly toxic reactive oxygen intermediates (ROIs) are generated, appears to be responsible for most intracellular killing. However, PMNs and eosinophils also contain a number of toxic proteins, of which the cationic proteins of the eosinophil are the best understood because of their effects in damaging parasitic helminths. It has also been realized in recent years that phagocytic cells, and especially macrophages, carry out many of their effects via secreted molecules, several of which show anti-microbial
22.4 activity (Fig. 22.7).

Innate & adaptive immune systems

	Innate	Adaptive
Resistance	not improved by repeated infection	improved by repeated infection
Soluble factors	lysozyme, complement, acute phase proteins (e.g. CRP), interferon	antibody
Cells	phagocytes natural killer (NK) cells	T lymphocytes

Fig. 22.5 There is considerable reaction between the two systems. Immunity due to soluble factors is sometimes termed humoral immunity.

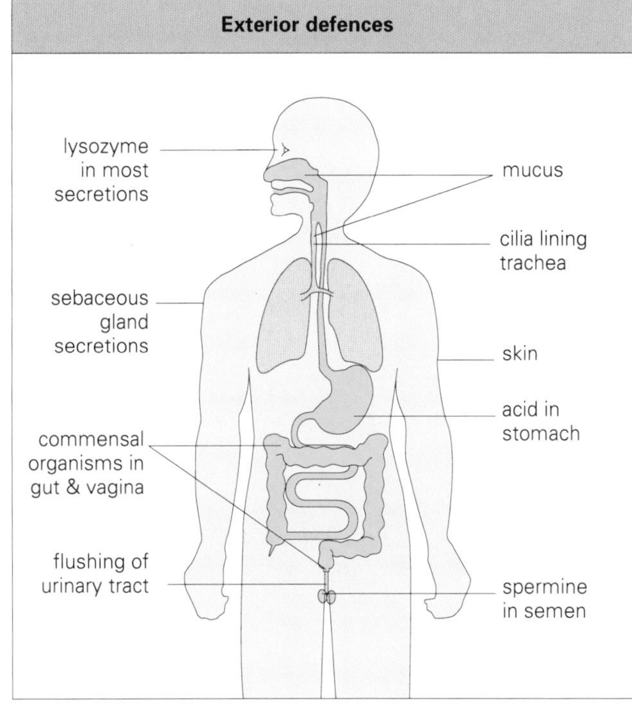

Fig. 22.6 Most of the infectious agents which an individual encounters do not penetrate the body surface, but are prevented from entering by a variety of biochemical and physical barriers. The body tolerates a number of commensal organisms which compete effectively with many potential pathogens.

Complement

Among the most sophisticated elements normally present in the serum are the components of the complement pathway, which interact with certain micro-organisms, with antibodies, and with each other to enhance phagocytosis and promote the vascular permeability changes of the inflammatory response (Fig. 22.8). Judged by the effects of

Cytotoxic secretory molecules		
Host component		**Effective against**
major cell source	**molecule**	
liver macrophage	complement C1–3 C5–9 C-reactive protein	bacteria, fungi *Neisseria* streptococci
macrophage neutrophil	reactive oxygen intermediates (& peroxidase)	bacteria, fungi malaria
macrophage	lysozyme IFN α, β TNF	Gram +ve bacteria viruses viruses, bacteria, malaria
	arginase reactive nitrogen intermediates	schistosome worms
neutrophil	defensins cathepsins lactoferrin	bacteria, fungi bacteria, fungi bacteria, yeasts
eosinophil	cationic proteins	worms
lymphocyte (T) NK cell	cytokines perforins	viruses viruses
lipids	high density lipoprotein low density lipoprotein (oxidized)	trypanosomes malaria
kidney	urea	

Fig. 22.7 Some secretory molecules with cytotoxic activity.

isolated complement deficiencies, it is the splitting of C3 which is the central event, though the later 'lytic' pathway is important in disposing of certain organisms such as *Neisseria*.

Cytokines

Another group of molecules that will be considered here, although they also show some features of adaptive immunity, are the interferons. Originally defined by their antiviral properties and later subdivided according to their principal cell of origin (α: leucocyte, β: fibroblast, γ: T lymphocyte), these are now seen as part of the larger system of cytokines, or intercellular mediators, which also includes the interleukins, tumour necrosis factor (TNF), and the haemopoietic growth factors. Nonetheless, antiviral activity remains one of their most remarkable effects, and is carried out through several quite separate pathways, including the induction of intracellular proteins that block viral replication, the induction of MHC expression on the surface of the infected cell, and the enhancement of macrophage and NK cell function. Interferon-γ (IFNγ) has recently been shown to be active against the liver stage of malaria, and it is possible that other non-viral infections may be susceptible. It is also likely that many roles for other cytokines in infection will be uncovered; well known examples are the effects of interleukin-1 (IL-1) and TNF in fever, and of TNF in stimulating PMN and eosinophil cytotoxicity.

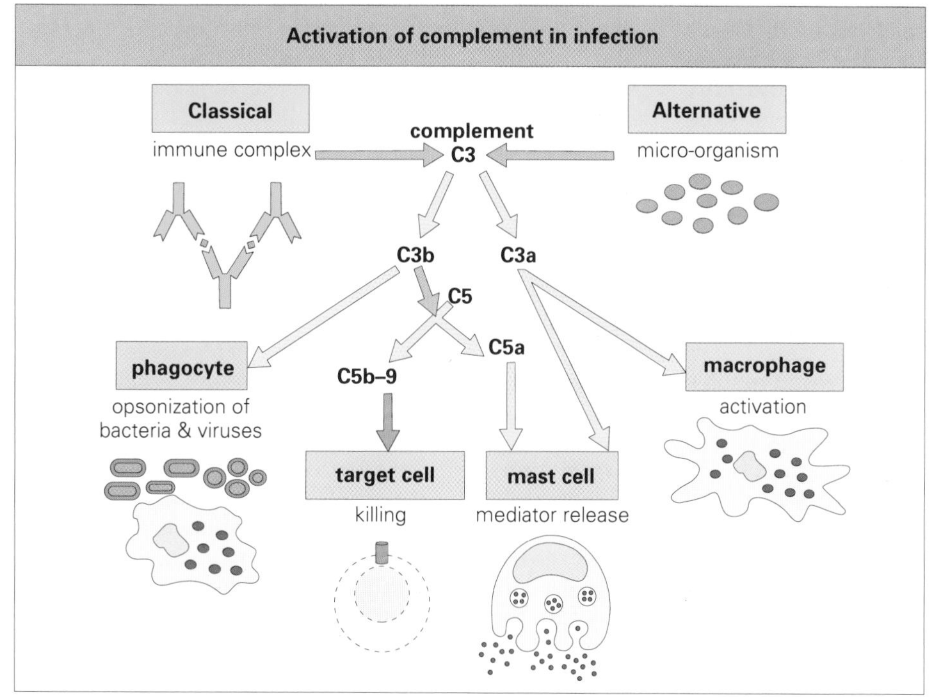

Fig. 22.8 The classical complement pathway is activated by immune complexes, whilst the alternative pathway is promoted by the lipopolysaccharide (LPS) component of the cell wall of Gram-negative bacteria. Both result in conversion of C3 to C3b, which activates the terminal lytic complement sequence.

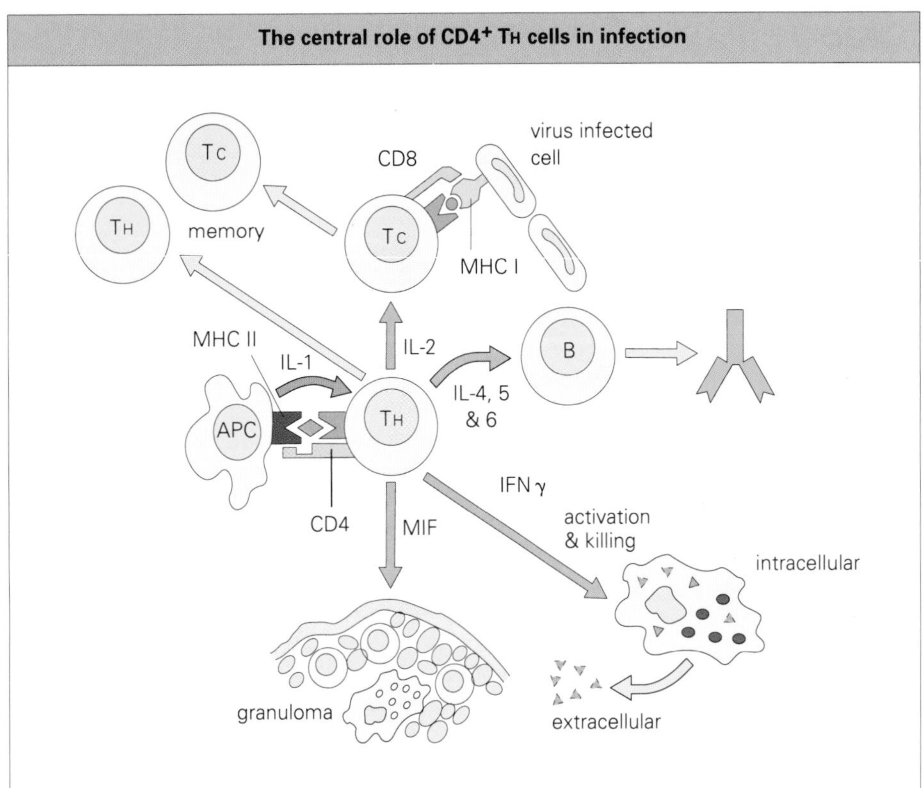

Fig. 22.9 The major secreted products of the $CD4^+$ cell and their targets.

ADAPTIVE IMMUNITY

Here the lymphocytes (T and B) are the key cells, their individually rearranged receptors and almost unlimited potential for clonal proliferation conferring on the 'immune response' the crucial elements of specificity and memory. Because the first response to an infection usually involves recognition of only a few antigens, and therefore only a small number of precursor lymphocytes, it can take several days to develop; for example the antibody response to the common cold appears after the virus has been controlled (probably by interferon). However secondary responses can be very rapid, and often dispose of micro-organisms before the host is aware of them; the usual immunity to second attacks of mumps and measles are good examples of this. Vaccines frequently induce equally good immunity, although living attenuated ones generally give more lasting protection than killed (see chapter 26).

Adaptive immune responses can be classified into three groups, depending on the principal effector cell:

- B cells (the antibody response);
- $CD8^+$ T cells (anti-viral cytotoxicity);
- macrophages and other myeloid cells (cell-mediated immunity).

The feature common to all is the helper activity provided by $CD4^+$ T cells in the form of various lymphokines (Fig.
22.6 22.9). Mention should also be made of the still controversial suppressor T cell, which appears to inhibit useful immunity (but also immunopathology) in some experimental infections and possibly in human diseases such as leprosy.

Cytotoxic T cells

Our understanding of cytotoxic T cell function is still far from complete; a recent surprise was the discovery that they often recognize not surface but nuclear antigens of viruses, peptides derived from which become associated with MHC class I molecules while still inside the infected cell. It has also been realized that cytotoxic T cells are involved in some non-viral diseases, for example theileriosis (East Coast fever) and liver-stage malaria; on the other hand not all the activities of $CD8^+$ cells involve killing, since they are also capable of secreting quite large amounts of IFNγ.

Cell-mediated immunity (CMI)

IFNγ is also thought to be the principal 'macrophage-activating factor' (MAF) secreted by helper T cells, but is probably not the only one. As regards this group of cell-mediated responses, it is worth stressing that they can take several forms, but are essentially concerned with persistent intracellular infections. It should also be remembered that the term 'delayed type hypersensitivity' really only applies to the skin test (for example the Mantoux reaction) often used to assess the strength of cell-mediated immunity; it has become evident that it does not correlate with protection as reliably as used to be thought.

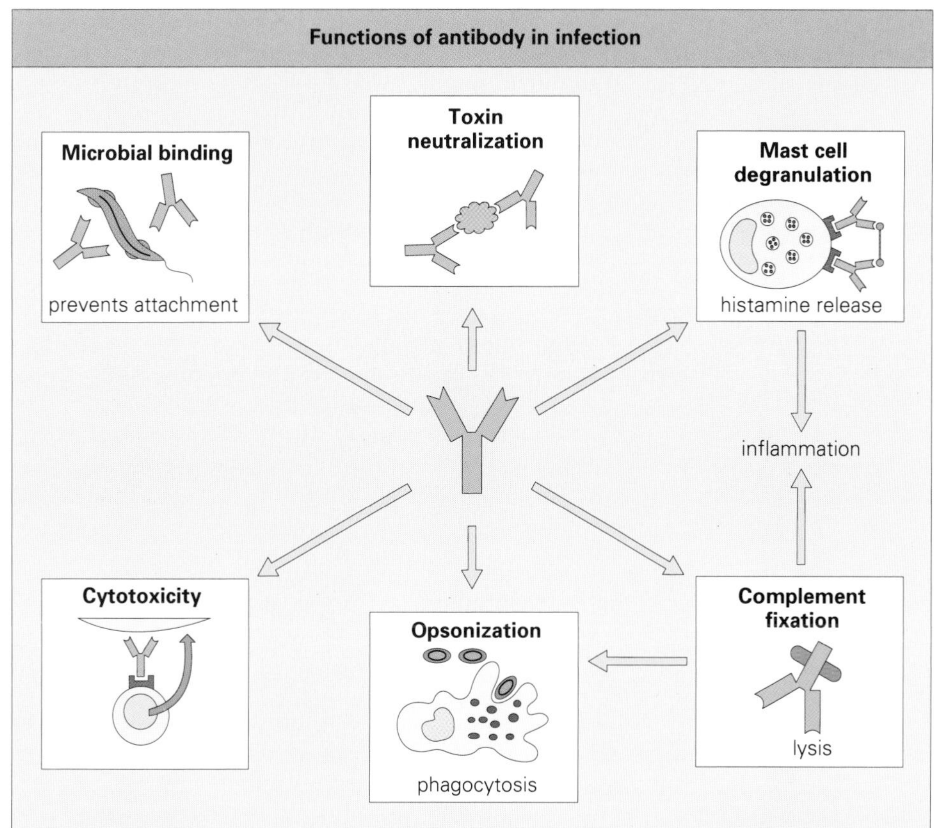

Fig. 22.10 The major anti-microbial functions of antibody.

Antibody

As described earlier, many of the functions of antibody also involve phagocytic cells and/or complement, which is why the effects of antibody deficiency and of PMN or complement defects are somewhat similar (see chapter 23). However in some cases antibody can act on its own, for example by blocking entry of viruses or immobilizing motile bacteria (Fig. 22.10).

IMMUNOPATHOLOGY

Adaptive immune responses are potentially dangerous to the host for two reasons. Firstly, the normal effector mechanisms may passively damage uninfected host tissue (hypersensitivity) and secondly, because of antigenic similarity between host and parasite, responses directed originally against the parasite may also be specifically targeted to host tissue (autoimmunity).

Autoimmunity

Most autoimmune diseases are still not entirely understood (see chapter 4), but there is a strong suspicion that an infectious organism is often involved at some level. This could be due to actual antigenic similarity between parasite and host tissue (Fig. 22.11), as has been shown for:

- Group A β-haemolytic streptococci and cardiac muscle (leading to rheumatic carditis);
- *Trypanosoma cruzi* and both cardiac and autonomic nerves (leading to the heart failure and mega-syndromes of Chagas' disease);
- an adenovirus and gliadin from wheat (possibly the basis of coeliac disease);
- *Klebsiella* bacteria and the class I MHC antigen B27 (which probably contributes to the remarkable susceptibility of B27 individuals to ankylosing spondylitis).

Some examples of parasite-host mimicry

Parasite	Host molecule
Bacteria	
Streptococcus	heart
Klebsiella	HLA-B27
M. tuberculosis	64kDa heat shock protein
N. meningitidis B capsule	embryonic brain
Protozoa	
malaria	thymosin α-1
T. cruzi	heart, nerve
Helminths	
Schistosoma	glutathione transferase

Fig. 22.11 Antigenic similarity between host and parasite may lead to host damage.

As more protein sequences and structures become available for comparison, further examples of cross-reaction will no doubt emerge.

Polyclonal activation. Another mechanism for autoantibody induction is polyclonal activation of B cells, some of which may produce antibodies against self components; malaria, bacterial lipopolysaccharides and some herpes viruses (EBV, CMV) are capable of such activation. More subtle induction via the idiotype network is also a possibility.

Hypersensitivity reactions

Hypersensitivity reactions are usually classified according to the mechanism of damage (Gell and Coombs' types I–IV; see chapter 1), and each category includes some examples due to infectious organisms (Fig. 22.12):

- Type I (allergic) reactions occur in certain worm infections where high levels of IgE are a common finding; typical examples are the tropical pulmonary eosinophilia of filariasis and the acute anaphylaxis that can follow rupture of a hydatid cyst.
- Type II (cytotoxic) reactions are, of course, a normal parasiticidal mechanism, and any damage to normal tissue is usually due to cross-reaction (see above).
- Type III reactions, in which immune complexes cause vascular damage, are probably the most common form of immunopathology in infection. This is seen in the glomerulonephritis of streptococcal and (quartan) malarial infection and the 'allergic alveolitis' of fungal infections such as aspergillosis.
- Type IV reactions are also an important complication of some infections. Here, a chronic inflammatory process culminating in granuloma formation and fibrosis is maintained by persistent infection. The organisms responsible are often parasites such as mycobacteria, fungi, and some protozoa (for example *Leishmania*) which survive inside macrophages, but may also be larger structures such as schistosome eggs which give rise to the portal or vesical cirrhosis of schistosomiasis.

In the conditions which prevail in type IV reactions, excessive T cell stimulation and lymphokine production may be modulated to some extent by suppressor T cells. The degree of this modulation may explain the contrasting patterns of response found at the ends of the 'immunological spectrum' typical of leprosy, with excessive CMI in the tuberculoid form and inadequate CMI in the lepromatous form.

PARASITE SURVIVAL MECHANISMS

If parasites are to survive the potent immune mechanisms already described, they must clearly take evasive action and it is often this which dictates the pattern of disease. To take two instances: mycobacteria and *Histoplasma* (a fungus) have both adapted to survival within the macrophage, and the resulting diseases, tuberculosis and histoplasmosis, are remarkably similar. The African trypanosome (a protozoan) and *Borrelia* (a bacterium) both

Hypersensitivity reactions in infectious disease		
Type I	IgE + mast cells	*Ascaris* (lung), hydatid cyst fluid
Type II	autoantibodies	*Mycoplasma* streptococcal myocarditis *T. cruzi*
Type III	immune complexes PMNs, complement disseminated intravascular coagulation (DIC)	streptococcus erythema nodosum glomerulonephritis meningococcus hepatitis B quartan malaria fungal allergic alveolitis septicaemia
Type IV	T cells & macrophages	TB granuloma tuberculoid leprosy schistosome egg granuloma ? *T. cruzi*
cytokine over-production	TNF, IL-1	Gram -ve bacteria (LPS) staphylococci (TSST1) mycobacteria (LAM) yeast malaria (exoantigens)

Fig. 22.12 Each type of hypersensitivity reaction includes some examples which are caused by infectious organisms. LPS=lipopolysaccharide; TSST1=toxic shock syndrome type 1; LAM=lipoarabinomannan.

22.8

evade the antibody response by varying their surface antigens, and as a result both give rise to an undulant or 'relapsing' pattern of fever. Not surprisingly, each successful parasite takes action against those components of the immune system which are most likely to eliminate it, so that there are almost as many survival as effector mechanisms. However they can conveniently be classified under three headings (Fig. 22.13):

- concealment
- variation
- suppression.

Parasite escape mechanisms	
Type	**Effector mechanisms**
concealment	intracellular capsules cysts privileged site mimicry of host host antigen coating
variation	mutation gene switching recombination
suppression	non–specific specific (tolerance) by: macrophages T suppressor cells parasite products

Fig. 22.13 Parasite escape mechanisms.

Concealment

All immune mechanisms, whether natural or adaptive, depend initially on recognition of the parasite either by a cell receptor (macrophage surface receptors, B cell immunoglobulin, the T cell receptor), or by a free molecule (complement components, C-reactive protein). Many parasites have succeeded in avoiding this type of contact (Fig. 22.14). At one extreme is the tapeworm *Echinococcus*, living in its hydatid cyst. Here, it is out of reach of the serum antibody which, if injected into the cyst, can destroy it. At the other extreme are the capsulated bacteria, with polysaccharide capsules that prevent contact with macrophages. Thus phagocytosis is only possible when antibody has been made against the capsular antigens, allowing attachment via macrophage Fc receptors. Antibodies to carbohydrate reside largely in the IgG2 subclass, and so patients deficient in this particular subclass may have excess respiratory tract infections with organisms such as pnuemococcus and *Haemophilus influenzae.*

Intracellular survival. This also represents an effective way of avoiding contact with antibody but, particularly when the cell involved is the macrophage, considerable ingenuity is required for the parasite to avoid destruction. This may take the form of inhibition of phagosome-lysosome fusion (for example *Toxoplasma*), escape into the cytoplasm (for example *Leishmania*) or simply a tough cell wall (for example mycobacteria). However it is frequently possible for the cell to transport antigenic fragments of the parasite to the surface, where they are displayed in association with MHC molecules. This brings the parasite to the attention of T cells, which can then sometimes tip the balance by enhancing macrophage microbicidal function, as occurs in the killing of *Leishmania*, or *T. cruzi*, under the influence of IFNγ.

Uptake of host molecules. Another rather specialized form of concealment is the uptake of host-derived

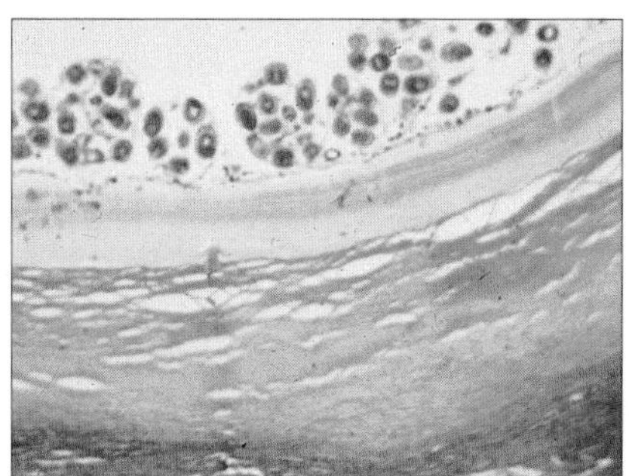

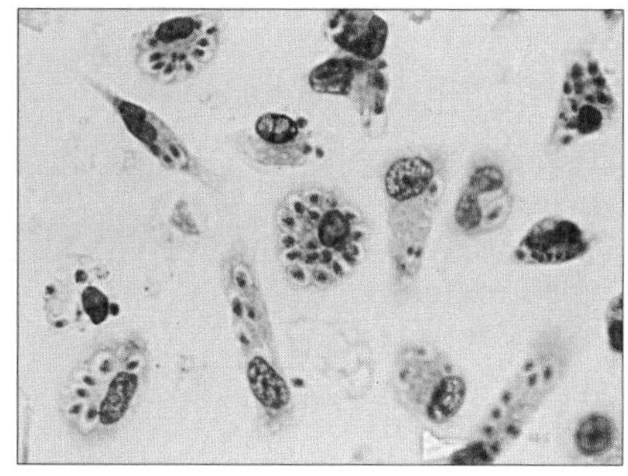

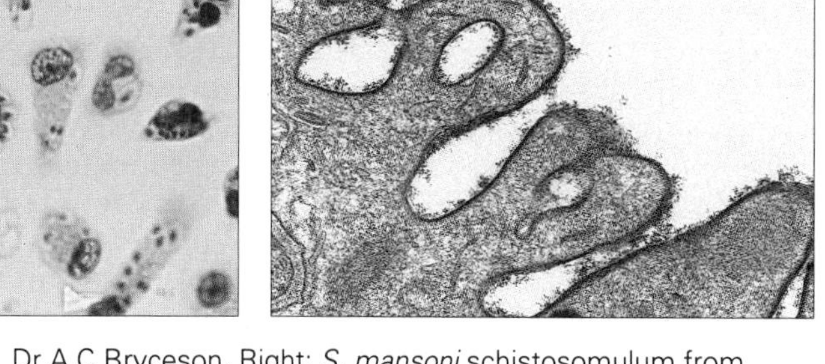

Fig. 22.14 Concealment of parasites. Left: section of hydatid cyst showing fertile germinal membrane which is releasing protoscolices into the cyst fluid. Courtesy of Dr R Muller. Middle: monolayer of blood monocytes containing large numbers of the amastigote form of *Leishmania*. Courtesy of Dr A C Bryceson. Right: *S. mansoni* schistosomulum from mouse lung labelled with ferritin-conjugated anti-murine RBC antiserum. Ferritin deposits on the parasite membrane indicate the presence of mouse RBC antigens at the worm surface. X 78000. Courtesy of Dr D J McLaren.

molecules onto the surface of the parasite. This is most vividly shown by the schistosome, the surface of which eventually becomes covered with red cell glycolipids, MHC antigens and immunoglobulin fragments, making it virtually 'invisible' to the immune system. One would predict that this mechanism would be more appropriate for non-dividing extracellular organisms such as worms, which have a relatively slow surface turnover.

Variation

Rapidly dividing organisms wishing to survive extracellularly in the presence of antibody (for example in the blood) can do so by repeatedly varying their surface antigens. The classical example is the African trypanosome, which contains about 1000 genes coding for separate complete surface glycoprotein coats. Switching from one gene to another results in totally new surface antigens (Fig. 22.15), which requires a new antibody response; thus, the majority of antibody is wasted and the host never achieves effective immunity. It is tempting to assume that antibody itself induces the switch, but in fact switching is a feature of free-living protozoa too. Whatever the reason, it certainly poses a great problem for the development of vaccines.

In some cases the variation evolves more slowly, over months or years rather than days, so that individuals already immune to one variant are susceptible to the next epidemic; this is the pattern in influenza. In other cases large numbers of variants or 'strains' co-exist and immunity, to be effective, must be developed against all or most of them; this is the case with pneumococci, staphylococci, streptococci, malaria, and many upper respiratory viruses. The possession of a complex life cycle with different antigens expressed at different stages (for example malaria and some worms) can also be thought of as antigenic variation.

Suppression

In those cases where the parasite cannot conceal its existence from the immune system, it often succeeds in inhibiting the expected response or neutralizing the damaging component. Examples range from the almost complete immunosuppression of AIDS (see chapter 24), due mainly to the progressive loss of $CD4^+$ T helper cells, to the local production by staphylococci of toxins that damage PMNs, of a factor which prevents PMN chemotaxis, and of a protein (protein A) which immobilizes IgG.

In many diseases there is fairly severe generalized suppression of immune responses but the precise cause is not known. In trypanosomiasis and malaria, for instance, the ability to make antibody against unrelated antigens is impaired and polyclonal B cell activation, disruption of lymphoid organ architecture, prostaglandins, anti-lymphocyte autoantibodies and suppressor T cells have all been incriminated. Whatever the cause, the immunosuppression of even quite mild malaria is sufficient to impair the response of patients to meningococcal and pneumococcal vaccines, with important economic consequences. However, it should be remembered that immunosuppression may in some cases be of value to the host by reduc-
22.10 ing the immunopathology.

HOST-PARASITE BALANCE AND IMBALANCE

With strong effector mechanisms ranged against sophisticated evasion strategies, an infection can have several possible outcomes (Fig. 22.16). The ideal from the host's viewpoint is complete elimination of the micro-organism

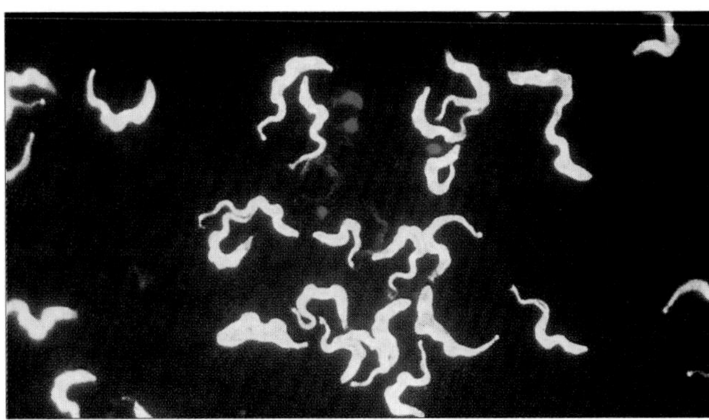

Fig. 22.15 African trypanosomes in immunofluorescence with antibodies specific for variant surface glycoprotein. The 2 negative trypanosomes, counterstained red, have undergone antigenic variation and are expressing an immunologically distinct surface glycoprotein. Courtesy of Dr J D Barry.

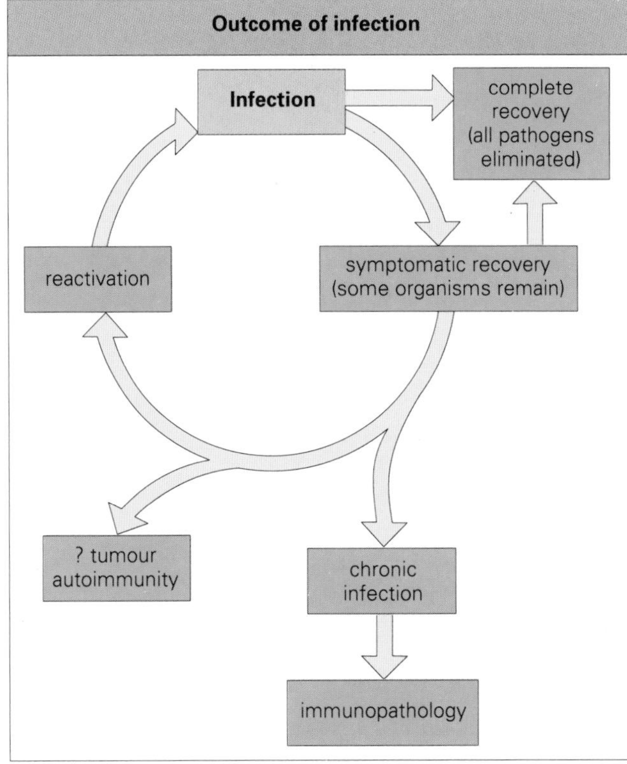

Fig. 22.16 Recovery from infection does not always mean that the organism has been eliminated. Patients can be asymptomatic carriers or organisms may surive in restricted sites.

Common opportunistic infections		
Defect		**Characteristic infections**
skin defences		staphylococci
mucus		*Pseudomonas*
phagocytosis, oxidative killing		staphylococci
complement C1–3		pyogenic bacteria
complement C5–9		*Neisseria*
antibody		pyogenic bacteria *S. pneumoniae* enteroviruses
T cells	viruses	vaccinia, herpes, measles, CMV
	bacteria	TB
	fungi	*Candida, Aspergillus, Pneumocystis carinii*
	protozoa	*Toxoplasma*
	worms	*Strongyloides*

Fig. 22.17 With normal immune function, infectious agents are rigorously controlled; immunosuppression allows opportunists to become established and cause disease.

Zoonotic infections		
Infection		**Animal host**
Viruses	yellow fever	monkey
	equine encephalitis	horse
	rabies	dog, fox, etc.
	lassa fever	rodents
Bacteria	*B. anthracis* (anthrax)	sheep
	Brucella	goat
	Borrelia (lyme disease)	rat, deer
	Yersinia pestis (plague)	rat
	Rickettsia (typhus)	rodents
	Listeria	rodents, birds
	Chlamydia (psittacosis)	birds
Fungi	*Histoplasma*	birds
Protozoa	*Babesia*	cattle
	Leishmania	dog
	Toxoplasma	cat
	Cryptosporidium	cattle
Worms	*Taenia*	cattle, pig
	Echinococcus (hydatid)	dog
	Toxocara	dog
	Trichinella	pig

Fig. 22.18 Zoonotic infections are important examples of host–parasite imbalance.

with resistance to reinfection; this is the usual sequence with the childhood viruses (although the apparently life-long immunity is probably maintained by annual boosts), and with bacteria such as *S. pneumoniae* (but here the immunity is strain specific and there are over 80 strains).

However recovery, in terms of disappearance of symptoms, does not always mean that all the organisms have been eliminated, and survival in restricted sites may occur. This can have two consequences. Firstly, the disease may reappear under circumstances in which immunity is weakened, well-known examples being the cold sores of herpes simplex and the zoster ('shingles') of varicella; in both cases the virus remains latent, often for many years, in dorsal root ganglia. Alternatively, the patient may remain well but be able to infect others; this 'carrier' state is a feature of infections such as hepatitis B, typhoid and amoebiasis. In malaria essentially all patients are carriers, immunity being of a slowly-developing and incomplete kind known as 'premunition'. Another type of partial immunity is seen in schistosomiasis, where mature worms survive in the presence of effective immunity against the young infecting form. This is known as 'concomitant' immunity and has obvious survival value for the parasite as well as the host.

Opportunistic infections

When the immune system is seriously weakened, as in transplant patients treated with immunosuppressive drugs or in AIDS, infections may develop apparently for the first time. These are the 'opportunists' (Fig. 22.17) and represent infections which become established without causing any obvious symptoms, to flare up when immunity is suppressed. This implies that normally their numbers are rigorously controlled by immune mechanisms, but the manner in which this is achieved is not known in most cases. Several mechanisms are probably involved, because different opportunists tend to dominate in different forms of immunodeficiency, for example CMV in the bone marrow transplant patients treated with total body irradiation and *Pneumocystis carinii* in AIDS. An opportunistic form of yeast infection, chronic mococutaneous candidiasis, is interesting in that some cases appear to respond to transfer factor but the mechanism of this has never been explained.

Zoonoses

A final example of host–parasite imbalance is the zoonotic infections, which include some of the most severe and rapidly fatal infections (Fig. 22.18). The micro-organisms are maintained in, and adapted to, some non-human species, so that human infection is sporadic and insufficient to have stimulated the evolution of adequate resistance. Some life-threatening diseases, such as African trypanosomiasis and *P. falciparum* ('malignant') malaria may represent an intermediate stage where evolution of the human–parasite balance is only in its early stages.

FURTHER READING

Beutler B, Cerami A. The biology of cachectin/TNF — a primary mediator of the host response. *Ann Rev Immunol.* 1989; **7**:625–655.

Damian RT. Molecular mimicry revisited. *Parasitol Today.* 1987; **3**:263–266.

Khardori N. Host–parasite interaction in fungal infections. *Eur J Clin Microbiol Infect Dis.* 1989; **8**:331–351.

Mims CA. *The pathogenesis of infectious disease (3E).* London: Academic Press, 1987.

Nathan CF. Mechanisms of macrophage anti-microbial activity. *Trans Roy Soc Trop Med Hyg.* 1983; **77**:620.

Root RK, Sande MA, eds. *Septic shock.* New York: Churchill Livingstone, 1985.

23

Congenital Immunodeficiency Syndromes

INTRODUCTION

The best characterized forms of congenital immunodeficiency are those with a simple Mendelian inheritance, such as the X-linked recessive form of immunoglobulin deficiency. The underlying gene defects of these syndromes are now being defined and some biochemical understanding of their pathogenesis should follow. Interim classifications of immunodeficiency syndromes on clinical or pathological grounds tend to be confusing, largely because of the heterogeneity of laboratory results. Examples of this heterogeneity include the plasma immunoglobulin concentrations in antibody deficiency or the number of blood lymphocytes in severe combined immunodeficiency. The approach to classification taken in this chapter is based on the type of immunological response that is deficient, as summarized in Fig. 23.1. As new primary immunodeficiency syndromes are recognized their classification is reviewed by an expert panel (WHO Special Report Series).

ANTIBODY DEFICIENCY SYNDROMES

The classification of antibody deficiency is summarized in Fig. 23.2.

CONGENITAL AGAMMAGLOBULINAEMIA

The X-linked form of congenital agammaglobulinaemia is a convenient prototype for antibody deficiency syndromes. Affected boys have undetectable or very low serum levels of IgM, IgD, IgE and IgA. IgG levels are usually between 40–100mg/dl. Pre-B cells are present in the bone marrow and produce the cytoplasmic form of μ chain. Further development of the B cell series appears to be arrested and B lymphocytes in the blood are absent or very rare. Recent DNA hybridization studies suggest that there may be more than one molecular defect which is clinically expressed as X-linked agammaglobulinaemia. Until the primary gene defect is defined, an affected male relative on the maternal side is required for a confident diagnosis.

Clinical course

The affected boys are usually in good health for the first month or two of life (while they are protected by maternal IgG) but by the time they have reached one year of age most have had frequent upper respiratory tract infections (typically colds and ear infections), progressing to

Classification of congenital primary immunodeficiency syndromes
Affecting specific immunity
antibody deficiency syndromes
selective immunoglobulin deficiencies
selective defects of cell-mediated immunity
combined immunodeficiencies
Affecting non-specific effector mechanisms
complement defects
neutrophil defects

Fig. 23.1 Classification of congenital immunodeficiency syndromes.

Classification of antibody deficiency
Panhypogammaglobulinaemia syndromes
congenital X-linked agammaglobulinaemia
acquired hypogammaglobulinaemia
X-linked immunodeficiency with IgM
hypogammaglobulinaemia with thymoma
immunodeficiency syndromes affecting mainly antibody formation
Selective antibody deficiencies
selective IgA deficiency
IgG subclass deficiencies
Transient hypogammaglobulinaemia

Fig. 23.2 Classification of antibody deficiencies.

pneumonia. As the children get older and their sinuses develop, these also become important sites for infection (Fig. 23.3). Common infections at other superficial sites are cellulitis and paronychia, and these sometimes spread systemically, leading to osteomyelitis or meningitis. The infections are caused mostly by streptococci, staphylococci, *Haemophilus influenzae*, mycoplasma and ureaplasma species and Gram-negative bacteria.

Complications

Affected individuals are at risk of developing three major complications:

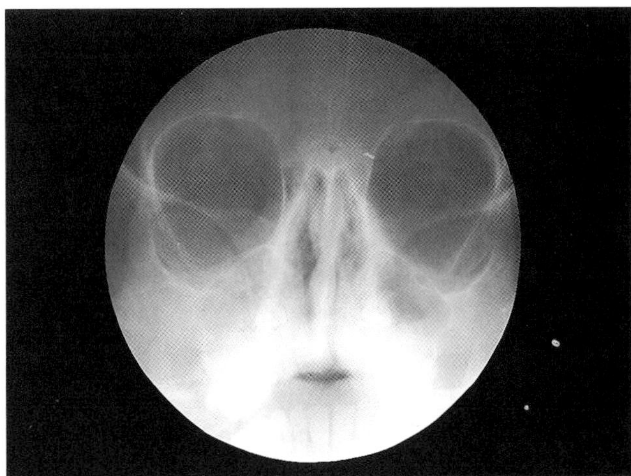

Fig. 23.3 Maxillary sinusitus in a boy with X-linked agammaglobulinaemia. The sinuses are one of the most common sites of infection in patients with antibody deficiency, and in many cases the underlying disorder is recognized only after a series of acute infections and surgical interventions.

- Arthritis affecting the ankle and knee is common before treatment starts but usually resolves rapidly when immunoglobulin replacement is given.
- Severe diarrhoea leading to weight loss occurs in about 20% of patients. In most cases it is caused by *Giardia lamblia* and resolves with metronidazole treatment. Cryptosporidia infection, which is difficult to treat, has been recognized more recently as a cause of intractable diarrhoea in antibody deficiency. Both types of diarrhoea may interfere with nutrition to such an extent that they can cause secondary defects in cell-mediated immunity, which resolve when nutrition is improved.
- Encephalitis is a third serious complication. It is often caused by echovirus 11 and is usually resistant to treatment with conventional amounts of immunoglobulin.

Treatment

Treatment of antibody deficiency is mostly by replacement of IgG. Even small amounts given by intramuscular injection, for example 25mg/kg body weight/week, which is enough to raise serum IgG to about 200mg/dl, greatly reduces the risk of severe infection. The injections are painful and most patients greatly prefer intravenous infusions of specially prepared, aggregate free, IgG. Much greater amounts can be given (400mg/kg or more) at four week intervals (Fig. 23.4), and there is some suggestion that this gives better protection against infection. Immunoglobulin for replacement is prepared from large pools of donors by ethanol fractionation. These have been proven to be remarkably free from the risk of transmitting AIDS or hepatitis.

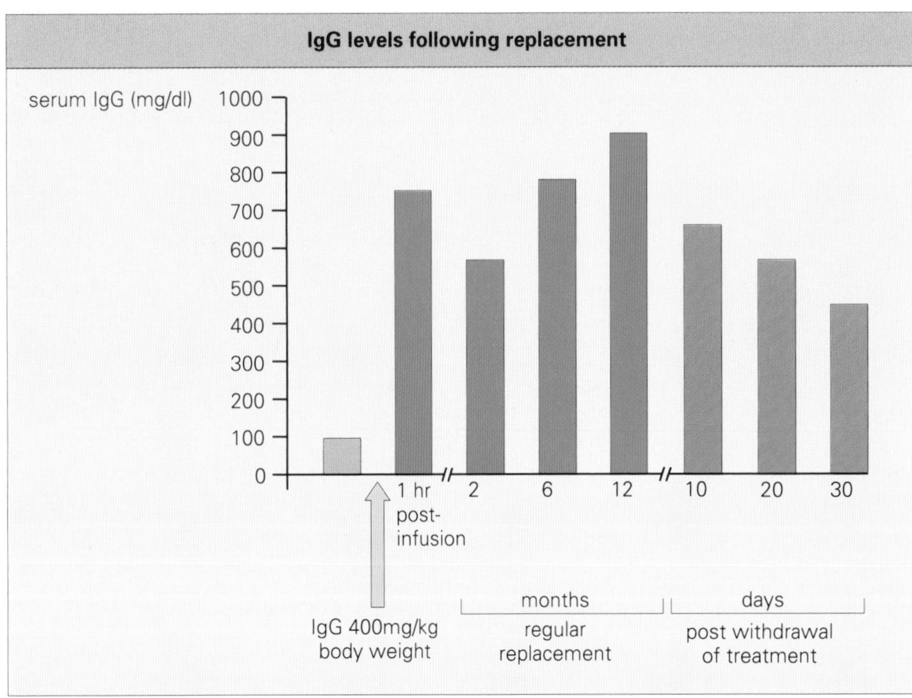

Fig. 23.4 Serum IgG concentrations after intravenous infusions in a boy with X-linked agammaglobulinaemia. The first two bars show levels before and one hour after loading with 400mg/kg body weight of IgG. Levels at 2, 6 and 12 months were obtained after institution of regular replacement of 400mg/kg every 3 weeks. Levels at 10, 20 and 30 days were obtained after the last iv infusion, and illustrate the half-life of IgG.

X-LINKED IMMUNODEFICIENCY WITH IgM

This generally appears in infants and children with symptoms of antibody deficiency but with the additional finding of normal or high serum IgM (Fig. 23.5). Thrombocytopenia and neutropenia are common associated problems and some subjects develop haemolytic anaemia. Epstein-Barr virus infections occurring in an immunodeficient host probably account for the elevated IgM level in many of these subjects. The severity and frequency of infections is reduced by IgG replacement unless the neutropenia is severe.

VARIABLE HYPOGAMMAGLOBULINAEMIA SYNDROMES

Both children and adults with otherwise unclassified types of antibody deficiency are included under this heading. Some of these individuals have B cells in their blood: others do not. Their serum immunoglobulin levels are very variable. IgG is usually below 200mg/dl and IgA below 50mg/dl; some IgM is usually detectable. In some cases, the immunoglobulin deficiency is detected in childhood but adult onset also occurs. An increased incidence of autoimmune disease, and sometimes selective IgA deficiency, in first degree relatives suggests that predisposition to acquired hypogammaglobulinaemia has a polygenic inheritance.

Pathogenetic mechanism

Possible pathogenetic mechanisms include maturation defects restricted to B cells and suppression of immunoglobulin production by T cells. While each of these can be demonstrated in some patients by laboratory tests, there is no clear evidence that either is responsible for the impaired antibody production *in vivo*. Plasma cells are reduced in number in the spleen and gut and the lymph nodes are usually small, unless the patient develops an Epstein-Barr virus infection. With increasing age many of these subjects develop defects of cell-mediated immunity, detected as reduced numbers of T cells in blood and impaired proliferative responses to mitogens.

Complications

The range of infections experienced by these individuals is similar to that in congenital X-linked agammaglobulinaemia, with an additional risk of opportunistic infection such as *Pneumocystis carinii* pneumonia, and of recurrences of herpes zoster. Enlargement of intestinal and bronchial lymphoid tissue is common. In the gut this causes filling defects in contrast X-rays, producing an appearance described as nodular lymphoid hyperplasia (Fig. 23.6). A similar lesion occurs in the lung. Adults with long-standing hypogammaglobulinaemia syndromes often develop B_{12} deficiency and macrocytic anaemia. This is probably secondary to chronic gastritis and reduced intrinsic factor production.

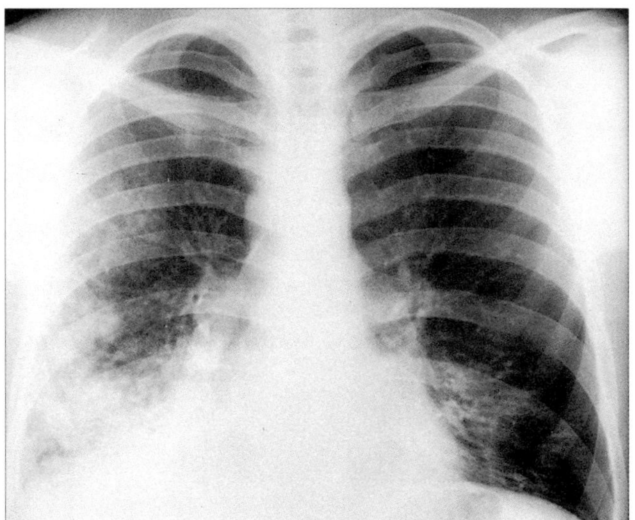

Fig. 23.5 X-ray of pneumococcal pneumonia in a 26-year-old man with hypogammaglobulinaemia with IgM. The respiratory tract is the site which is most often infected in antibody deficient subjects and *Strep. pneumoniae* is one of the most common causal organisms.

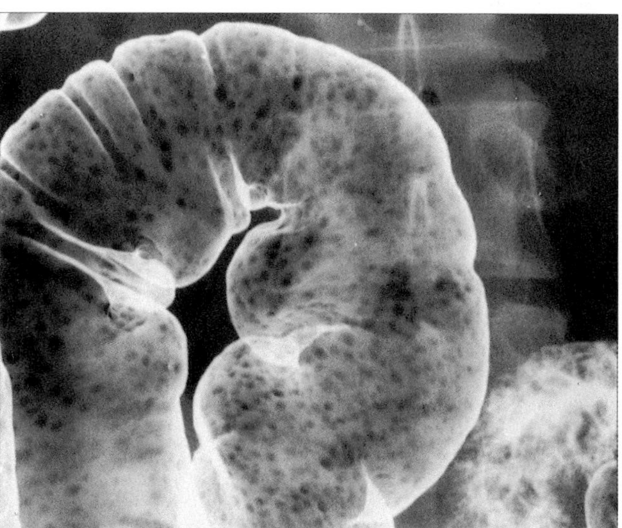

Fig. 23.6 Nodular lymphoid hyperplasia of the large bowel shown by double contrast enema. The lymphoid nodules are seen as filling defects. Comparable degrees of lymphoid hyperplasia occasionally occur in the bronchial tree. In both cases, continued antigenic stimulation with an ineffective antibody response is thought to contribute to the pathogenesis.

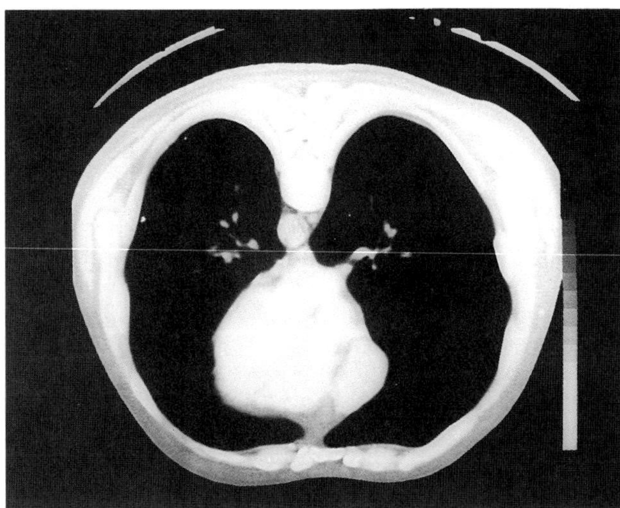

Fig. 23.7 Axial tomogram showing a thymoma in the anterior mediastinum of a 56-year-old man who had developed recurrent pneumonia. The thymoma was removed uneventfully and the hypogammaglobulinaemia persisted, as is the usual case in this condition.

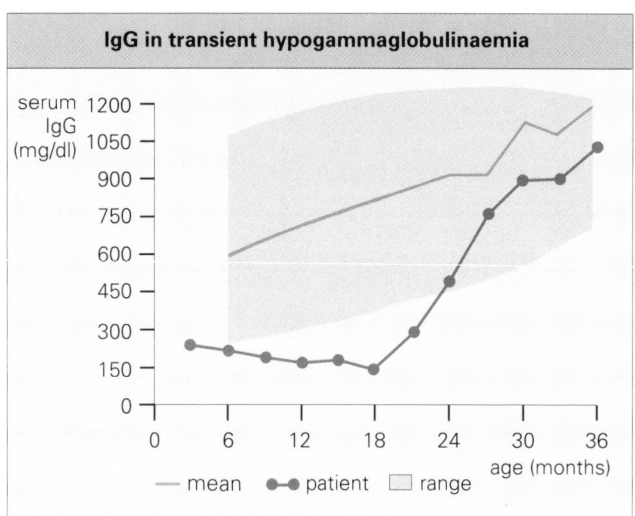

Fig. 23.8 Serum immunoglobulin levels in a boy with transient hypogammaglobulinaemia compared with a healthy control. The subject developed mild paralytic polio following immunization at four months of age, but his IgG did not reach normal levels until he was two years old, suggesting the diagnosis of transient hypogammaglobulinaemia.

Antibody deficiency with thymoma

Although rare, thymic tumours (thymomas) (Fig. 23.7) are of great interest because of their association with myasthenia gravis, red cell aplasia and, in about 10% of cases, hypogammaglobulinaemia. In most instances the thymoma is of the benign spindle cell type. Eosinophils are absent from the bloodstream and serum IgM and IgG levels are very low; IgA may persist, particularly in the secretions. These changes are reflected in the blood lymphocyte populations, where μ- and δ-bearing B cells are absent and α-bearing cells persist. Pre-B cells are lost from the marrow and an autoimmune response to B cell precursors is a possible mechanism which may account for the immunodeficiency. Removal of the thymoma does not reverse the immunoglobulin deficiency and these patients need continued IgG replacement to protect them from infection.

Transient hypogammaglobulinaemia

Serum immunoglobulin levels normally fall during the first five months of life as maternally derived IgG is catabolized and diluted; the nadir is about 250mg/dl, and levels subsequently rise as the infants begin to produce their own IgG. Infants who have low IgG levels and frequent infections (mostly of the respiratory tract) at or following the normal trough are possible cases of transient hypogammaglobulinaemia. The diagnosis can only be made when serum immunoglobulin concentrations have returned to normal (Fig. 23.8): in most cases this occurs within 12 months. During the period of hypogammaglobulinaemia blood lymphocyte counts are normal, as is the frequency of T and B cells. Although IgG levels are low it is usually possible to obtain some antibody response to immunization with toxoid antigen. Infants with transient hypogammaglobulinaemia usually thrive normally and do not require IgG replacement. A few cases of paralysis following spread of vaccine strain poliovirus to the central nervous system have been reported but apart from this, infants with transient hypogammaglobulinaemia do not have problems with virus infections.

OTHER IMMUNOGLOBULIN DEFICIENCY SYNDROMES

SELECTIVE IgA DEFICIENCY

This is the most common primary immunodeficiency with a prevalence between 1:500 and 1:1,200 amongst healthy blood donors. Affected individuals have serum IgA concentrations of 10mg/dl or lower and they lack IgA in secretions. All have B lymphocytes in the blood with cell surface IgA, but for reasons which are not understood they fail to switch their B cells to IgA secretion. Selective deficiency of the IgG2 subclass commonly accompanies IgA deficiency, and such individuals tend to have the greatest problems with infection.

Clinical symptoms

Symptoms of IgA deficiency are variable. At least as many as 50% of the subjects have no problems with infection, perhaps because they are able to protect their mucous membranes with secreted IgM and IgG antibodies. Symptoms, where present, result from infection, allergy and autoimmunity. Infections are mainly of the upper respiratory tract, particularly sinusitis and otitis. Diarrhoea is

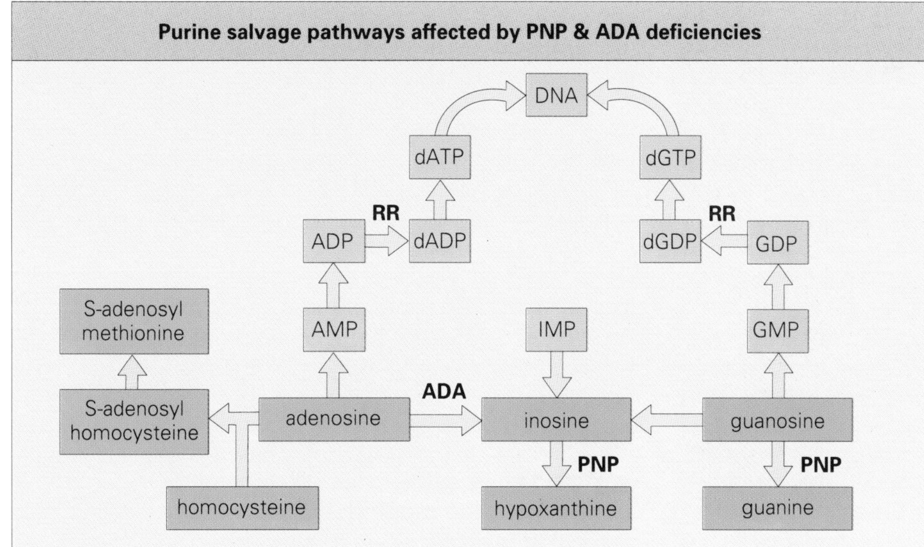

Fig. 23.9 Purine nucleoside phosphorylase (PNP) converts inosine and deoxyinosine to hypoxanthine, so it is the enzyme which follows adenosine deaminase (ADA) in the purine utilization pathway. Absence of either enzyme activity increases intracellular levels of deoxyguanosine triphosphate or d ATP respectively, which inhibits ribonucleotide reductase (RR) and, consequently, DNA synthesis.

the main gut symptom, and is sometimes severe enough to cause weight loss. The allergic symptoms are mainly of asthma and hay fever and there is an increased incidence of serum antibodies to food constituents such as cow's milk. Many autoimmune diseases are associated with IgA deficiency, including SLE, rheumatoid arthritis, haemolytic anaemia, thyroiditis and type I diabetes.

SELECTIVE DEFICIENCIES OF IgG SUBCLASSES

The IgG heavy chain genes are on chromosome 11, where the IgG1 gene is close to that of IgG3 and the IgG2 gene close to that of IgG4. Most serum IgG is IgG1 and most viral and protein antigens elicit antibody of IgG1 and IgG3 subclasses. Low levels of one or more IgG subclasses are common among subjects with an excess of bacterial infections who have no other defined immunodeficiency. IgG2 is the best characterized subclass deficiency and is associated with IgA or IgG4 deficiency in some affected individuals. Symptoms in these cases are mainly an excess of upper respiratory tract infections and the pattern of infection is consistent with the finding that IgG2 is the subclass with greatest antibody activity to bacterial polysaccharides, such as those of *Haemophilus influenzae*. IgG1 and IgG3 subclass deficiencies are also reported although there is less agreement on the infections to which they increase susceptibility. The mechanisms responsible are poorly understood but most probably involve factors regulating immunoglobulin isotype switching in antigen triggered B cells.

DEFECTS OF CELL-MEDIATED IMMUNITY

Effective cell-mediated immunity (delayed type hypersensitivity, graft rejection, lysis of virus infected cells and antigen specific help to B cells) requires contributions from mononuclear phagocytes, T cells and, often, natural killer cells. Of the congenital immunodeficiencies, selective defects of T cells are the best defined. A complete deficiency of T cells abolishes both antibody and cell-mediated immune responses: this is one of the causes of a clinical syndrome called severe combined immunodeficiency. Selective loss of cell-mediated immunity with continued antibody production is very rare and is best exemplified by the immunodeficiency which results from purine nucleoside phosphorylase deficiency (see below).

SELECTIVE DEFECTS OF T CELLS

Congenital defects which interfere completely with T cell development usually give rise to a severe combined immunodeficiency in which there is some immunoglobulin production but no useful antibody response. Partial deficiencies of T cells give a more complicated clinical syndrome in which there is preservation of some antibody response but control may be inadequate, leading to autoantibody production. In these instances, T cell function may be sufficient to prevent severe malabsorption but not to protect the subject against viral pathogens such as varicella, herpes simplex or vaccinia. The best example of this rare combination is an inborn error of metabolism, purine nucleoside phosphorylase deficiency.

PURINE NUCLEOSIDE PHOSPHORYLASE DEFICIENCY

The gene for purine nucleoside phosphorylase (PNP) is on chromosome 14 and symptoms develop only in individuals homozygous for the defect, in whom DNA synthesis by lymphocytes is inhibited (Fig. 23.9). This is a very rare defect, with fewer than 50 families known to be affected.

Presentation of purine nucleoside phosphorylase deficiency
severe herpes virus infections
reduced T cell numbers
reduced T cell proliferation
normal immunoglobulin levels
antibody responses generally present
autoantibody production: haemolytic anaemia

Fig. 23.10 Presentation of purine nucleoside phosphorylase (PNP) deficiency.

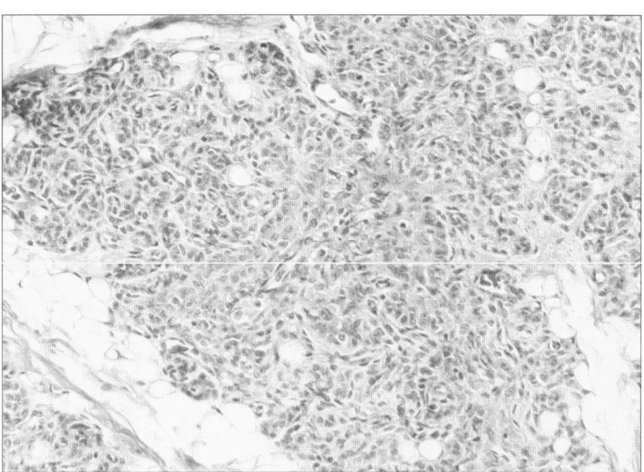

Fig. 23.11 Thymus histology in severe combined immunodeficiency. This child died of *Pneumocystis carinii* pneumonia aged four months. He had previously had blood lymphocyte counts of less than 800mm^3 and a serum IgM of less than 10mg/dl. The thymus shows disorganized epithelial cells with very few lymphocytes and no Hassall's corpuscles.

Clinical presentation and laboratory findings

Affected individuals have severe infections, mainly of herpes viruses, occurring after the first year of life. Developmental retardation, spasticity and behavioural disorders also occur, perhaps as a consequence of defects of CNS purine transmitters. Autoimmune haemolytic anaemia has developed in some cases. Laboratory findings include a low serum uric acid, reduced numbers of circulating T cells, reduced lymphocyte proliferative responses to mitogens with normal immunoglobulin concentrations, and the presence of some antibodies (Fig. 23.10). Treatment has been unsatisfactory because stem cell grafts have generally been rejected.

COMBINED IMMUNODEFICIENCY SYNDROMES

Severe combined immunodeficiency (SCID) syndromes have in common a failure of antibody-mediated and cell-mediated immunity. There are at least three different congenital forms of SCID, two with autosomal recessive inheritance and one with an X-linked inheritance. About 25% of cases of autosomal recessive SCID syndromes are due to adenosine deaminase deficiency, which is the best characterized form.

ADENOSINE DEAMINASE DEFICIENCY

Adenosine deaminase (ADA) catalyses the conversion of adenosine and deoxyadenosine to inosine. The gene is on chromosome 20 and only infants homozygous for the deficiency are symptomatic. There are several biochemical mechanisms which may account for the immunodeficiency. Adverse effects of increased intracellular deoxyadenosine include a fall in intracellular NAD which, when experimentally induced, kills resting and dividing T cells after about eight hours. Another is the inhibition of ribonucleotide reductase by dATP. This enzyme is the rate limiting step in the synthesis of nucleoside triphosphates, and its inhibition blocks further nucleic acid synthesis. Both of these processes may also contribute to the pathophysiology of purine nucleoside phosphorylase deficiency (see Fig. 23.9).

An additional factor in ADA deficiency is interference with the recycling of S-adenosyl homocysteine, leading to inhibition of methylation reactions. The particular susceptibility of T cells to purine toxicity may result from their need to remain as resting cells for long periods, retaining the ability to proliferate rapidly following antigen stimulus. Infusions of ADA conjugated to PEG give some improvement in T cell function and reconstitution by gene therapy is to be tested next.

Clinical features of SCID

Infants with SCID commonly have superficial infections in the first month of life, and by three months of age almost all have diarrhoea and are failing to gain weight. Respiratory tract infections are common, usually in the form of pneumonia caused by opportunists such as *Pneumocystis carinii* (Fig. 23.11). Without effective reconstitution affected infants lose weight and die in the course of 1–2 years.

Treatment

This is primarily by stem cell grafting using either unseparated bone marrow from an HLA matched sibling or T cell-depleted marrow from a parent. Unseparated sibling grafts are generally successful in reconstituting both antibody and cell-mediated immunity: T cell-depleted grafts often reconstitute only cell-mediated immunity.

OTHER TYPES OF SCID

Lack of expression of class II MHC products (HLA-DR, -DP and -DQ) occurs in one rare type of SCID, also called 'bare lymphocyte syndrome'. This is described separately because it may constitute a definable disease entity. Most of the remaining infants with less well characterized forms of SCID (with X-linked recessive or autosomal recessive inheritance which is not due to ADA deficiency) have normal or high numbers of B cells in their blood but they lack T cells. Differences in symptoms or the presence of leucopenia or of some immunoglobulin have been used as a basis for classification, but this approach is at best provisional.

Class II expression deficiency

Abnormalities of HLA antigen expression on the cell surface fall broadly into two groups. Individuals with low amounts of class I HLA determinants generally have no major problems with infection. Subjects lacking class II MHC expression have a SCID syndrome which is difficult to recognize because they have normal numbers of lymphocytes and normal T cell subsets in blood, together with normal T cell proliferative responses to mitogens.

Treatment of SCID

Pending transplantation

IgG replacement and iv hyperalimentation

co-trimoxazole for *Pneumocystis* prophylaxis

ketoconazole for candidiasis, if present

Transplant

matched sibling donor & unseparated marrow if available

T-depleted parental marrow if no matched sibling

T-depleted HLA-matched donor if parents unsuitable

Fig. 23.12 Treatment of SCID.

Nevertheless, their T cells do not proliferate in antigen stimulated cultures and antibody responses are impaired.

Some infants with SCID lack any mature T or B cells: failure of development of a common stem cell may account for this in some patients, in others an enzyme which is essential for both B and T cell development may be lacking. Mice homozygous for a SCID gene are a possible example of the latter as their marrow and thymic cells lack a recombinase which would be needed for gene rearrangement for the generation of cell surface receptors.

The undoubted occurrence of partial engraftment with maternal T or non-T cells in some infants with SCID adds to the heterogeneity of laboratory findings. Some of these chimeras have a mild chronic graft-versus-host disease and the clinical presentation may resemble histiocytosis-X. Difficulty in transplantation with bone marrow due to graft rejection is an important consequence of maternal T cell engraftment.

TREATMENT OF SCID SYNDROMES

Intravenous infusion of bone marrow cells obtained from an HLA-matched sibling is the simplest and most consistently successful treatment for SCID. Mature T cells appear in the recipient after 2–3 weeks, diarrhoea (if present) stops 1–2 weeks later and antibody responses develop after 2–3 months (Fig. 23.12)

Most infants with SCID do not have HLA-matched siblings. For them, the best approach is to infuse parental bone marrow (Fig. 23.13) which has been depleted of T cells using either monoclonal antibodies or rosetting procedures. Engraftment is much slower under these circumstances and an important hazard is the development of a lymphoproliferative disease caused by EBV transformed B lymphoblasts. Recipients who escape or survive this develop normal numbers of circulating T cells after 6–12 months. Most develop normal numbers of circulating B cells but antibody responses remain deficient in about 50% of cases.

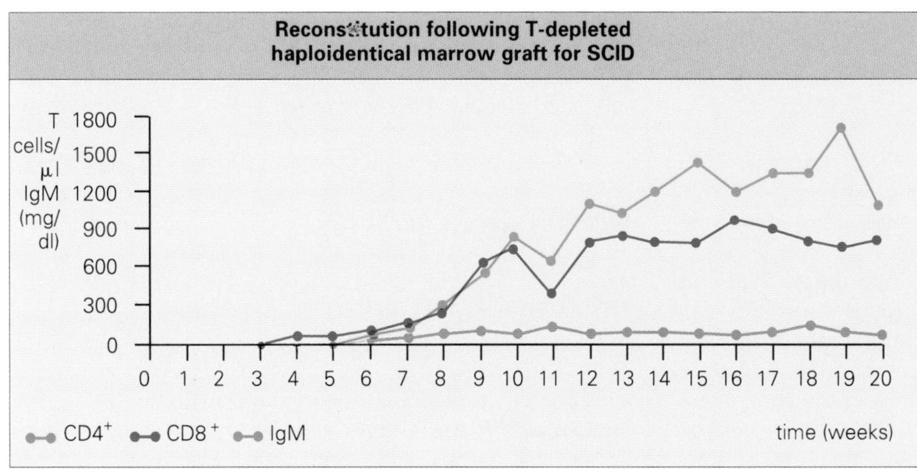

Fig. 23.13 Immunological reconstitution following a graft of T cell-depleted parental bone marrow into an infant with SCID. Increasing numbers of $CD4^+$ and $CD8^+$ T cells appeared in the circulation eight weeks after the graft and serum IgM was detected after nine weeks. Lymph nodes were palpable after four months. This is a rapid course for reconstitution after a T cell-depleted graft, perhaps because the recipient remained in good health.

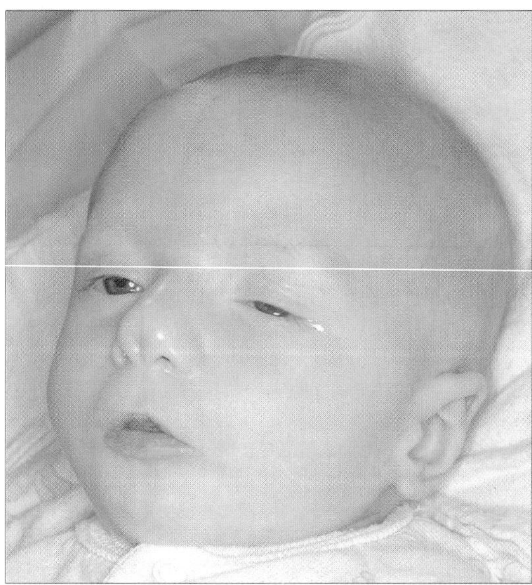

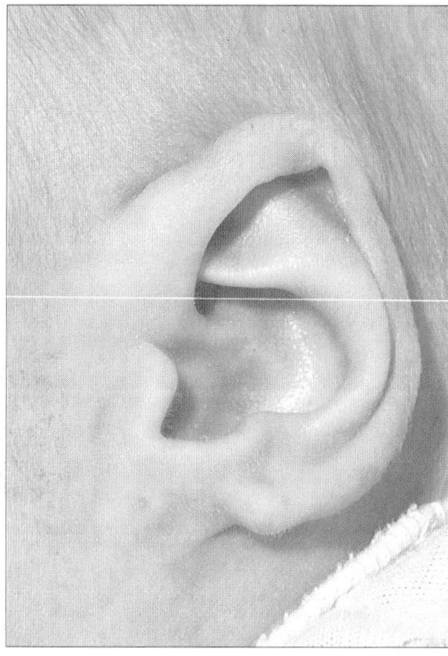

Fig. 23.14 Di George syndrome. Facial features vary in this syndrome. This infant presented with a small jaw and small ears.

OTHER PRIMARY IMMUNODEFICIENCY SYNDROMES

WISKOTT-ALDRICH SYNDROME

Characteristic features are thrombocytopenia, eczema of atopic distribution, and recurrent infections. The platelets are small and function abnormally, as well as being reduced in number. The result of these changes is bruising, neurological stroke in childhood and blood loss with diarrhoea. Infections are mostly of the upper respiratory tract, causing otitis, but the frequency of septicaemia is increased. Serum IgG levels are usually normal, IgA is often increased and IgM reduced, particularly in older children. The disease has an X-linked recessive transmission and the immunodeficiency tends to progress so that older children are most at risk of developing severe infections. Lymphoma is an additional risk as the patient ages. The aetiology is incompletely understood, however, blood lymphocytes, platelets and monocytes have defective expression of sialophorin, which is apparently necessary for normal function.

ATAXIA TELANGIECTASIA

Affected infants are normal at birth with the first symptom, usually ataxia, developing around 2–4 years of age. Accompanying neurological changes include cerebellar atrophy and subsequent axonal neuropathy and muscle denervation. Telangiectases develop over the next few years. They are most easily seen on the conjunctivae but also occur on the nose, ears and shoulders. Infections are mostly of the upper respiratory tract, and sometimes progress to pneumonia. Immunological changes include a reduced number of circulating T cells and reduced T cell proliferative responses to mitogens. These abnormalities tend to get worse with increasing age and few patients survive beyond the age of 25. Common causes of death include pneumonia and malignancy, particularly lymphoma and epithelial cancers. Other abnormalities include raised serum α-fetoprotein levels, impaired glucose tolerance and both reduced and erroneous DNA repair following irradiation induced damage. The latter defect is probably the most consistent laboratory abnormality and may underlie the whole syndrome, although the mechanisms involved are not understood.

CHRONIC MUCOCUTANEOUS CANDIDIASIS

The mucous component of the candidiasis usually involves the mouth and sometimes the oesophagus, and cutaneous involvement may be widespread or restricted to the nails. Other skin infections are common, particularly those caused by staphylococci which occur around the eyelash follicles or as boils on the scalp. Mucocutaneous candidiasis may occur as an isolated condition, or in association with other immunodeficiencies (such as thymoma) or autoimmune syndromes (hypoparathyroidism, hypopituitarism, Addison's disease). Immune function tests are very variable in this condition. Their return to normal after eradication of *Candida* is consistent with the view that mannan, a sugar released by the yeast, is itself immunosuppressive.

ENVIRONMENTAL DEFECTS

THYMIC HYPOPLASIA (DI GEORGE SYNDROME)

Di George described a combination of hypoparathyroidism, thymic hypoplasia and abnormalities of the aortic arch occurring in children with recurrent *Candida* infections (Fig. 23.14). These organs develop in parallel and

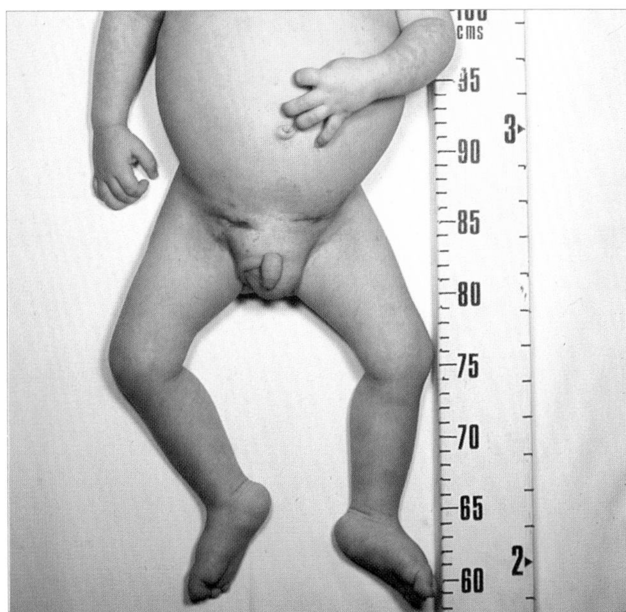

Fig. 23.15 Bilateral draining inguinal lymph nodes in an 18-month-old boy with chronic granulomatous disease. Both groins had developed abscesses caused by *Staph. aureus* and had to be surgically drained.

the syndrome is thought to result from damage to the fetus around the eighth week of gestation. There are a few reports of familial occurrence, associated with abnormalities of chromosome 22. The clinical consequences of the defect are very variable. Severely immunodeficient infants, who are rare, have low numbers of T cells in blood, small hypoplastic lymph nodes, moderately reduced serum immunoglobulin concentrations and failure to make antibody following immunization. *Candida* infections in these infants are usual and herpes simplex and zoster infections may be severe. Those with deficient antibody responses suffer from recurrent upper respiratory tract infections, particularly sinusitis.

Partial hypoplasia. Partial impairment of thymic function is much more common than the complete defect. These infants are usually identified during corrective cardiac surgery because they lack a thymus. When tested, they may have low numbers of T cells in the blood but these show a normal distribution between $CD4^+$ and $CD8^+$ cells. In most instances there are no problems with infection in relation to the cardiac surgery, and the number of T cells in the blood increases over the ensuing six months.

Treatment

Treatment of thymic hypoplasia with grafts of fetal thymus is reported to result in rapid increases in the number and responsiveness of circulating T cells. For severely immuodeficient infants, grafting with fetal thymus carries the theoretical risk of graft-versus-host disease. Other approaches to treatment, such as injections with putative thymic humoral factors, have not been regularly successful.

PHAGOCYTE DEFECTS

Useful phagocyte function involves at least four major steps:

- adherence to the vascular endothelium;
- migration through tissues to sites of inflammation (chemotaxis);
- phagocytosis of opsonized particles;
- intracellular killing of ingested organisms.

LFA-1 OR iC3b RECEPTOR DEFICIENCY

This condition is also known as LAD (leucocyte adhesion deficiency syndrome). Affected individuals fail to make the common β subunit (CD18) which associates with different forms of CD11 to form LFA-1, MAC-1 and the p150, 95 membrane protein. The inheritance of the defect is autosomal recessive and increased susceptibility to infection occurs in the first month of life. Typical early infections include peri-umbilical abscesses, progressing to cellulitis and tissue necrosis. Wound healing is delayed. Multiple cell lines are affected and the consequences in granulocytes are defective cell adherence, with delayed phagocytosis of organisms.

CHRONIC GRANULOMATOUS DISEASE

This syndrome is characterized by recurrent infections with catalase-positive organisms, such as staphylococci, *Serratia marcescens* and opportunists such as *Aspergillus*. The first infections are usually staphylococcal lymph node abscesses which, without treatment, both drain externally (Fig. 23.15) and tend to metastasize via the bloodstream to give liver and bone abscesses. Microabscesses in the gut wall result in diarrhoea and interfere with nutrition.

Most affected individuals are boys and the inheritance is X-linked recessive. Their granulocytes do not show a respiratory burst following phagocytosis, and ingested staphylococci are not killed. (Figs 23.16 & 23.17). In families with X-linked recessive transmission, the biochemical defect is of neutrophil cytochrome-b; rare families with autosomal recessive transmission may have defects of a smaller protein which provides oxidase function together with cytochrome-b. Daily treatment with antibiotics reduces the frequency of infections in CGD.

CHEDIAK-HIGASHI SYNDROME

This very rare autosomal recessive syndrome is characterized by the presence of large cytoplasmic granules in many cell types (B cells, NK cells and neutrophils). Recurrent infections result from failure of NK and neutrophil function, with impaired chemotaxis and killing. Bone marrow transplantation has been tried to avoid the death which otherwise usually occurs before the age of 20.

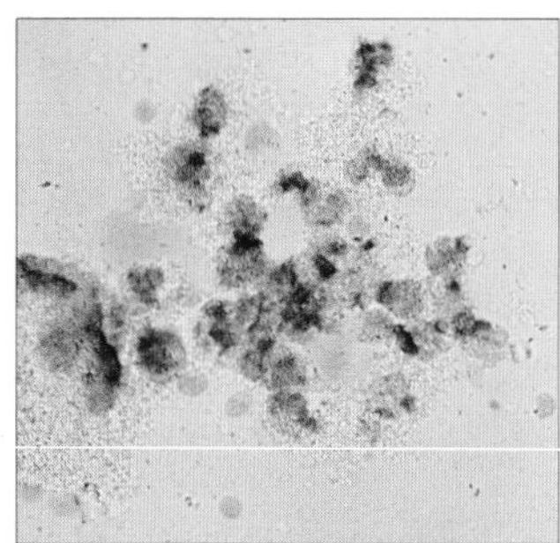
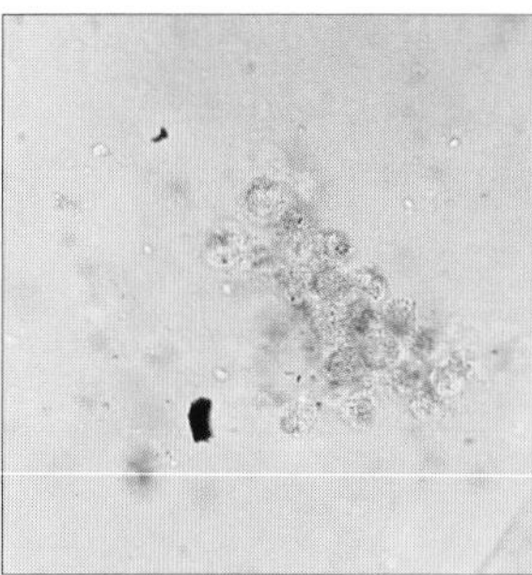

Fig. 23.16 Nitro blue tetrazolium (NBT) test. Left: in normal polymorphs and monocytes, reactive oxygen intermediates are activated by phagocytosis and the yellow NBT is converted to blue formazan. Right: this does not occur in CGD because of a defect in cytochrome-b245 and the dye stays yellow.

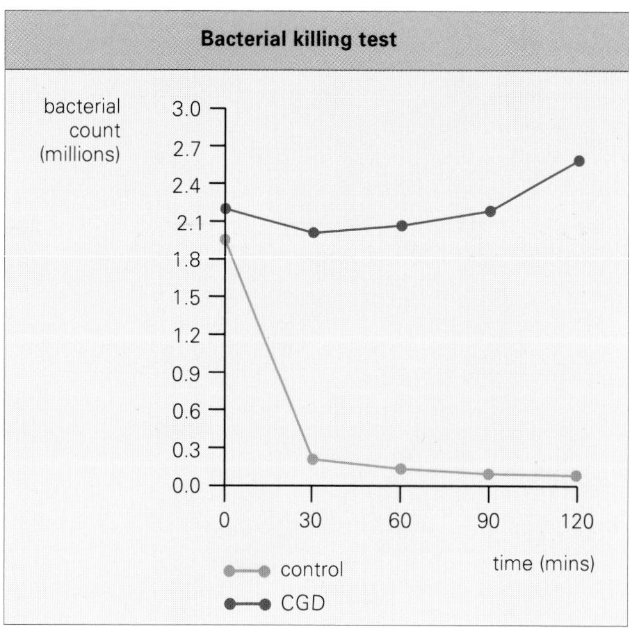

Fig. 23.17 Abnormal bacterial killing test by neutrophils from a boy with chronic granulomatous disease (CGD). The test organism is *Staph. aureus*, which is killed rapidly by normal cells but not by the patient's cells.

LAZY LEUCOCYTE SYNDROME

The leucocytes of two children with respiratory tract infections and gingivitis were described as 'lazy' because of their reduced mobility in a chemotaxis test. This phenomenon has also been found in LFA-1 deficiency, hyper IgE syndrome and Job's syndrome. The latter two are characterized by recurrent staphylococcal abscesses, dermatitis and raised IgE levels.

COMPLEMENT DEFECTS

Deficiencies of each of the complement components occur with an autosomal recessive inheritance. Most are very rare and increased susceptibility to infection results mainly from C3 deficiency. Selective deficiency of C1 components and C4 is associated mainly with SLE-like syndromes. Antibody dependent complement-mediated lysis in these individuals can be provided by the alternative pathway of complement activation. Individuals with C2 deficiency may have an increased susceptibility to *Haemophilus influenzae* septicaemia in infancy but other pyogenic infections are handled normally.

C3 deficiency results in an increased susceptibility to bacterial infection, which resembles that seen in antibody deficiency. Although these individuals make normal antibody responses following immunization, their serum lacks opsonizing activity for neutrophils. C3 replacement is not practical and so antibiotic treatment is employed. Deficiency of the later complement components (C5,6,7,8) increases susceptibility to disseminated or recurrent neisserial infection but usually not to other organisms.

FURTHER READING

Alarcon B, Terhorst C, Arnaiz Villena A, Perez Aciego P, Ramon Regueiro J. Congenital T cell receptor immunodeficiencies in man. *Immunodefic Rev.* 1990;**2**:1–16.

Carson DA, Carrera CJ, Immundeficiency secondary to adenosine deaminase deficiency and purine nucleoside phosyphorylation deficiency. *Semin Hematol.* 1990;**27**:260–269.

Eibl MM, Wedgwood RJ. Intravenous immunoglobulin: A review *Immunodefic Rev.* 1989;**1**:1–42.

Marcy TW, Reynolds HY. Pulmonary consequences of congenital and acquired primary immunodeficiency states. *Clin Chest Med.* 1989;**10**:503–519.

Pachman LM, Lynch PA, Silver RK, Ozog DL, Poznanski AK. Primary immunodeficiency disease in children: An update. *Curr Probl Pediatr* 1989;**19**:1–64.

24

AIDS & HIV Infection

INTRODUCTION

The acquired immune deficiency syndrome (AIDS) and its causative virus, the human immunodeficiency virus (HIV), have emerged in the last ten to fifteen years, coinciding with an upsurge in our understanding of cell-mediated immunity and an ability to measure several of its most important cells and humoral mediators. AIDS is perhaps unique among acquired immunodeficiencies in the specificity of the underlying biological defect, and has provided the anvil upon which many current concepts of human cellular immunity have been forged.

EPIDEMIOLOGY

Nearly two hundred thousand cases of AIDS had been reported to the World Health Organization by the end of 1989. WHO estimate the number of those infected to be between 5 and 10 million.

Essentially two patterns of spread of HIV (and hence of AIDS) have been seen in the emerging pandemic (Fig. 24.1). The first to be identified affected particularly homosexual or bisexual men, intravenous drug users, haemophiliacs and other transfusion recipients, and the heterosexual partners and children of these groups. The second pattern, which was occurring contemporaneously even though it was not initially recognized, appeared essentially as a disease of the young heterosexually active population, transfusion recipients and children of affected women. Broadly speaking, the first pattern is seen in developed countries, for example the United States, Western Europe and Australasia, and the second in developing countries, such as parts of Africa and the Caribbean. Some regions, for example South America, show a mixed pattern.

In certain areas of the developed world, such as the East coast of the USA, Southern Europe, Scotland and Ireland, the prevalence among intravenous drug users approaches or exceeds that among homosexual men. The major determinant of these different patterns is the prevalent social, and specifically sexual, anthropology with the superimposition of injected drug abuse.

WHO identifies a third group of affected regions, where HIV appears to have been introduced more recently; these show varying spread according to the risk behavior outlined in the first two patterns. Such countries include those of Eastern Europe, North Africa, the Middle East and most countries in Asia and the Pacific.

A related virus, HIV-2, has been found in West Africa and shows a similar epidemiological pattern of spread to that seen elsewhere in Africa.

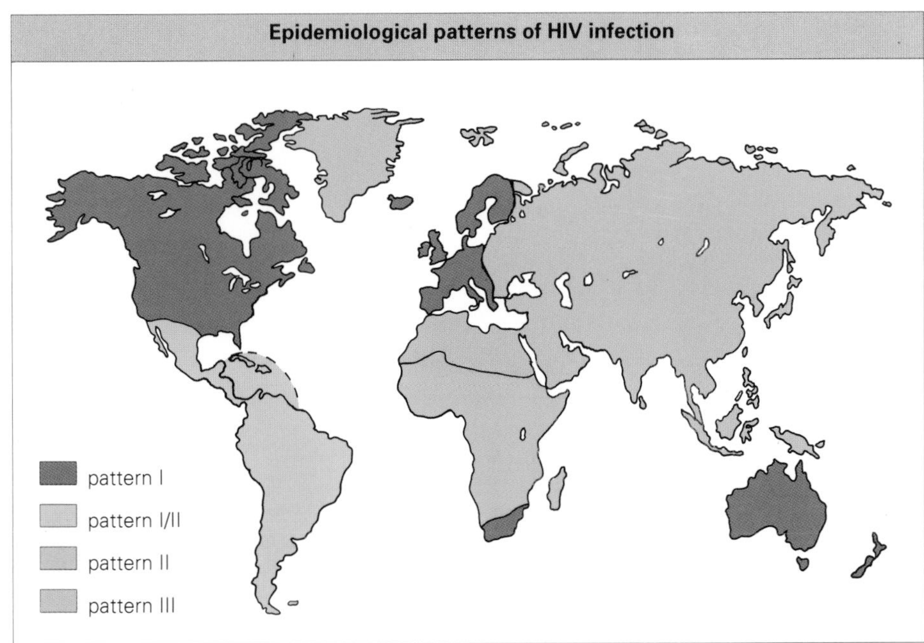

Fig. 24.1 In pattern I, 80–90% of cases are homosexual or bisexual men, or intravenous drug users; in pattern II the ratio of male to female cases is almost equal. The pattern in Latin America is changing from I to II, and is now classified separately as I/II. Pattern III is used to describe areas in which few cases to date have occurred. Modified from Sato, Chin & Man (1989).

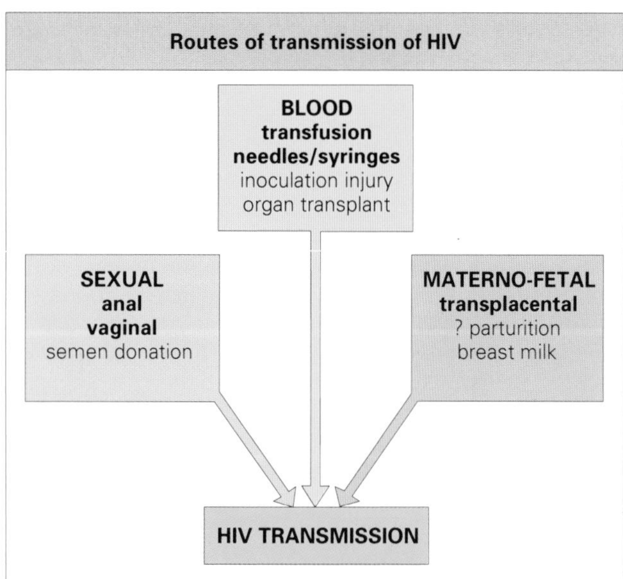

Fig. 24.2 Routes of transmission of HIV, as established by epidemiological evidence or case report. Sexual transmission may be male to male, female to male or male to female.

Factors influencing ease of transmission	
HIV–infected person	**HIV–exposed person**
type of contact phase of infection early (before seroconversion) with progressive disease activation of T cells	route of exposure quantity of HIV inoculum size genital ulceration activation of T cells? genetic factors?

Fig. 24.3 Factors that may influence ease of HIV transmission in the source and contact.

TRANSMISSION

The epidemiological patterns clearly show that HIV is a sexually transmissible, blood-borne or transplacentally transmitted viral infection (Fig. 24.2). There is no evidence for spread through casual contact, despite many studies on such exposure. Exposure to HIV by one of these routes may or may not result in infection. Regular sexual partners, whether homosexual or heterosexual, needle-sharing drug users, recipients of HIV-contaminated factor VIII, and children of HIV-infected women all show roughly 50% infection rates. Factors affecting the transmission of HIV in these settings (Fig. 24.3) include the infectiousness of the source of infection (the inoculum) and the state of the exposed host.

It appears that infectiousness may become greater as disease progresses, as indicated by both epidemiological studies and higher prevalence of HIV antigenaemia in progressive disease. Although it is clearly not essential, genital ulceration may facilitate sexual spread of HIV. Genetic factors may also play a part as there appear to be varia-
24.2 tions in individual or group susceptibility, even where behavioural features and HIV prevalence are similar. Whether or not other host factors, such as T cell activation due to intercurrent events, can increase susceptibility is unclear.

Epidemiologically, it is hard to separate evidence for such factors from their role as markers of exposure to persons at high risk of HIV infection. There is no clear evidence that any recognized form of immunodeficiency increases susceptibility to HIV infection. It would appear that the factors that affect the ease of infection are relative rather than absolute.

CLINICAL FEATURES

SPECTRUM OF OUTCOME

Of those who do become infected with HIV, a substantial proportion show no signs of progression to immunodeficiency disease in the 10 years of follow up that are the limit of most current prospective studies (Fig. 24.4). There is a spectrum of clinical outcomes (Fig. 24.5), and although the natural history of HIV infection is still emerging, it is clear that these outcomes are distinctive, both clinically and biologically. HIV-2 infection has a similar clinical profile, although some evidence suggests that the associated disease is less severe and progression is slower than for HIV-1. The great majority of infected subjects seroconvert for HIV antibodies within four to six months of infection and some 10–15% have a discernible clinical illness at this stage, which is transient, acute, and glandular

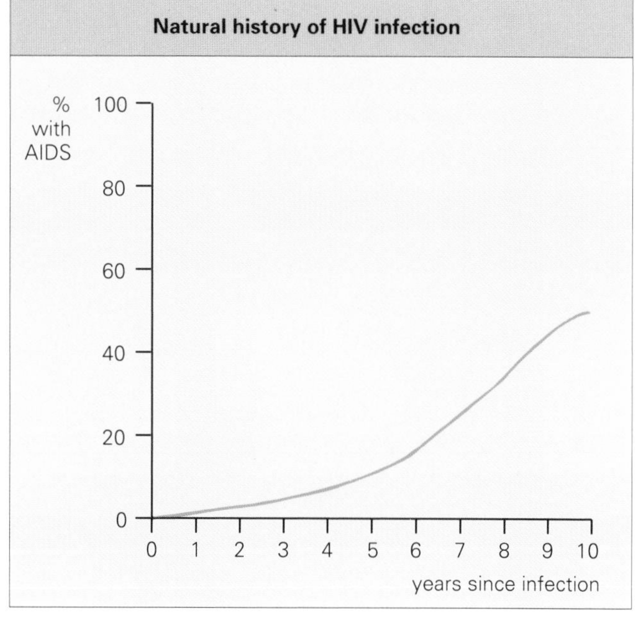

Fig. 24.4 The proportion of homosexual men developing AIDS correlated with the estimated duration of HIV infection (derived from the San Francisco City Clinic Cohort Study).

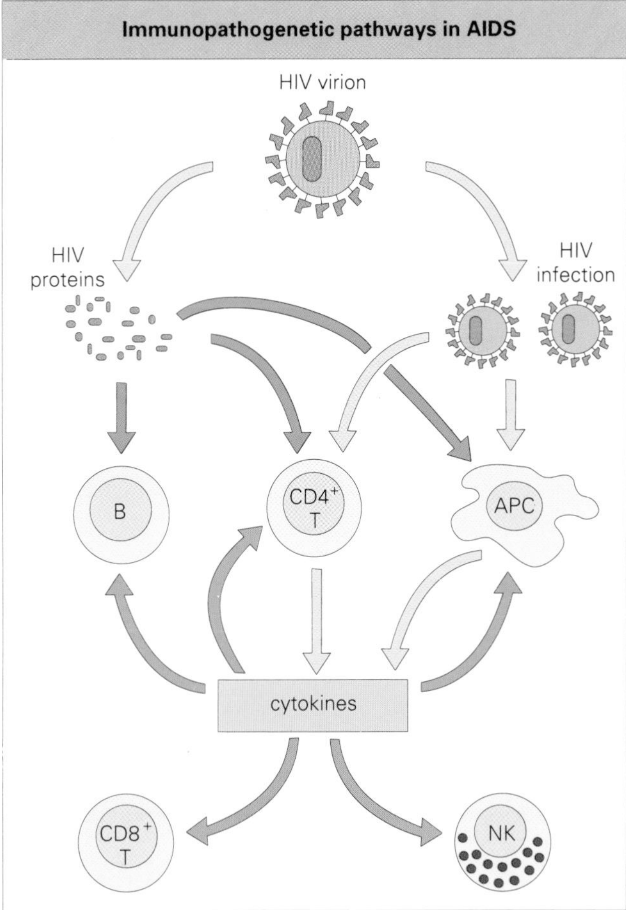

Fig. 24.15 HIV can infect CD4+ cells and, to a lesser extent, antigen presenting cells (APCs), which as a result show decreased cytokine production. The low level of cytokines leads to impaired induction of cytotoxic cells and reduced help for Ig production. HIV proteins can also exert a direct suppressant effect (red arrows) on CD4+ cells, B cells and APCs.

Many of the other observed immunological defects can be ascribed directly or indirectly to the primary attack on CD4+ cells (Fig. 24.15). Nevertheless it has become increasingly apparent that macrophages and other accessory cells, such as dendritic and follicular dendritic cells, may also become infected. This may be a result of low levels of expression of CD4 antigen, or may occur through other means such as Fc binding. While these cells appear to be less frequently destroyed as a result of infection, they do show some functional changes, but more importantly, appear to serve as a major reservoir of HIV infection.

It seems likely that the neurological effects of HIV are mediated by infection of microglia and other cells of the monocyte/macrophage lineage in the nervous system with consequent release of HIV or macrophage products, which then affect neuronal function. However it is also possible that some glial or even neuronal cells are directly
24.6 infected.

Destruction of CD4+ lymphocytes

An issue that remains far from being resolved is how HIV leads to the destruction of CD4+ lymphocytes (Fig. 24.16). Certainly HIV is a cytopathic virus, with the capacity to cause lysis and syncytium formation, but it is unlikely that this alone would cause loss of the bulk of CD4+ cells.

The low level of latency of HIV among remaining cells, variously estimated as between 1 in 100 and 1 in 10,000, has prompted theories to explain the elimination of uninfected cells. However, it is perhaps unwise to assume that the remaining cells are representative, in terms of their frequency of HIV infection, of those that have been eliminated.

Apart from direct virus cytotoxicity, it is probable that host mechanisms are involved in the elimination of CD4+ cells that express viral antigen, whether by antibody-dependent cytotoxicity or by MHC-restricted cytotoxic T cells, or even by non-specific host mechanisms. It is still possible, however, that uninfected CD4+ cells are also eliminated by fusion in syncytia with infected cells, or by adherence of HIV glycoprotein gp120 to the CD4 molecule leading to host-mediated elimination. It is probable that several of these mechanisms act together to produce the profound depletion of CD4+ cells found in patients infected with HIV.

Functional effects of CD4+ cell destruction

CD4+ T cells mediate helper and inducer functions and cooperate with macrophages in the elimination of facultative intracellular pathogens and related organisms (Fig. 24.17 & Appendix 24.3). Thus it follows that loss of this subset of cells affects these functions, many of which are mediated by the release of lymphokines such as interleukin-2 (IL-2), interferon-γ and other macrophage activating lymphokines. There has been some evidence that a particular subset of CD4+ cells is affected to a greater degree than others, leading to a functional imbalance, but evidence that Leu8 or 4B4 positive populations are more susceptible is not consistent.

Some of the functional defects cannot be explained just by HIV induced loss of CD4+ cells and hence of their lymphokines. Evidence has shown that HIV infected cells release gp120 and possibly other products that cause suppression of T cell responses. This may result from chronic activation of signal transduction pathways (inositol polyphosphate) rendering cells refractory to further stimulation. Furthermore, antigen presenting cells are slightly reduced in number and their function and expression of HLA class II antigens is severely reduced; these abnormalities are likely to contribute in part to the observed functional immunological changes.

Effect on B lymphocytes

Another characteristic feature of HIV infection and AIDS is polyclonal activation and increased immaturity of B cells, with polyclonal hypergammaglobulinaemia, leading to striking increases in IgG (subclasses I and 3), IgA and IgD; IgM is also raised in children with AIDS and there is

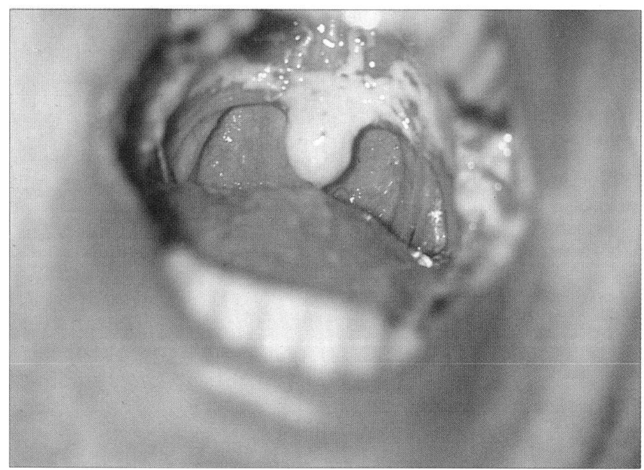

Fig. 24.10 Severe oral candidiasis in AIDS patient.Courtesy of St. Mary's Hospital Audio-Visual Dept.

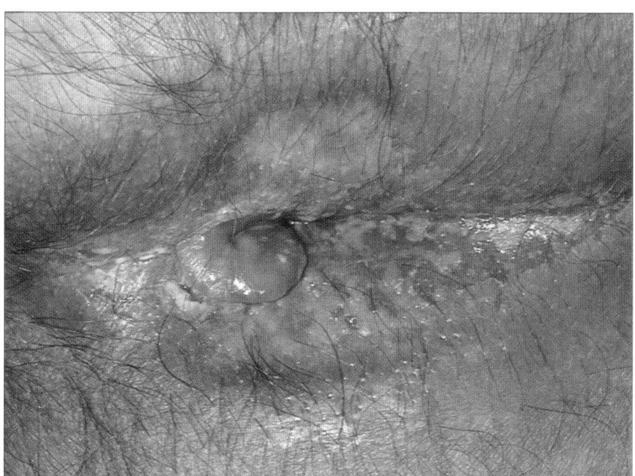

Fig. 24.11 Severe ulcerative perianal herpes simplex infection. This may be the presenting sign in patients with AIDS. Courtesy of St. Mary's Hospital Audio-Visual Dept.

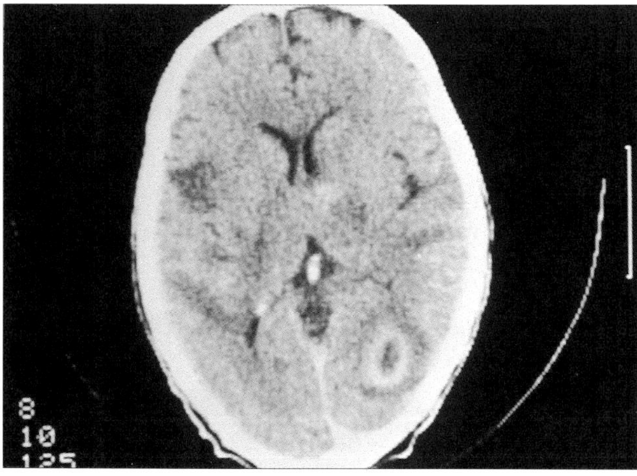

Fig. 24.12 CT brain scan of AIDS patient with toxoplasmosis showing cerebral abscesses.Courtesy of St. Mary's Hospital Audio-Visual Dept.

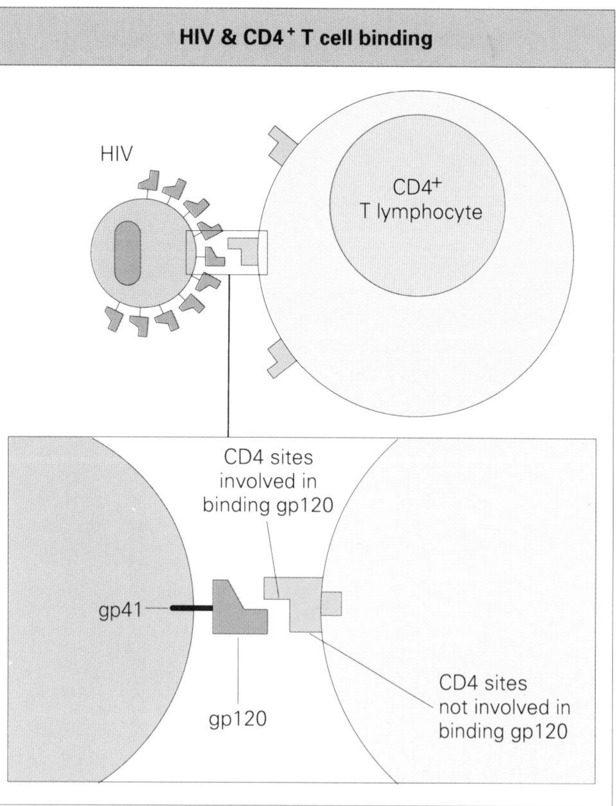

Fig. 24.13 The gp120 molecule on the surface of HIV binds with the CD4 antigen on the surface of T cells.

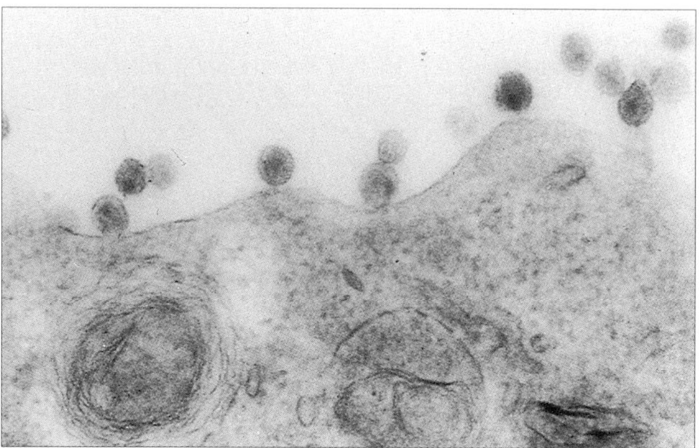

Fig. 24.14 Electron micrograph of HIV virions budding from the surface of a $CD4^+$ cell.

striking reduction in lymphocytes of the $CD4^+$ (T4) phenotype, both in peripheral blood and in the tissues. Once HIV had been identified, it was soon established that the virus showed a specific tropism for these cells and that the CD4 molecule itself served as the receptor for HIV (Fig. 24.13). New virions may bud from $CD4^+$ cells which have become infected by the virus (Fig. 24.14); most are destroyed, and the remaining cells, which rarely show evidence of HIV latency, show functional defects.

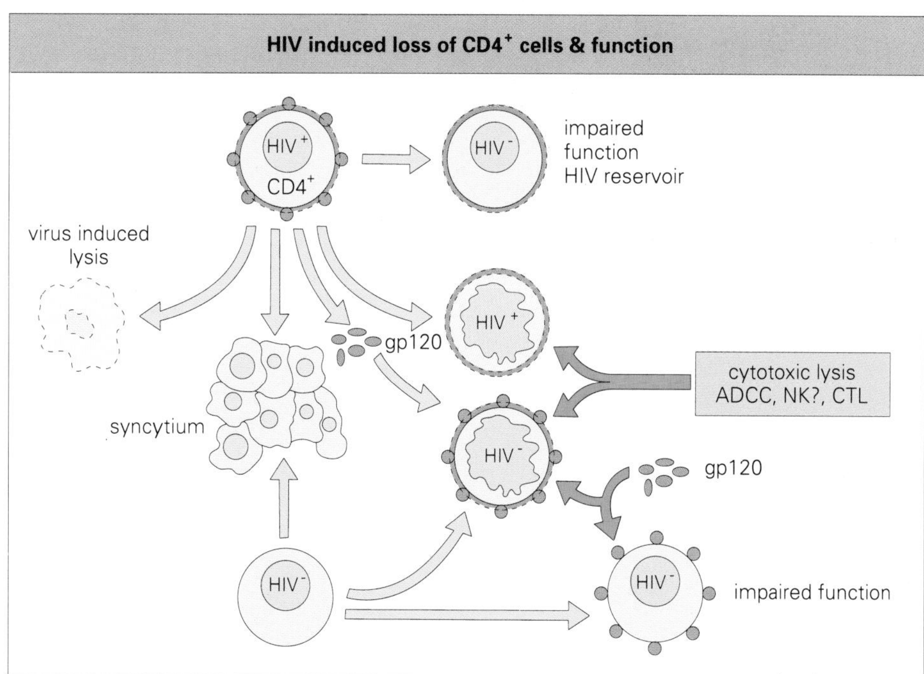

Fig. 24.16 Possible mechanisms of HIV induced CD4+ lymphocyte depletion and dysfunction. HIV infected cells (HIV+) may be killed directly by the virus or become susceptible to virus specific cytotoxic cells. These cells may form syncytia with other cells, thereby removing them or impairing their functions. The action of uninfected cells (HIV−) may be impaired by gp120, which may also sensitize these cells for cytotoxic killing.

Cellular defects in HIV infection

Cells	Abnormality	Main effects
T cell	↓CD4+ cells ↓function	anergy in DTH ↓mitogen proliferation ↓antigen proliferation ↓Tc activity ↓cytokine release ↓IL-2 receptors
antigen presenting cell	↓IL-1 & IFNα ↑acid-labile IFNα	↓intracellular killing ↓Fc receptors ↓chemotaxis ↓HLA class II ↓antigen presentation
B cell	polyclonal activation immaturity	↓neo-antigen responses ↑IgG1, IgG3, IgA, IgD, ↑IgE ↓IgG2, IgG4 ↑IgM (children) ↑immune complexes
NK cell	↓killing	defective killing

Fig. 24.17 Main cellular defects seen in HIV infection.

some elevation of IgE. However IgG2, and sometimes IgG4, is reduced. The latter, combined with loss of responsiveness to neoantigens, probably underlie the humoral immunodeficiency seen in some AIDS and ARC patients, especially children. While the B cell defects may to some extent reflect the loss of CD4+ cell regulation, they also appear to be due to the effect of HIV proteins as polyclonal activators of B cells; this may in part be T cell dependent.

HIV GENES AND PATHOGENICITY

The main genes of HIV and their functional interactions are shown in Fig. 24.18. The principal genes are gag, pol and env, encoding core proteins (p24, p17, and p15), polymerases (reverse transcriptase, protease, endonuclease) and the envelope proteins (gp160, which comprises the transmembrane protein, gp41, and outer membrane component, gp120) respectively. HIV-1 and HIV-2 show similar gene structure and have strong homologies at the gag and pol regions, but have major variations in env; the CD4 recognition sites are, however, conserved. gp41 appears to influence infectivity and cell fusion capacity. However, increasing attention is being paid to smaller gene segments that appear to play a major regulatory role in viral replication.

Viral replication

The tat gene encodes a 14kDa protein which is essential for viral replication, acting as a transactivating factor both for transcription and post-transcriptional modification of all viral proteins. Tat enhances viral replication by acting on the HIV LTR (long terminal repeat) promoter sequence. Another gene, rev encodes a 13kDa protein which enhances synthesis by promoting active translation of viral mRNA and facilitating transport of RNA from nucleus to

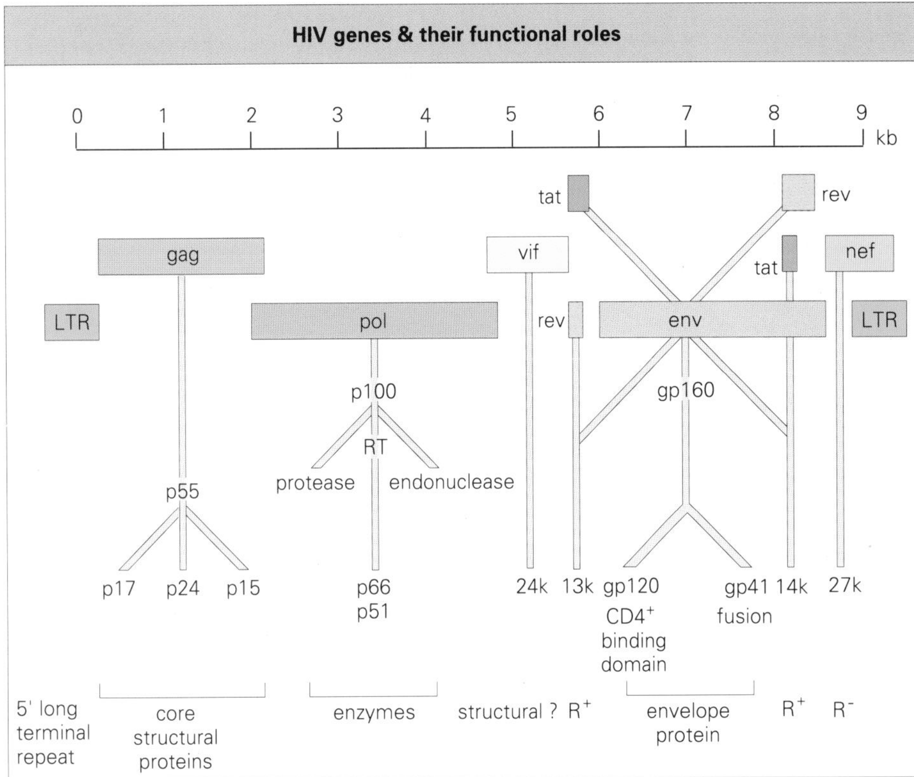

Fig. 24.18 Principal genes of HIV-1 and their functional roles. R=regulatory gene; RT=reverse transcriptase; gag and pol encode core proteins and enzymes; env encodes the envelope proteins, and tat, nef and rev encode regulatory proteins.

cytoplasm. Differences between HIV-1 and HIV-2 have been shown in their tat specificities and LTR function and these may underlie the apparently lesser cytopathic effect and lower pathogenicity of HIV-2.

Enhancing LTR

It has been shown that transactivating gene products from other viruses such as herpes simplex, CMV, HHV-6 and HTLV-1 can also enhance LTR promoter function, suggesting a precise molecular means whereby other specific virus infections can enhance HIV replication and hence progression. Furthermore, T cell activation by mitogens appears to enhance LTR promoter function *in vitro* through the NFkB region, suggesting that this is a point of convergence for multiple cofactors which can enhance viral replication. On the other hand, the nef gene seems to exert negative regulation of HIV expression and may also act to reduce CD4 expression in chronically infected cells. The other open reading frame gene, vif, is probably structural; vif deletion mutants may produce lower HIV titres and appear to be required for efficient virus transmission *in vitro*.

FACTORS AFFECTING NATURAL HISTORY

So far, natural history studies have largely been reported using cohorts of homosexual men with HIV infection.
24.8 While the overall rate of progression to AIDS in subjects who were asymptomatic HIV seropositive at recruitment is about 10–15% at 3 years, 20–25% at 6 years and 50% at 10 years (see Fig. 24.4), it has become increasingly apparent that certain factors are associated with higher rates of progression in subsets of HIV-infected subjects.

Intercurrent sexually transmitted diseases

Several studies have shown that intercurrent sexually transmitted infections in homosexual men increase the risk of progression. However, an African cohort has shown a similar rate of progression, suggesting that cofactors that apply amongst homosexual men are balanced by others affecting Africans infected with HIV, for example parasitic or other infections.

Intravenous drug use

Continued intravenous drug use is associated with an increased risk of progression. This may be caused either by direct effects of the drug on immune responses or, more likely, by intercurrent infections introduced by continued intravenous injections.

Pregnancy and infancy

Pregnancy in HIV-infected women who have borne two or more infants subsequent to infection seems to increase the risk of progression, although no such effect can be discerned in first pregnancies with HIV. Neonates and infants show high rates of progression, with perhaps as many as 50% of perinatally infected children developing AIDS within two years.

Cell activation

In vitro studies have shown that activation of lymphocytes or macrophages harbouring HIV promotes viral replication in the cells by switching on the HIV LTR. Herpes viruses and HTLV-I may be especially effective in promoting viral replication because their own transactivating mechanisms can also act directly on the HIV LTR gene segment (see Fig. 24.18). Foreign antigens, whether from infecting organisms, the fetal graft or the whole range of exogenous antigens to which the infant is exposed, could thus activate HIV replication in latently infected cells. In all of these settings, the increased HIV replication will lead to a greater burden of infection in immunocompetent cells and hence a more rapid progression to the threshold of immune impairment for overt immunodeficiency disease.

Other factors

By adding their similar immunosuppressive effects to that of HIV, it is also thought that malnutrition, some immunosuppressive drugs and immunosuppressive organisms such as cytomegalovirus may exacerbate the clinical susceptibility. Thus in the HIV-infected host, both activation and suppression of $CD4^+$ cells can enhance the pathogenetic mechanisms of immune impairment, emphasizing the critical balance in which such individuals coexist with HIV (Fig. 24.19).

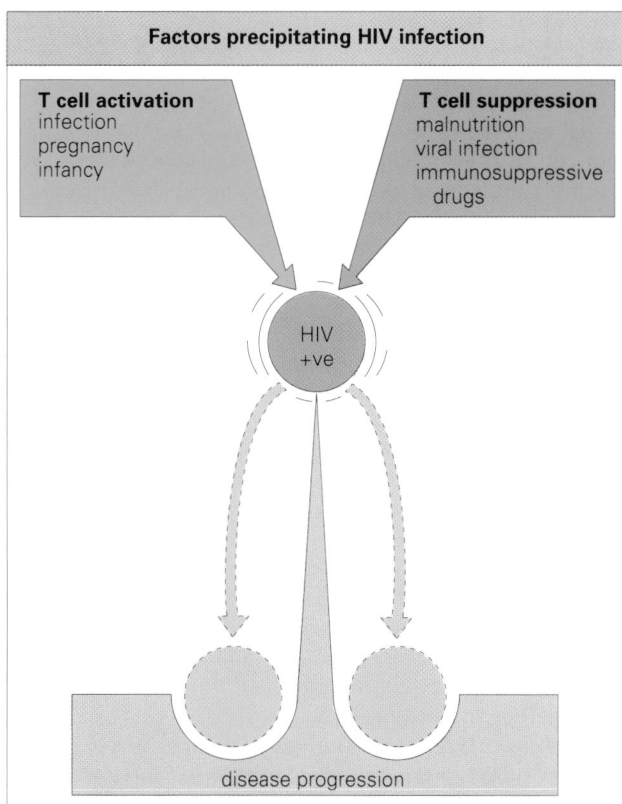

Fig. 24.19 The cofactors that can precipitate disease in an HIV-infected subject may do so by either activating or suppressing cell-mediated immunity.

Genetic factors

Genetic susceptibility to disease amongst infected subjects seems to be as important as it is for other infections, but only limited evidence is available so far. HLA-DR5 is associated with Kaposi's sarcoma and PGL in some ethnic groups, while HLA-B35 appears to be associated with progression from PGL to AIDS. The HLA-A1, B8, (DR3) complex is also associated with enhanced risk of progression to HIV disease. Other genetic factors are likely to emerge in due course.

LABORATORY MARKERS FOR HIV INFECTION

From an early stage of the HIV epidemic, many studies have sought ways to identify people infected with HIV and, amongst these, the ones most likely to progress to more severe disease. Similarly, there have been attempts to find tests that can determine the current immunological state of the patient, although few are more informative than taking a good history and performing an adequate physical examination. The serological profile of HIV infection is now becoming clearer (Fig. 24.20).

HIV ANTIBODY

Identifying the great majority of those infected has been readily achieved by the use of HIV antibody tests. It is usual to screen first with an ELISA (antiglobulin or competitive) and to confirm the result with another test, the most commonly used being the Western blot, largely to exclude false positives. The false positive rate has been diminished by the use of recombinant envelope antigens for ELISA assays rather than the virus infected cell lysates used in the first generation assays.

Although early assays seemed to show a significant false negative rate in advanced disease, the currently available assays are much better. The problem still exists, however, in those that detect predominantly core-specific antibodies (p24 or p17), since a declining anti-core antibody titre is associated with disease progression.

HIV ANTIGEN

The use of antibodies to identify any infection obviously has the limitation that an antibody response takes some time to develop; in the case of HIV this may take up to several months. The supplementation of antibody tests with those for HIV antigen has helped somewhat in identifying some early infections, antigenaemia preceding antibody development by several weeks.

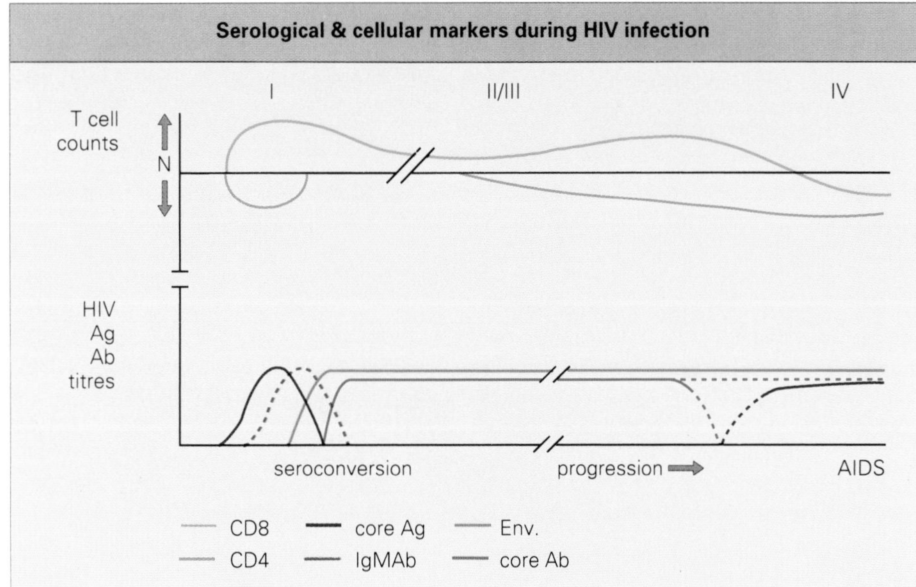

Fig. 24.20 Serological and cellular markers during HIV infection. Events after the broken lines (//) occur in those patients showing progression. A fall in core antibody and subsequent rise in core antigen is seen in some but not all patients progressing to HIV disease.

PROGNOSTIC MARKERS FOR PROGRESSION

CD4+ CELL COUNT

The most obvious prognostically valuable test to identify people at higher risk of early progression to AIDS was the $CD4^+$ cell count. While this indicates an overall trend for decline in people showing progression, there is considerable variability in members of high risk groups due to intercurrent events, and a distinctive downward trend due to HIV is not always evident for some time. Moreover, responses over time are quite heterogeneous. Thus, although some studies have shown some positive predictive value of a low or falling $CD4^+$ cell count in cohorts of HIV infected people, it may be of limited value in individuals, especially if based on a single observation.

SKIN AND LYMPHOCYTE FUNCTION TESTS

Lymphocyte function tests, such as cutaneous anergy or mitogen/antigen responses have been used. There is, however, a high incidence of anergy in HIV positives who do not progress rapidly and in uninfected members of risk groups. Proliferative responses to antigen or to pokeweed mitogen and the production of interferon-γ in response to such stimuli have been proposed for testing, but have not gained wide acceptance; this may be partly due to their relative complexity for serial study in large numbers of subjects. Others have proposed the use of β_2-microglobulin, acid-labile interferon-α, neopterin and several other serological markers.

SPECIFIC HIV ANTIGENS AND ANTIBODIES

The development of antibody assays to specific HIV antigens and of antigen assays have offered a more valuable and straightforward approach. It has been shown that loss or falling titres of antibodies to the p24 or p17 core proteins of HIV are reliable predictors of early adverse outcome in subjects in developed countries; this fall is not, however, seen in African cohorts. It is still unclear whether the fall in anti-core antibody represents a selective loss of protective responses to core antigens (leading to a secondary increase in virus activity), or a primary increase in viral replication and antigen production, with consequent consumption of anti-core antibodies in immune complexes. The persistence of HIV antigenaemia beyond the initial phase of infection is associated with a high risk of progression to AIDS. In longitudinal studies, it seems that p24 antigen-specific antibody titres fall before serum antigen becomes detectable (see Fig. 24.20). The use of two assays together will probably prove a more sensitive marker of prognosis, perhaps combined with enumeration of $CD4^+$ cell numbers.

Assays of $CD4^+$ cell numbers and function, HIV antigen (where present) and anti-core antibody responses are also likely to be of considerable value in assessing immunological and virological responses to therapeutic intervention. Useful *in vivo* markers include cutaneous delayed type hypersensitivity responses, changes in the stage of HIV-associated disease, the incidence and severity of opportunistic events, neurological disease progression and survival.

IMMUNE RESPONSES TO HIV

In general, antibody responses to HIV infection do not seem to confer protection against disease or containment of virus, since they are found both in those who do and those who do not progress. However, it has been postulated that progressive loss of anti-core antibodies could represent loss of protective antibodies involved in antibody-dependent cellular cytotoxicity (ADCC).

Neutralizing antibodies are produced in relatively low titres compared with other retroviruses; there is no clear association between their presence or titre and disease progression, although they could in theory affect fluid phase transmission of HIV from cell to cell. Cytotoxic lymphocytes or ADCC could in principle offer some protection against HIV and HIV-associated disease although, as indicated above, they could equally contribute to pathogenesis by the elimination of HIV-infected $CD4^+$ cells (see Fig. 24.16). Recent studies on HIV-infected subjects have shown some evidence of HLA-restricted cytotoxicity against HIV-infected cells, as well as of ADCC. However, it has yet to be determined whether such responses play any significant role in protection against HIV-associated disease.

TREATMENT

STRATEGIES

There are four basic strategies that may be used in treating HIV disease:

- general management;
- treatment and prophylaxis of opportunistic infections and tumours;
- anti-retroviral therapy;
- immunorestorative approaches.

General maintenance includes counselling and other support, and a medical care structure in the hospital and community with open access. Health maintenance is also important, and should include advice on nutrition, stopping smoking, avoidance of infections and other cofactors. Anti-microbial therapies are available for many of the opportunistic diseases, except cryptosporidiosis and progressive multifocal leucoencephalopathy. Optimal prophylactic strategies have yet to be established, although their desirability for the more common infections is evident. Tumour therapy is improving, but cerebral lymphoma still shows little response. It is clear that in advanced AIDS, diminishing cell-mediated immune responsiveness renders anti-microbial and anti-tumour therapies less and less effective.

Anti-retroviral therapy

Nucleoside analogues. Anti-retroviral therapy is a main focus of attention at present, especially in the light of the benefits of the prototype drug Zidovudine (AZT). This interferes with the process of reverse transcription and hence suppresses viral replication and cell-to-cell spread *in vivo*. It reduces the rate of disease progression in symptomatic HIV disease, decreasing the frequency and severity of opportunistic infection, improving or delaying HIV encephalopathy and roughly doubling expected survival time. Its main toxicities are bone marrow suppression and myopathy. Some of the newer nucleoside analogues such as di-deoxyinosine and di-deoxycytidine appear to have similar benefits in early studies, but show peripheral neurotoxicity.

Other anti-retrovirals. A number of other anti-retroviral approaches are being explored (Fig. 24.21), but clinical benefits are not yet established. These include the use of soluble CD4, in an attempt to decoy HIV gp120 away from cell-bound CD4, but this would depend on fluid phase transmission, which may not be the main route of cell-to-cell spread *in vivo*. Also, CD4 is rapidly excreted and, in order to ensure high levels with a longer half-life, the molecule has been bound to part of an immunoglobulin molecule to create an 'immunoadhesin'. This clever approach may, however, reduce the impact of CD4 therapy in the nervous system. A further limitation is that some infection in macrophages and related cells may be via the Fc receptor.

Protease inhibitors specific for the HIV aspartate protease are now being developed and look promising in pre-clinical studies, as do some compounds of the amino-sugar class that interfere with glycoprotein processing. Interferon-α shows some modest anti-HIV activity *in vitro* but studies in vivo are not convincing. Future developments include approaches to modify the effects of the regulatory genes, but these remain at a very preliminary stage of development.

Immunorestoration

Although a logical approach to the management of this immunodeficiency disease, immunological therapy has been disappointing to date. Bone marrow transplantation, initially without, but more recently with anti-retroviral drugs has proved generally ineffective. Several cytokines have been used, including IFNα and IFNγ, IL-2 and GM-CSF. Without anti-retroviral therapy, these have shown minimal clinical benefit, but some *in vitro* measures on treated patients have suggested a degree of amelioration of the biological defects, notably with low dose IFNγ. Combinations of cytokines, used in conjunction with anti-retrovirals would seem a logical next step. Immunostimulation has also been largely disappointing, as in other disorders, although recent reports suggest that di-thioethylcarbamate (Imuthiol) may have clinical activity. Inosine pranobex (Isoprinosine) has been ineffective in all but one study and its role remains uncertain.

Gamma-globulin therapy has proved especially valuable in children, in whom the antibody repertoire is more limited and who suffer proportionately more bacterial

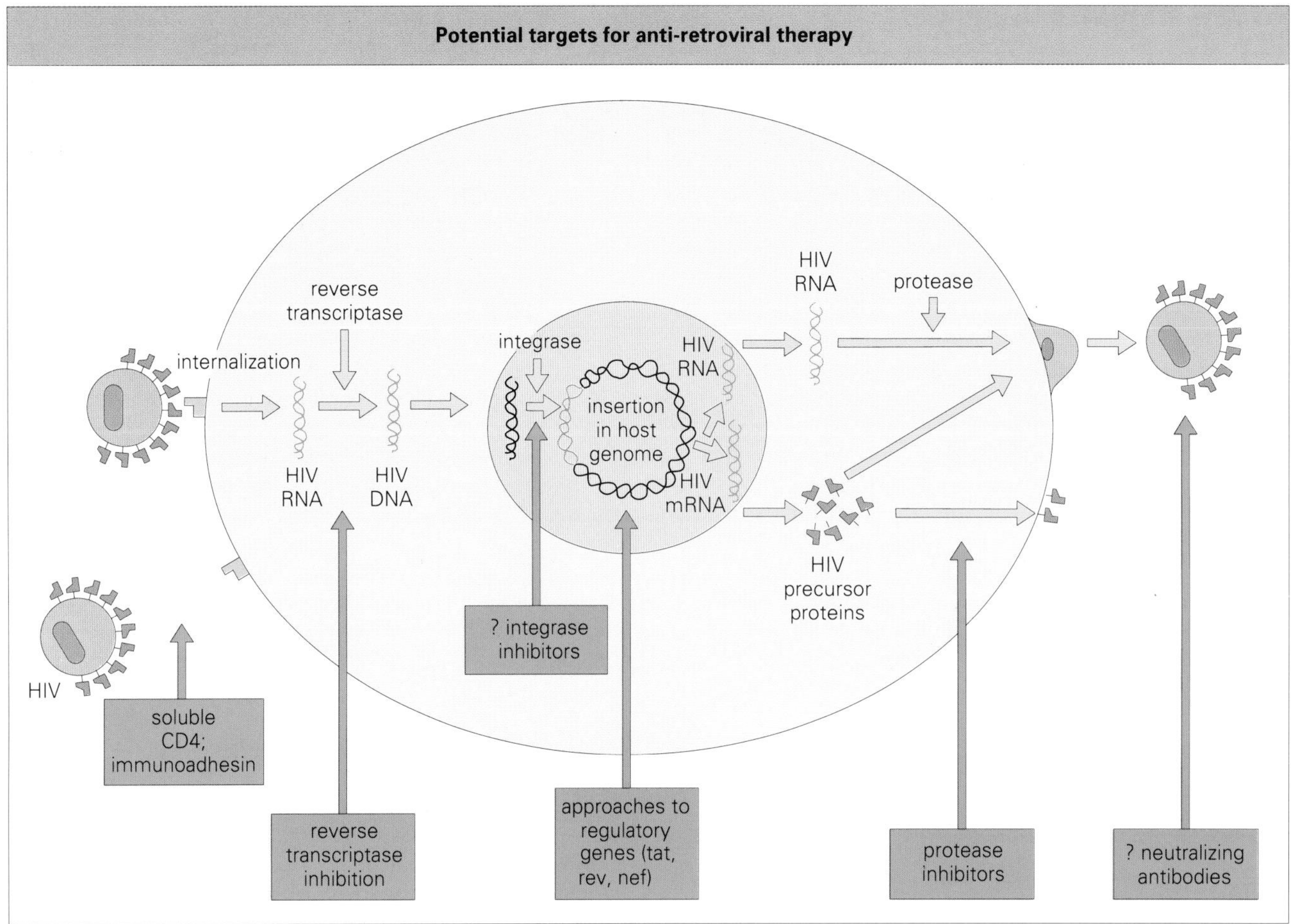

Fig. 24. 21 Replication cycle of HIV, showing points at which anti-retroviral therapies might be employed.

infections. It has also helped some adults with secondary IgG2 defiency. The use of high titre HIV (neutralizing) antibody from asymptomatic HIV-infected subjects in the treatment of AIDS has been advocated but no convincing clinical benefit has been reported.

Vaccine development

Much work is now being done to develop anti-HIV vaccines, mainly to protect against primary HIV infection, but they might also be used to stem progression in those already infected. A variety of vaccine strategies are being explored using HIV components, vectors and adjuvants. While immunogenicity for both B and T cell specificities has been clearly demonstrated, none of the candidate vaccines have been able to show protective effects in susceptible animals.

Recent evidence that immunization with inactivated whole simian immunodeficiency virus (SIV) may lead to protection against subsequent SIV challenge in most animals offers some hope that vaccination against HIV can be achieved, but the relevance of these experiments to HIV in man is uncertain.

Symptomatic HIV infection (group IV)

A Constitutional symptoms

Persistent unexplained fever
Unexplained weight loss (>10%)
Persistent unexplained diarrhoea

B Neurological disease

Encephalopathy
Myelopathy
Peripheral/autonomic neuropathy
Myopathy

C1 Major opportunistic infection

Pneumocystis pneumonia
Chronic cryptosporidiosis
Toxoplasma cerebral abscess
Extraintestinal strongyloidiasis
Isosporiasis
Oesophageal/bronchial candidiasis
Cryptococcosis
Histoplasmosis
Atypical mycobacterial infection
Cytomegalovirus infection
Herpes simplex ulceration or disseminated herpes
Progressive multifocal leucoencephalopathy

C2 Minor opportunistic infection

Oral candidiasis
Hairy oral leukoplakia
Multidermatomal herpes zoster
Salmonella bacteraemia
Nocardiosis
Tuberculosis

D Opportunistic tumours

Kaposi's sarcoma
B cell lymphoma
Cerebral lymphoma
Hodgkin's disease

E Other HIV – associated diseases

Lymphocytic pneumonitis

Appendix 24.1 These types of infection may occur concurrently. The AIDS-related complex incorporates sub-groups A and C2, and AIDS as originally defined is sub-groups C1 and D.

Major opportunistic events in AIDS by organ system

Pulmonary
Pneumocystis carinii pneumonia
Mycobacterium tuberculosis
Atypical mycobacterial infection
Cytomegalovirus pneumonitis
Cryptococcal pneumonitis
Nocardiosis
Pneumococcal pneumonia
Staphylococcal pneumonia
Haemophilius influenzae
Branhamella catarrhalis

Neurological
Toxoplasma cerebal abscess
Cryptococcal meningitis
Cytomegalovirus
PML
Mycobacterium tuberculosis

Cutaneous
Herpes simplex ulceration
Herpes zoster
Cutaneous mycoses
Molluscum contagiosum

Gastrointestinal
Oesphageal candidiasis
Mycobacterium tuberculosis
Atypical mycobacterial infection
Cytomegalovirus colitis
Herpes simplex ulceration
Salmonellosis
Cryptosporidiosis
Isosporiasis

Opportunistic tumours in AIDS
Kaposi's sarcoma
- Cutaneous
- Lymphadenopathic
- Gastrointestinal
- Pulmonary

Lymphoma (B cell or Hodgkin's)
- Cerebral
- Lymphadenopathic
- Disseminated extranodal

Appendix 24.2 The major opportunistic events occurring in patients with AIDS by organ of predominant presentation. Many of these infections may be disseminated.

Main immunological abnormalities in HIV infection & AIDS	
T Cells	**B cells**
↓CD4 count	polyclonal activation of B cells
↓Leu8 subset (?)	↑plaque forming cells
↓4B4 subset (?)	↓B cell mitogen responses
↓proliferative response to soluble antigen	↑transferrin receptor expression
↓proliferative response to T cell mitogens (PHA, ConA)	↓Leu8 expression
↓proliferative response to T cell – dependent B cell mitogen (PWM)	↑CD10 expression
↓allogeneic and autologous MLR	↓humoral response to primary immunization
↓mitogen/antigen induced release of IL-2, IFN γ, MAF	polyclonal hypergammaglobulinaemia
↓expression of IL-2 receptors	↑IgG1 and IgG3
anergy to delayed type hypersensitivity antigens	↓IgG2 and IgG4
↓help for immunoglobulin production (PWM-induced)	↑IgA, IgM, (children) IgD, IgE
impaired induction of cytotoxic T cells	immune complexes
↓cytotoxicity for virally infected cells	
Antigen presenting cells	**Natural killer cells**
↓HLA Class II expression	↑Leu7 cells
Impaired killing of intracellular pathogens	↓Leu11 cells
↓induced release of IL1(?)	defective target cell killing (normal binding)
↓release of normal IFN α	
↑release of acid labile IFN α	
↓chemotaxis of monocytes	
↓Fc receptors on monocytes	
↓Fc and C3b clearance	

Appendix 24.3 Many of the observed defects are due to the loss of CD4+ cells and their mediators, to defective antigen presenting cell (APC) function, or to polyclonal B cell activation. Each of these is largely due to the effects of HIV infection of CD4+ cells and APCs or of HIV proteins on cellular function. PHA=phytohaemagglutinin; ConA=concanavalin A; PWM=pokeweed mitogen; MAF=macrophage activating factors; IL-2=interleukin-2; MLR=mixed lymphocyte reaction.

FURTHER READING

AIDS 1989 — A Year in Review. *AIDS* 1989; **Suppl. 1**:S1–S307.

Friedland GH, Klein RS. Transmission of the human immunodeficiency virus. *New Eng J Med.* 1987;**317**:1125–1135.

Gottlieb MS *et al*, eds. *Current Topics in AIDS I.* Chichester: John Wiley, 1987.

Gottlieb, M S *et al*, eds. *Current Topics in AIDS II.* Chichester: John Wiley, 1989.

Ho D, Pomerantz RJ, Kaplan JC. Pathogenesis of infection with human immunodeficiency virus. *New Engl J Med* 1987; **317**:278–286.

Pinching AJ, ed. AIDS and HIV infection. *Clinics in immunology and allergy 6.* London: Saunders, 1986. 441–687.

Pinching AJ, Weiss RA, Miller D, eds. AIDS and HIV infection: the wider perspective. *Br Med Bull* 1988; **44**:1–234.

Seligmann M, Chess L, Fahey JL *et al.* AIDS — an immunologic reevaluation. *New Engl J Med* 1984; **311**: 1286–1292.

Seligman M, Pinching AJ, Rosen FS *et al.* Immunology of HIV infection and AIDS — an update. *Ann Int Med* 1987; **107**: 234–242.

Spickett GP, Dalgleish AG. Cellular immunology of HIV infection. *Clin Exp Immunol* 1988; **71**:1–7.

25

Nutrition & immunity

INTRODUCTION

An effective host protective system consists of various physical barriers, and both innate and acquired immunity. Breakdown of any of these mechanisms leads to immunodeficiency and its sequelae, for example increased incidence and severity of infection, infection by atypical organisms, malignancy, and collagen vascular and autoimmune diseases. Immunodeficiency can occur due to congenital, often inherited, defects of development of the immune system, or it may be acquired secondary to a variety of systemic disorders. In the acquired group, nutritional disorders are the most common cause of immunodeficiency, affecting at least 400 million people worldwide.

Nutritional status

There are several factors, often interacting, that influence an individual's nutritional status, such as food quality and quantity, efficiency of digestion and biochemical individuality. To these may be added the effects of chronic infection which, in the presence of an abnormal nutritional state, may further impair host defence and immune function.

Food quality. Food grown on nutrient-poor soil may be deficient in certain elements such as minerals and trace elements. Pesticides and other chemicals added to crops enter the food chain and can have further damaging effects on metabolic processes.

Quantity of food. In developed countries under-nutrition is rarely a problem, although malnutrition can be prevalent because of abnormal food choice or a highly refined food intake.

Digestive efficiency. The presence of gut parasites, chronic diarrhoea and enzyme deficiency, malabsorption and achlorhydria can all impair digestive efficiency and lead to malnutrition.

Biochemical individuality. Each person has unique nutritional requirements depending on factors such as age, activity level, concurrent illness and pregnancy. Other factors that can impair absorption of nutrients include competing chemicals (drugs) and other foods (for example wheat, which can inhibit absorption of calcium, iron and zinc through the formation of insoluble phytate salts).

Minerals

The major minerals — potassium, sodium, calcium, phosphorus and magnesium — are present in large amounts in the body. The trace elements such as zinc, iron, chromium and copper are required in very small quantities (in the order of milligrams or micrograms a day). Their importance far outweighs their low concentration in serum as there are several hundred metalo-enzymes in which the mineral is crucial to the enzyme's function.

Some trace elements are also important for the anti-oxidant activity of a number of enzymes, for example glutathione peroxidase and superoxide dismutase. Thus, enzyme and metabolic function may be significantly reduced by subtle deficiencies in nutrition. This must, of course, be contrasted with the gross changes seen in protein-energy malnutrition (PEM).

Studies in developing countries have shown that children suffering from severe undernutrition epitomized as PEM, have a profound depression of several facets of immunity. Infection occurs as a consequence and is facilitated by the network of interacting factors that also cause malnutrition (Fig. 25.1).

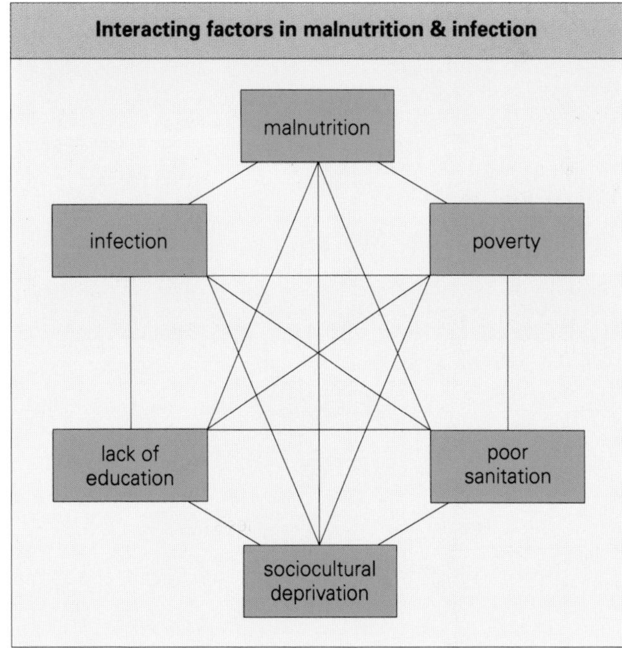

Fig. 25.1 Network of interacting factors causing malnutrition and infection. Undernutrition can be the result of poverty, contaminated environments, socioeconomic deprivation and lack of education. Infection occurs as a sequel to the immunodeficiency that occurs in malnutrition, and is contributed to by some of the factors that cause malnutrition.

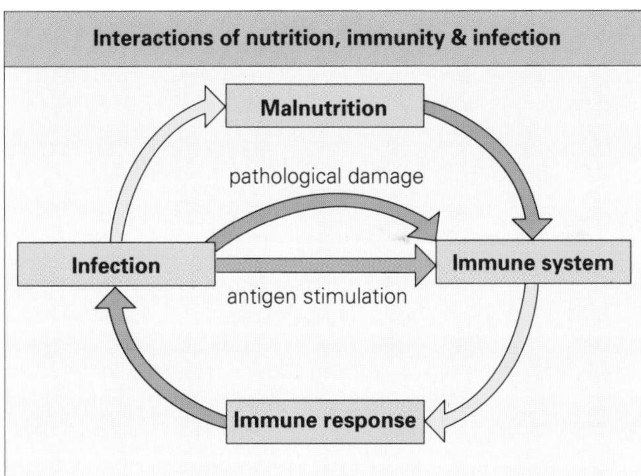

Fig. 25.2 Nutrition, immunity and infection are closely related to one another. Malnutrition impairs immune responses and is associated with increased prevalence and severity of infection. At the same time, infection itself suppresses immune responses and depletes the body of nutrients.

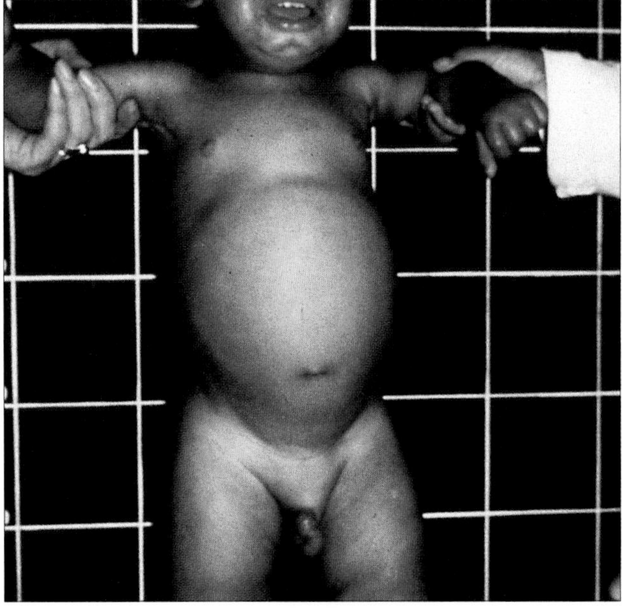

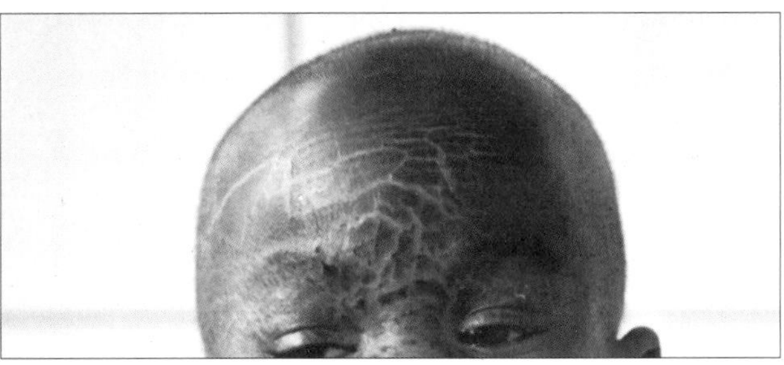

Fig. 25.3 Kwashiorkor. Upper: the condition is typified by a protruding abdomen accompanied by oedema. Courtesy of Dr J. Carlton Gartner Jr. Lower: skin involvement is also common, the characteristic presentation being a weeping dermatitis which subsequently ulcerates and desquamates. Courtesy of WHO and Paul Almay.

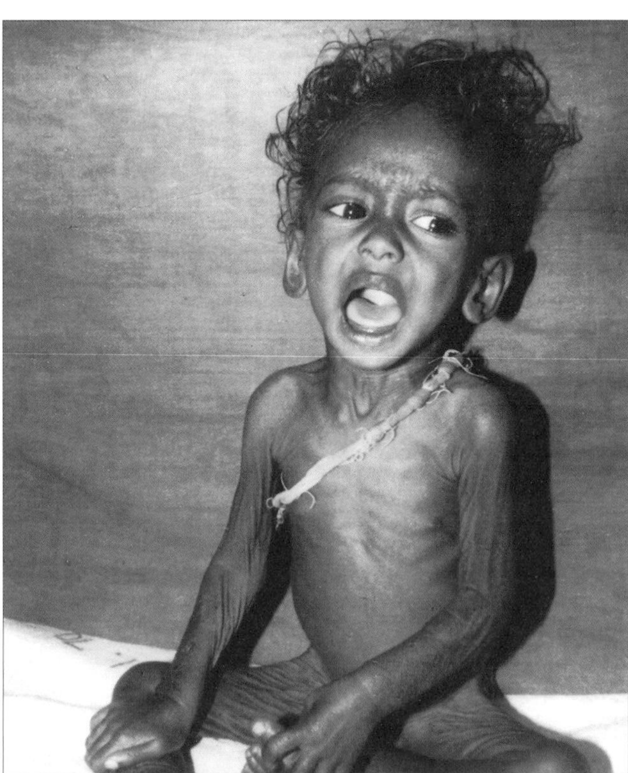

Fig. 25.4 Marasmus. This 13-month-old child shows the gross wasting and wrinkled skin which is characteristic of this disorder. Courtesy of WHO and W Cutting.

Human studies and laboratory experiments have confirmed the existence of immunodeficiency in PEM, and showed that isolated deficiencies of some nutrients impair immune functions — the most thoroughly studied are zinc, iron, copper, selenium, and vitamins A, B6, and E. If nutritional deficiency occurs during fetal life when the immune system is immature, the effects on immunity are severe and long lasting. At the other end of the age spectrum, impaired immune responses in old age are due in part to associated nutritional deficiencies.

Paradoxically, immune functions are also compromized in overnutrition, including obesity, and selective excess of nutrients like lipids, zinc and iron. Furthermore, infection itself can deplete the body of nutrients and contribute to immunodeficiency. It is of fundamental and practical importance to recognize these interactions between nutrition, immunity and infection (Fig. 25.2).

PROTEIN-ENERGY MALNUTRITION (PEM)

Protein-energy malnutrition (PEM) covers a wide spectrum of disorders between the two polar entities of kwashiorkor (Fig. 25.3) and marasmus (Fig. 25.4). In PEM, multiple nutritional deficits are present, and the observed immunological defects constitute the sum total of the effects of

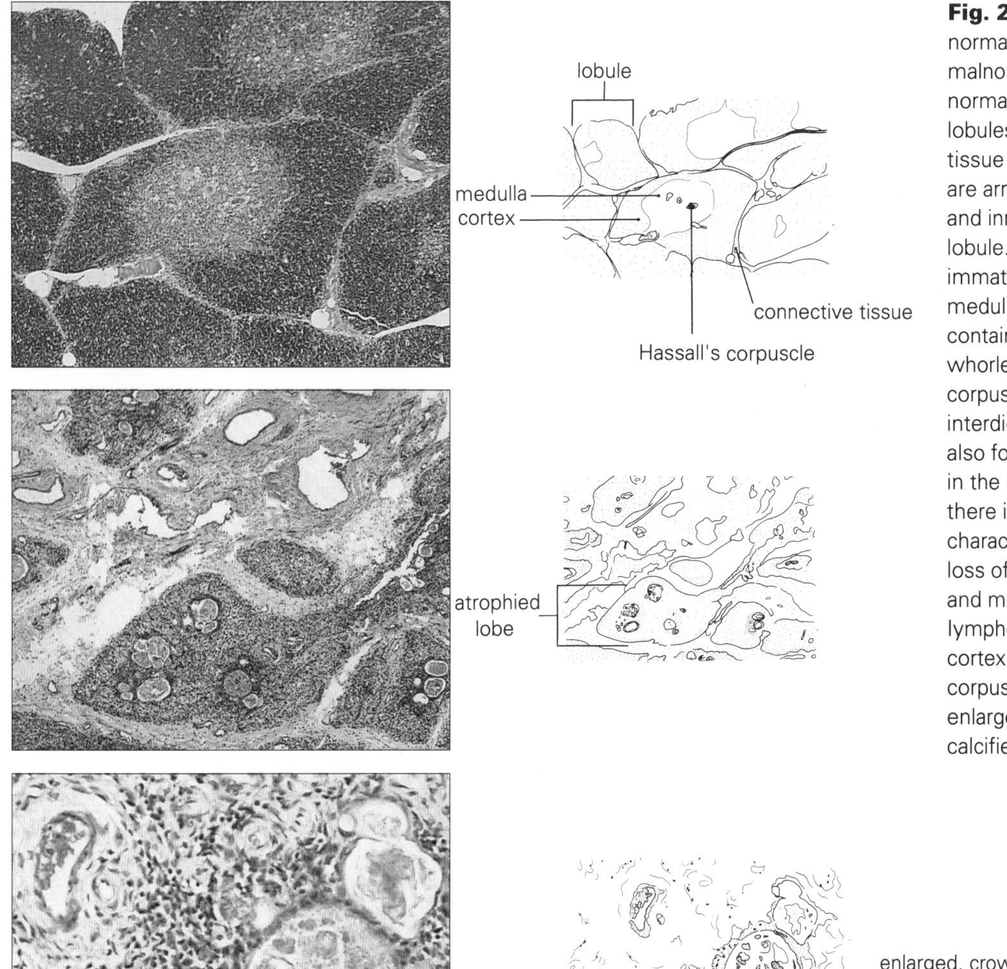

Fig. 25.5. Thymic histology in normal and protein-energy malnourished children. Upper: the normal thymus is composed of lobules separated by connective tissue trabeculae. Lymphoid cells are arranged into an outer cortex and inner medulla within each lobule. The cortex contains immature proliferating cells; the medulla is less cellular and contains more mature cells, and whorled structures called Hassall's corpuscles. Epithelial and interdigitating dendritic cells are also found in the lobules, especially in the medulla. Middle: in PEM, there is acute involution characterized by lobular atrophy, loss of distinction between cortex and medulla, and depletion of lymphocytes (particularly in the cortex). Lower: the Hassall's corpuscles appear degenerate, enlarged, crowded and are often calcified.

these deficits. Although dietary factors are known to affect the structure and function of all cells of the body, the lymphoid tissues are particularly susceptible due to their rapid rate of turnover and synthesis of immunomodulating proteins.

LYMPHOID ORGANS

In PEM the thymus, as well as other lymphoid tissues such as the spleen, lymph nodes and Peyer's patches in the gut, is altered in size and structure. The thymus from children with PEM often weighs less than half the expected normal weight and gross structural alterations are seen on histological examination (Fig. 25.5). The spleen, lymph nodes and gut-associated lymphoid tissues also involute in PEM, the thymus dependent areas being more affected than others. Similar changes are seen in zinc deficiency, but are less marked. The factors involved in the histomorphological effects on lymphoid tissues in PEM include reduced cell proliferation due to decreased protein and DNA synthesis, cytolysis due to increased levels of unbound glucocorticosteroid, and possibly the effects of microbial products.

CELL-MEDIATED IMMUNITY

Delayed hypersensitivity skin responses

Skin tests are a common and useful *in vivo* measure of cell-mediated immunity. In PEM, both the number of positive responses and the size of induration is reduced, and there is often complete anergy to a battery of different antigens. Impaired skin test responses are also seen in moderate deficiencies. There is a significant positive correlation between the size of induration in skin sensitivity

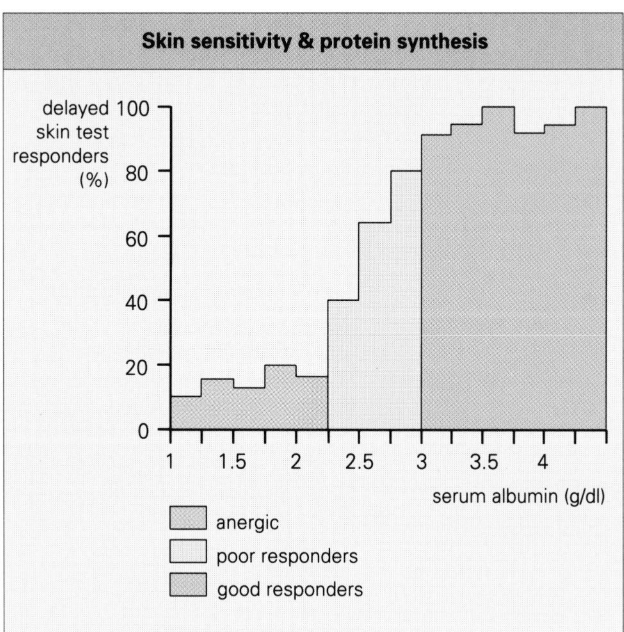

Fig. 25.6 Frequency of positive cutaneous delayed hypersensitivity response compared to serum albumin concentration. Fifty one adults were tested for sensitivity to six standard skin test antigens. An induration of 5mm or greater at 72 hours was counted as positive. Individuals with serum albumin levels less than 2.25 g/dl were often anergic, whereas those with levels above 3.0 g/dl generally showed positive responses.

and body protein synthesis, as judged by serum albumin concentration (Fig. 25.6). The impaired response is probably due to loss of memory T cells. Primary sensitization of the afferent limb may also be involved, as undernourished individuals show depressed responses to chemical sensitizing agents in addition to reduced reaction to the common recall antigens.

Lymphocyte counts and T cell subpopulations

The total lymphocyte count is generally decreased in PEM. The proportion and absolute number of circulating T cells, recognized by the classical technique of rosette formation with sheep red blood cells, is decreased; B cells are unaltered or slightly increased, and null cells (which lack the conventional markers of mature lymphocytes) are elevated (Fig. 25.7). Recent studies using monoclonal antibodies and cell sorting techniques have confirmed the above findings and demonstrated alterations of T cell subsets in PEM. Cells bearing the mature T cell antigen, CD3, are decreased. Studies of T cell sub-populations show a profound reduction of $CD4^+$ helper/inducer cells and moderate reduction of $CD8^+$ suppressor/cytotoxic cells. The $CD4^+$: $CD8^+$ lymphocyte subset ratio is decreased, in some cases falling below 1.0, however the proportions return to normal when the patients recover.

Helper T cell function. Co-culture experiments with the reverse haemolytic plaque technique for the enumeration

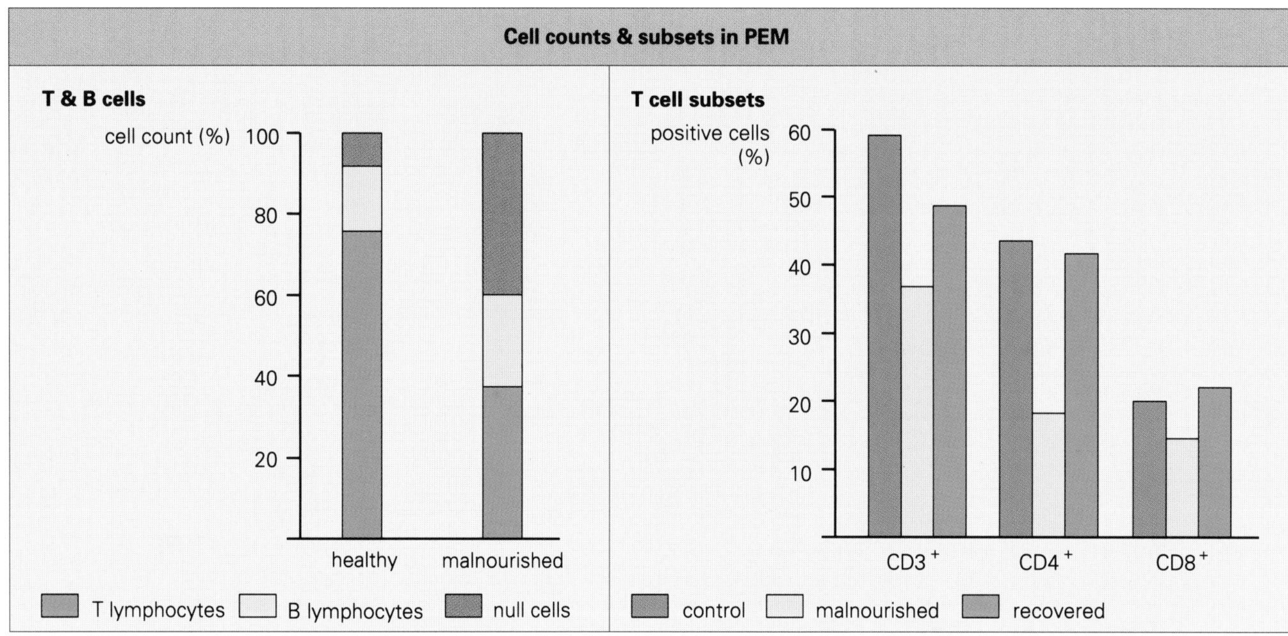

Fig. 25.7 Left: the proportion of circulating T cells, determined by rosetting with sheep red blood cells (OKT II^+ cells) or anti-T3 antibody ($CD3^+$ cells), is decreased in malnourished patients compared to healthy individuals. The B cell count is usually unaltered, and null cells are increased. Right: studies on T cell subpopulations using anti-CD4 and anti-CD8 antibodies and the fluorescence-activated cell sorter show a profound reduction of $CD4^+$ cells and a moderate reduction in $CD8^+$ cells. The proportion returns to normal after 4–8 weeks of nutritional therapy.

of IgG producing cells *in vitro* show abnormalities of TH cell function in PEM (Fig. 25.8). B lymphocytes from PEM patients in the presence of T cells from well-nourished controls function normally, whereas the combination of B and T cells from PEM patients, or B cells from well-nourished controls and T cells from PEM patients yield very few IgG-forming cells. The molecular mechanisms and the probable influence of cytokines have not yet been fully evaluated. These changes in number and function of distinct T lymphocyte subsets explain, to a large extent, the consistent alteration of cellular immune functions in PEM.

Terminal deoxyribonucleotidyl transferase (TdT). The activity of TdT, a marker of immature lymphocytes, is increased in PEM (Fig. 25.9). Increased numbers of null cells in peripheral blood together with increased leucocyte TdT points to impaired maturation and differentiation of lymphocytes in this condition.

Thymic hormone activity

The thymus produces several factors or hormones that are important in T cell maturation and differentiation within the thymus, and in their maintenance in the secondary lymphoid tissues. The activity of these hormones is reduced in PEM and also in selective deficiencies of some other nutrients (Fig. 25.10). Zinc deficiency has the greatest demonstrable effect on the activity of facteur thymique serique (FTS), which is largely dependent on zinc as a

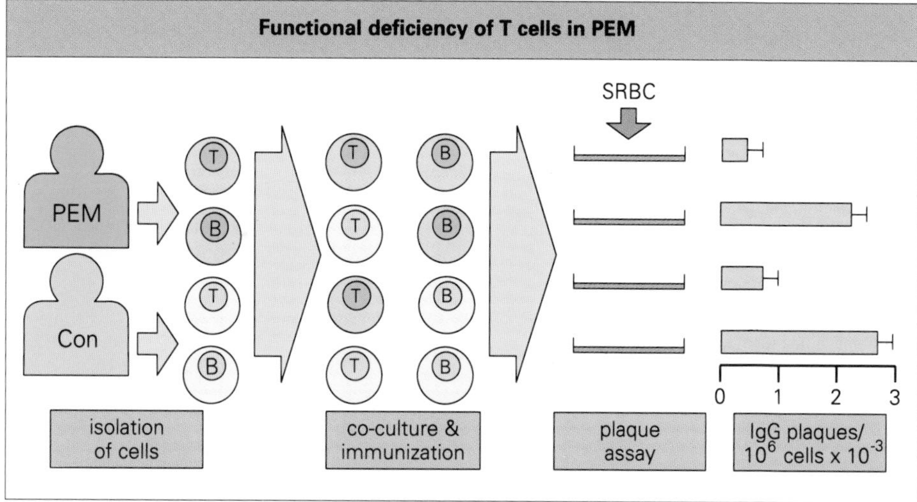

Fig. 25.8 Functional deficiency of TH cells in PEM. T and B cells from PEM patients and well-nourished subjects (Con) were isolated and co-cultured in four possible combinations. Each culture was immunized *in vitro* with sheep RBC and layered on molten agar also containing sheep RBC. Diluted anti-human rabbit IgG and guinea-pig complement were added to the mixture and caused lysis of RBC around IgG-producing lymphocytes. These plaque-forming cells were enumerated. The results show an abnormality of TH cell function in PEM.

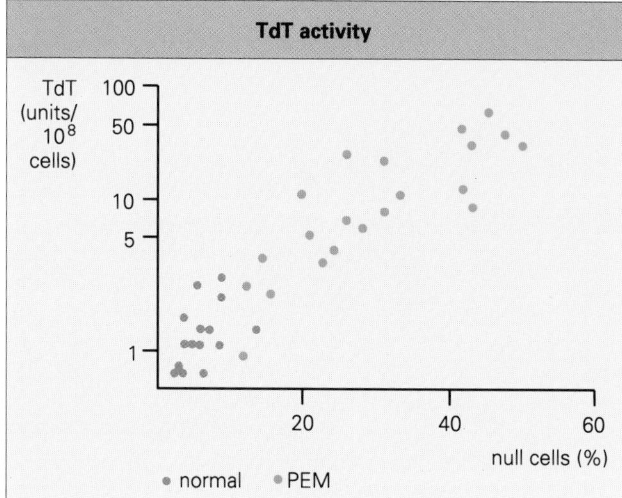

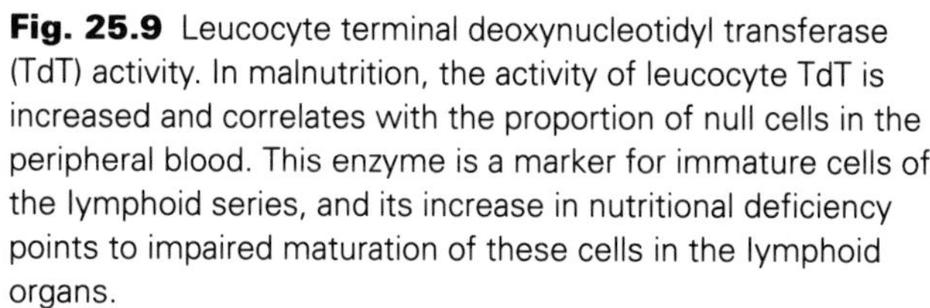

Fig. 25.9 Leucocyte terminal deoxynucleotidyl transferase (TdT) activity. In malnutrition, the activity of leucocyte TdT is increased and correlates with the proportion of null cells in the peripheral blood. This enzyme is a marker for immature cells of the lymphoid series, and its increase in nutritional deficiency points to impaired maturation of these cells in the lymphoid organs.

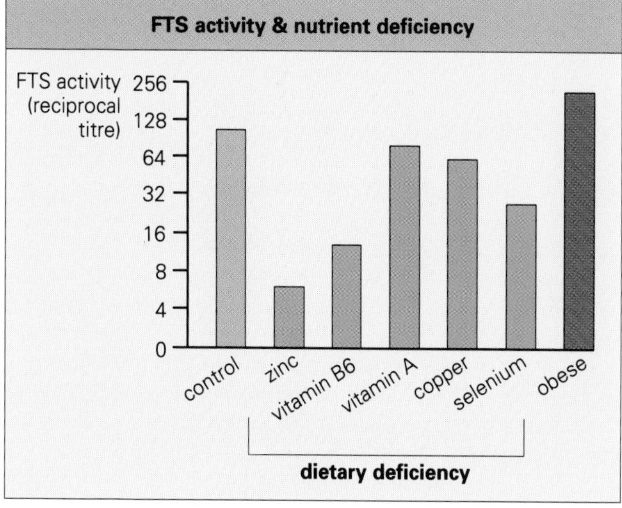

Fig. 25.10 Serum thymic hormone activity. Rats fed a calorie restricted diet have lower facteur thymique serique (FTS) activity than animals fed a standard laboratory diet. Animals fed a diet deficient in zinc or vitamin B6 also have reduced FTS activity, but vitamin A, copper, and selenium deficiency have little demonstrable effect. Genetically obese animals have high thymic hormone activity.

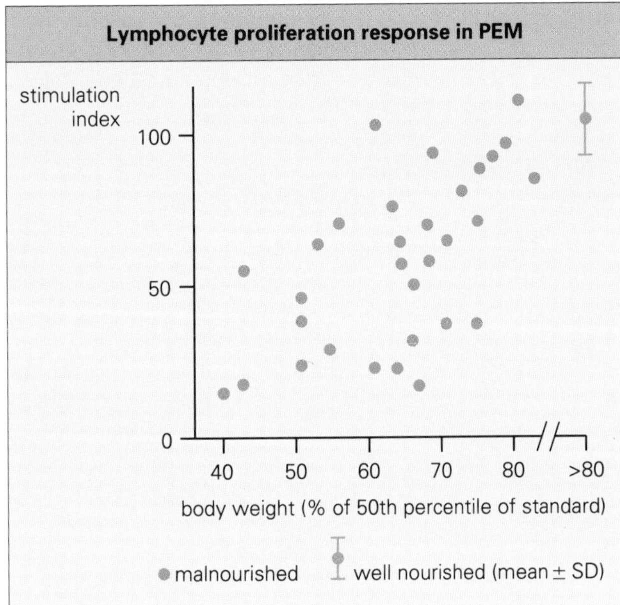

Fig. 25.11 Lymphocyte transformation related to deficit in body weight. The lymphocyte stimulation response to phytohaemagglutinin is reduced in undernourished individuals as compared to healthy subjects. The response is reduced even in marginal undernutrition, although not consistently. In those with weight-for-height between 70–80% of standard, the lymphocyte stimulation index can vary from very low to well within the normal range.

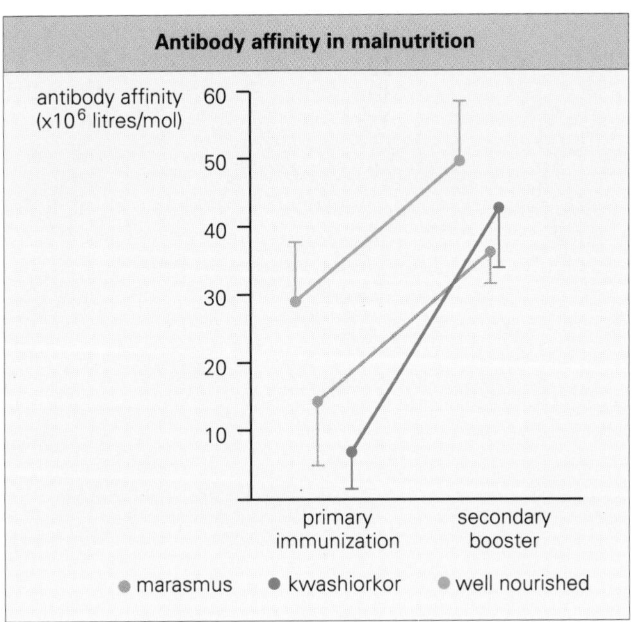

Fig. 25.12 Tetanus toxoid was administered twice, 6 weeks apart, to groups of marasmic, kwashiorkor and well-nourished children and blood was collected 14 days after each immunization. None of the children was previously immunized against tetanus. The affinity of the antibody produced against the immunizing antigen was lower in malnourished groups, both after primary and booster immunization, but more so after primary immunization.

cofactor; other trace elements and some vitamins may also influence its activity. This explains the finding of increased null cells bearing TdT in the peripheral circulation in PEM.

Lymphocyte proliferative response

Lymphocytes from PEM patients respond poorly to mitogens *in vitro* (Fig. 25.11). Various factors may be involved in reducing this response. Protein restriction reduces the number of cells in mitosis and prolongs the cell cycle. Furthermore, the plasma of malnourished patients, who are often infected, contains inhibitory factors such as C-reactive protein, endotoxin, and α-fetoprotein, and also lacks nutrients essential for cell proliferation

Lymphokine production. Production of various lymphokines, such as interferon-γ, interleukin-2, and macrophage migration inhibition factor, is reduced in PEM. Activated monocytes from malnourished donors produce less interleukin-1, a soluble mediator required for T cell activation, compared with normally nourished donors.

ANTIBODY RESPONSES

In PEM, the concentration of serum immunoglobulins of all classes is generally elevated, although one class often predominates. High IgA levels are the likely consequence of repeated gastrointestinal and/or respiratory tract infections, and high IgE levels are usually found with parasitic infestations. In the absence of concomitant or recent infection, serum levels of IgG, and occasionally IgM and IgA, are low. Serum antibody responses to common immunization antigens are generally adequate in PEM patients, however the presence of infection can act as an immunosuppressant and reduce the antibody response. Moreover, the affinity of antibody for antigens is decreased, being more marked after primary immunization (Fig. 25.12).

In contrast to the situation with serum immunoglobulin, the degree of secretory and mucosal IgA response to specific antigen challenge is depressed (Fig. 25.13). The appearance of these antibodies is also often delayed.

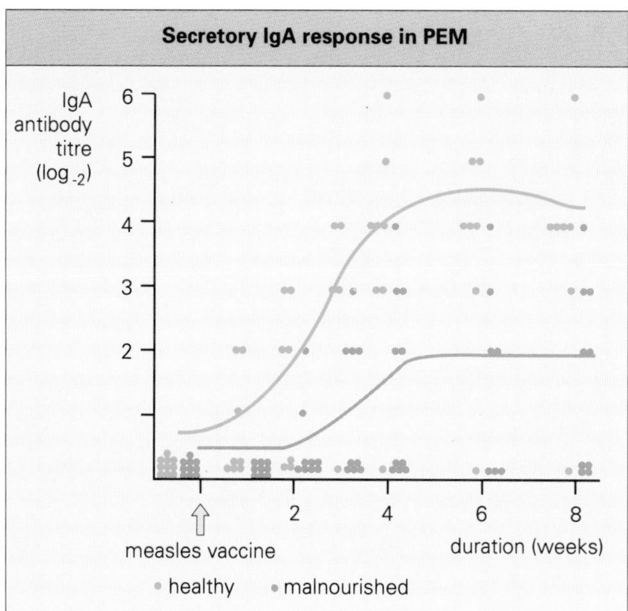

Fig. 25.13 A group of protein-energy malnourished and age-matched healthy children were given a single dose of live attenuated measles virus vaccine and the level of neutralizing IgA antibody in nasopharyngeal secretions was measured for 8 weeks. The level of antibody was lower in malnourished children and its appearance was delayed.

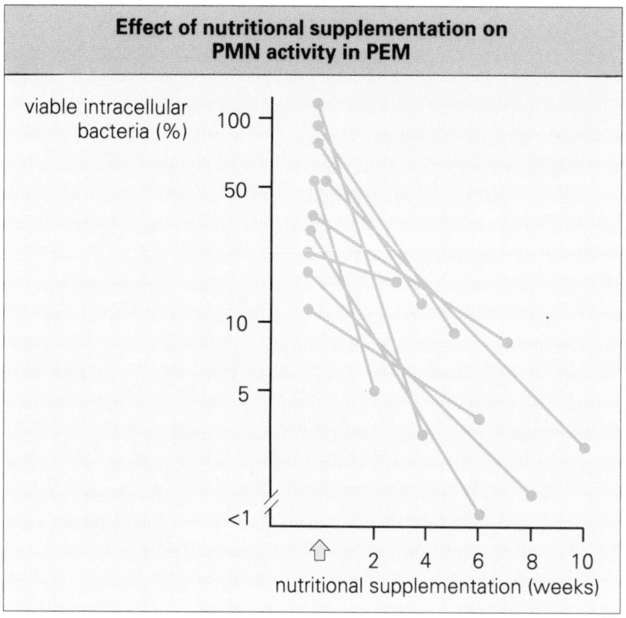

Effect of nutritional supplementation on PMN activity in PEM

viable intracellular bacteria (%)

100

50

10

5

<1

2 4 6 8 10

nutritional supplementation (weeks)

Fig. 25.14 Polymorphonuclear leucocytes (PMNs) and *Staph. aureus* were mixed in the ratio of 1: 5 and incubated at 37° C in the presence of 20% normal plasma. At 140 minutes viable intracellular bacteria were estimated by surface colony count on nutrient agar, and expressed as a percentage ratio of a similar count at 20 minutes. The bactericidal capacity of polymorphs from malnourished individuals was increased following a short period of nutritional supplementation with a diet adequate in calories, proteins and all micronutrients. Following this, there were reduced numbers of viable intracellular bacteria remaining after 140 minutes' incubation.

PHAGOCYTIC CELLS

Polymorphonuclear leucocytes and macrophages recognize foreign proteins, either via non-specific receptors or bound antibody, and show chemotaxis towards them if they activate the complement system (C5a) or cause the release of other chemotactic mediators. Attachment is augmented by opsonins, such as immunoglobulins and complement component C3b, and phagocytosis is followed by the release of lytic enzymes into the phagolysosomes: this is accompanied by a post-phagocytic increase in metabolic activity.

Various steps of this process are affected in PEM. Chemotactic migration of neutrophils is sluggish, particularly in the presence of infection. The opsonic function of serum at lower concentrations is reduced; this will reduce phagocytosis in extravascular compartments, as the concentration of opsonins is low at these sites under normal circumstances. The post-phagocytic metabolic burst is also reduced. The severity of these deficits varies according to the degree of malnutrition, the relative proportion of nutrients affected, and the presence of concomitant infection. Appropriate nutritional supplementation and treatment of infection reverses the abnormality (Fig. 25.14).

COMPLEMENT SYSTEM

Almost all components of the classical and alternative complement pathway are reduced in PEM. The most marked reduction is observed in the level of C3. Changes in complement proteins are more pronounced when infection complicates nutritional deficiency, in contrast to the findings in well-nourished subjects, in whom complement levels rise in the presence of infection. The reduced protein intake in PEM largely accounts for the reduced levels of complement proteins. Altered function of monocytes-macrophages, and of the gastrointestinal and urinary tracts may contribute to the deficit. Demonstration of an increased amount of C3 breakdown products in PEM also suggests that the consumption of complement proteins is increased.

IMMUNOLOGICAL EFFECTS OF FETAL MALNUTRITION

The development of the immune system begins in early gestation and continues into the first few months of life. Nutritional deprivation during this critical period of

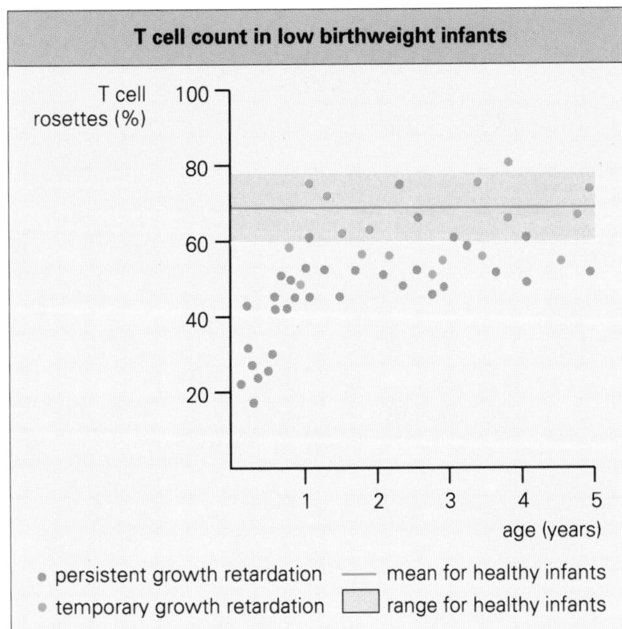

Fig. 25.15 T cell count in low birthweight infants. Rosette-forming T lymphocytes in small-for-gestational age infants were examined for several months after birth. In infants with persistent growth retardation, the proportion of T cells was lower than in those who had caught up in weight and height.

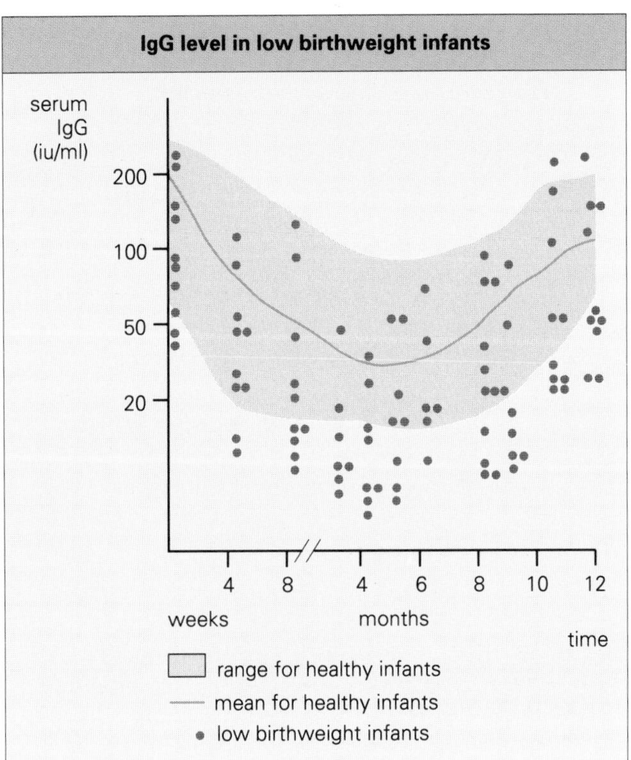

Fig. 25.16 IgG level in low birthweight infants. Serum IgG concentrations of 10 low birthweight children were followed up for 12 months. There was a wide scatter of values, but most of the estimations were either in the lower end of the normal range or below it.

ontogeny has severe and long-lasting effects on immunity. Small-for-gestational-age (SGA), low birthweight infants who suffer from undernutrition during the fetal stage subsequently have reduced T cell numbers and impaired cell-mediated immunity which persists for several months to years, particularly in those who fail to achieve a 'catch-up' growth (Fig. 25.15). Immunoglobulin production is similarly affected (Fig 25.16). In contrast, appropriate-for-gestational-age (AGA), low birthweight infants resulting from preterm delivery also have depressed immunocompetence, but recover within three months after birth. In animal models of intra-uterine malnutrition, depressed cell-mediated immunity is seen to continue even beyond the first generation offspring to the second generation (Fig. 25.17). This further emphasizes the importance of fetal growth on subsequent immune function.

NUTRITION AND IMMUNE COMPETENCE IN OLD AGE

Impaired immune responses are a frequent finding in old
 age. Cell-mediated immunity is reduced and facteur thymique serique activity is almost undetectable; phagocytic dysfunction has also been observed.

Many studies have confirmed the presence of nutritional deficiencies in the elderly. Besides general undernutrition due to reduced calorie intake, a reduced intake and lower blood levels of iron, zinc, vitamin C, B vitamins, and vitamin E have also been found. Socioeconomic deprivation, physical disability, isolation, dental problems, and increased nutrient needs due to disease, are common causes of nutritional problems in this group.

Recent data suggest that nutritional deficiencies may contribute to the decline in immune responses seen in old age. Interventional trials that attempted to correct nutritional deficiencies in the elderly demonstrated an improvement in immune responses, including antibody titres after prophylactic vaccination.

Given the established role of nutrition in the modulation of immune responses, the frequent prevalence of nutritional deficiencies in the elderly, and the commonly observed reduction in immune competence in old age, it is logical to expect that nutritional status is critical in old age and that correction of nutritional abnormalities will improve immunity and decrease the risk of illness.

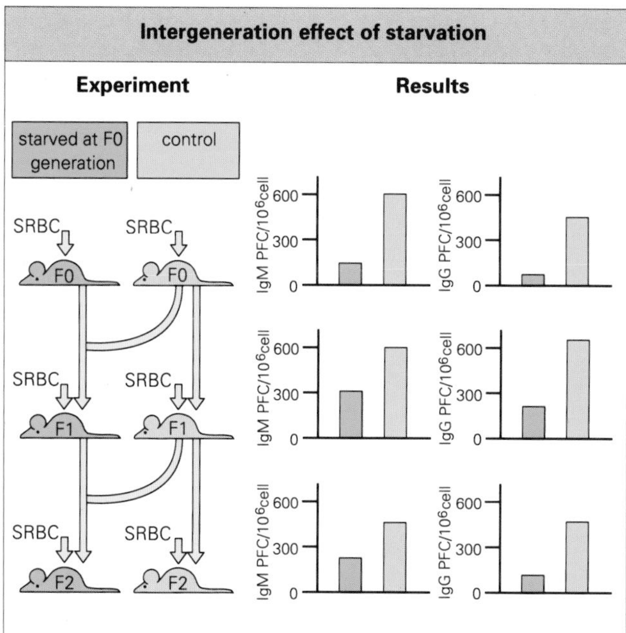

Fig. 25.17 Three-week-old rats were subjected to partial starvation for 6 weeks by restricting their food intake to 25% of the optimal amount fed to control animals. One batch of starved and control animals (Fo generation) were immunized with sheep RBC and the IgM- and IgG-plaque forming cells (PFC) assayed at 10 days post-immunization. Another batch of starved and control rats were mated with control animals. The F1 generation was given free access to feed; some were immunized with sheep RBC and studied for IgM- and IgG-PFC response, and others were mated with control animals and the F2 progeny studied as above. Results show that antibody-forming cell response is reduced in F1 and F2 offspring of starved F0 mothers.

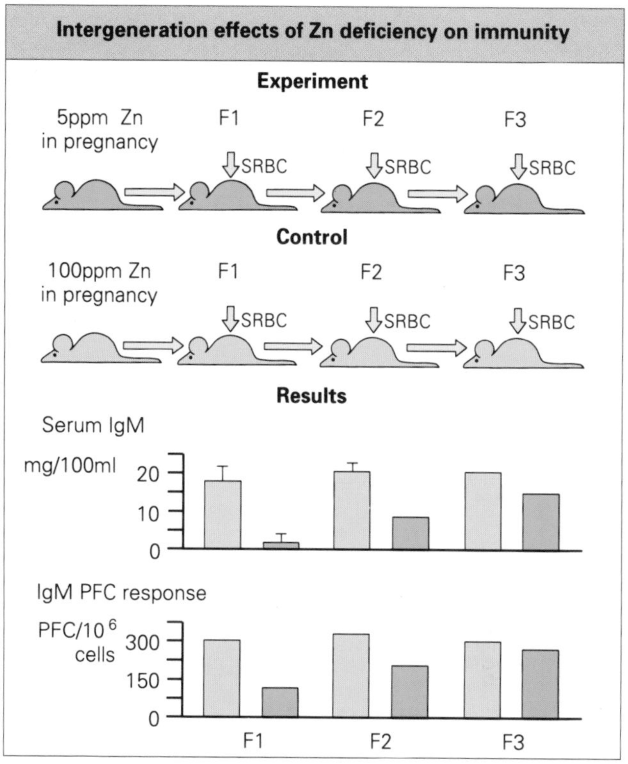

Intergeneration effects of Zn deficiency on immunity

Experiment

5ppm Zn in pregnancy — F1 — F2 — F3 — SRBC

Control

100ppm Zn in pregnancy — F1 — F2 — F3 — SRBC

Results

Serum IgM mg/100ml (0, 10, 20)

IgM PFC response PFC/10⁶ cells (0, 150, 300)

F1 F2 F3

Fig. 25.18 An experimental group of animals was fed a Zn-deficient diet (5ppm Zn) during the later two-thirds of pregnancy and a control group was fed a Zn-adequate diet (100ppm Zn) during the same period. The former regime reduced serum Zn to 60–70% of control values. F1, F2 and F3 generations were fed sufficient Zn throughout. Both the PFC response and serum concentration of IgM were assessed at 6 weeks. Results showed that both were low in at least 3 generations of offspring.

SINGLE NUTRIENT DEFICIENCIES AND IMMUNE FUNCTION

The immune system dysfunction observed in PEM may be the combined result of deficiency of multiple nutrients. Recently, studies of laboratory animals deprived of one dietary element and of rare patients with single nutrient deficiencies has elucidated the role of several trace elements and vitamins in the immune system.

TRACE ELEMENTS

Iron

Among the trace elements, iron and zinc have been studied extensively. Worldwide, iron deficiency is the most common single nutrient deficiency, occurring in both developed and underdeveloped countries. Iron deficiency is characterized by reduced intracellular killing of bacteria by phagocytes and by decreased T cell numbers, lymphocyte transformation to mitogens and lymphokine production. These immunological alterations occur before a drop in haemoglobin concentration is detectable. The cellular basis of these effects is reduced activity of ribonucleotide reductase (necessary for DNA synthesis), and myeloperoxidase and hydroxyl radical production (required for intracellular killing of bacteria by phagocytes).

Zinc

Zinc deficiency results in lymphoid atrophy and lower FTS activity. Various immune functions, such as antibody production against heterologous antigens, lymphocyte transformation response to mitogens, neutrophil function, and natural killer cell and T cell mediated cytotoxicity are depressed. These result in anergy to skin sensitization and frequent infections by opportunistic organisms. As in generalized undernutrition, zinc deficiency early in fetal ontogeny results in a severe and prolonged effect on immune functions (Fig. 25.18). 25.9

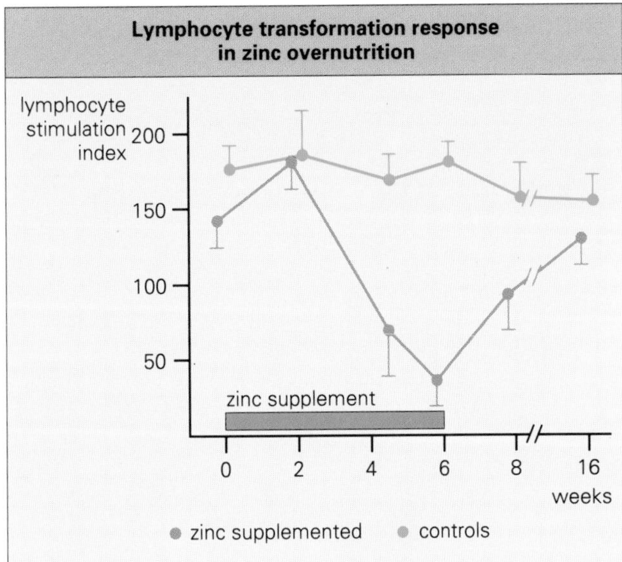

Fig. 25.19 Lymphocyte transformation response to phytohaemagglutinin in zinc overnutrition. 11 healthy young adults were given 300mg elemental Zn daily for 6 weeks and their lymphocyte stimulation was measured. Data shown are optimum results obtained on dose-response curves. In the Zn-supplemented group, the response was lower than in untreated controls at 4 and 6 weeks of treatment. The stimulation index rose 2 weeks after cessation of treatment, and was comparable to the control value after 10 weeks.

Vitamins

Deficiency of certain vitamins also adversely affects immune functions. Vitamin A deficiency depresses cell-mediated immunity and T cell dependent antibody responses. Secretory IgA production and anti-tumour activity are also impaired. Vitamin E deficiency reduces antibody production and cell-mediated immunity if accompanied by deficiency of other anti-oxidants, particularly selenium. In extreme vitamin C deficiency phagocytic function is depressed. Among the B vitamins, pyridoxine and folic acid deficiency reduces T cell function and T cell dependent antibody responses. In addition, pyridoxine deficiency causes thymic epithelial dysfunction and reduction in FTS.

IMMUNOLOGICAL ALTERATIONS IN OVERNUTRITION

GENERALIZED OVERNUTRITION

T cell function

Generalized overnutrition resulting in obesity is the most common nutritional disorder in industrialized countries. Limited human studies show that in obese persons T cell functions, such as delayed cutaneous hypersensitivity, response to antigens and lymphocyte proliferation to mitogens are slightly reduced. Animal studies on genetically obese mice are in agreement with the human observations and also show that T cell number, T cell dependent antibody production, natural killer cell activity, and antibody dependent cell-mediated cytotoxicity are reduced. These immunological alterations are probably related to the effects of lipids on membranes. Lipids are an essential constituent of cell membranes, and excess probably alters membrane composition and hence function. Excess lipoproteins of low density also directly inhibit protein and DNA synthesis in many cells including lymphocytes.

EXCESS INTAKE OF SINGLE NUTRIENTS

Zinc

This has also been shown to alter immune functions. Daily intake of large supplements of zinc for prolonged periods decreases lymphocyte transformation to mitogens (Fig. 25.19), polymorphonuclear leucocyte cell migration and bactericidal capacity. Alterations of leucocyte membrane lipid composition by zinc is probably responsible for the altered immune functions as large doses of zinc are known to increase low-density and decrease high-density lipoprotein levels in serum.

Iron

Excess iron also has deleterious effects on host defence mechanisms. Iron is essential for all organisms, including human pathogens. It is usually chelated by iron-binding proteins, such as transferrin, so that very little is available for microbial needs. In severe undernutrition, when iron-binding protein levels are low, large doses of iron can saturate the binding proteins and increase the availability of free iron for microbial growth thus increasing susceptibility to infections.

CONCLUSIONS

The alteration of immune function in nutritional disorders has several practical implications.

- Nutritional status is a significant determinant of morbity and mortality of hospitalized and debilitated patients.
- Immunological changes occur early in the course of nutritional deficiencies. Thus altered immunocompetence can be used as a sensitive functional index of malnutrition and can predict the outcome after therapeutic intervention.
- In countries where undernutrition is rampant, immunization in seasons when nutritional status is likely to be better will elicit a better immune response.
- The response to prophylactic immunization in the elderly can be improved even by short term nutritional support before and after the administration of vaccine.

FURTHER READING

Beisel WR. Single nutrients and immunity. *Am J Clin Nutr* 1982;**35:**17–468.

Chandra RK. *Immunology of nutritional disorders.* London: Edward Arnold, 1980.

Chandra RK. Nutrition, immunity, and infection: Present knowledge and future directions. *Lancet* 1983;**i**:688–691.

Chandra RK. *Nutrition, immunity and illness in the elderly.* New York: Pergamon, 1985.

Chandra RK. Trace element regulation of immunity and infection. *J Am Col Nutr* 1985;**4**:5–16.

Chandra RK. *Nutrition and Immunology.* New York: Alan R Liss, 1988.

Fraker PJ, Gershwin ME, Good RA, Prasad AS. Interrelationships between zinc and immune function. *Fed Proc* 1986; **45**: 1474–1479.

Gross RL, Newberne PM. Role of nutrition in immunologic function. *Physiol Rev* 1980;**60**:188–302. 25.11

26

Vaccines

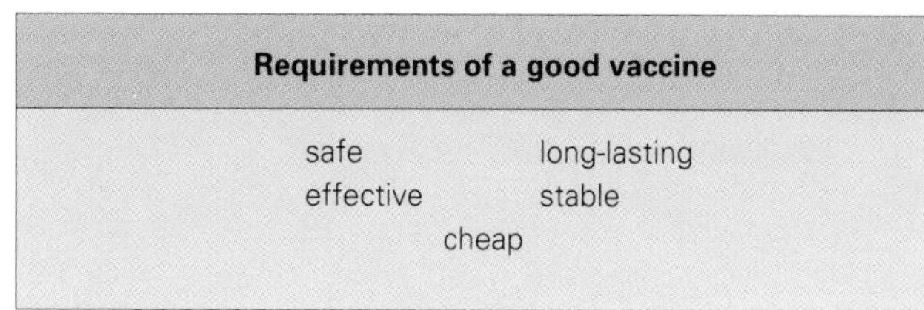

Fig. 26.1 Requirements of a good vaccine.

Existing vaccines

INTRODUCTION

The use of vaccines to prevent disease is one of the oldest, yet one of the most lasting success stories in medicine. It had long been recognized that individuals who recovered from their first attack of a disease developed resistance to that disease. This lead to early experiments with smallpox, in which small amounts of material were given by an abnormal route under controlled circumstances in the hope that the recipient would develop immunity but not disease. There were extreme side-effects from using the fully virulent virus, and vaccination became an established principle only after the work of Edward Jenner in the late eighteenth century. He took advantage of the cross-protection afforded by using a related organism — cowpox virus — which was relatively non-pathogenic for man.

A vaccine is defined as a preparation administered to an individual which induces an immunologically specific resistance to an infectious disease. This need not involve complete resistance to infection. The requirements of a good vaccine are shown in Fig. 26.1.

VACCINE ADMINISTRATION

A government policy exists to cover the administration of all of the widely used vaccines, with on the one hand, mass immunization programmes (for example whooping cough, polio) which aim to raise the level of herd immunity and diminish, or eliminate, the transmission of the disease in the community, and on the other, selective immunization being offered to those who are likely to be exposed, for example because of occupation or foreign travel.

Immunizing schedule

It is often worth giving multiple vaccines at a single visit. Individuals are capable of responding to multiple antigens administered simultaneously, although there is a period of about 4–14 days after the administration of one vaccine when individuals will respond poorly to others. Where multiple doses of vaccine are required, the optimum interval between first and second doses is 6–8 weeks, and a third (if required) after an interval of 4–6 months.

Route of administration

This depends on the nature of the vaccine. Oral polio vaccine must always be given by mouth and BCG must always be given intradermally. It is usually recommended that all other injectable vaccines are given by the intramuscular or deep subcutaneous route, however, some may be given intradermally. By this route, a much smaller dose is usually sufficient to produce the desired effect, which is an important advantage with expensive vaccines (for example rabies) and those with which systemic reactions sometimes occur (for example typhoid).

SYSTEMIC VERSUS MUCOSAL INFECTIONS

Cholera and typhoid

There is a remarkable contrast between diseases which have been relatively easily and effectively controlled by immunization and those which have not. The contrast between the typhoid and cholera vaccines is a good example. Both consist of killed bacteria and are administered by injection. Typhoid vaccine gives 70–90% protection for about three years (except in the face of a massive infecting dose) whereas cholera vaccine only gives about 50% protection for around 6 months (Fig. 26.2).

Polio

Inactivated poliovirus vaccines are effective since they stimulate circulating antibody which blocks the viraemic spread of the virus from the portal of entry, the gastrointestinal tract, to the main target organ, the central nervous system and can also be used in those subjects where live vaccines are contraindicated. Even though some countries have controlled poliovirus infection with inactivated vaccines, it has been more usual for developed western countries to use live-attenuated vaccines administered orally, by the natural route. This has the advantage of adding gut mucosal immunity to the barrier of circulating antibody induced by inactivated vaccines (Fig. 26.3).

26.2

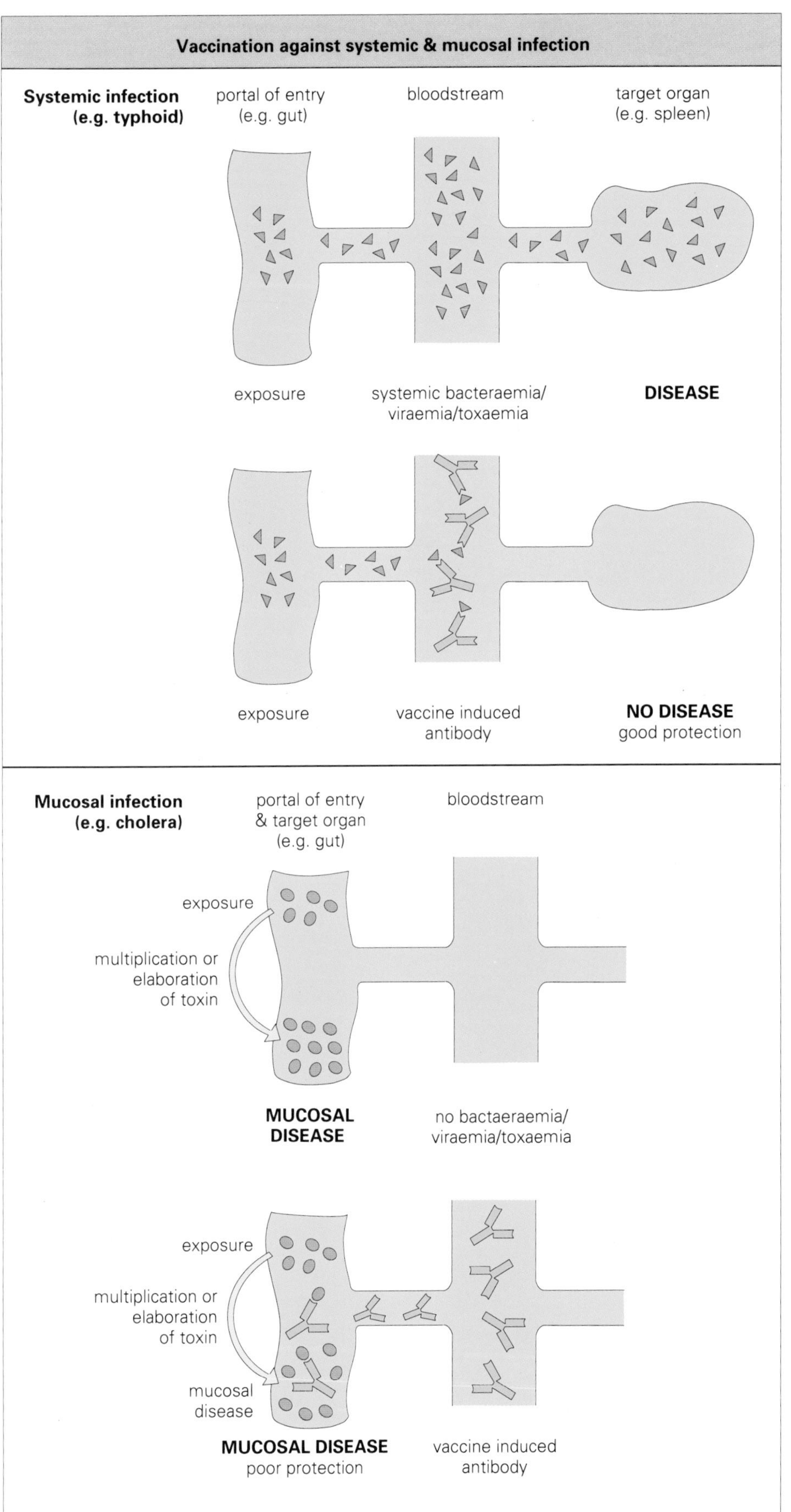

Fig. 26.2 Typhoid vaccine induces production of circulating antibodies which are likely to be effective against typhoid fever, in which bacteraemia is an essential component of the disease. Circulating antibodies are also produced following cholera vaccination, but are less effective in preventing the disease, which is confined to the gut and caused by the direct action of bacterial toxin on intestinal mucosal cells.

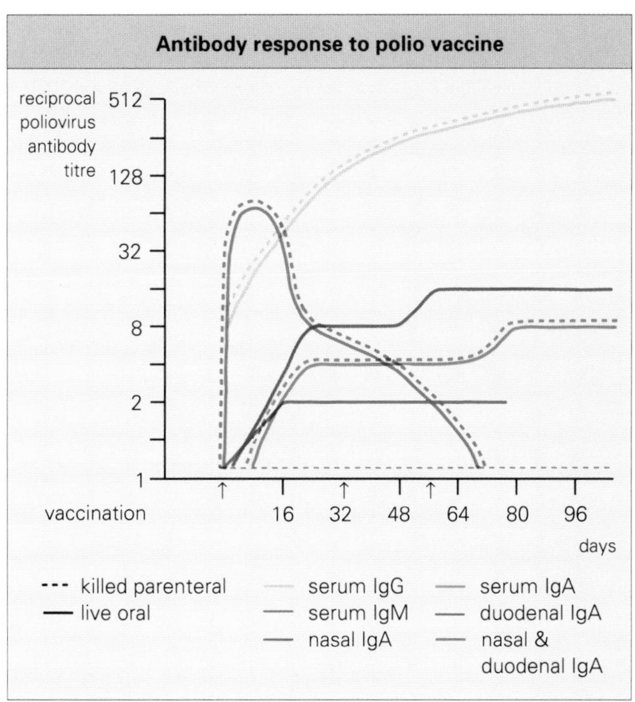

Fig. 26.3 Antibody response to orally administered live-attenuated polio vaccine (solid lines) and to intramuscularly administered killed polio vaccine (broken lines). Note that the former induces production of secretory IgA in addition to serum antibodies. Modified from Fields, BN (1985).

Relative merits of live versus killed vaccines

	Live	Killed
doses	often single	multiple
relative amounts of antigen in vaccine	small	large
possible inclusion of viable adventitious agents	+	-
posssible reversion to virulence	+	-
automatic contraindications (pregnancy/immunosuppression)	+	-

Fig. 26.4 Relative merits of live versus killed vaccines showing some of the problems with live viruses.

Influenza

Immunity gained from inactivated influenza vaccines injected into a peripheral site is short lived, even in the absence of a major antigenic shift, as little virus specific antibody can be detected in respiratory tract secretions. However live virus vaccines administered into the upper respiratory tract do induce substantial titres of secreted antibody, and when some of the persistent problems of attenuation are resolved this may be the most effective approach.

INACTIVATED VERSUS LIVE-ATTENUATED VACCINES

Vaccine induced protection can be achieved with either killed or live-attenuated organisms (Fig. 26.4). Most bacterial vaccines are killed (BCG is the exception) and, by contrast, viral vaccines are live (although there are exceptions). In contrast with killed vaccines, current live virus vaccines induce long-lasting immunity after a single dose (except live poliovirus vaccine, which requires three doses to ensure protection against all three types). With less initial antigen load there is multiplication in the recipient. Bacterial vaccines are often killed, since the organisms can be grown readily in culture and relatively large concentrations can be incorporated into the vaccines. Viruses are more difficult to replicate in the laboratory and therefore live vaccines are preferred. If a particular virus (for example hepatitis) cannot be replicated in the laboratory or a satisfactory attenuation cannot be achieved (for example rabies, influenza), then viral vaccines must also be inactivated.

Drawbacks of live virus

There is the possibility that attenuated strains will revert to full virulence on passage through a human host. Poliovirus type 3 can revert in this circumstance, but in practice this has not led to the occurrence of disease. Adventitious agents can be incorporated into a live vaccine, as happened with simian virus 40 when polio vaccine was manufactured in monkey cell lines, but again there was no apparent adverse effect. Finally, the attenuation and control of injected virus is judged in immunocompetent individuals and therefore live virus vaccines are very often contraindicated in immunocompromised hosts and during pregnancy.

TYPES OF IMMUNIZATION

PASSIVE IMMUNIZATION

Passive immunization involves the transfer to one individual of antibodies formed in another. Animal antisera have been used in the past with all the attendant risks of serum sickness, but all immunoglobulins currently used to prevent microbial disease are of human origin. Passive immunization gives protection which is rapid in onset, significant plasma levels of the transferred antibody being achieved 24–28 hours after intramuscular injection and within minutes of intravenous injection. Unfortunately it is not long lasting, since the injected immunoglobulin (almost all IgG) will be eliminated with a half-life of about 21 days and protection against an infectious disease lasts for around 4–6 months (Fig. 26.5).

Normal human immunoglobulin

This is made from the supernatant of unselected pooled plasma packs after the removal of cryoprecipitate. It is particularly rich in those specific antibodies which are common in the population and is of proven and recommended use in the prevention of measles and hepatitis A. A normal human immunoglobulin preparation with a specific content of measles antibody and one with a reduced content are available for specific uses. Normal human immunoglobulin has also been used to protect pregnant women against rubella but it should be emphasized that it will not reliably prevent either maternal or fetal infection.

Hyperimmune globulins

These are made from a pool or units of blood which have been selected because they have a relatively high titre of a particular anti-microbial antibody. Such preparations are available for the prevention of tetanus, hepatitis B, rabies and chickenpox. They can be used as the sole preventative agents or, more often, with a specific vaccine in combined prophylaxis (see below).

ACTIVE IMMUNIZATION

Active immunization involves the stimulation of an individual's own immune system by the administration of killed or live-attenuated micro-organisms, their components (subunit vaccines) or their inactivated products (toxoids). Vaccine induced protection is relatively slow in onset, often taking 2–4 weeks or longer to develop. However the protection is long lasting, often for a period of years, and even when it has waned it can be restored rapidly with a booster dose of vaccine.

It is possible to combine both active and passive immunization and take advantage of the best features of each, so that passive immunization protects in the immediate post-exposure period until lasting active immunity develops. In addition, immunoglobulin may be given at the same time as vaccine to diminish the possibility of unwanted side-effects of live vaccines.

For each vaccine there are precise recommendations for use and these are summarized in Fig. 26.6.

26.4

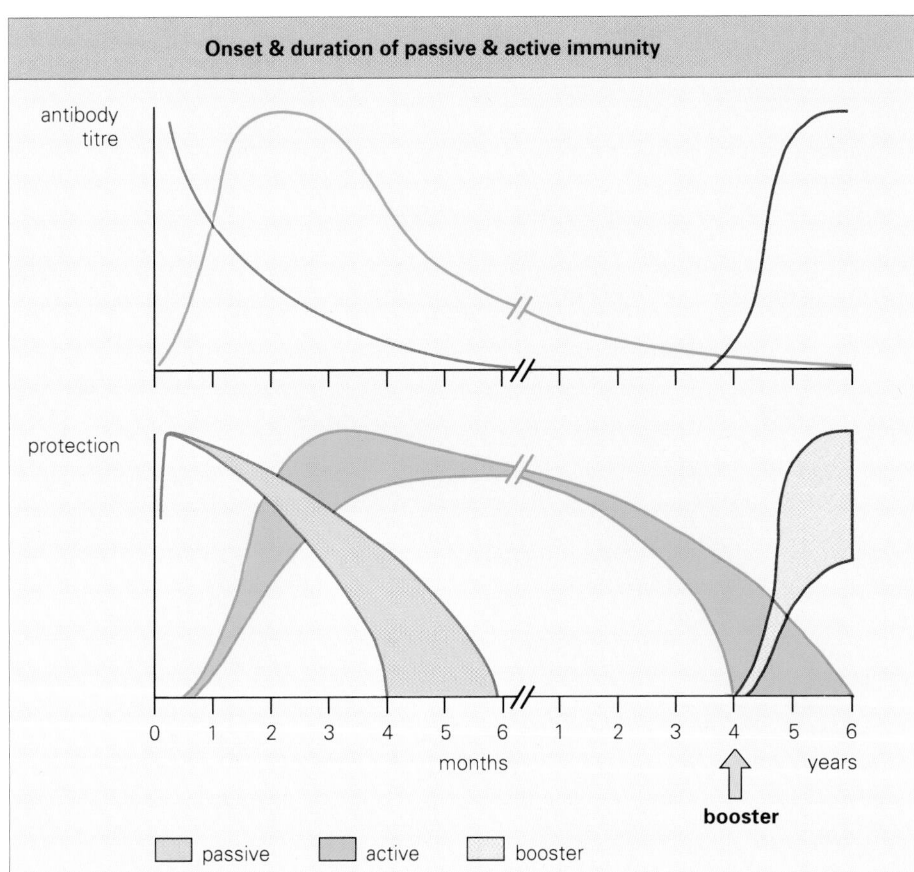

Fig. 26.5 Antibody levels decline during the six months following passive immunization (at time 0), eventually becoming undetectable; protection wanes similarly. After active immunization there is a lag period, followed by a rise in antibody titres, which peak between 1–3 months. Protection is high during this period and persists after the decline in antibody titre because the immune system retains the ability to mount a rapid secondary response to the antigen. Protection is shown in ranges to represent variations with different vaccines and in different individuals.

Toxoids

The serious nature of diphtheria and tetanus is due to the action of bacterial exotoxins, infection at the site of invasion usually being trivial in itself. The most effective protection against disease is therefore provided by immunization with toxoids, which are cell-free preparations of toxins treated with formaldehyde. Used alone, toxoids are weak antigens and are adsorbed onto aluminium salts which act as adjuvants.

Bacterial vaccines

Pertussis. The virulence factors are not well understood, although it is clear that the majority of complications and deaths occur in infants, particularly those under the age of six months. Accordingly, whooping cough vaccine is a suspension of killed *B. pertussis* organisms and contains all three varieties of the principal surface antigens, and is given as part of triple vaccine in the first year of life.

Pertussis vaccine may cause permanent brain damage, and in the past this has lead to a marked fall in the number of people accepting vaccine, with a consequent increase in incidence of whooping cough. The overall benefits of vaccination greatly outweigh the risk of serious neurological side-effects which vary from an isolated febrile convulsion, through a prolonged screaming attack, to a severe encephalopathy resulting in permanent brain damage. The latter probably occurs at a rate of 1/100,000 given a full course of three injections. In an attempt to minimize this the vaccine should not be given to anyone with a history of cerebral irritation at birth or fits, and the balance of risk and benefit should be carefully considered in those with neurological disease or a family history of epilepsy.

Immunization schedule		
Vaccine	**Timing**	**To whom given**
Mass programmes		
Triple vaccine: Diphtheria, Tetanus, Pertussis; Polio	3 doses at 3 months, 6 weeks later, 6 months later & boosters at school entry & leaving (tetanus & polio only)	everybody
Measles (& mumps & rubella in some countries)	second year of life	everybody
Selective large scale programmes		
BCG	10 – 14 years of age	tuberculin negative individuals
Rubella	10 – 14 years of age	all girls
Influenza	annually in the Autumn	elderly, chronically sick
Travellers to developing countries		
Cholera, Typhoid, Yellow fever	during the month or so prior to travel	
Exposure (occupational or accidental)		
Hepatitis B	pre-exposure	health care personnel
	post-exposure	neonates of carriers
Rabies	pre-exposure	some laboratory & kennel workers
	post-exposure	individuals bitten or licked by infected animals

Fig. 26.6 Immunization schedule. Mumps and rubella vaccines are given at the same time as measles vaccines in some countries. In addition to those mentioned here, normal human immunoglobulin and tetanus and polio boosters should be considered for travellers to developing countries.

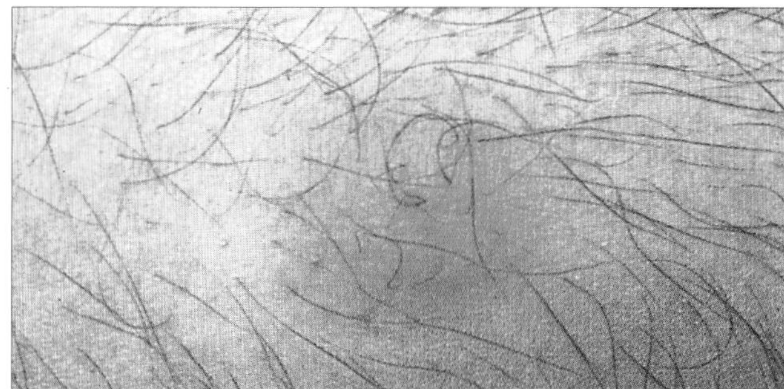

Fig. 26.7 Mantoux test showing cell-mediated hypersensitivity to tubercle bacillus, characterized by induration and erythema. Courtesy of Professor J H L Playfair.

Tuberculosis. Effective protection (about 70% for 15 years) against tuberculosis can be achieved by an intradermal injection of the live avirulent mycobacterium Bacille Calmette-Guérin (BCG) in individuals who are not already sensitized. All potential recipients of BCG should first be tested for hypersensitivity to the proteins of *M. tuberculosis* by a skin test involving a single intradermal injection (Mantoux test) (Fig. 26.7) or the multiple puncture inoculation (Heaf test) of purified protein derivative. Only those with a negative skin reaction require BCG. It is recommended that the following groups are tested and vaccinated if negative:

- school children aged 10–14 years;
- health service staff;
- contacts of cases of active respiratory disease.

Cholera. This vaccine has limited effectiveness and the World Health Organization (WHO) no longer recommends cholera vaccine for travel. Some countries still require a certificate of vaccination issued within the previous six months for entry and a degree of personal protection is provided by two doses of vaccine separated by one month.

Typhoid. Enteric fever is the name given to the systemic disease caused by *Salmonella typhi, S. paratyphi* A, B & C, and very occasionally other *Salmonella* species. In the past, a combined typhoid/paratyphoid A and B (TAB) vaccine was used to generate protection. However, since the A and B components were of doubtful efficacy and increased the incidence of side-effects, a monovalent typhoid vaccine is now recommended. This gives relatively good protection after primary immunization, with two doses of vaccine administered 4–6 weeks apart, and is reinforced every three years in individuals who are continually exposed.

Diphtheria and tetanus. In these cases, vaccines have had a major impact on the frequency of the disease. Before the Second World War there were up to 75,000 notifications of diphtheria annually. Immunization was introduced in 1940s and by the early 1950s the disease had been virtually eradicated (Fig. 26.8).

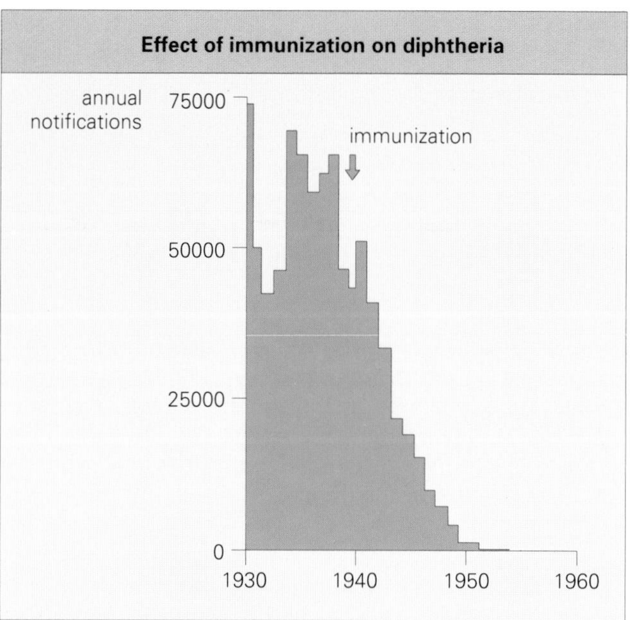

Fig. 26.8 Annual notifications of diphtheria from 1930. The number of cases reported dropped dramatically after the immunization programme was introduced in 1940.

Viral vaccines

Most viral vaccines in use today are directed against infections in which an extracellular viraemia is an essential component of the pathogenesis of disease. Inducing serum antibody can therefore be expected to generate protection.

Polio. Many recipients are protected after a single dose, but a full course of three doses is required to produce long lasting immunity to all three types in over 95% of recipients.

Inactivated vaccines may also have to be used in developing countries where the results of oral polio vaccines have been disappointing, probably due to interference from other enteroviruses circulating in the community. Clinical poliomyelitis occurs very rarely (about 2–3 per million children immunized) in those given oral polio vaccine or their contacts.

Measles. This is also a live-attenuated virus vaccine, and following its introduction in the UK in 1968, the number of cases reported fell rapidly (Fig. 26.9). It is given later than polio vaccine because maternal antibody leads to failure of immunization in children under 12 months of age. It should be given in the second year of life in developed countries. Only one dose is required since there is only a single antigenic type and the multiplication of the live virus in the recipient generates antibody which persists for at least 15 years in over 95% of those vaccinated. The contraindications are the usual ones for a live virus vaccine, but if it is needed, immunoglobulin should be given at the same time as the vaccine. The most common

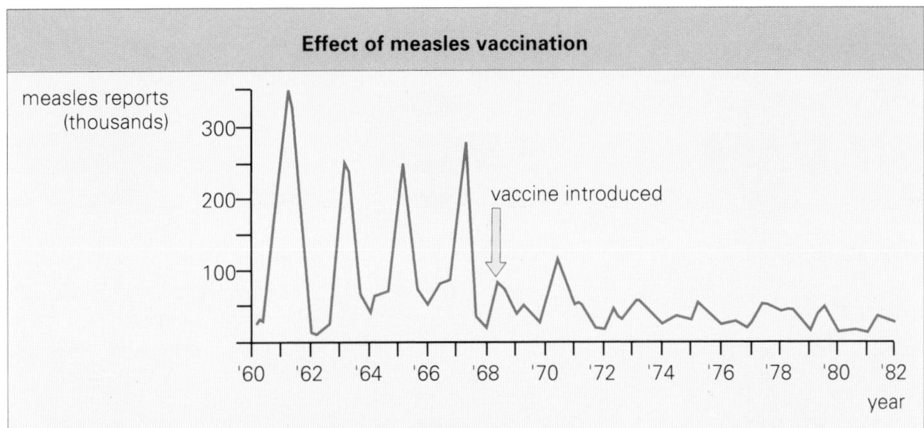

Fig. 26.9 Effect of measles vaccination on the number of cases reported quarterly in England and Wales. The biennial epidemics are evident and, whilst the number of cases fell dramatically after 1968, the pattern of epidemics remains. Modified from Zuckerman *et al.* (1987).

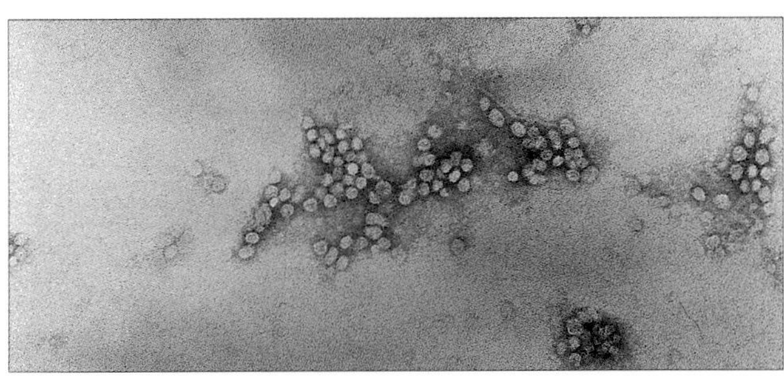

Fig. 26.10 Electron micrograph of purified 22nm hepatitis B surface antigen particles expressed in yeast cells.

side-effect is fever and malaise. Serious side-effects such as convulsions and encephalitis occur ten times less frequently with the vaccine than with the natural infection.

Rubella. A live-attenuated rubella vaccine is used to prevent the only serious consequence of rubella virus infection, namely congenital rubella. The policy is to vaccinate young children of both sexes in order to reduce and eventually eliminate rubella from the community. In the UK, females aged 10–14 years and all seronegative women of childbearing age are also given vaccine, provided they are not pregnant. The latter is still judged to be an absolute contraindication to rubella vaccination and should be avoided for three months following vaccination.

Mumps. The mumps vaccine is very safe and effective and has been widely used in the USA and Scandinavia. It is usually given as a combined formulation with measles and rubella vaccines in the second year of life. It is likely that other countries in the developed world will use this formulation in future.

Yellow fever. The live-attenuated yellow fever vaccine is one of the most effective and safe formulations currently available and is used principally in relation to foreign travel. As well as providing personal protection, the vaccine is necessary because many countries require entrants coming from an area in which yellow fever is endemic to have an internationally valid certificate of immunization. For these reasons the vaccine is administered only at WHO approved centres. The certificate becomes valid from the tenth day after primary immunization and boosters are required every 10 years. The only significant side-effect is encephalitis in infants, and therefore vaccine should not be given to anyone under nine months of age.

Hepatitis B (Fig. 26.10). The most widely used vaccine at the present time consists of a suspension of inactivated, adjuvant-adsorbed 22nm surface antigen particles purified from the plasma of chronic carriers as it cannot be grown in cell cultures. Over 95% of healthy individuals develop high levels of hepatitis B surface antibody after three doses of vaccine, which are given at times zero, 1 month and 6 months. Protection against natural infection by this vaccination regimen has been demonstrated and side-effects are minimal and local. Hepatitis B is the first human vaccine for which a genetically engineered alternative is now available.

Influenza. The surface antigens of influenza virus (haemagglutinin, H, and neuraminidase, N) continue to change in major (antigenic shift) or minor (antigenic drift) steps, and thus the antigenic formulation of the vaccine has to be continually updated; at present it contains two influenza A strains (an H3N2 strain and an H1N1 strain) and a recently isolated influenza B strain. The inactivated vaccines produce protection which lasts for one influenza season only and individuals at risk such as the chronically sick (chest, heart and renal disease), the immune suppressed and the elderly in residential homes must be immunized each Autumn.

Rabies. This vaccine has developed through a number of formulations since it was introduced by Pasteur about a hundred years ago. It was originally made in animal brains, but proved too reactogenic (Fig. 26.11). A duck embryo vaccine was then developed but this proved to be relatively weak antigenically. The present vaccine consists of virus grown in human diploid cells (Fig. 26.12) and inactivated with β-propiolactone. It is used for pre-exposure prophylaxis (two doses, four weeks apart with a booster at 12 months) in those at special risk, for example workers in quarantine kennels, and also for post-exposure prophylaxis of those in contact with rabies. In the latter circumstance the treatment of choice is human diploid cell vaccine on days 0, 3, 7, 14, 30 and 90 in combination with human rabies immunoglobulin.

COMBINED ACTIVE AND PASSIVE IMMUNIZATION

There are a number of situations in which the most effective prophylaxis against an infectious disease involves a combination of active and passive immunization. This approach is used when exposure has, or probably has, already taken place. With tetanus-prone wounds in individuals who are not known to have been actively immunized it is recommended that human tetanus immunoglobulin be given. The first dose of a course of active immunization is given at the same time. Children born to mothers who are high-risk hepatitis B carriers (HBe antigen positive) should be given hepatitis B immunoglobulin within 48 hours of birth and a course of vaccine during the first six months of life. Passive immunization with human rabies immunoglobulin should be given in combination with vaccine after exposure to rabies since the protection afforded by immunoglobulin is immediate and covers the delay in the development of active immunization. Up to half the dose is locally infiltrated into the wound and the remainder is given intramuscularly.

The alternative use for combined active and passive immunization is in preventing side-effects of measles vaccine. Children with a history of convulsions or a family history of epilepsy should be immunized in the second year of life but only if the specially diluted human normal immunoglobulin for use with measles vaccine is given simultaneously.

Side-effects of vaccines

Almost all vaccines have some side-effects. These range from relatively minor local reactions, which are common, to more generalized non-specific illness. For example, most recipients of typhoid vaccine will have some local reaction of redness and swelling and some will feel feverish with myalgia and general malaise. A variety of immunopathological mechanisms may also lead to side-effects, for example allergy (commonly to egg proteins with vaccines manufactured in eggs), hypersensitivity (sometimes induced by multiple doses of tetanus toxoid) and cross-reactivity of antigens (the encephalopathy of early rabies vaccines). Finally, with live vaccines there is the possibility of organ-specific disease in rare instances (for example vaccine induced poliomyelitis). Consequently live vaccines are contraindicated in the immunosuppressed and in any group in which the risk of side-effects is known to be high (for example yellow fever vaccine under the age of one year).

Diseases without vaccines

In some instances immunization has been spectacularly successful in preventing disease. In the case of smallpox the disease has been entirely eliminated, although it is worth remembering that it was not mass vaccination that achieved this, but accurate identification of cases and the vaccination of the population in contact with them.

In spite of this success new vaccines and new approaches to vaccination are the subject of intense research and development. Fig. 26.13 lists some of the important diseases for which there is no satisfactory vaccine.

Evolution of rabies vaccine

Origin	Immunogenicity	Reactogenicity
rabbit brain	++	++
duck embryo	+	+
human cells	++	-

Fig. 26.11 Evolution of rabies vaccine.

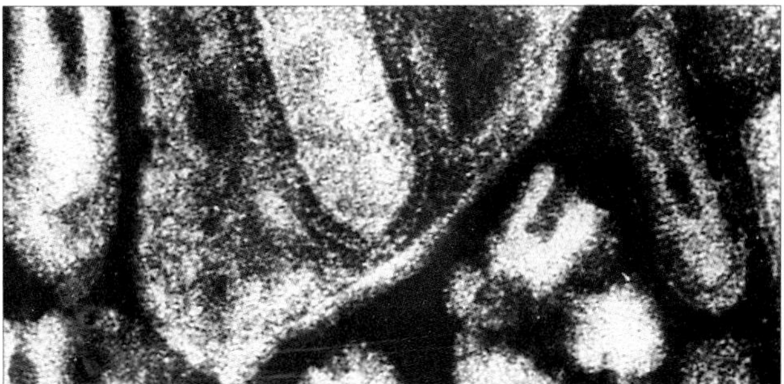

Fig. 26.12 Electron micrograph of rabies virus, showing characteristic bullet-shaped virions. Courtesy of Dr G M Scott.

Important infections or parasitic diseases for which there is no satisfactory vaccine

Micro-organism/parasite	Disease
HIV	AIDS
herpes simplex virus	genital infection
cytomegalovirus	effect on fetus
EB virus	glandular fever
varicella zoster virus	shingles (zoster)
Neisseria gonorrhoeae	gonorrhoea
Mycobacterium leprae	leprosy
Treponema pallidum	syphilis
Chlamydia trachomatis	trachoma
Plasmodium sp.	malaria
Trypanosoma sp.	trypanosomiasis
Schistosoma sp.	schistosomiasis

Fig. 26.13 Important infections or parasitic diseases for which there is no satisfactory vaccine.

Trends in new vaccines

INTRODUCTION

The great majority of the vaccines in use today were developed by empirical methods and without the benefits of the advances in our understanding of the structure and functioning of both the pathogens and of the mammalian immune system that have been made in recent years. Despite this they have had an enormous and highly cost-effective impact on the control of disease. Vaccines can be broadly separated into two categories:

- replicating, in which a live, attenuated strain of the pathogenic organism is used to infect the vaccinee;
- non-replicating, in which the pathogen (or toxic products thereof in the case of bacterial toxins) is inactivated by chemical or physical treatment while retaining its immunogenic properties.

There are a number of ways in which the new technologies developed in the last few years may lead to significant improvements in vaccine design. These include:

- development of vaccines against diseases for which none currently exist;
- reducing harmful side-effects caused by occasional reversion to increased virulence of live-attenuated organisms, or by contaminating impurities in inactivated vaccines;
- increasing stability during storage;
- overcoming the problems caused by antigenic variation exhibited by many pathogens;
- improving presentation so that, for example, fewer doses are required.

LIVE VACCINES

DIRECTED ATTENUATION

Among the drawbacks associated with live-attenuated virus vaccines are their frequent physical instability or their reversion to a more virulent form during replication in the vaccinee. This can also place non-immune contacts at risk of contracting disease. Although the incidence of vaccine related complications is extremely low, their importance far outweighs their statistical significance. Not only is a rare vaccine related condition, such as poliomyelitis, a tragedy for the individual concerned, it can also adversely influence the public attitude to vaccination when control programmes have reduced the incidence of natural disease.

Directed attenuation of bacteria

Considerable progress in the development of new attenuated bacterial vaccines has been achieved by the deletion, or introduction of non-reverting mutations into genes coding for key enzymes in metabolic pathways which are essential for the normal growth of the organisms in standard culture conditions or *in vivo*. Supplementation of the medium with metabolites which occur downstream in the pathway from the product normally produced by the mutated enzyme allows bacterial growth to continue.

Directed attenuation of viruses

Since viruses are obligate cell parasites and are almost entirely dependent on the host metabolic machinery the methods of attenuating bacteria mentioned in the previous section are, in general, not appropriate to viruses. Some of the more complex DNA viruses (for example herpes and pox viruses) do code for their own DNA-metabolizing enzymes, such as thymidylate kinase; inactivation of this enzyme has an attenuating effect on virulence, but little has been done to explore the potential of such modification for vaccine purposes.

Sabin polio vaccine. Only 10 nucleotide changes distinguish the attenuated polio 3 vaccine strain from its virulent progenitor and, only three of these result in amino acid substitutions.

The nucleic acid genomes of positive strand RNA viruses (for example poliovirus and human rhinovirus) are infectious in the free form. Full length clones of cDNA or RNA transcribed *in vitro* from such clones are also infectious and so it is possible to construct specific recombinations between cloned cDNA copies of different virus genomes and recover the corresponding mutated viruses (Fig. 26.14). Cloned cDNA is essential for these purposes since specific manipulations are virtually impossible with RNA molecules. Since only two mutations are responsible for the attenuation, one in the non-protein coding region at the 5′ end of the virus RNA, the function of which is not understood, and one in the virus capsid protein VP3, it is not surprising that vaccine related disease caused by reversion to virulence is most commonly associated with the polio 3 component. Considerably more mutations distinguish polio type 1 and 2 vaccine components from the wild type viruses.

Such detailed knowledge of the factors responsible for attenuation should facilitate the design and incorporation of attenuating changes which will less easily revert to the virulent phenotype.

LIVE VECTORS

The advantages of live vaccines make them attractive vectoring systems for the delivery of foreign antigens. This has been achieved by introducing genes coding for appropriate proteins into vaccine strains of bacteria or viruses by genetic engineering techniques.

Bacterial vectors

Considerable advances have been made in the development of stably mutated bacterial vaccine strains, especially *Salmonella*. Following oral administration, these organisms

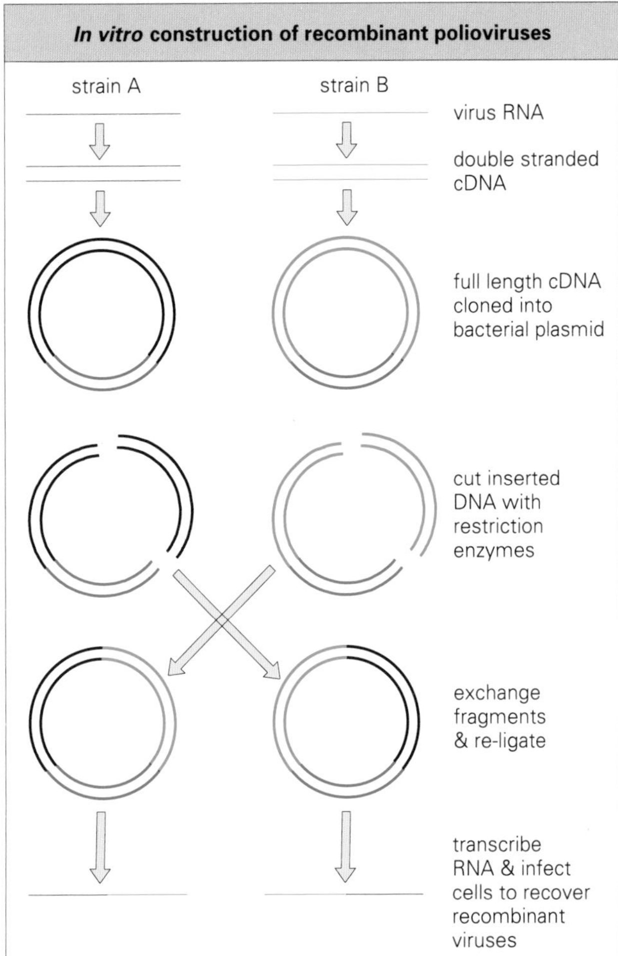

Fig. 26.14 *In vitro* construction of recombinant polioviruses. The RNA genomes of two strains of virus (e.g. polio) are converted to double stranded cDNA copies and cloned into bacterial plasmids. Specific fragments of the inserted DNAs are excised with appropriate restriction enzymes, purified by gel electrophoresis and re-joined (using DNA ligase) to produce recombinant plasmids. These are recovered by transfecting cells with the plasmids directly or, for greater efficiency, with RNA copies of virus sequences. To transcribe into RNA copies of the virus sequences *in vitro*, an appropriate promoter is incorporated into the plasmid, adjacent to the viral cDNA.

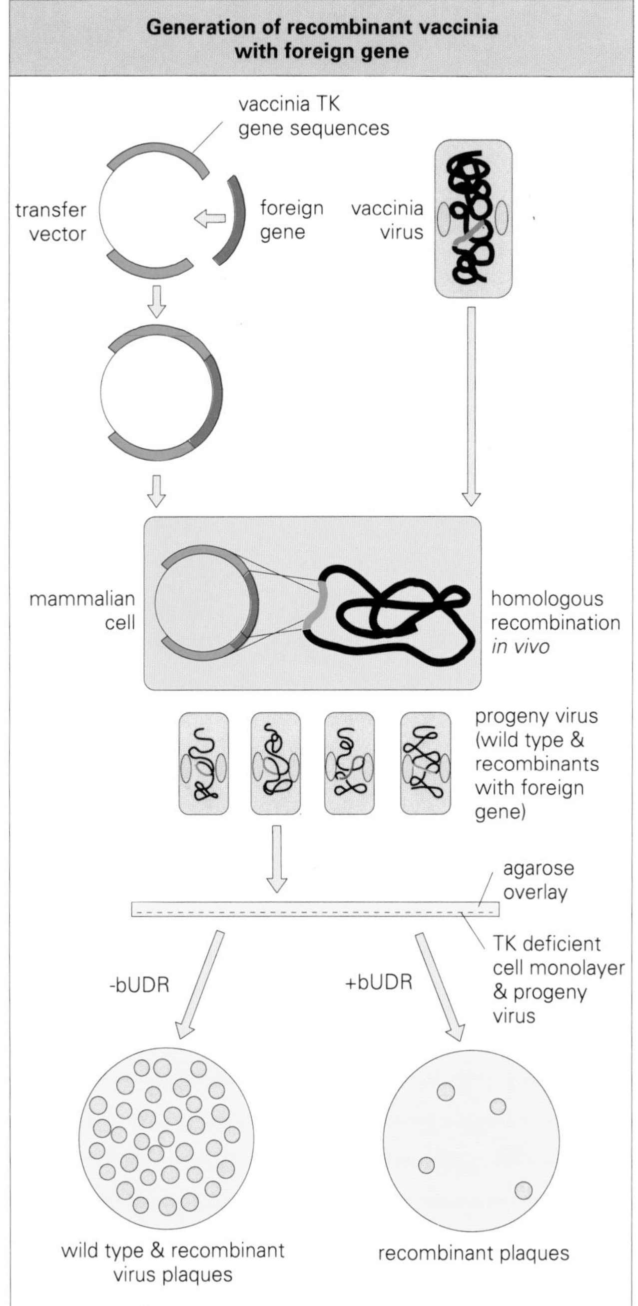

Fig. 26.15 Generation of recombinant vaccinia virus for the expression of a foreign gene. A foreign gene is inserted into the vaccinia genome so that immunization can be effected by both the vaccinia virus and recombinant antigen.

are taken up at the Peyers patches in the gut and reside in macrophages wherein they appear to undergo very limited replication. These properties make them ideal candidates as live carriers for the expression of antigenic proteins from other pathogenic organisms. Foreign genes can be incorporated into bacteria either as expression plasmids or in a more genetically stable form by insertion into the chromosome using homologous recombination.

Viral vectors

Vaccinia. The most widely explored live virus vectoring system involves insertional mutation of the vaccinia virus genome. Moss and Paoletti and their colleagues first described a method by which foreign genes could be incorporated by *in vivo* recombination into the viral DNA (Fig. 26.15). Bacterial plasmid vectors containing a foreign gene to be expressed, which is flanked by sequences of the thymidine kinase (TK) gene of vaccinia virus, can be introduced into cells infected with vaccinia virus. Occasionally homologous recombination occurs between the TK sequences in the plasmid and in the virus DNA,

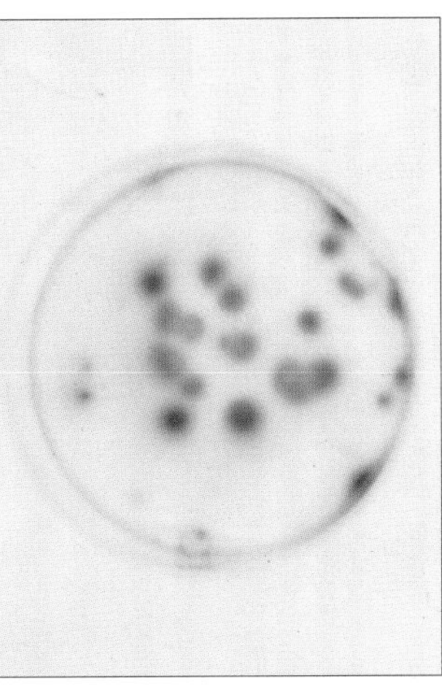

Fig. 26.16 Visualization of plaques formed by recombinant vaccinia virus expressing β-galactosidase. Monolayers of cells were infected with wild-type virus (left) or recombinant virus expressing the bacterial enzyme β-galactosidase (right). When plaques had developed, the presence of β-galactosidase was detected by the substrate X-gal, which is hydrolysed by the enzyme to form a blue product.

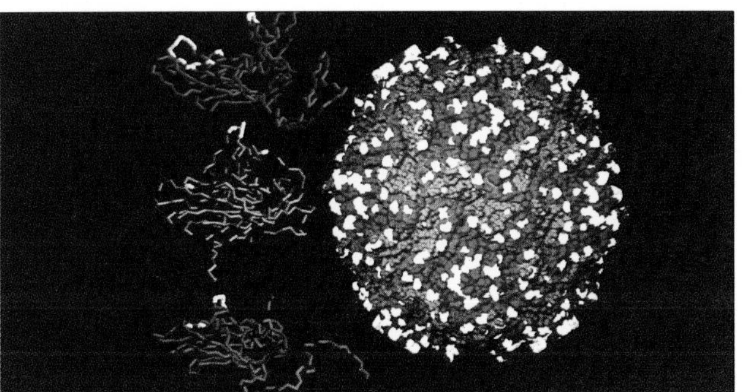

Fig. 26.17 Location of the antigenic determinants on poliovirus. The left side of the figure shows the folding of the back bone chains of the three major capsid proteins of poliovirus: VP1 (blue), VP2 (yellow) and VP3 (red). The positions of amino acid substitutions found in viruses which escape neutralization by a variety of monoclonal antibodies are highlighted in white. On the right is a representation of the surface of the virus particle using the same colour codes. The substituted amino acids are clustered into a number of antigenic sites which correspond to the most exposed regions on the virus. Courtesy of Dr J Hogle

resulting in insertion of the foreign gene and inactivation of the TK gene of the recombinant virus genome. The progeny virus is plated onto monolayers of cells deficient in TK activity. In the presence of bromodeoxyuridine (bUDR) wild-type virus with a functional TK gene does not replicate, since the nucleoside is phosphorylated and incorporated into DNA, resulting in inactivation. Consequently only recombinant or spontaneous TK mutant viruses survive to form plaques (Fig. 26.16).

Many proteins have been expressed in this way; and the method has become a useful research tool as well as a potential way of developing vaccines. An example of a specific application is the immunogenic rabies glycoprotein gene which has been incorporated into vaccinia virus. The recombinant has been shown to protect a number of mammalian species against challenge with a lethal dose of rabies virus.

Major obstacles

There is a relatively high frequency of side-effects associated with vaccinia virus itself. The most widely used site for insertion of foreign genes is into the sequence coding for thymidylate kinase. However, although this functionally inactivates the enzyme and appears to further attenuate the virus, there is still concern over the potential side-effects of the recombinant viruses. The validity of such concerns can only be determined by carefully monitored field trials. Recombinant virus vectors have also been constructed using adenoviruses, but again their usefulness in humans has yet to be established .

Recently, a live vectoring system has been developed by producing chimeric polioviruses. The antigenic sites of poliovirus (and a few other viruses) have been identified by a combination of epitope mapping and X-ray crystallography (Fig. 26.17). This has facilitated the construction of mutant viruses, in which antigenic loops have been replaced by sequences from foreign proteins (Fig. 26.18), and which thus express the antigenic properties of the foreign sequence as well as the unmodified poliovirus epitopes.

NON-REPLICATING VACCINES

EXPRESSION OF IMMUNOGENIC PROTEINS BY GENETIC ENGINEERING

With most microbial diseases protective immunity is correlated with the production of antibodies directed against a few, or sometimes just one protein of the outer coat of the pathogen. Consequently it was hoped that the production and purification of large amounts of immunogenic proteins would allow the rapid development of new vaccines, and with the advent of gene cloning and expression techniques, such an approach is feasible.

Expression in bacteria

Bacterial cells were first used for the large scale production of heterologous proteins. The key elements involved are:

- a source of DNA coding for the protein in question;
- a vector system in which the foreign DNA can be integrated and subsequently transferred into bacterial cells as a stable element replicating with the bacteria;
- genetic control elements which allow transcription and translation of the foreign gene to be switched on or off by manipulation of culture conditions.

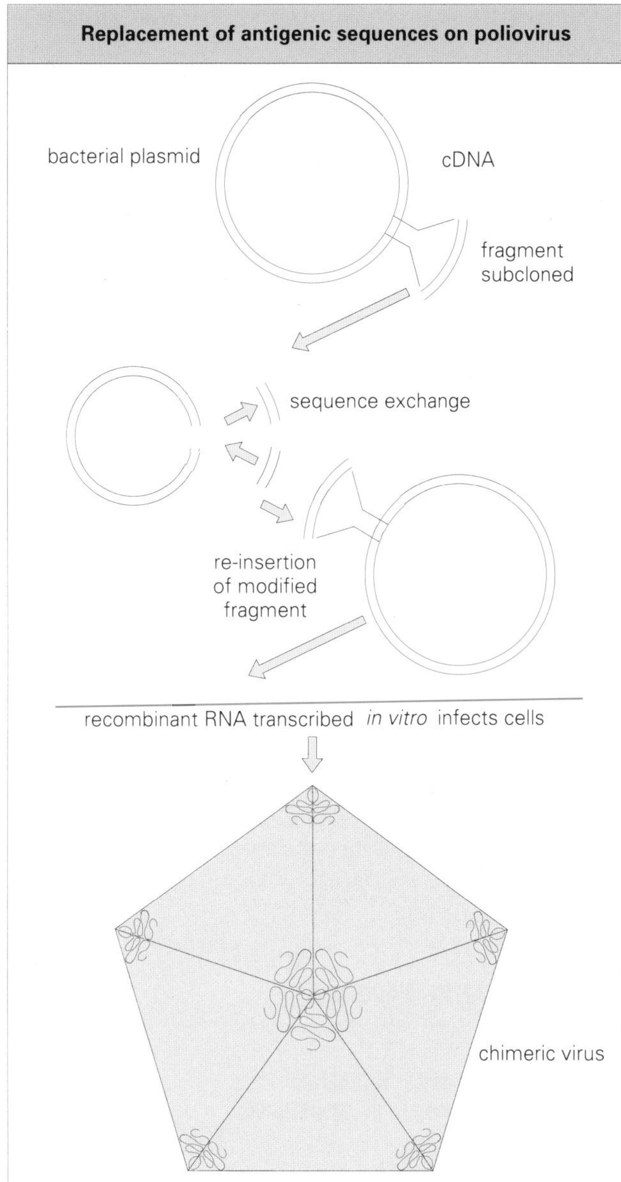

Fig. 26.18 Replacement of antigenic sequences on poliovirus. Chimeric viruses are produced in a similar way to recombinant viruses (see Fig. 26.14) except that the appropriate region of the virus cDNA is subcloned to facilitate the detailed genetic manipulations involved. The modified fragment is then re-inserted into the full length cDNA-bearing plasmid and the chimeric virus recovered by transfection of cells with the plasmid or *in vitro* transcribed RNA.

A combination of sophisticated bacterial genetics and nucleic acid manipulation has resulted in bacterial strains which produce up to 20% of their total protein as foreign gene product in a tightly controlled manner.

Problems with production of cloned protein. Most proteins of potential value as vaccines are membrane glycoproteins, characterized by specific hydrophobic sequences which are involved in directing and anchoring the proteins to lipid membranes. They also contain numerous glycosylation sites on the portions of the structure located outside the membrane and the folding of the molecules is stabilized with disulphide bonds. Such signal sequences , glycosylation sites and disulphide bonds do not generally occur in prokaryotic proteins and when eukaryotic membrane proteins are expressed in bacteria they are usually either toxic to the expressing cells or are proteolytically degraded and therefore inactive.

Foot and mouth disease virus (FMDV). A chimeric protein composed of FMDV VP1 fused to a bacterial protein (TrpE) has been shown to elicit virus neutralizing antibody and protects cattle from challenge with live virus in the same way as does VP1 produced from virus particles. However, the isolated VP1 protein is a very inefficient immunogen, being many orders of magnitude less effective than intact virus particles in inducing a protective response.

Expression in yeast cells

Yeasts combine ease of bulk culture with protein synthesis and processing machinery which shares features of mammalian cells. It is possible to produce biologically active protein products in yeast cells which cannot be expressed in a native form in bacteria.

Hepatitis B. The yeast derived surface antigen protein of hepatitis B virus (HBsAg), has been commercially available since 1985 and is the first vaccine product of genetic engineering technology to reach the marketplace.

One drawback of yeast-derived vaccines is the sensitivityof some vaccinees to minute quantitiesof yeast products in the vaccine.

Expression in mammalian cells

Proteins produced in mammalian cells resemble those present on normal virus particles. The steps involved in the synthesis, transport and post-translational modification of a typical membrane glycoprotein are shown in Fig. 26.19. The important features of a typical membrane glycoprotein are the presence of hydrophobic sequence domains at each end of the protein and a number of sequences which signal the covalent addition of complex carbohydrate structures to the protein. Most surface glycoproteins are anchored at the cell membrane via a carboxyl terminal sequence of hydrophobic amino acids which span the lipid bilayer. Deletion of the anchor sequence gives rise to a protein which is secreted into the medium and this can have great advantages in the purification of the product. A number of systems are available for the expression of proteins in mammalian cells.

Expression in insect cells

A more recent addition to the genetic engineer's armoury of expression systems capitalises on particular features of a group of viruses of invertebrates, the baculoviruses. One of the gene products of these viruses, the protein polyhedrin, forms insoluble aggregates (polyhedra) within infected cells and newly formed virus particles become

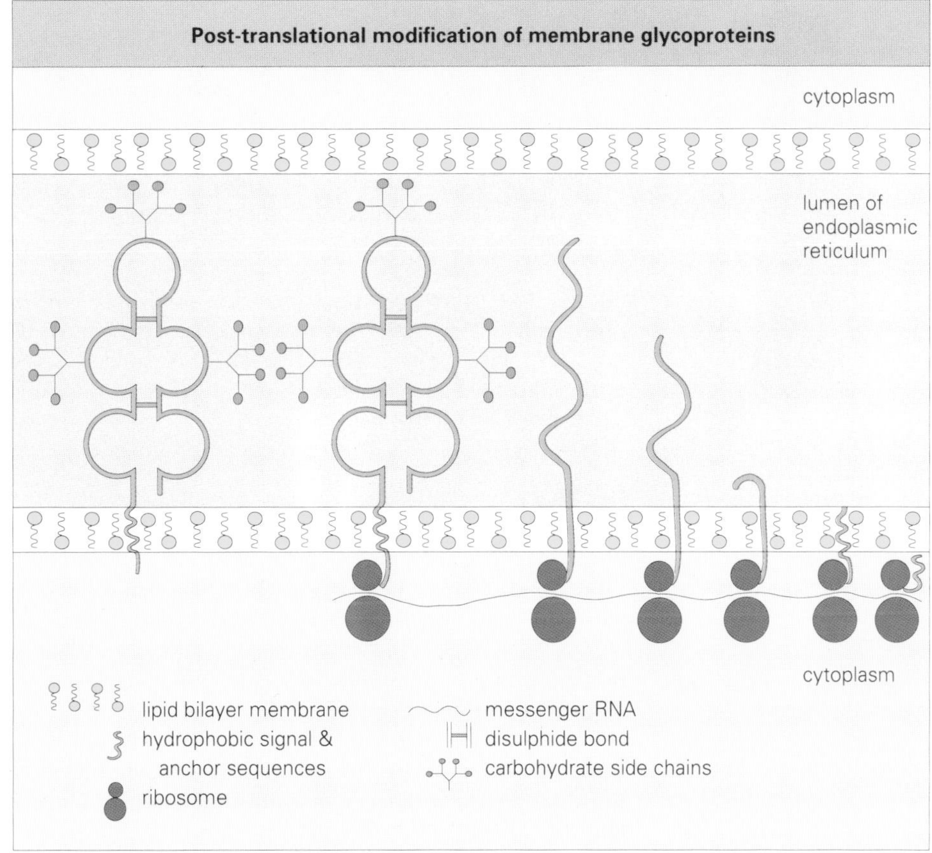

Fig. 26.19 Post-translational modification and translocation of membrane glycoproteins. The hydrophobic domain at the amino (N) terminus of the protein associates with the lipid membrane of the Golgi apparatus before translation of the protein is completed. The remainder of the protein chain is inserted through the membrane during synthesis and is anchored by the carboxyl (C) terminal hydrophobic sequence which spans the lipid bilayer. The N terminal signal sequence is cleaved off from the mature polypeptide chain. A complex and specific series of side-chain glycosylation events and disulphide linkages occur before the completed glycoprotein is transported to the plasma membrane of the cell.

embedded, or occluded, within these aggregates (Fig. 26.20). The natural function of polyhedra is to protect the virus particles from environmental damage, for example from UV light, before they are ingested by a new host insect. Polyhedrin is expressed in extraordinarily large amounts due to the strength of the promoter controlling transcription of the polyhedrin gene. This promoter is, therefore, a very attractive candidate as a control element for the production of foreign proteins.

Many proteins have now been produced in insect cells using recombinant baculovirus vectors, and in some cases very high levels of expression have been achieved (Fig. 26.21).

SYNTHETIC PEPTIDE VACCINES

Short peptide sequences can induce antibodies that recognize the protein from which they are derived. This was first shown by Anderer in 1963, who derived a peptide from the coat protein of tobacco mosaic virus which, when coupled to a protein carrier, induced antibodies that neutralized the virus. This approach was further explored by Sela and his colleagues using sequences from the coat protein of the bacteriophage MS2. The application of this technology to the development of novel vaccines for animal and human diseases could not proceed further until the advent of nucleic acid cloning and sequencing in the 1970s made it readily possible to predict the amino acid sequences of relevant proteins.

Solid phase technique

The most commonly used method for chemical synthesis of peptides is the solid phase technique pioneered by Merrifield. Peptides of 15-20 amino acids synthesized in this way and coupled to a carrier protein frequently

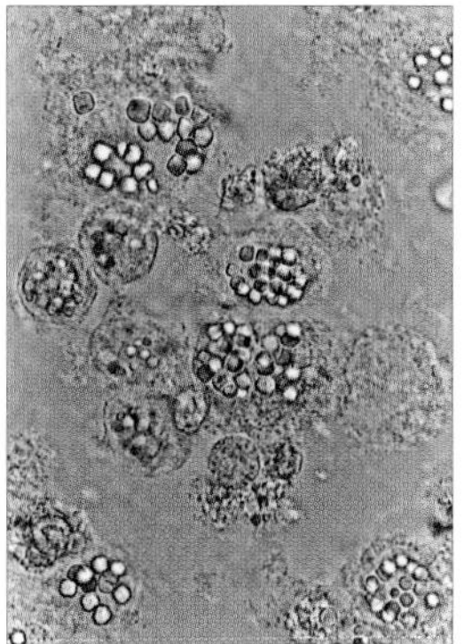

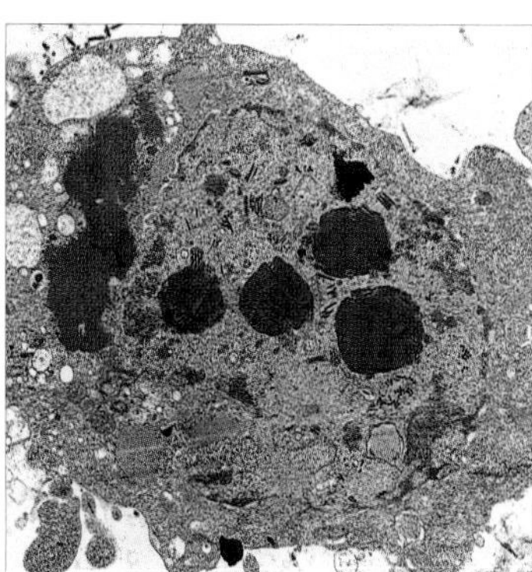

Fig. 26.20 Baculovirus polyhedra. Left: polyhedra can be seen in the nuclei of insect cells infected with baculovirus. Right: high power view of infected insect cell showing the inclusion of virus particles within polyhedrin.

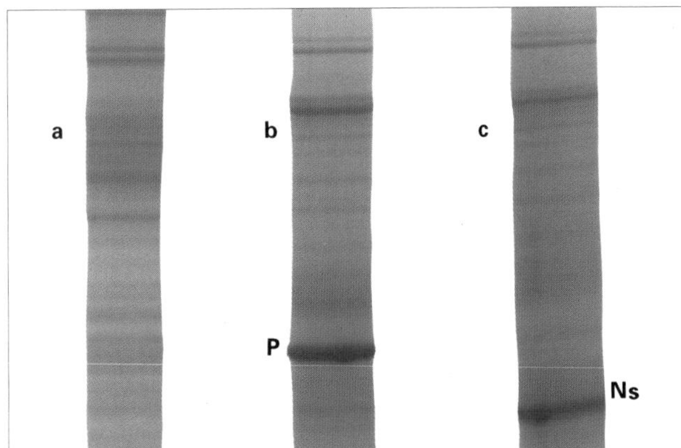

Fig. 26.21 High-level expression of a foreign protein by a recombinant baculovirus. Protein extracts of a) uninfected insect cells, b) wild-type baculovirus, and c) recombinant baculovirus, in which the gene for the Ns protein of Puntatora virus was inserted in the baculovirus polyhedrin gene, are separated by polyacrylamide gel electrophoresis and the proteins stained. P is polyhedrin protein.

induce antibodies which recognize the denatured form of the protein from which their sequence was obtained. The induction by peptides of antibodies capable of recognizing the native form of a protein is more difficult Firstly, only those amino acids which are represented at the surface of the protein can be expected to be involved in antibody binding; furthermore, some regions of a protein surface are more important than others in terms of their immunodominance and biological significance of antibody binding, for example neutralization of infectivity.

Antigenic sites

It is not sufficient to determine the sequence of a protein in order to produce immunogenic peptides; the location of the important antigenic sites must be determined. The methods that have been used to locate such sites include:

- determination of the position of amino acid substitutions conferring resistance to neutralization by monoclonal antibodies;
- comparison of the sequences of naturally occurring antigenic variants;
- predictions of physicochemical features such as hydrophilicity;
- determining the immunogenicity of defined fragments of the protein.

Even with linear antigenic sites, a short synthetic peptide will not necessarily adopt the secondary structure which the same sequence has when it forms part of a native protein. Determination of the preferred structure of short peptides and the exploration of methods of inducing defined structural features in synthetic peptides are currently receiving much attention.

Tertiary structure

26.14 The majority of antigenic sites on proteins are not linear

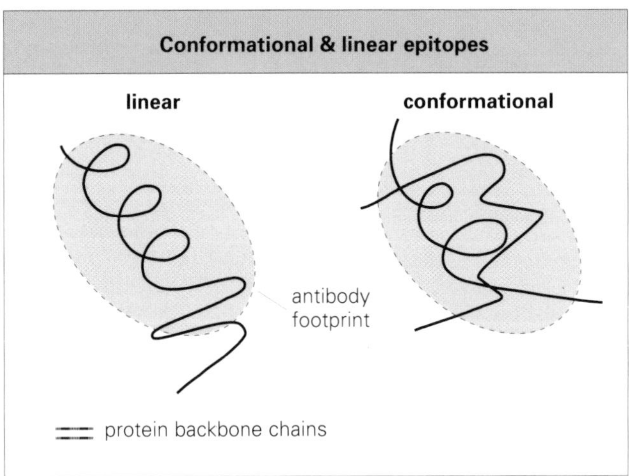

Fig. 26.22 Conformational and linear epitopes. A linear epitope is composed of amino acids comprising a continuous stretch of protein sequence. A conformational epitope is formed from amino acids from different regions of a protein, separated on the linear sequence, or from different polypeptide chains, which are brought together in the tertiary or quaternary structure of the protein. Very few antigenic epitopes on native proteins are entirely composed of linear sequences.

but complex, composed of amino acids brought into juxtaposition by the folding of the protein chain (Fig. 26.22). There is therefore a problem in synthesizing linear sequences which mimic the activity of the whole complex.

Protective function

Synthetic peptides have been shown to elicit neutralizing, and in some cases protective, responses in a number of systems. The most promising at present is that from foot and mouth disease virus. A synthetic sequence of VP1 can induce protective responses in laboratory animals when linked to carrier protein or injected as free peptide (Fig. 26.23). The uncoupled peptide is active because it includes sequences capable of inducing TH activity, which is required in the development of an antibody response (Fig. 26. 24).

ANTI-IDIOTYPE VACCINES

The anti-idiotype approach to novel vaccine development relies on the complementary nature of the interaction between an antigen and the combining site of antibody recognizing that antigen (Fig. 26.25). The antigen binding site (idiotope) of an antibody (Ab1) is effectively a mirror image of the epitope on the antigen recognized by that antibody. Consequently antibodies (Ab2) recognizing the idiotope of Ab1 resemble the original antigen and can, therefore, act as surrogate antigens capable of inducing antibodies (Ab3) of similar specificity to Ab1, (i.e. Ab1 and Ab3 both recognize the original antigen). Although induction of antibodies capable of combining with the original antigen by injecting anti-idiotypic antibodies has

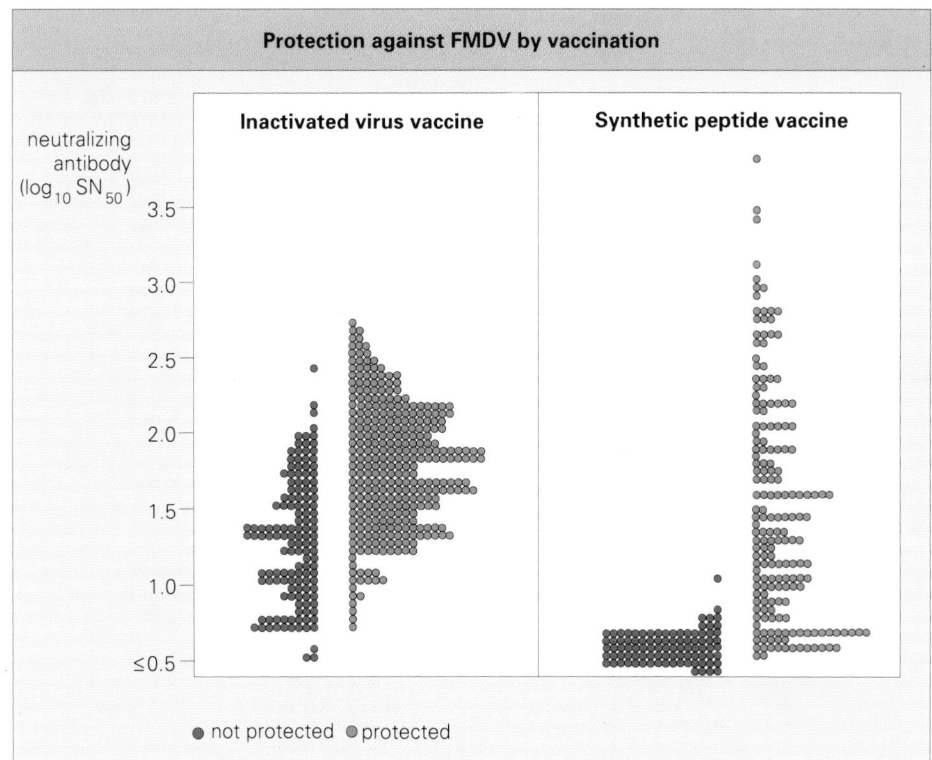

Fig. 26.23 Protection of experimental animals (guinea pigs) against challenge with foot and mouth disease virus after vaccination with inactivated virus or synthetic peptide. Each point represents a single animal. The vertical scale represents the neutralizing antibody titre of sera at the time of challenge. Protection induced by the synthetic peptide vaccine correlates better with the neutralization titre than that induced by whole virus, suggesting that the peptide induces a more uniform spectrum of protective antibodies.

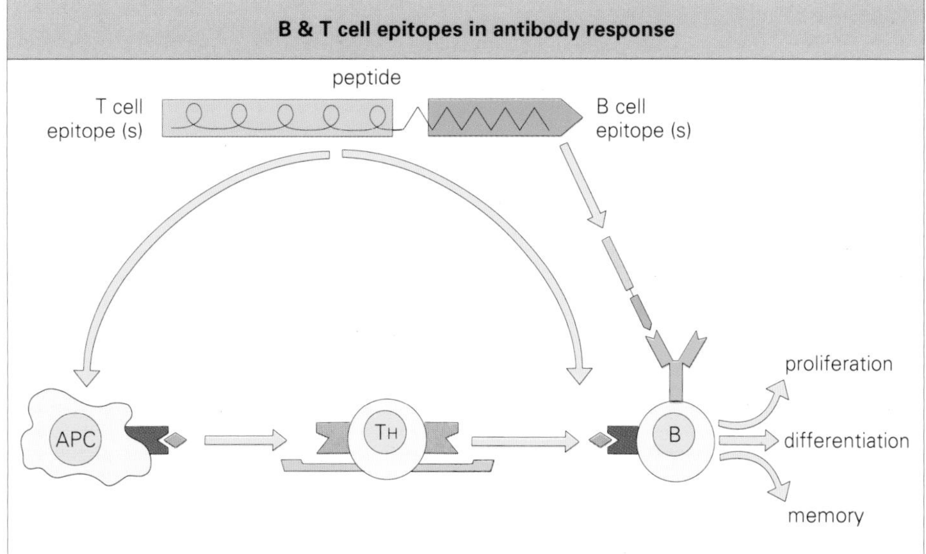

Fig. 26.24 The role of B and T cell epitopes in the induction of an antibody response to a synthetic peptide vaccine. Amino acid sequences capable of eliciting antibodies of a desired specificity (B cell epitopes) are non-immunogenic in the absence of sequences which can bind the MHC class II proteins (T_H epitopes) and elicit a response. The primed T cells recognize the T_H epitope presented by B cells, which trap the peptide via their surface immunoglobulin. T_H cells provide the signals required to stimulate B cell proliferation and differentiation into antibody-secreting plasma cells.

been demonstrated in several systems, the responses are low and often critically dependent on the dose of anti-idiotypic antibody. In practice this approach will probably have more impact in the therapeutic area (e.g. autoimmunity) than in the development of vaccines .

ANTIGEN PRESENTATION

Ideally, a vaccine should induce high levels of humoral antibody of the appropriate specificity, a long-lasting memory response, secretory antibody, and possibly a cytotoxic T cell response. Generally antibodies are important for the prevention of infection and cytotoxic cells are involved in the eradication of established infections. Non-replicating antigens, such as killed virus particles, need to be formulated with adjuvants to induce a good antibody response and are generally unable to induce a cytotoxic response mediated by $CD8^+$ lymphocytes.

Adjuvants

The mode of action of adjuvants is complex and poorly understood but two main features seem to be important.

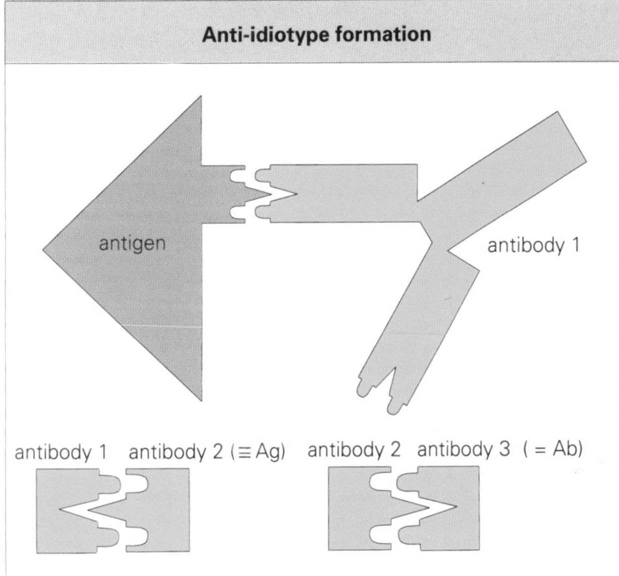

Fig. 26.25 Anti-idiotype formation. This relies on the fact that the unique structure of the hypervariable region of an antibody represents a novel feature (idiotope) to the immune system. It is therefore not seen as self and elicits the formation of antibodies (anti-idiotypes) which recognize this domain. A part of the hypervariable region (idiotope) will represent the antigen combining site (paratope) of the antibody and anti-idiotype antibodies recognizing the paratope of antibody 1 will, in effect, be surrogate antigens. A repetition of the cycle using antibody 2 as antigen results in the production of antibody 3, which is functionally equivalent to antibody 1.

First, a depot of antigen is produced resulting in its slow release and second, a local inflammatory response is induced by stimulation of lymphokine production, resulting in the recruitment of lymphocytes to the site of injection (see chapter 28).

The most effective is Freund's complete adjuvant, in which the antigen is emulsified with an oil in the presence of *Mycobacterium* cell walls, but the side-effects caused by this adjuvant precludes its use for practical vaccines. The acceptable adjuvant for human vaccines is aluminium hydroxide gel. Since subunit vaccines are less immunogenic than whole organisms it is particularly important to develop methods to enhance responses if genetically engineered or synthetic vaccines are to be developed, and a variety of systems are being studied.

Polymeric presentation

Incorporation of proteins or peptides into larger polymeric structures generally improves their immunogenicity. For example virus glycoproteins elicit better responses when incorporated into liposomes (Fig. 26.26) or complexed in a micellar form with the glycoside Quil A (Fig. 26.27). The immunogenicity of peptides is considerably enhanced by incorporation into synthetic polymeric constructs or by including them in biosynthetic fusion constructions with proteins capable of self-assembly into particles (Fig. 26.28) .

Slow-release systems

Effective responses to vaccines usually require a primary injection followed by boosters. Incorporation of part of

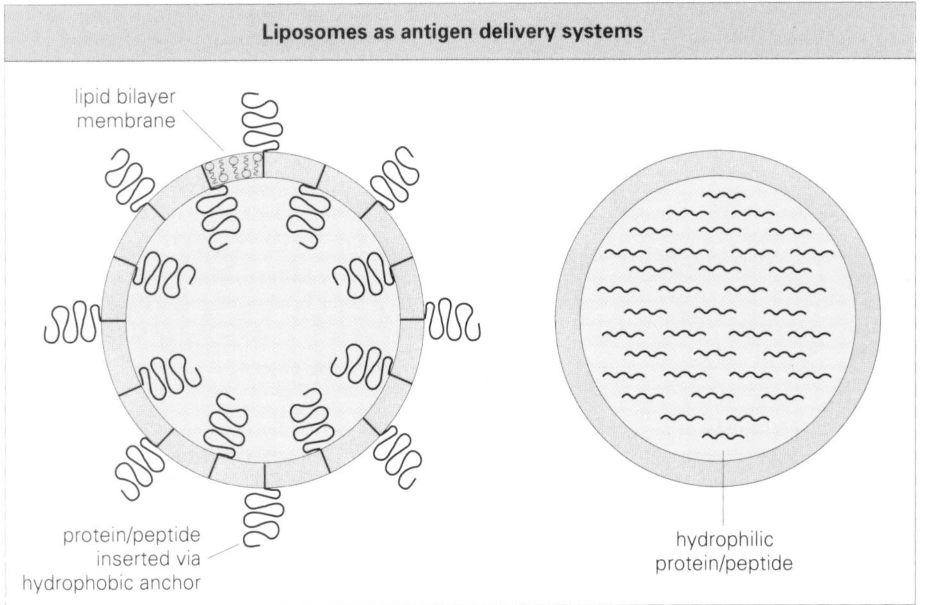

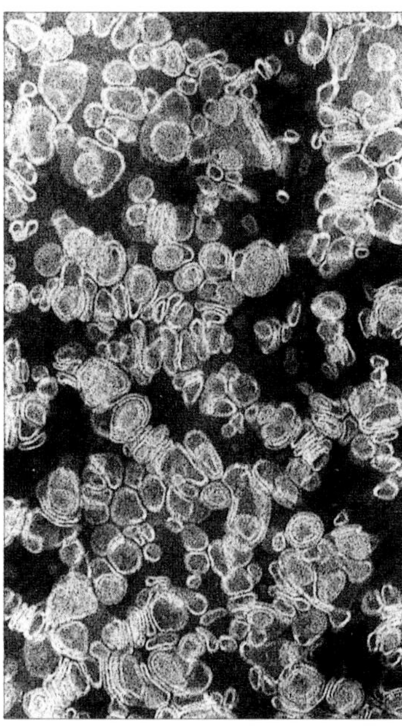

26.16 **Fig. 26.26** Liposomes as antigen delivery systems. Antigens containing hydrophobic domains, such as membrane glycoproteins or synthetic peptides linked to a fatty acid, can be inserted into the lipid bilayer membranes of liposomes to increase the size and epitope density of the immunogenic structure. Alternatively, hydrophilic antigens can be incorporated within the fluid lumen of liposomes. The latter method has obviated the requirement for conventional adjuvants in experimental peptide vaccines. The electron micrograph shows the appearance of unilamellar liposomes.

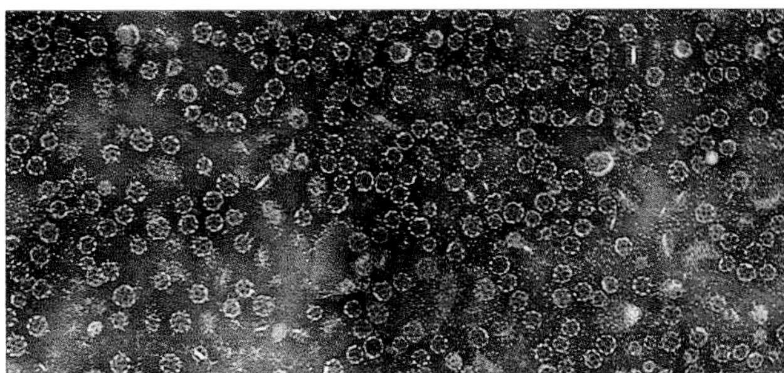

Fig. 26.27 Electron micrograph of immune stimulatory complexes (ISCOMS). These cage-like structures are formed by complexing protein with the glycoside Quil A, and have been shown to greatly enhance the immune response to the complexed protein.

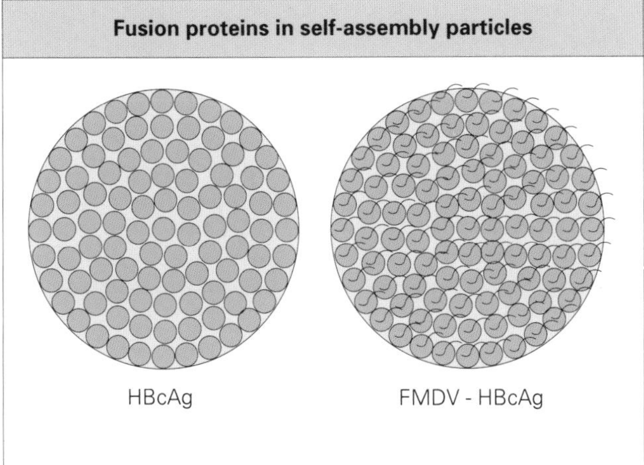

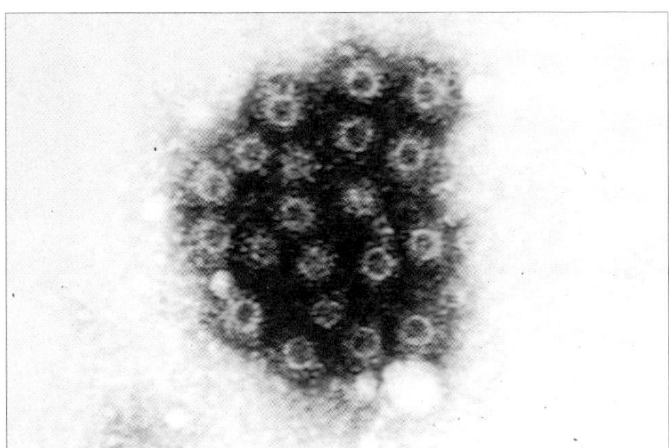

Fig. 26.28 Expression of fusion proteins capable of assembly into polymeric structures. Some virus proteins have the innate property of self assembly into spherical particles (e.g. the core protein of hepatitis B virus — HBcAg). Antigenic sequences can be fused to the termini or inserted within such proteins, without interfering with their assembly properties, resulting in particles displaying a high density of the added epitopes at their surfaces. Lower: EM of hepatitis B core particles carrying a peptide sequence from foot and mouth disease virus (FMDV). The particles are complexed with anti-FMDV antibody.

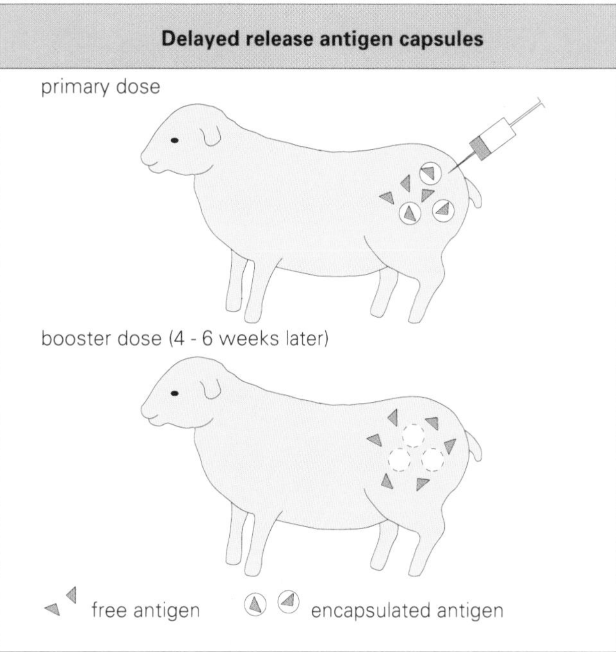

Fig. 26.29 Delayed antigen release capsules. The capsules are injected with free antigen as the primary dose. Ideally, the capsules should dissolve 4-8 weeks after vaccination to provide optimal boosting of the antibody response.

the antigen in the primary dose in a slow or pulsed release form may allow priming and boosting doses to be included in a single injection (Fig. 26.29). Peptide vaccines are ideally suited to this approach since they would not be thermally inactivated in the body prior to release. Examples of materials which are suitable for constructing slow release capsules are biodegradable polymers (e.g. lactic and glycollic acid co-polymers) and soluble glass.

Targeting

The immunogenicity of antigens may be increased by directing them to specific cells of the immune system. Encouraging results have been obtained by linking antigens to monoclonal antibodies recognizing MHC class II proteins. As more is learned about the surface proteins specific to certain cell types it may be possible to design synthetic ligands for targeting purposes.

Topical application

Non-replicating vaccines which are effective when applied to mucosal surfaces (e.g. oral or intranasal) would have logistic advantages and may induce secretory immunity. Some success has been reported but the problems of designing an antigen which can efficiently traverse the mucosal membrane without damage are great. Although an attempt has been made here to categorise the approaches to improvements of vaccine immunogenicity this is too simplistic. Most 'adjuvanting' systems work by a combination of mechanisms .

FURTHER READING

Battle JL, Murphy FL, eds. *Vaccine biotechnology*. London: Academic Press, 1989.

Fields BN, ed. *Virology*. New York: Raven Press, 1985.

Zuckerman AJ, Banatvala JE, Pattison JR, eds. *Principles and practice of clinical virology (2E)*. Chichester: John Wiley & Sons, 1990.

Modern vaccines. 1. *Lancet*. 1990; **i**: 448–451.This is the first of 17 weekly articles covering all aspects of modern vaccines.

Coldspring Harbor Meetings. *Vaccines: 1984. Modern approaches to vaccines. Vaccines: 1985. Vaccines 1986*, etc.

Synthetic peptides as antigens. Ciba symposium. 1986; 119.

27

Immunosuppression

INTRODUCTION

The clinical necessity to suppress immune responses applies both to the prevention of graft rejection in organ and tissue transplantation and to the treatment of autoimmunity. Indeed, as our understanding of the immune system improves, an immune aetiology is incriminated in more and more diseases.

It is not difficult to suppress the immune system. One thousand rads whole body irradiation will satisfactorily eradicate most immune responses. Such treatment, however, inevitably leads to the death of the recipient from overwhelming and multiple infections, often from the most innocuous of micro-organisms (Fig. 27.1).

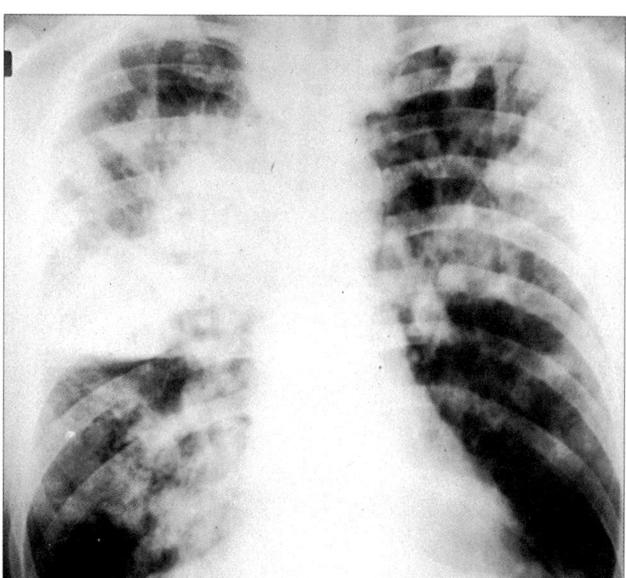

Fig. 27.1 Aspergillus pneumonia. This immunosuppressed patient developed increasing breathlessness and bilateral shadowing was found on radiographic investigation. *A. fumigatus* was detected in sputum samples and autopsy showed extensive invasive aspergillosis. Courtesy of Dr I D Starke.

The skill in successfully managing clinical immunosuppression is to be able to suppress the undesired immune response while leaving the patient enough immune competence to combat successfully such overwhelming infections. Attempts to maintain this balance between infection and rejection (Fig. 27.2) have led to the development of more and more specific immunosuppressive protocols, each designed to maximize the efficiency with which one component of the immune system is compromised while minimizing the effect on the other components of our immunological repertoire.

IRRADIATION

The application of immunosuppression induced by ionising irradiation was first attempted in the late 1950s when prospective renal allograft recipients were treated with whole body irradiation. However, it was found that the irradiation dose required to produce allograft prolongation caused such severe bone marrow and gastrointestinal damage that this form of treatment was abandoned when pharmaceutical immunosuppression was introduced.

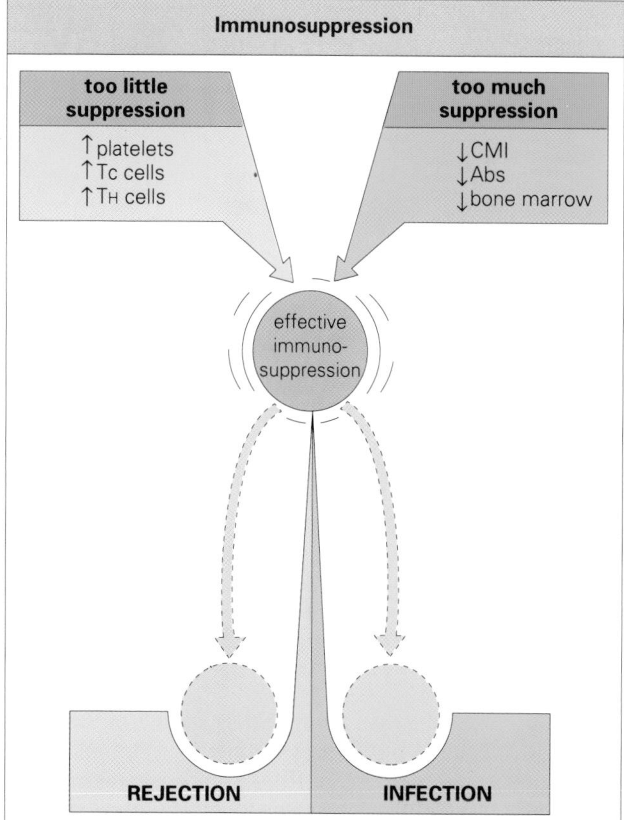

Fig. 27.2 Effective immunosuppression is difficult to achieve. Too much will lead to infection, while not enough allows rejection of the graft.

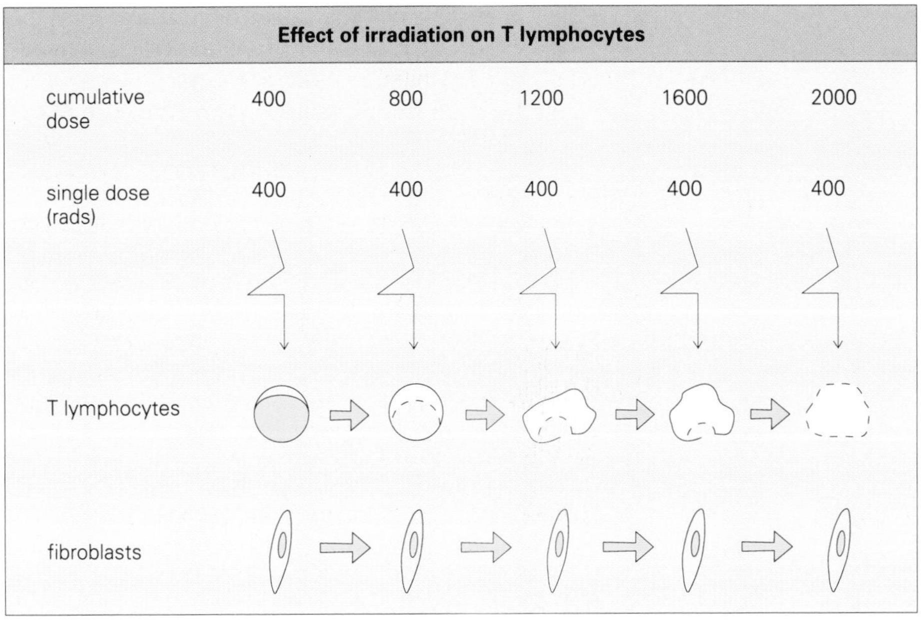

Effect of irradiation on T lymphocytes

cumulative dose	400	800	1200	1600	2000
single dose (rads)	400	400	400	400	400
T lymphocytes					
fibroblasts					

Fig. 27.3 Repair of radiation damage occurs between each exposure in non-lymphoid cells (e.g. fibroblasts). T lymphocytes receive effectively a cumulative dose which results in their destruction. The mechanism by which this cell death is induced is not yet fully understood.

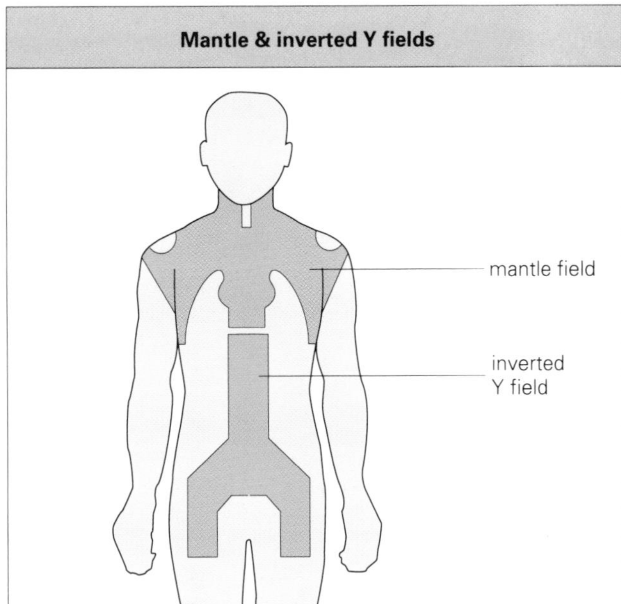

Fig. 27.4 The inverted Y and mantle fields consist of a series of lead aprons placed over the sternum, part of the pelvis and gonads, shielding the minimal amount of bone marrow to allow repopulation of the lymphoid system after irradiation.

Over the intervening years, our understanding of the fundamental biological mechanisms underlying the effect of ionising irradiation on cells, tissues and organisms has improved considerably. Most cells killed by ionising irradiation die as a result of lesions produced in DNA which cause death during attempted mitotic divisions. Many of these lesions, notably base damage and single strand breaks, may be repaired by enzymes in advance of any attempted division. Radiation damages large and small molecules indiscriminately and has no selective effect on DNA; it is the unique role of this molecule in cell replication that confers a particular significance to the lesion induced in it.

Radiosensitive lymphocytes

There is a population of highly radiosensitive cells, including the small resting lymphocyte, which die as a result of radiation damage during interphase (Fig. 27.3). Thus, although radiation doses fractionated over several days allow repair to occur in most cells between successive exposures, no such repair occurs in the radiosensitive cell population and an almost linear dose–response curve can be achieved. This peculiar characteristic of the small lymphocyte led to treatment by fractionated radiation therapy of Hodgkin's disease; this has proved a highly effective procedure for an otherwise fatal condition. The necessity of treating all involved lymph nodes, however, required an expansion in the size of the field irradiated, which resulted in the use of the 'mantle field' (Fig. 27.4); this shields the protected areas from which the lymphoid system is subsequently repopulated. It was found that most patients could tolerate the very high doses of irradiation (up to 4,000 rads total dose) remarkably well and such total lymphoid irradiation (TLI) made it possible to offer a cure for at least 70% of all patients with a once invariably fatal disease.

Total lymphoid irradiation

There has been no clinical evidence that patients treated with TLI have any overall impairment of their immunity. However, it has been demonstrated that patients receiving this treatment have a severe and substantial deficiency in their T cell function (Fig. 27.5).

The clinical use of TLI has been restricted to a few centres, where it is used either to prevent graft rejection or as a therapy for intractable rheumatoid arthritis. Side-effects from this treatment are common and can be severe (Fig. 27.6). Despite these risks and the substantial costs involved, however, the use of TLI as a therapy should not be dismissed out of hand. There are certain poorly understood characteristics of the treatment which may prove to be of value. Although the clinical role for this regimen is unclear, once the initial conditioning phase is completed, TLI is thought to produce a long-lasting, selective effect on the function (and possibly the number) of T helper cells. It is also associated with the appearance of non-specific suppressor cells.

Effects of TLI on immune function
↓circulating T cells
reversal of $CD4^+$: $CD8^+$cell ratio
↓mixed lymphocyte reaction
↓responses to mitogens
loss of delayed type hypersensitivity responses

Fig. 27.5 These observations have led to the use of TLI as an immunosuppressive treatment.

Side-effects of TLI
↑risk of infection
leucopenia
thrombocytopenia
nausea
vomiting
↑risk of lymphoma

Fig. 27.6 The non-specific nature of the conditioning phase can lead to a high risk of infection.

It has been reported that TLI can be used to establish chimerism prior to organ grafting when donor type bone marrow is infused (Fig. 27.7). It is a curiosity that TLI can prevent graft-versus-host disease from occurring in such a situation since the grafted marrow has not undergone any therapeutic procedure. If reproduced reliably in the clinic, such chimerism could have major implications for the treatment of a variety of different conditions.

PHARMACOLOGICAL IMMUNOSUPPRESSION

PURINE ANALOGUES

In 1959 Schwartz and Damashek demonstrated that the purine analogue anti-metabolite 6-mercaptopurine (6-MP) suppressed the immune response in rabbits to foreign proteins. Subsequently Calne showed that 6-mercaptopurine profoundly immunosuppressed kidney graft rejection in the mongrel dog but, in contrast to the observation of Schwartz and Damashek, the effect did not persist after withdrawal of drug therapy.

In an effort to modify the toxic effects of 6-mercaptopurine, azathioprine was developed by Hitchings and Ellion (Fig 27.8). This is a combination of 6-MP to which an imidazole ring has been added (Fig. 27.9). This imidazole ring is cleaved from the inactive compound by the

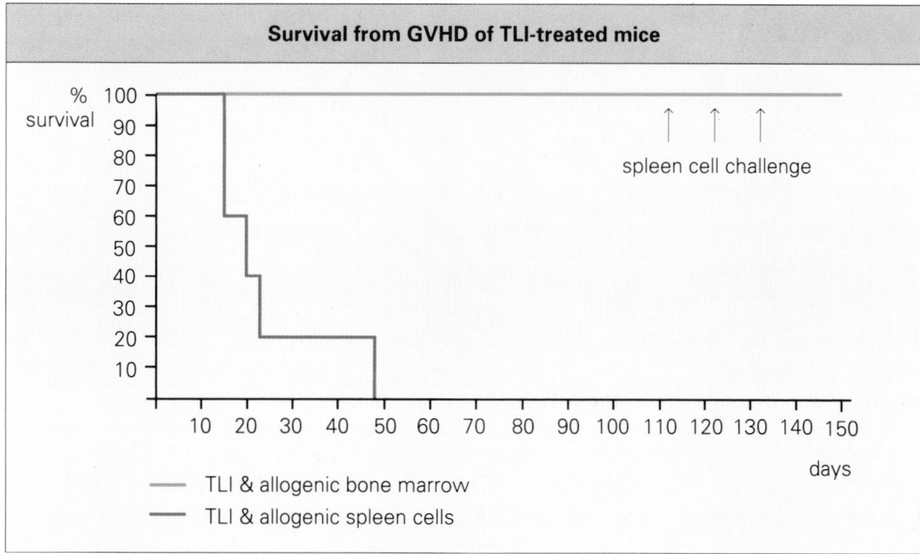

Fig. 27.7 Mice treated with TLI (3400 rads) were given either allogeneic bone marrow or spleen cells. Those given spleen cells died of graft-versus-host disease (GVHD): those given bone marrow survived. Subsequent challenge of these chimeric mice with allogeneic spleen cells failed to induce GVHD.

action of liver enzymes, thus releasing active 6-MP. Azathioprine has been actively marketed as an immunosuppressive and as such has been preferred to the 'cytotoxic' 6-MP. However, there is little evidence to suggest that in man one drug offers significant advantages over the other.

It must of course be appreciated that a given dose of azathioprine releases approximately 50% by weight of active 6-MP, so that doses must be adjusted accordingly before comparison can be made. 6-MP is said to exert its immunosuppressive effect by transforming into thioinosinic acid, which then blocks DNA synthesis in the actively dividing cell.

Target cells

Although the target for azathioprine is the small lymphocyte, the blockade of the actively dividing cell is ubiquitous. This gives rise to the major toxic effects of azathioprine — leucopenia, hepatotoxicity, and hair loss. With large doses myelotoxicity can be substantial, otherwise the side-effects are dose dependent and controllable. However, there is now a considerable amount of data to show that 6-MP can cause malignancy.

Thus, in principle, the drug works by killing only the activated lymphocyte clones. It can, however, produce profound leucopenia and doses are often determined by monitoring white blood cell counts. Azathioprine has also been reported to possess an anti-inflammatory component but this seems to be linked to the severity of the leucopenia.

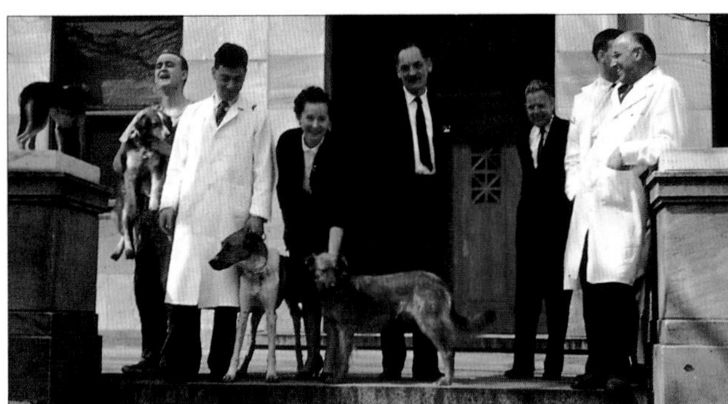

Fig. 27.8 Professors Calne and Murray and Drs Ellion and Hitchings with some of the first dogs to have successful renal transplants with azathioprine treatment.

STEROIDS

Corticosteroids form an important and often the sole component of most immunosuppressive regimens. In support of the axiom that today's medicine is tomorrow's science, and despite the extensive clinical experience with these drugs, the mode of action of steroids in immunomodulation remains largely unresolved.

Part of the reason for this lack of understanding is the large number of different biological functions which corticosteroids possess. Thus for any given clinical condition, it can be difficult to evaluate which action or combination of actions is responsible for any beneficial effects observed. In addition to their well-known anti-inflammatory properties, corticosteroids have a stabilizing effect on membranes which can reduce the ability of the immune system to present antigen. This can also cause changes in patterns of cell traffic. In particular, there are marked changes in T cell distribution, with a greatly diminished number appearing in the circulation. Steroids can also slow down cell division and may influence the overall size of the lymphocyte pool. It should be stressed, however, that extensive studies have failed to identify consistent sub-set deficiencies which could be accounted for by steroid treatment. The major effects of the various immunosuppressive drugs are shown in Fig. 27.10.

Choice of steroid

There are a variety of different steroid preparations available of which the most commonly used is prednisone and its derivative prednisolone (Fig. 27.11). Long-acting preparations such as dexamethasone and beta-methasone may be of use for short-term therapy but need to be avoided in chronic treatment because of their tendency to induce adrenal atrophy. There is some evidence to suggest that fluocortolone is less likely to produce as marked a Cushing's syndrome as an equipotent dose of prednisone (Fig. 27.12). Hydrocortisone and methyl-prednisolone are favoured for intravenous administration. Adrenocorticotropic hormone (ACTH) is rarely used because the amount of steroid release that it stimulates is unreliable and varies from patient to patient.

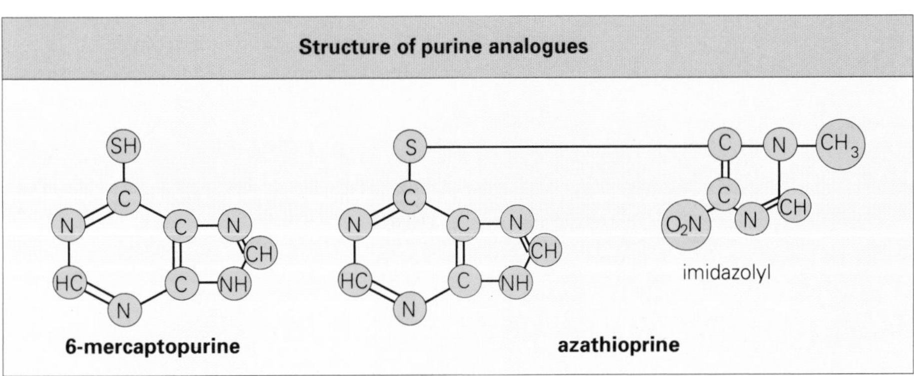

Fig. 27.9 6-MP proved an effective immunosuppressant in dogs with kidney transplants, but was found to be toxic to liver and bone marrow. Azathioprine is as immunosuppressive as 6-MP, but less toxic.

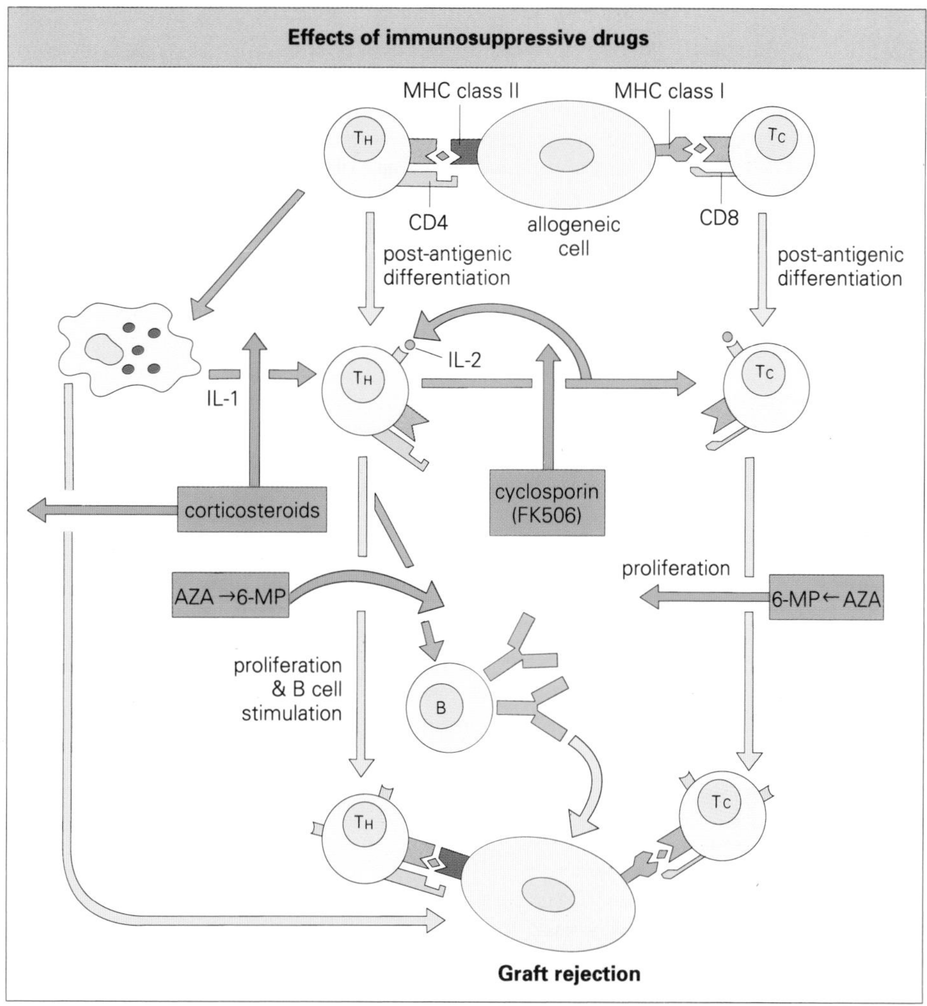

Fig. 27.10 The effects of pharmacological immunosuppressants in the process of rejection. Allogeneic cells stimulate CD4+, MHC class II restricted TH cells and CD8+ TC cells. These differentiate into mature cells, which interact by cytokines (including IL-2) and develop further into effector cells capable of graft rejection. Cyclosporin blocks release of IL-2 by TH cells. Corticosteroids interfere with mononuclear phagocyte and APC function, causing reduced TH stimulation (e.g. by IL-1). Azathioprine (AZA) and its derivative, 6-mercaptopurine (6-MP) interfere with effector cell development.

Pharmacological properties of corticosteroid preparations

	Anti-inflammatory potency	Equivalent dose (mg)	Sodium-retaining potency	Approximate plasma half-life (min)
Hydrocortisone (cortisol)	1.0	20.00	2+	90
Cortisone	0.8	25.00	2+	30
Prednisone	4.0	5.00	1+	60
Prednisolone	4.0	5.00	1+	200
Methylprednisolone	5.0	4.00	0	180
Triamcinolone	5.0	4.00	0	300
Betamethasone	20–30	0.60	0	100–300
Dexamethasone	20–30	0.75	0	100–300

Fig. 27.11 Pharmacological properties of corticosteroids.

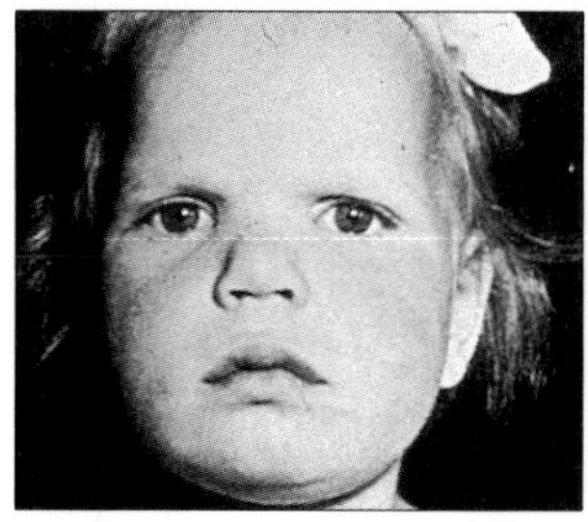
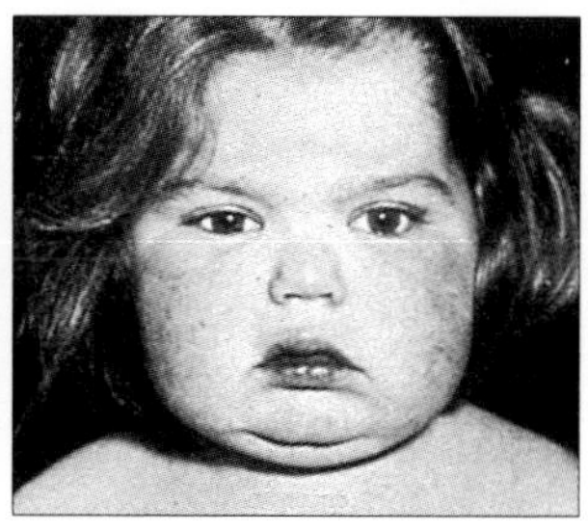
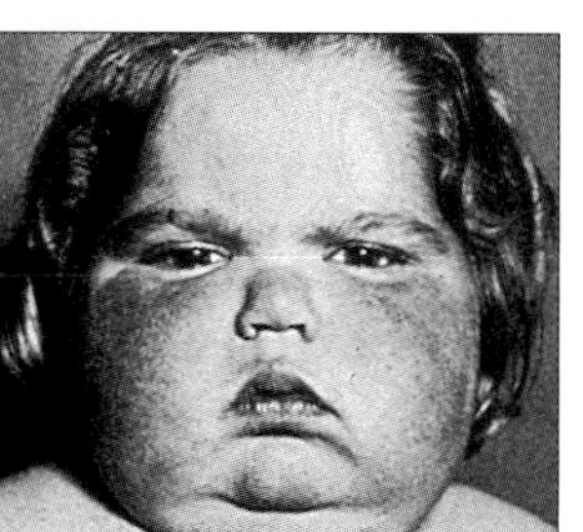

Fig. 27.12 The effect of large doses of steroids. This child developed severe Cushing's syndrome during long-term exposure to steroids. The introduction of new immunosuppressive agents, particularly cyclosporin A, has allowed much smaller doses to be used.

Combination therapy

The combination of the immunosuppressive and anti-inflammatory properties of adrenocorticosteroids makes these drugs very valuable in preventing untoward immune reactions either in autoimmunity or graft rejection. However, their use is limited by the severe side-effects with which they are associated (Fig. 27.13). Thus the selection of steroids as a therapy, the type of steroid chosen, the dose, and the pattern of dosing are all dictated by a need to avoid or limit these side-effects. In particular the inclusion, where possible, of drug-free days into the immunosuppressive regime is widely advocated.

Much research into immunosuppressive drugs is directed towards avoiding or reducing the dependence on steroid therapy. This has led to the proliferation of 'non-steroidal anti-inflammatories' (NSAIDS), much used in the treatment of rheumatic and other inflammatory disorders.

ANTIBODIES AS IMMUNOSUPPRESSANTS

The combination of azathioprine with prednisolone provided the pharmacological basis for immunosuppression in organ transplantation. It was in this group of patients that the need to avoid side-effects became most apparent.

Side-effects of steroid immunosuppression
increased risk of infection
impaired wound healing
growth suppression in childhood
diabetes
gastric ulcers
psychological disturbances ± insomnia
oedema
aseptic bone necrosis
hypertension
Cushing's syndrome

Fig. 27.13 Side-effects of steroid immunosuppression.

Unlike the treatment of autoimmune diseases, the cessation of immunosuppression in these patients meant loss of the graft and, in heart and liver transplants, loss of the patient's life. Thus, after the initial rush of heart transplants stimulated by the work of Dr Christian Barnard, the transplant surgeons and their colleagues found the balancing act between under and over-immunosuppression too difficult and, with the exception of one or two notable centres, withdrew from the unequal contest. With the development of new immunosuppressants, the transplantation programmes have restarted and are now developing rapidly (Fig. 27.14).

The idea of using antibodies against lymphocytes to suppress the immune system originated with the late Sir Peter Medawar. However, the execution of this concept is fraught with difficulties. The main problems were:

- choosing the most relevant antigen;
- how to avoid antibodies against other blood products;
- what species to make the antibody in;
- how to avoid batch variation.

Only when these questions were resolved could the question of efficacy be addressed. Animal studies demonstrated that the principle itself was valid. The use of an anti-lymphocyte globulin (ALG) in the Stanford heart programme has been attributed with giving that group their success. Recent studies have suggested that in kidney transplantation at least, ALG does not so much prevent graft rejection as postpone its onset for the length of time for which the globulin is used.

Anti-species antibodies

An additional problem confronting the use of antibodies as immunosuppressants is that most recipients make antibodies against the serum of the animal from which the ALG is derived. These rapidly complex with and inactivate the ALG, thus requiring either larger and larger doses or a switch in species. Despite these disadvantages, however, ALG has been shown to have therapeutic benefit in a range of conditions, of which idiopathic thrombocytopenia and organ grafting are the best documented.

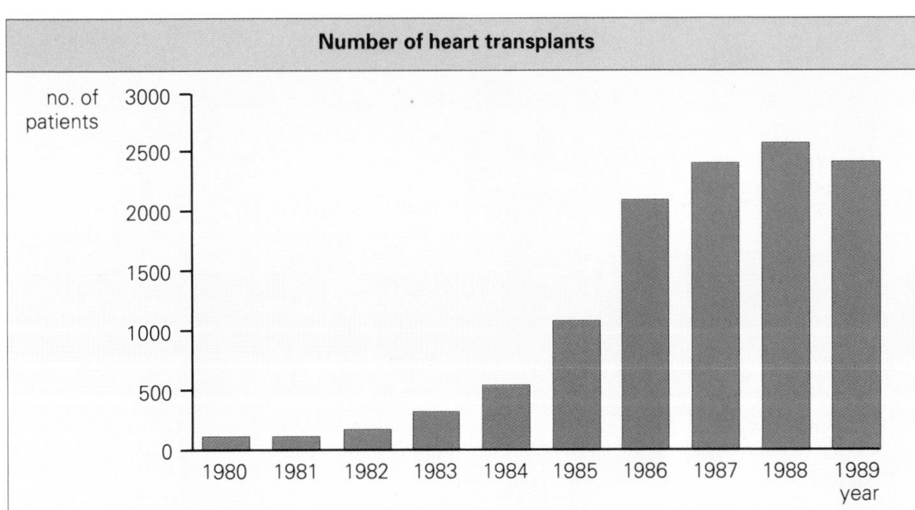

Fig. 27.14 Heart transplant activity has increased dramatically in the last decade. However, the rate is now limited by the supply of donors. Courtesy of J M Kriett and M P Kaye. *The Journal of Heart Transplantation*. Jul – Aug 1990.

Monoclonal antibodies

Many of the problems in the production of immunosuppressive antibodies have been resolved by the introduction of monoclonal antibodies (see chapter 3) to replace the old polyclonal anti-lymphocyte serum (ALS) and ALG. This technology allows a reliable never-ending source of antibody to be produced in a less agricultural style than that used for the old polyclonal antibodies. Moreover, batch variation and contaminating anti-red cell antibodies can be avoided. However, it has also posed as many problems as it solves.

Currently, there are no suitable alternative monoclonals to those produced in rodents, and so species switching to avoid host antiglobulins has been lost as an option. Thus monoclonal antibody treatment must be regarded as a 'one shot' therapy. Happily, this problem may shortly be resolved by the humanizing of monoclonal antibodies, that is, the attachment of the rodent variable to human Ig constant region (see chapter 20).

The very nature of monoclonal antibodies has forced researchers to consider which specificities on the lymphocyte surface are the most appropriate targets for control of the immune response. Thus, is it appropriate to kill the entire lymphocyte population, just T cells, the T helper subset, or even just activated T helper cells? Furthermore, it is unresolved whether antibodies must lyse their target cell to be effective, or whether blocking an appropriate receptor or specific idiotype and causing it to be modulated from the cell surface is sufficient. Will it be necessary to produce mixtures of monoclonals to get the best immunosuppressive recipe, or should monovalent antibodies be used to increase Fc density (Fig. 27.15)? Clinical trials designed to answer these questions are currently in progress in different centres around the world, but it will be many years yet before it is possible to achieve the full potential which monoclonal antibodies offer for controlling the immune system.

Theoretical advantage of monovalent antibodies

divalent — antigen cross-linking & modulation

monovalent — increased Fc density

Fig. 27.15 By using hybrid monoclonals with only one specific Fab region (monovalent), the Fc density can be increased for the same number of antigenic sites, and antigenic modulation is avoided.

The attraction which these antibodies have as immunosuppressants is their specificity, which allows selective suppression of only part of the immune system, leaving the rest free to fight infection. One form of selective pharmacological immunosuppression is the drug cyclosporin.

CYCLOSPORIN

Cyclosporin was isolated from cultures of the fungal species *Tolypocladium inflatum*. It is a neutral, extremely hydrophobic cyclical polypeptide comprised of eleven amino acids, one of which is unique to the cyclosporins (Fig. 27.16). The drug preferentially affects the activated but not the resting T cell at an early stage in the cell activation process, inhibiting lymphokine production.

Various clinical trials have led to some important

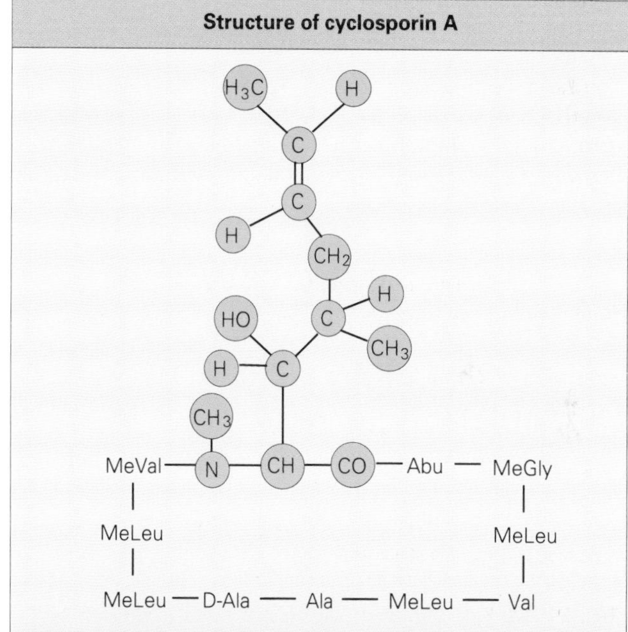

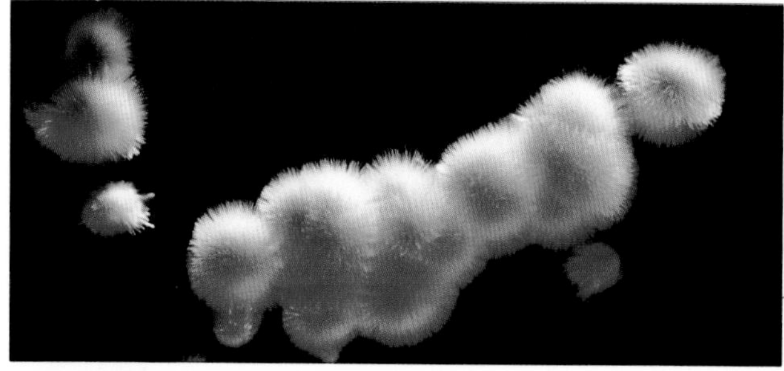

Fig. 27.16 Cyclosporin A. Upper: cyclical structure of cyclosporin A showing the c. nineonene amino acid, which is unique to the cyclosporins. The molecule is highly N-methylated and N-ethylated, rending it insoluble in aqueous solution. It must therefore be administered dissolved in oil. Lower: crystals of cyclosporin N-methyl-C-9-amino acid. Courtesy of Dr R Wenger.

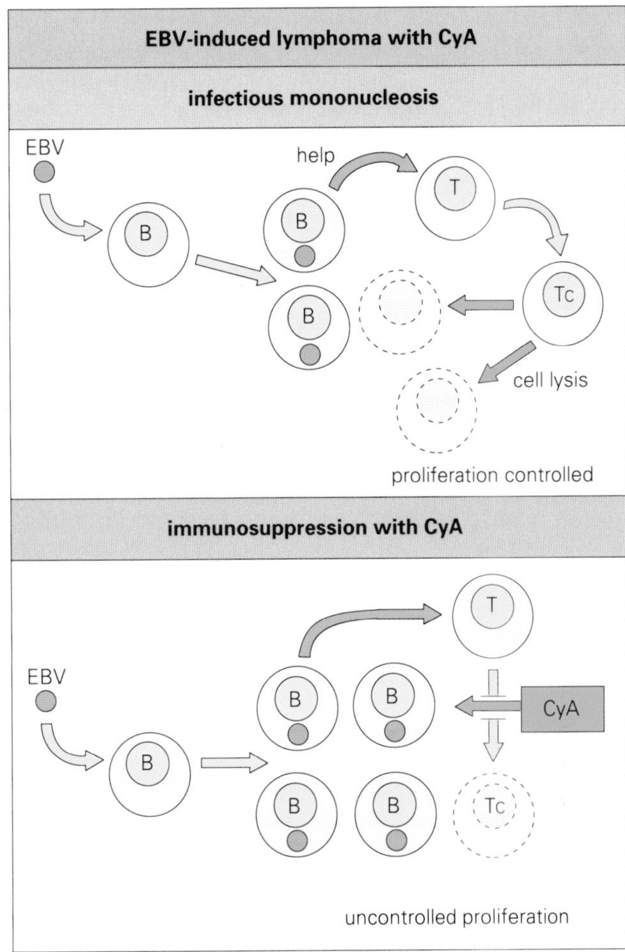

Fig. 27.17 Epstein-Barr virus (EBV)-induced B cell proliferation is usually kept in check by cytotoxic T cells. Cyclosporin A inhibits the formation of Tc cells and can lead to uncontrolled B cell proliferation resulting in lymphoma formation. This condition has been sucessfully treated with acyclovir in the polyclonal phase.

conclusions on the use of this immunosuppressant. First, cyclosporin is a powerful T cell immunosuppressive. Second, the addition of cyclosporin to other immunosuppressives can produce drug cocktails that may be excessively immunosuppressive. Thus, the risk of life-threatening infection and the occurrence of Epstein–Barr virus-induced lymphomata may become unacceptably high, anti-lymphocyte globulins being particularly incriminated as a dangerous additive to cyclosporin (Fig. 27.17). Third, and perhaps most importantly, the drug is nephrotoxic to man at normal immunosuppressive doses, although this is not so in most animals. This last factor makes the drug difficult to manage, particularly in renal transplantation, because the differential diagnosis between rejection and nephrotoxicity can be almost impossible to make and this may lead to unnecessary immunosuppression or delayed identification and treatment of rejection episodes. Despite this, the introduction by Calne and co-workers of cyclosporin A into clinical transplantation is one of the most important developments in recent years.

The drug has been tested in a number of multi-centre and single-centre trials for its efficacy in preventing kidney graft rejection. These trials established that immunosuppression with azathioprine and prednisolone invariably produced inferior results when compared to cyclosporin.

Combination with other drugs

The use of cyclosporin A in combination with other immunosuppressive agents is controversial. Every combination of cyclosporin with prednisolone, azathioprine and ALG (and/or its monoclonal counterparts) has been advocated by different authorities. In no case has an advantage over cyclosporin alone been demonstrated by appropriately-designed controlled trials. In contrast, several controlled trials have failed to demonstrate improved results from the addition of steroids to cyclosporin immunosuppression. While there is evidence that cyclosporin and steroids can produce a highly immunosuppressive cocktail, benefits accruing from this may well be counter-balanced by steroid complications and an increased incidence of infection.

The current trend in clinical immunosuppression is to use triple therapy (Fig. 27.18) in which cyclosporin, steroids and azathioprine are used together in relatively modest doses thereby, in principle, reducing the side-effects of all three while maintaining a high degree of immunosuppression. This regimen is undoubtedly efficient, particularly in the reduction of the nephrotoxic side-effects of cyclosporin. However, several centres are now using low-dose (6–8mg/kg) cyclosporin therapy alone, apparently with equally good results.

Serum levels and metabolism

The clinical management of cyclosporin therapy is greatly aided by the availability of blood or serum level measurements. These can be performed either by radioimmunoassay (RIA) or high-pressure liquid chromatography (HPLC). The latter provides a selective determination of the whole-drug concentrations only, while RIA, until recently, would also detect some metabolites. This problem with the RIA has now been resolved by the introduction of monoclonal antibody based assays in which whole drug can be distinguished from metabolites.

Of the drug concentration, 40–60% is bound to erythrocytes in the blood and the remaining amount is associated with lipoproteins. Drug–RBC binding is temperature dependent, and so the plasma must be separated from the erythrocytes at 37°C to obtain reproducible plasma levels. Thus, for convenience, most centres now determine the drug concentration of lysed whole blood since this approach avoids the temperature dependent erythrocyte binding phenomenon (Fig. 27.19).

Because cyclosporin is metabolized primarily by the liver and excreted in bile, liver dysfunction can cause significant accumulation of both whole drug and metabolites, and management of cyclosporin therapy can be much more difficult in patients with poor liver function.

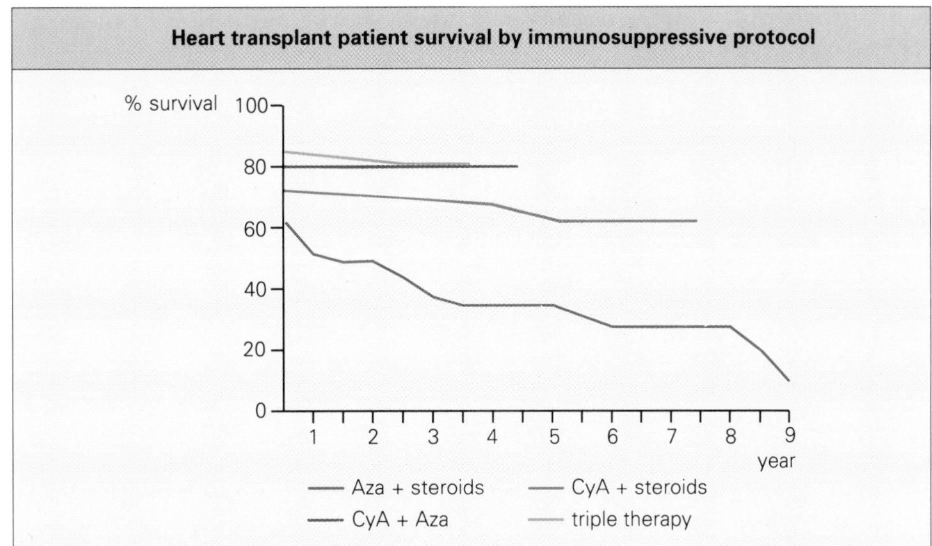

Fig. 27.18 Heart transplant patient survival with different immunosuppressive protocol. Courtesy of Mr T English.

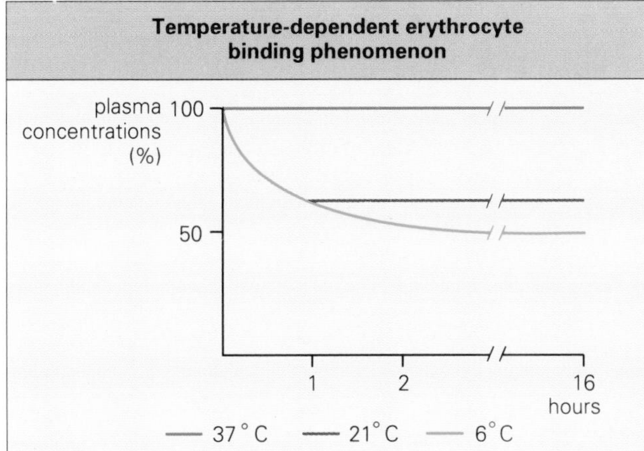

Fig. 27.19 Plasma levels of CyA measured when blood is allowed to cool to room temperature or placed in a fridge prior to separation are significantly lower than if the blood is maintained at 37°C. The red cells take up the cyclosporin as they cool over a period of 1–2 hours.

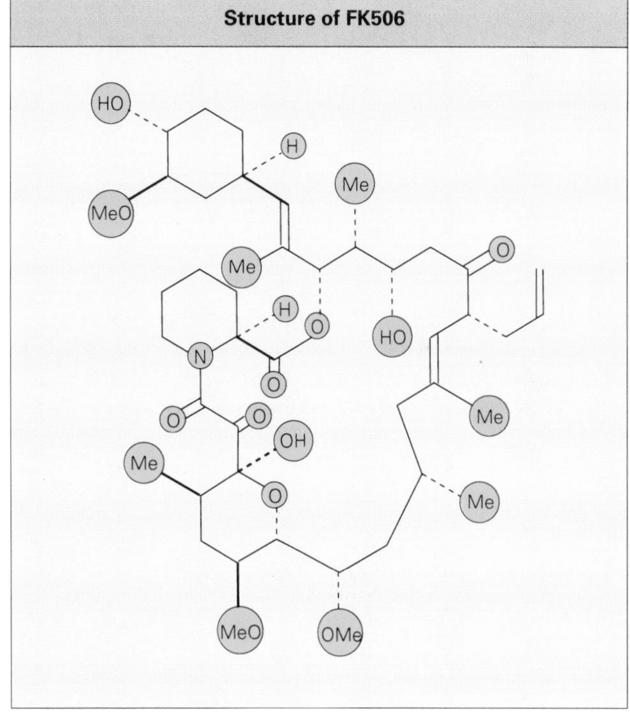

Fig. 27.20 FK506 exerts similar effects to cyclosporin A but at significantly lower molar doses.

Over the years, the recommended therapeutic window for whole blood or serum levels of cyclosporin has been decreasing so that most centres now aim their therapy at producing whole blood trough levels of 200–300ng/ml range.

Catabolism of the drug is accelerated by coincident administration of rifampicin or phenytoin, which activate the cytochrome p450 pathway to increase the speed of degradation. Cyclosporin and prednisolone interact with each other by competing for this route of secretion. Concurrent therapy with aminoglycosides, trimethoprim, ketoconazole or amphotericin-B also elevate cyclosporin blood levels and can result in increased nephrotoxicity.

FK506

In recent years much interest has centered around the development of a new immunosuppressive compound developed in Japan. While the structure of this drug is very different from that of cyclosporin A (Fig. 27.20), its mode of action appears to be similar.

FK506 is a macrolide isolated from *Streptomyces tsukubaensis*. It prevents the activation of T lymphocytes in response to antigenic or mitogenic stimulation *in vitro*; this is almost certainly achieved by inhibiting the production of IL-2. Early animal studies in the dog suggested that FK506 was toxic, causing widespread vasculitis. However initial clinical studies at the University of Pittsburgh, using doses considerably below those studied in the dog experiments (0.15mg/kg versus 1mg/kg), have suggested that in man the drug may have few significant side-effects in the short term. A particular advantage would appear to be its lack of nephrotoxicity compared with cyclosporin A.

Extensive clinical studies on the efficacy of FK506 are currently in progress. Initial studies have been on recipients of liver transplants and although follow-up of these cases is still relatively short, results of the immunosuppressive potential of this drug have been encouraging in an experience which now exceeds 60 patients. These studies are now being extended to include recipients of kidney, heart and heart-lung transplants.

If the initial promise of this drug is fulfilled, it will enable the side-effects of immunosuppression to be further reduced and should allow the use of powerful T cell immunosuppression to be applied to a range of conditions in which, at present, the risks of side-effects makes the use of current immunosuppressive drugs unacceptable.

Indications for use of cyclosporins

The list of indications for the use of cyclosporin is steadily growing (Fig. 27.21). Its controversial use in the treatment of type I insulin dependent diabetes mellitus deserves special mention. The pioneering work of the group in the University of London, Ontario has demonstrated that where cyclosporin therapy is started soon enough (certainly within 6 weeks) after diagnosis, a substantial portion of these patients recover enough islet cell function to re-establish an insulin-free carbohydrate control. However, in many cases, cessation of cyclosporin therapy within a few months post onset results in recurrence of disease. Insufficient data exist to resolve the issue of whether the immune activity against islets will wane after several years' cyclosporin therapy. Nor is it possible to assess accurately the comparative risk of the side-effects from a lifetime's insulin versus a lifetime's cyclosporin.

As more specific and less toxic methods of suppressing the immune system are developed, such issues will undoubtedly confront most clinicians.

Use of cyclosporin in autoimmune diseases
Efficacy demonstrated in:
rheumatoid arthritis
posterior uveitis
Behçet's disease
psoriasis
myasthenia gravis
Crohn's disease
nephrotic syndrome
systemic lupus erythematosus
polymyositis/dermatomyositis
aplastic anaemia, pure red cell anaemia
endocrine ophthalmopathy
insulin dependent diabetes
scleroderma
Efficacy unknown in:
multiple sclerosis (chronic progressive)
amyotrophic lateral sclerosis
primary biliary cirrhosis
vasculitis syndromes
pulmonary sarcoidosis
Not effective in:
multiple sclerosis (remitting-relapsing)

Fig. 27.21 The manufacturers do not recommend that cyclosporin is used in insulin dependent diabetes and scleroderma. Modified from Borel *et al.* (1989).

FURTHER READING

Borel JF, ed. Cyclosporin. In: Ishizaka K, Kallós P, Lachmann PJ, Waksman BH, eds. *Progress in allergy. Volume 38.* Basle, New York: Karger, 1986.

Calne, RY, ed. *Transplantation immunology. Clinical and experimental.* Oxford: Oxford University Press, 1984.

Flye MW. *Principles of organ transplantation.* Philadelphia: WB Saunders Company, 1989.

Morris PJ, Tilney NL, eds. *Progress in transplantation. Volume 2.* Edinburgh: Churchill Livingstone, 1985.

Waldmann H, ed. Monoclonal antibody therapy. In: Ishizaka K, Kallós P, Lachmann PJ, Waksman BH, eds. *Progress in allergy. Volume 45.* Basle, New York: Karger, 1988.

28

Immunopotentiation

INTRODUCTION

The use of adjuvants to increase cell-mediated and humoral immune responses to vaccine antigens and for laboratory experimentation has a long history. Two strategies have been employed, one based on dispersion of antigens on the surface of oil or lipid particles, and the other based on the adsorption of antigens on precipitates. In 1916 Le Moignac and Pinay found that suspending heat-killed *Salmonella typhimurium* in mineral oil increased antibody responses to the bacterium. Mineral oil formulations have since been used in several veterinary vaccines. Mineral oil was also used to increase the efficacy of influenza vaccination in American armed forces personnel. Some recipients developed severe haemorrhagic lesions or persistent granulomas, which is the main reason why regulatory authorities have not approved mineral oil for regular use in human vaccines.

ADJUVANTS

Freund's adjuvants

In 1945 Freund incorporated the detergent Arlacel A (mannide monoleate) in his incomplete adjuvant (FIA) to facilitate emulsification of mineral oil. Killed mycobacteria were added to produce Freund's complete adjuvant (FCA). FIA is sufficient to elicit the formation of antibodies to many antigens; when the same antigens are administered in FCA, cell-mediated immunity is also elicited, as shown by delayed hypersensitivity, and the isotype of the antibodies is changed. Following administration of antigens to guinea pigs in FIA, most of the antibodies detected are of the IgG1 isotype, whereas when FCA is used, antibodies of the IgG2 isotype predominate.

FCA has been the adjuvant most widely used in laboratory animals for the past forty years. However, it produced granulomatous reactions at injection sites (Fig. 28.1), which precluded its use in human and veterinary vaccines. These reactions can be severe in laboratory, domestic and farm animals, and the use of this adjuvant has already been banned in some large research institutions, a trend which is likely to spread. For this and other reasons there has been a need to develop an adjuvant formulation with the efficacy of FCA, but lacking its undesirable effects.

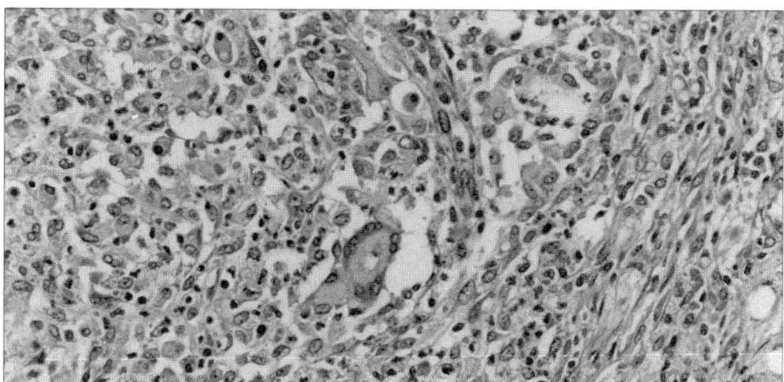

Fig. 28.1 Granulomatous lesion at the site of subcutaneous injection of Freund's complete adjuvant in a guinea pig. This section was taken two weeks after a single injection. x500.

Aluminium salts

The second most widely used adjuvant is alum (aluminium hydroxide or aluminium phosphate). In 1926, Glenny precipitated diphtheria toxoid with potassium alum and found that the precipitate elicited the formation of antitoxin more effectively than the unprecipitated toxoid. Sixty years of application have confirmed the usefulness of alum as an adjuvant (Fig. 28.2), and it is the only one generally approved by regulatory authorities for human vaccines.

The efficacy varies: alum is satisfactory when used in bacterial toxoids, when moderate levels of antibodies of any isotype are sufficient for neutralization, but it is less satisfactory in the currently used vaccine for hepatitis B virus (HBV). Three doses of alum-precipitated surface antigen (HBsAg) are required to elicit the formation of antibodies in the majority of normal adults. However vaccination is less effective in infants and in persons predisposed for genetic or other reasons to be low responders to the antigen. In experimental animals other adjuvants are more efficacious than alum in HBsAg vaccines. Alum is ineffective with other antigens, for example influenza virus haemagglutinin (HA), so that influenza vaccine is currently

Effect of aluminium hydroxide (alum) as adjuvant

Antigen		Anti-DNP titres by radioimmunoassay		
injection	dose (μg)	DNP-BSA	DNP-FGG	DNP-KLH
saline	1	5	5	10
saline	10	10	10	160
alum	1	320	640	40
alum	10	5120	2560	2560

Fig. 28.2 Effect of aluminium hydroxide on antibody responses to a hapten (dinitrophenol, DNP) conjugated to bovine serum albumin (BSA), fowl gamma-globulin (FGG) and keyhole limpet haemocyanin (KLH). Data from R Bomford.

Structure of dimethyldioctadecyl ammonium bromide (DDA)

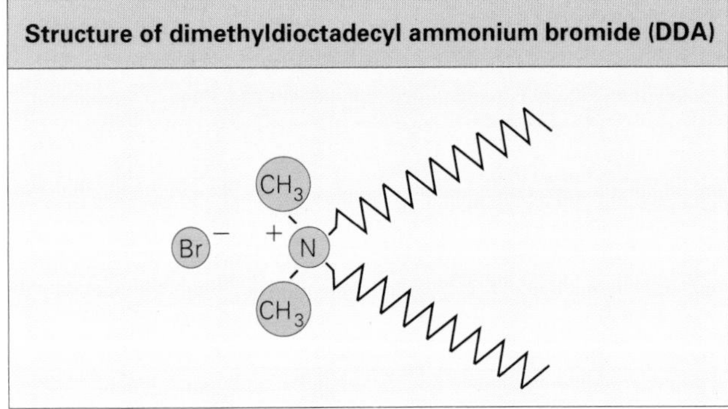

Fig. 28.3 Structure of dimethyldioctadecyl ammonium bromide, showing the quaternary amine and the carbon chains.

Structure of triterpene ring from *Quillaia saponaria*

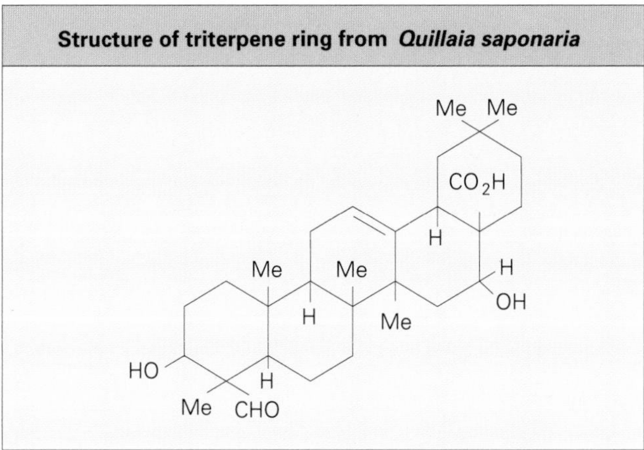

Fig. 28.4 The triterpene ring from the saponin of *Quillaia saponaria*. The sugar chains, which are not shown, are attached to the two hydroxyl groups. Me = methyl group

administered in saline. Under these conditions influenza HA is in the form of micelles, which are not optimal for immunogenicity. This may explain why the vaccine has rather low efficacy, as outlined in the last section of this chapter.

A NEW GENERATION OF VACCINES

Influenza HA

Influenza HA is one of the best known immunogens: the three-dimensional structure of the molecule, the major epitopes and their variations, both naturally occurring and laboratory-produced, have all been defined. Despite the accumulation of this academic information, influenza vaccines are much less effective than they should be. However, recently developed adjuvants have greatly improved responses to these vaccines.

Adjuvants could, therefore, be used to optimize vaccines already in use, including those for influenza and hepatitis B. The need is even greater with the new vaccines made possible by recombinant DNA technology and the synthesis of glycoconjugates and peptides (see chapter 26). Using appropriate expression systems it has been possible to produce antigens of several viruses, bacteria and other infectious agents with three-dimensional structures which closely resemble those of the naturally-occurring subunits. HBsAg produced in yeast was the first recombinant vaccine to be approved by regulatory authorities. This antigen cannot be produced efficiently in *Escherichia coli*, but the core antigen of the virus, HBcAg, can be produced in this bacterium in the form of particles which are like those found in serum; denaturation converts HBcAg into HBeAg, indicating the importance of the three-dimensional configuration.

Glycosylation of antigens

Glycosylation of antigens can also influence antigenicity. Surface glycoproteins of herpes simplex virus, gB and gD, can be expressed in their correctly glycosylated form in mammalian cells and used to elicit protective immunity. Studies with inactivated virus are being superceded by those with recombinant antigens, which make possible a new generation of vaccines. However their promise will only be realized if some of the recently developed adjuvants are approved for human use.

Surface-active agents and iscoms

Many cationic and non-ionic surface-active agents have shown adjuvant activity. A simple example is hexadecylamine, in which the sixteen carbon hydrophobic chain has the optimal length. Several quaternary amines have been employed as adjuvants, in particular dimethyldioctadecyl ammonium bromide (DDA) (Fig. 28.3) and N,N-dioctadecyl-N′,N′-bis(2-hydroxyethyl) propanediamine (Avridine). Again, the sixteen to eighteen carbon chain length is optimal.

The most widely used surface-active adjuvants have been saponins, plant-derived glycosides of triterpenes and sterols that bind cholesterol; these have been used in several veterinary vaccines. Recently, their ratio of efficacy to side-effects has been improved by purifying the saponins and defining which have the most potent adjuvant activity, for example Quil A, which is obtained from *Quillaia saponaria* (Fig. 28.4). However, saponins disrupt membrane structure and are cytolytic, and it was therefore desirable to obtain the adjuvant effect with the minimum free saponin. This was achieved when constructs of virus envelope glycoproteins were formed with membrane lipids and Quil A to produce immune-stimulating complexes (ISCOMs). These regular, multimeric complexes with antigen (Fig. 28.5) are highly immunogenic.

Liposomes

Liposomes are spherical structures in which a phospholipid bilayer encloses an aqueous compartment. The size, number of phospholipid bilayers (unilamellar or multilamellar), surface charge and the composition can all be varied. It has been shown that liposomes can function as adjuvants, increasing the formation of antibodies against diphtheria toxoid. The technology needed to produce

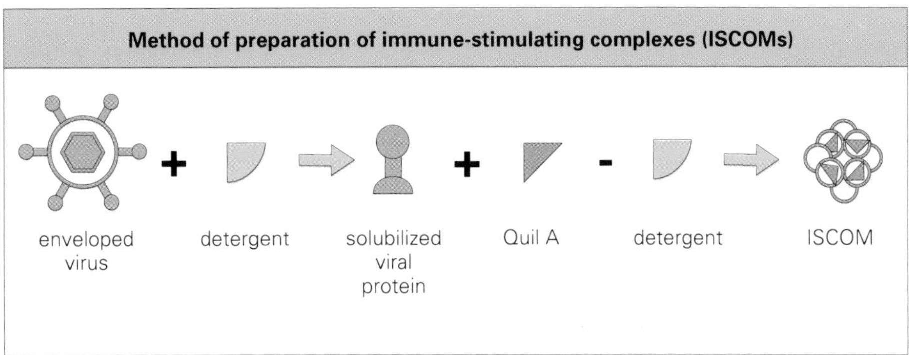

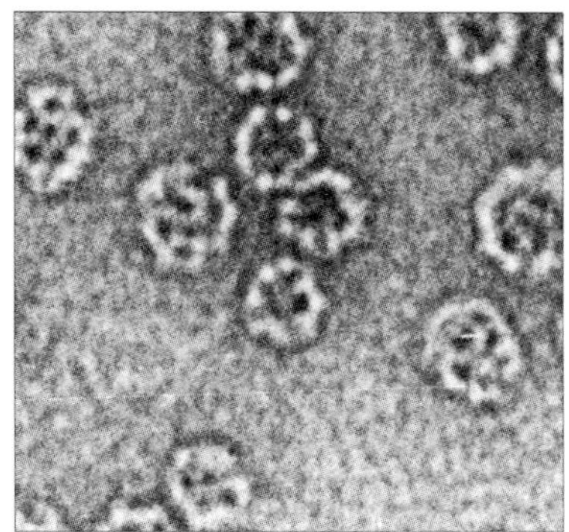

Fig. 28.5 Immune-stimulating complexes (ISCOMs). Left: method by which ISCOMs are prepared from an enveloped virus. Modified from K Dalsgaard. Right: electron micrograph of negatively stained (uranyl acetate) ISCOMs, which were constructed from a detergent-solubilized *Plasmodium falciparum* antigen and Quil A. x 218,600. Courtesy of K Dalsgaard & U Moslet).

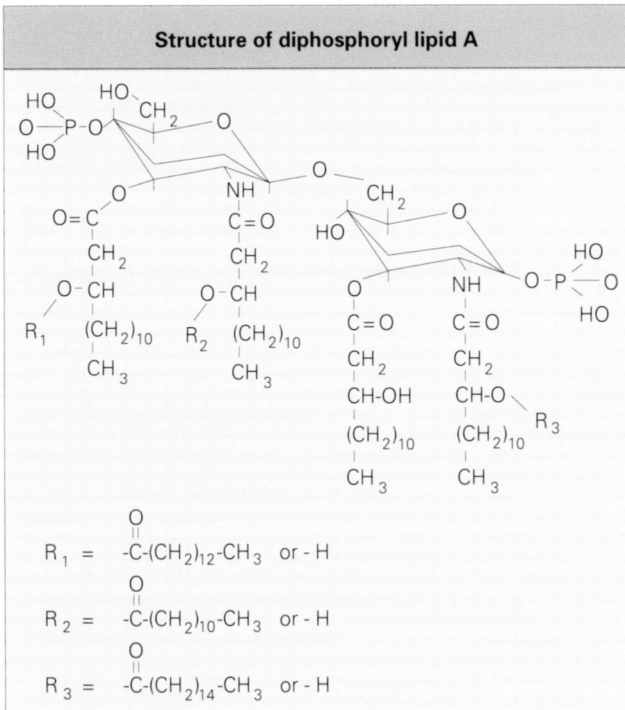

Fig. 28.6 Generalized structure of diphosphoryl lipid A. The most highly acylated form obtained from most Gram-negative bacteria corresponds to the hexa-acyl structure where R3 = H and R1 and R2 are tetradecanoyl and dodecanoyl groups respectively. In monophosphoryl lipid A the phosphate group on the right is removed. Courtesy of J Rudbach.

liposomes on an industrial scale has now been developed, and these structures have been found to be suitable for use with a variety of antigens. However, available evidence suggests that the composition of the liposomes may have to be optimized for each antigen. Lipopolysaccharide or lipid A added to liposomes increases their potency as adjuvants for laboratory immunization, but is unacceptable for human use.

Lipopolysaccharide and monophosphoryl lipid A

Lipopolysaccharide (LPS) endotoxins of Gram-negative bacteria are adjuvants, increasing antibody formation when administered with antigens. However, they have many undesirable effects, including pyrogenicity and the capacity to produce anterior uveitis. The adjuvant-active component of endotoxins is the lipid A core structure (Fig. 28.6). One phosphate group of lipid A is relatively acid labile and the residual compound, monophosphoryl lipid A (MPL), retains adjuvant activity with decreased side-effects. For immunization of laboratory animals, MPL is often used with trehalose dimycolate (TDM), the cord factor of mycobacteria. Since TDM has diverse biological activities, this combination may not be approved for human use. MPL is also used with squalane emulsions.

Muramyl dipeptide-based adjuvants

The cell wall of mycobacteria has been progressively degraded to define the minimal component with adjuvant activity. This proved to be muramyl dipeptide (MDP, N-acetylmuramyl-L-alanyl-D-isoglutamine). Natural or synthetic MDP added to the mineral oil emulsion of FIA, converted it to a complete adjuvant, able to elicit cell-mediated immunity and antibodies of the IgG2 isotype in the guinea pig. However, MDP has unacceptable side-effects: it is pyrogenic and induces anterior uveitis in the rabbit and adjuvant-type arthritis in the rat. It also acts on macrophage-type cells to induce non-specific immunity.

In an attempt to dissociate adjuvant activity from the capacity to induce side-effects, more than one hundred analogues of MDP were synthesized. It was found that substituting the central L-alanine residue by L-threonine provides the desired separation of activities: N-acetylmuramyl-L-threonyl-D-isoglutamine (Fig. 28.7) was therefore selected as the counterpart of the mycobacterial cell wall in an adjuvant formulation. Nuclear magnetic resonance analysis shows that the tertiary structure of MDP depends on intramolecular hydrogen bonding, and the threonyl residue has a hydroxyl group that provides an additional hydrogen bond.

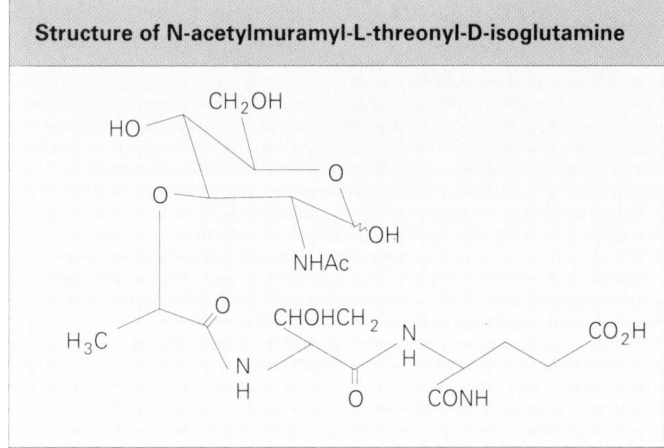

Fig. 28.7 N-acetylmuramyl-L-threonyl-D-isoglutamine, an adjuvant-active synthetic muramyl dipeptide analogue.

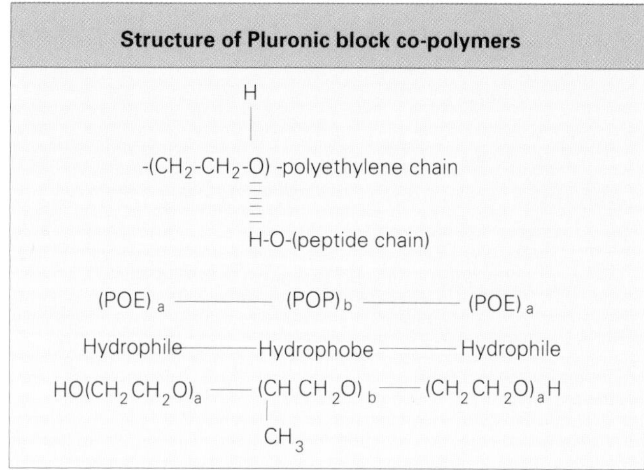

Fig. 28.8 Generalized structure of Pluronic block co-polymers. These have a central block of polyoxypropylene ether (POP), flanked by two blocks of polyoxyethylene ether (POE), which is hydrophilic because it can form hydrogen bonds with water. It can also form hydrogen bonds with peptides, as shown above. The symbols a and b denote different chain lengths.

MDP and analogues in saline have low adjuvant activity, and the next requirement was to develop a counterpart of the mineral oil emulsion of FCA that would be acceptable for human use. After much experimentation with liposomes, vegetable oils and surface-active agents, it was found that squalene or squalane emulsions, microfluidized with the Pluronic block co-polymer L-121 and a small amount of Tween 80 (sorbitan mono-9-octadecanoate poly(oxy-12)-ethanediyl) provided a versatile formulation for antigens (Fig. 28.8). The structure of L-121 associates with membranes, but it does not penetrate into membranes and disrupt their structure, unlike saponins which bind cholesterol and are cytolytic. Squalane is saturated and stable in formulation whereas squalene is unsaturated and becomes oxidized. The squalane-L-121 emulsion is remarkably stable, even when frozen. Mixtures of the emulsion and antigen kept at refrigerator temperature retain immunogenicity for at least six months.

MDP adjuvant formulation (MDP-A). The combination of the threonyl analogue of MDP and squalane-L-121 emulsion is termed MDP adjuvant formulation (MDP-A). Our interpretation of the effectiveness of the squalane L-121 emulsion as a vehicle for antigens is shown diagramatically in Fig. 28.9. Electron micrographs confirm that labelled protein antigens are concentrated on the surface of the squalane microspheres. A wide range of antigens are retained there, partly because they are amphipathic and partly by hydrogen bonding to L-121. The squalane L-121 emulsion system is therefore more efficient than squalane emulsions, which lack the block co-polymer, and more versatile than liposomes, the structure of which has to be optimized for each antigen. Squalane L-121 microsphere particles also activate complement and migrate from injection sites to lymph nodes of the drainage chain. The C3b on the surface of the microspheres should target them to follicular dendritic cells. A depot of antigen on follicular dendritic cells is more important for immunogenicity, as well as better for the patient, than a depot at the injection
28.4 site.

EFFECTS OF ADJUVANTS ON ELICITED ANTIBODIES

Quantity

Traditionally, the efficacy of adjuvants has been assessed by the levels of antibodies elicited, using a convenient test such as the enzyme-linked immunosorbent assay (ELISA) or haemagglutination. Although these assays have provided useful information, they should now be supplemented by other measures of the quantity and quality of antibodies elicited. Preferably, antibody levels should be quantified by tests relevant to function, such as neutralization of bacterial toxins or viruses. Because of potential problems with solid-phase assays, at least some measurements of antibody levels using fluid-phase assays should be made.

Affinity

In addition to the quantities of antibodies elicited by a vaccine, their affinity for antigen is also important for protection. To neutralize a virus or bacterial toxin, antibodies should bind them with sufficiently high affinity. If the complexes are not removed by phagocytic cells, antibodies must bind to a virus or toxin with an affinity at least of the same order as the natural receptor.

Isotype

Another important property of antibodies is their isotype. IgG antibodies pass from the vascular to the extravascular compartment more easily than those of the IgM class, and only the former are transferred across the placenta or by milk to fetuses and newborn animals. Antibodies of some

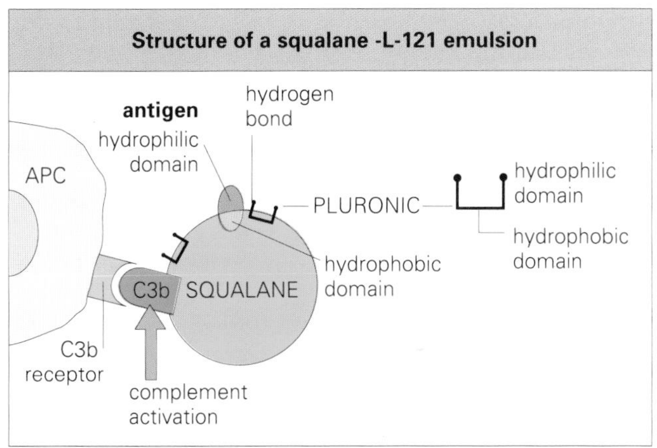

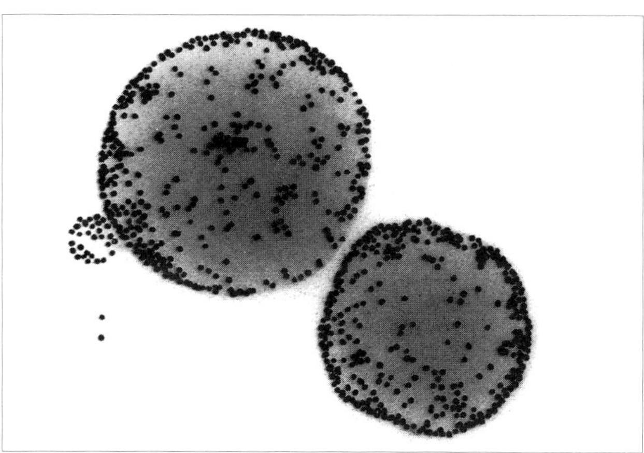

Fig. 28.9 Left: generalized representation of the structure of a squalane-L-121 emulsion, showing antigens retained on the surface of the lipid microspheres because of their amphipathic character and hydrogen bonding to L-121. Complement is also activated by the alternative pathway on the surface of the microspheres; C3b is retained on their surface and targets the complex to antigen presenting cells bearing C3b receptors. Right: electron micrograph of model antigen (ovalbumin labelled with colloidal gold) concentrated on the surface of squalane-L-121 emulsion microspheres. x25,000.

isotypes efficiently activate complement, bind to high-affinity receptors on monocytes, and act synergistically with antibody-dependent effector cells to produce cytotoxicity. Examples are IgG2a antibodies in mice and IgGl antibodies in humans, both of which bind to high-affinity Fcγl receptors. Studies with isotype-switch variants of murine monoclonal antibodies (which have the same Fab regions, so that binding to antigen is comparable) show that IgG2a antibodies confer better protection against tumors than those of other isotypes. Investigations with 're-shaped' human antibodies genetically constructed so that they have antigen-binding hypervariable regions like those of rodent monoclonals, confirm the superiority of the human IgG1 isotype in antibody-dependent cell-mediated lysis. The desirability of developing an adjuvant that preferentially elicits high-affinity antibodies of the IgG2a isotype in mice and IgG1 in humans is therefore apparent. Production of IgE antibodies should usually be avoided, although they might contribute to protection against some parasites.

Alum, lipopolysaccharide, monophosphoryl lipid A and saponins elicit antibodies mainly of the IgG1 isotype in the mouse, whereas the muramyl dipeptide formulation MDP-A increases the formation of IgG2a antibodies.

Cytokines selectively stimulate the production of antibodies of particular isotypes. Interleukin-4 increases the formation of IgE antibodies in both mice and humans; in mice IL-4 also increases the production of IgG1 antibodies. Interferon-γ in mice increases the formation of antibodies of the IgG2a isotype. This explains why adjuvants that elicit cell-mediated immunity and consequent production of IFNγ also preferentially stimulate the production of IgG2a antibodies. Examples of adjuvants with both effects are FCA and MDP-A.

ELICITATION OF CELL-MEDIATED IMMUNITY

Helper T lymphocytes are required for the formation of antibodies against most antigens. In addition, cytotoxic T lymphocytes can lyse infected cells or produce mediators, such as IFNγ, following interaction with antigen in a genetically restricted situation. Cytotoxic T lymphocytes able to lyse autologous cells expressing several antigens of human immunodeficiency virus (HIV) are demonstrable in infected persons, although it is not yet known whether they have a protective role.

It is therefore likely that optimal protection against some infectious agents, for example herpes viruses and possibly HIV, needs the elicitation of cell-mediated immunity (CMI). Tests for CMI should include not only delayed hypersensitivity but also proliferative responses to the antigen and the release of IL-2 and IFNγ. Cytotoxicity for autologous or syngeneic infected target cells should also be studied.

If mice or rats are used, syngeneic target cells are readily available. With outbred species, such as humans and subhuman primates, B cells transformed by Epstein-Barr virus, transfected with a vaccinia virus vector expressing the antigen under consideration, for example HIV antigens, can provide autologous target cells for studies of genetically restricted cell-mediated cytotoxicity.

It has long been believed that production of antigens within cells, for example by replicating viruses, is required to elicit cytotoxic T cells, and that this cannot be achieved by subunit antigens. However, the envelope protein of HIV or influenza virus HA in ISCOMs elicits $CD8^+$ T cells which specifically lyse target cells in a MHC class I-restricted fashion in mice; recombinant gD of herpes simplex virus in MDP-A elicits $CD4^+$ T cells which lyse target cells in a class II-restricted fashion in guinea pigs.

MODE OF ACTION OF ADJUVANTS

Delayed release of antigen

It was believed for a long time that adjuvants exert their effects at the injection site by allowing slow release of antigens which bind to macrophages migrating into the site. FCA elicits a strong granulomatous response (see Fig. 28.1) and even alum elicits some response of this type. If this were true it would not be possible to separate adjuvant effects from a granulomatous response, which would be unfortunate. However, sites of injection of antigens with FCA or alum can be excised quite soon after injection without impairing antibody responses. It is now thought to be more important to produce depots of antigen associated with antigen presenting cells (APCs) (Fig. 28.10).

Antigen presenting cells

Although many cell types can present antigens when suitably stimulated, for example during infections, three cell types do so efficiently under normal conditions, such as those which prevail during routine vaccination. One cell type originates from the bone marrow and migrates into the dermis and epidermis of the skin, where it sends out dendritic extensions; this is known as the Langerhans' cell. After about a week it migrates from the skin through afferent lymphatics (Fig. 28.11), to the paracortical areas of lymph nodes, where it extends its branches among T lymphocytes. In this site, it is termed an interdigitating dendritic cell (IDC). Dendritic cells in the spleen and their counterparts in peripheral blood (which may be of the same lineage as Langerhans' cells) have also been shown to present antigens efficiently to T lymphocytes.

Another type of dendritic cell is the follicular dendritic cell (FDC) which is present in the follicles of lymph nodes. Complement-activating immune complexes become localized on FDC (Fig. 28.12), which express C3b receptors. Antigens can form beaded immune-stimulating bodies (iccosomes) on the dendrites of FDC (Fig. 28.13 upper) which remain for a long time (months). In the absence of antigen, FDC have smooth dendritic extensions (Fig. 28.13 lower). Vehicles bearing antigens and C3b on their surfaces, for example emulsion particles in MDP-A or liposomes activating complement, can likewise be targeted to FDC, and this seems to be important for increasing the immunogenicity of associated antigens. FDC are major presenters of antigens to B lymphocytes, and these, in turn, can efficiently present antigens to T lymphocytes (Fig. 28.14). Thus the function of dispersing the antigen on the surface of particle is to facilitate targeting to presenting cells.

Cytokines

The complementary function of adjuvants is to increase the production of cytokines that are required to elicit

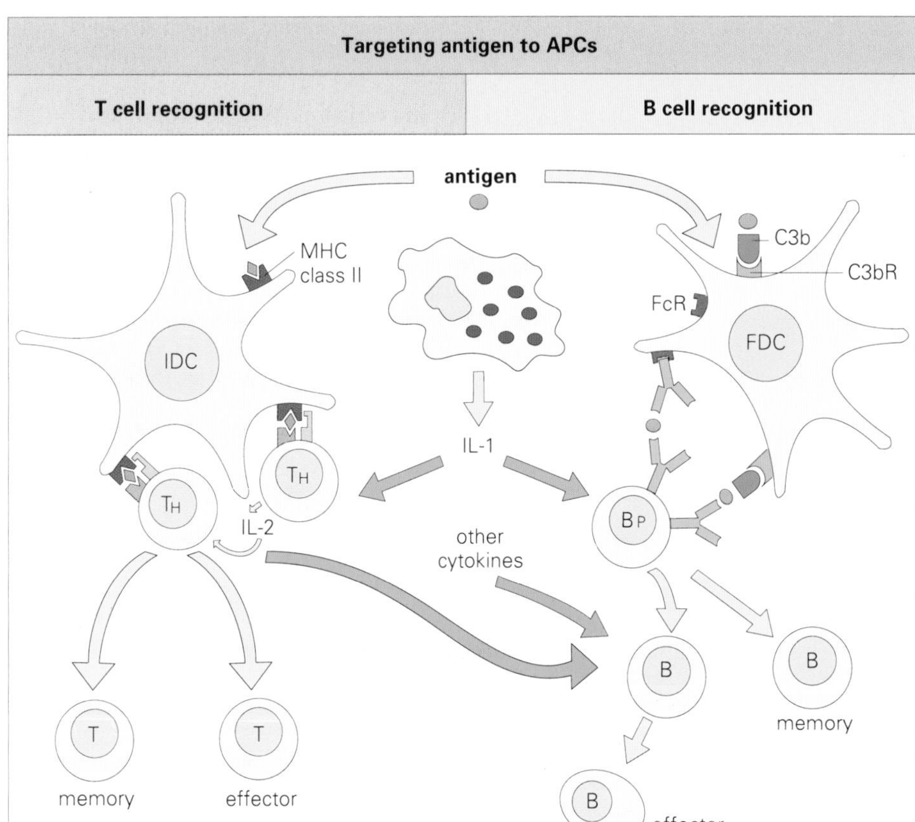

Fig.28.10. Antigent targeting through complement to follicular dendritic cells (FDC) and via MHC class II to interdigitating dendritic cells (IDC). FDC present antigen via the C3b or Fc receptor to B precursor lymphocytes (Bp), which proliferate or mature to become plasma (B effector) cells and generate B cell memory. B cells and IDC present antigens or fragments of them in association with MHC class II to T cells. T_H cells produce IL-2 which is needed for proliferation of other subsets of T effector cells, e.g. cytotoxic T cells as well as for the generation of T cell memory. Adjuvants acting on macrophages and other accessory cells induce production of IL-1, IL-6 and other cytokines.

immune responses efficiently. Adjuvants such as LPS and MDP are potent inducers of cytokine (IL-1α, IL-1β, TNFα, IL-6) production by macrophages and other accessory cells. Responding T lymphocytes produce IL-2 and IFNγ. IL-2 not only stimulates the proliferation of lymphocytes, but also the production of antibodies by B lymphocytes. IFNγ increases the expression of class II major histocompatibility antigens, which could facilitate antigen presentation. Moreover IFNγ is a co-factor in the formation of antibodies of some isotypes, for example IgG2a in the mouse. Co-administration of IL-2 or IFNγ with antigens augments antibody responses, which suggests that these cytokines are normally produced in small amounts that are limiting.

IL-Iβ and TNFα act on endothelial cells to increase attachment of lymphocytes. In lymph nodes draining sites of injection of adjuvants, homing of labelled lymphocytes from the circulation is increased. The augmented cell traffic in these lymph nodes raises the probability that lymphocytes bearing high-affinity receptors for an antigen will be exposed to that antigen on presenting cells. In the presence of the appropriate cytokines proliferation of specific clones of lymphocytes with receptors for antigen is favoured, resulting in primary immune responses and the generation of populations of memory cells able to respond rapidly on second exposure to the antigen.

IMMUNOPOTENTIATION FOR HUMAN VACCINES

Influenza

Human trials of an influenza vaccine in MDP-A are planned for the near future, and should establish whether the adjuvant formulation is safe and efficacious. If this proves to be the case, the opposition of regulatory authorities to the use of adjuvants other than alum in human vaccines may change. That should open the way for a new generation of vaccines.

As stated above, the first objective is to improve vaccines already in use, for example influenza and hepatitis B vaccines. These two illustrate the requirements for adjuvants, one of which is to improve sub-optimal immune responses which may be due to the age or genetic constitution of recipients, or to concurrent infections.

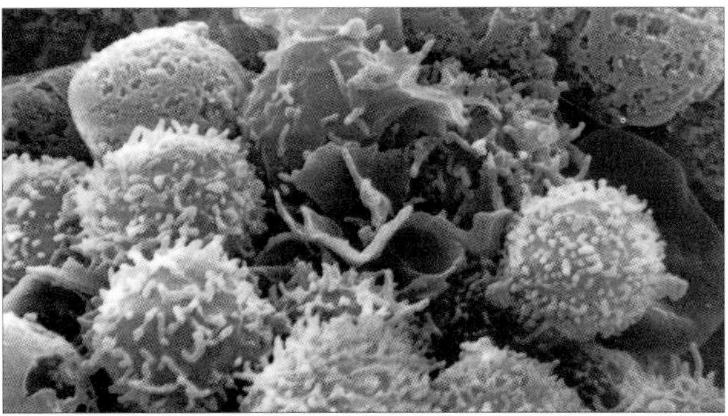

Fig. 28.11 Scanning electron micrograph of lymphocytes clustered around an afferent lymph dendritic (veiled) cell. x 1400. Courtesy of Dr S Knight.

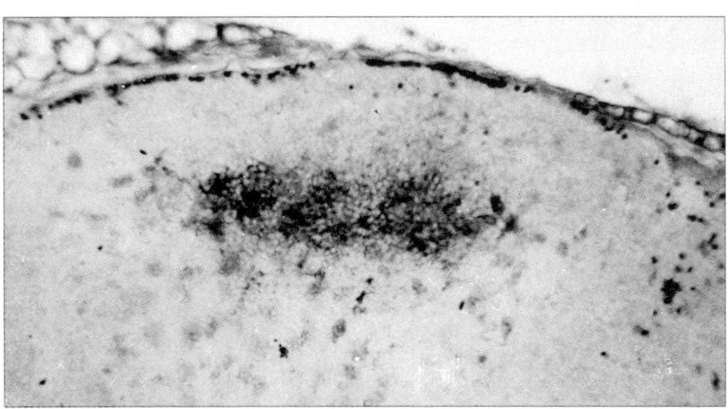

Fig. 28.12 Light micrograph of a popliteal lymph node showing the localization of antigen (horseradish peroxidase) 5 days after antigen injection in an immune mouse. Antigen in the form of immune complexes is retained in association with FDCs (dark area). x70. Courtesy of Dr P Szakal.

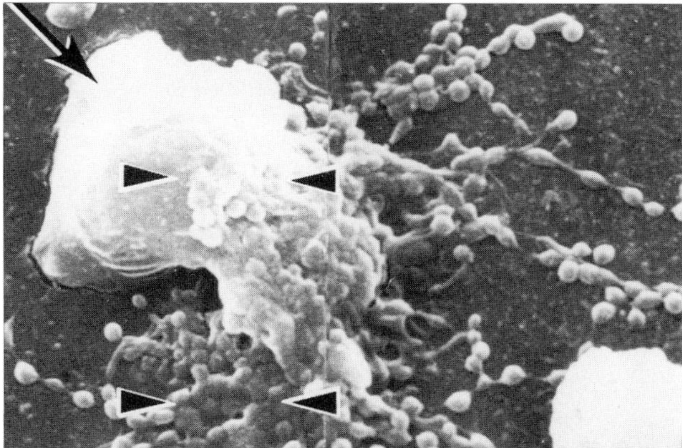

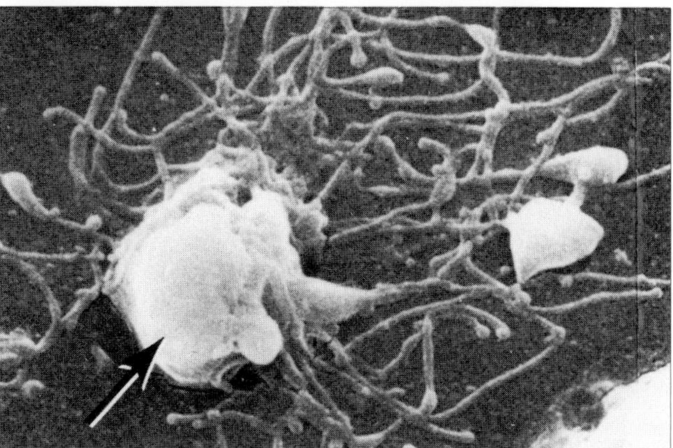

Fig. 28.13 Upper: scanning electron micrograph of a follicular dendritic cell (arrow) with iccosomes (arrow heads) x 2000. Lower: scanning electron micrograph of follicular dendritic cell (arrow) with smooth cytoplasmic extensions x 2000. Courtesy of Dr P Szakal.

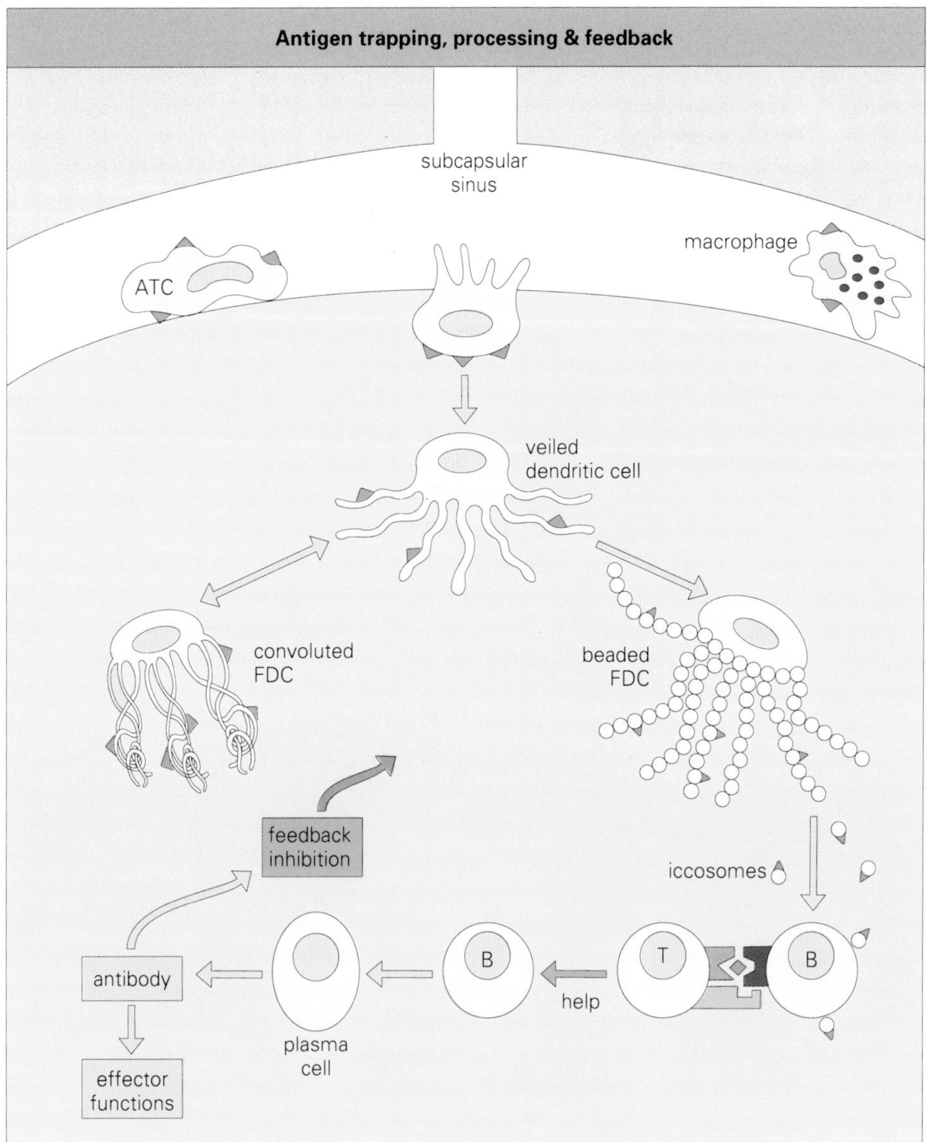

Fig. 28.14 Trapping of immune complexes by antigen-transport cells (ATC) in the subcapsular sinus (SS) of the lymph node. ATC migrate to follicles and become follicular dendritic cells (FDC), which retain beaded immune complex-coated bodies (iccosomes) on their surfaces. Antigen is transiently associated with macrophages in the subcapsular sinus. Antigen interaction with convoluted FDC is probably long term, where as that with beaded FDCs is short lived.

Hepatitis

Although infants respond poorly to many antigens, there are situations in which neonatal vaccination is desirable. In South-East Asia and Africa a high percentage of persons are persistent carriers of HBV (Fig. 28.15). The virus is often transmitted by mothers to offspring in the postnatal period, and this early infection leads to persistence, cirrhosis and hepatocellular carcinoma (Fig. 28.16). Conventional vaccination in the postnatal period can prevent early and persistent infection.

In normal adults three doses of alum-adjuvanted HBsAg induce antibody responses in the great majority of recipients. However, some individuals fail to respond to repeated doses of antigen; non-responders are frequently of the HLA-B8, SCOI, DR3 haplotype, suggesting that genetic restriction of responses to HBsAg epitopes is operative in humans, as it is in mice. MDP-A improves recombinant HBsAg vaccination in mice so that:

- two doses of antigen in adult animals are sufficient to elicit satisfactory antibody levels;
- the amount of expensive antigen in each dose can be reduced to one fifth;
- inherited low responsiveness can be overcome;
- very young mice can be induced to respond well.

If these observations can be extended to humans, a useful vaccine will be made even better.

The major cause of non-A, non-B hepatitis is hepatitis C virus (HCV), which has recently been identified by recombinant technology. It frequently produces persistent infections and chronic hepatitis, and is also associated with cirrhosis and primary hepatocellular carcinoma in South-East China. The possibility of vaccination with the recombinant major envelope glycoprotein of HCV in an effective adjuvant formulation is appealing. Systematic use of HBV and HCV vaccines in South-East Asia and

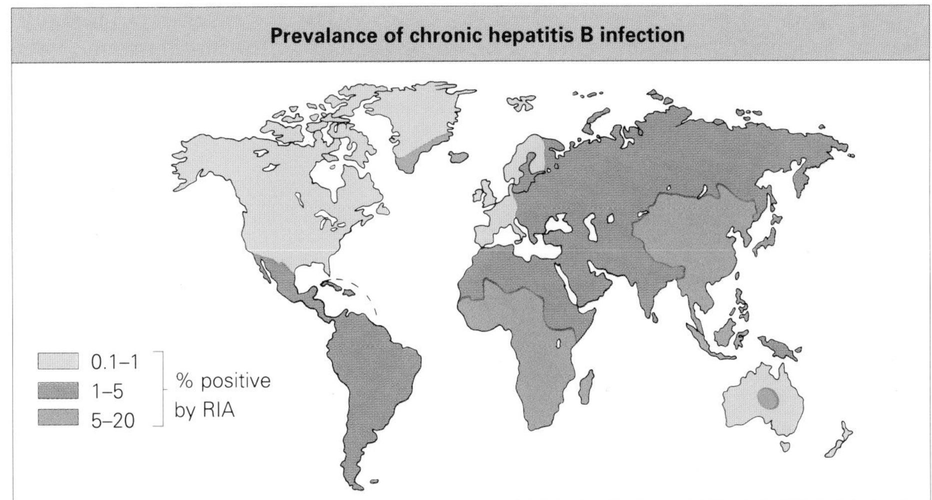

Fig. 28.15 Prevalence of chronic hepatitis B virus infection in the world, measured by the presence of HBsAg, detected by radioimmunoassay (RIA). Modified from Maupas & Melinck (1981).

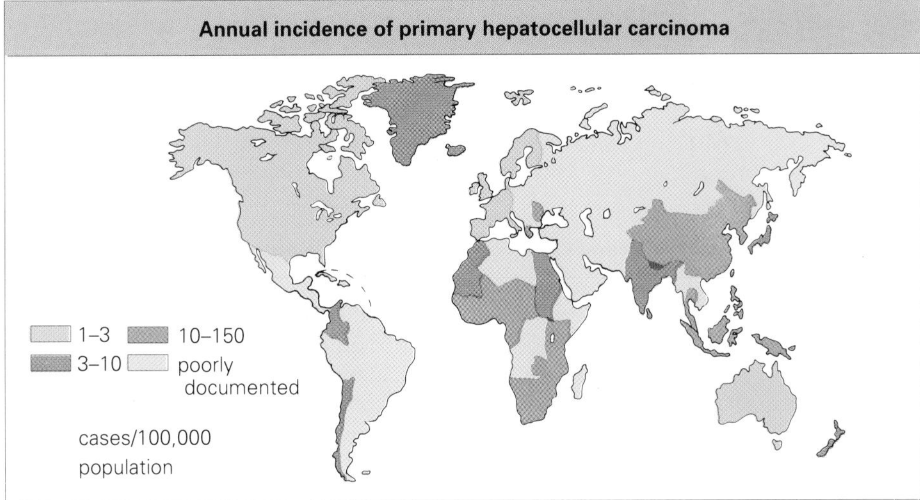

Fig. 28.16 Annual incidence of primary hepatocellular carcinoma in the world. Modified from Maupas & Melinck (1981).

Africa could prevent much illness and one of the commonest malignancies in these regions.

Influence of age

The age factor is also important in influenza vaccination. Persons aged 65 or over frequently have severe influenza infections, which represent the major cause of mortality from infectious disease in that age group. Annual vaccination is recommended in Europe and North America, but less than half of the recipients show the four-fold rise in antibody titre which indicates seroconversion. Old mice respond poorly and inconsistently to influenza vaccine, but the responses can be improved and made more consistent by the use of MDP-A. Again, if this is applicable to humans, the utility of influenza vaccine will be greatly extended because younger people will also choose to be vaccinated.

Herpes viruses

The feasibility of vaccination against herpes viruses using isolated or recombinant subunits in experimental animals has been demonstrated.

Epstein-Barr virus. In infected humans, Epstein-Barr virus (EBV) transforms B-lymphocytes into continuously proliferating cell lines; responding T lymphocytes limit that proliferation. Infectious mononucleosis is produced by the two responses, and can be a debilitating disease. When the T cell response is decreased for genetic reasons, or by chronic immunosuppression, B cell proliferation can continue to the extent of producing lymphomas. In subhuman primates termed cottontop tamarins (*Sanguinus oedipus oedipus*), the balance is also shifted in favour of B lymphocytes and against the responding T lymphocytes, so that lymphomas are produced in all recipients of a moderate dose of EBV. However, vaccination with the major surface glycoprotein of the virus (gp340) in MDP-A or ISCOMS protects all recipients against challenge with a 100% lymphomagenic dose of virus. It is reasonable to predict that in humans, with their more effective T lymphocytic response, vaccination will prevent infectious mononucleosis in Europe and North America.

Herpes simplex type 2. The guinea pig provides a good model of genital herpes simplex virus (HSV-2) infection. Vaginal infection produces severe local lesions, and the virus infects dorsal root ganglia, which results in recurrent infections in the great majority of recipients. Vaccination with a recombinant surface glycoprotein, gpD2, in MDP-A provides highly effective protection against challenge at the primary infection site. Very few vaccinated recipients develop dorsal root ganglion infections and recurrence. If these findings can be extended to humans, it should be possible to reduce the recurrence of this infection which is a cause of chronic discomfort and spread of the virus in the community. Genital herpes virus infections are also hazard in childbirth. Vaccination of infants against HSV, mainly type 1, may also reduce the severity of the primary stomatitis and probability of nerve–ganglion infection, recurrence and transmission in the community.

Varicella-zoster virus. The live, attenuated varicella-zoster virus vaccine cannot be safely used in children or other persons with immunodeficiency; a subunit vaccine would be safe. The importance of generating a population of memory cells (presumably T lymphocytes) is illustrated by the observation that when immunosuppressed persons (for example bone marrow or organ graft recipients) have primary cytomegalovirus (CMV) infections, they are frequently severe. If the CMV infection occurs before the period of immunosuppression, serious infections are rare. Effective immunization with a CMV subunit vaccine before transplantation would be a useful strategy, as would vaccination of women of child-bearing age.

HIV. Perhaps the greatest present need is for a vaccine against the human immunodeficiency viruses, HIV-1 and HIV-2. Simian immunodeficiency virus (SIV) is related to HIV and produces an AIDS-like disease in *Macaca mulatta* monkeys. Inactivated virus administered with MDP-A to monkeys provides highly effective protection against virus challenge, so that by analogy the development of a vaccine against HIV may be feasible.

BACTERIAL VACCINES

Bacterial capsular polysaccharides are poorly immunogenic, and coupling to a protein carrier increases immunogenicity. This has been done with *Haemophilus influenzae* polysaccharide to produce a vaccine which is safe and efficacious in children aged 15 months or older.

Inactivated *Bordetella pertussis* vaccine has demonstrated efficacy against the infection, but produces neurological complications in a few recipients (perhaps 1 in 300,000). This has led to litigation against vaccine manufacturers and given vaccines in general a bad name. The complications are attributed to residual active pertussis toxin, a potent ADP ribosylating protein with many biological effects. Unlike diphtheria or tetanus toxins, pertussis toxin cannot easily be inactivated while preserving immunogenicity. However, a recombinant pertussis toxin has been produced, and site-specific mutagenesis inactivates the enzyme while preserving its capacity to elicit neutralizing antibodies. Fimbrial proteins mediating attachment of *Bordetella* bacteria to cilia have also been identified. Circulating antibodies against this protein reduce colonization of the respiratory tract mucosa, and antibodies against the toxin can neutralize it before it damages distant organs including the brain. The combination of attachment protein, recombinant mutagenized toxoid and an efficacious adjuvant could provide the defined, acellular pertussis vaccine that has long been needed.

FURTHER READING

Allison AC, Byars NE. Antigens and adjuvants for a new generation of vaccines. *Mol Immunol.* 1990; in press.

Gregoriadis G, Allison AC, Poste G, eds. Immunological adjuvants and vaccines, NATO ASI series. *Adv Life Sci*, 1989; **79**: 1–244.

29

Plasmapheresis

HISTORY

The term plasmapheresis was coined by John Abel of Johns Hopkins Medical School in 1914 to describe a technique by which blood was removed from an animal, separated into its cellular and plasma components, the cells then being returned to the animal but the plasma retained. The word literally means withdrawal of plasma and has nothing to do with electrophoresis, which comes from an altogether different Greek root.

The therapeutic use of plasmapheresis derives from the practice of blood letting, a supposedly toxic substance in the plasma being efficiently removed without consequently killing the patient with anaemia. Between the wars, Whipple used the technique to study the turnover of plasma proteins, and during World War II plasmapheresis was evaluated as a means of providing the large quantities of donor plasma demanded by the military.

The first effective therapeutic use of plasmapheresis was in treating the hyperviscosity syndrome of Waldenström's macroglobulinaemia but further applications had to await the development of automated cell separators which made large-volume plasmapheresis feasible and cost-effective.

TECHNIQUES

Two methods of plasma separation are in current use: centrifugation and filtration.

CENTRIFUGAL TECHNIQUES

Blood consists of several components with different specific gravities which will separate on standing and do so more rapidly when centrifugal force is applied (Fig. 29.1). Early methods of plasmapheresis involved the withdrawal of a pint of blood from the donor into a bottle or plastic bag, centrifugation of this vessel at a point remote from the donor, removal of the supernatant plasma, and reinfusion of the packed cells. These methods are still in use for plasma donations in blood banks but are too cumbersome for therapeutic use and have been superseded by techniques using automated devices.

Large-volume plasmapheresis requires the removed plasma to be replaced by a suitable fluid, and when this is done the technique is often known as plasma exchange.

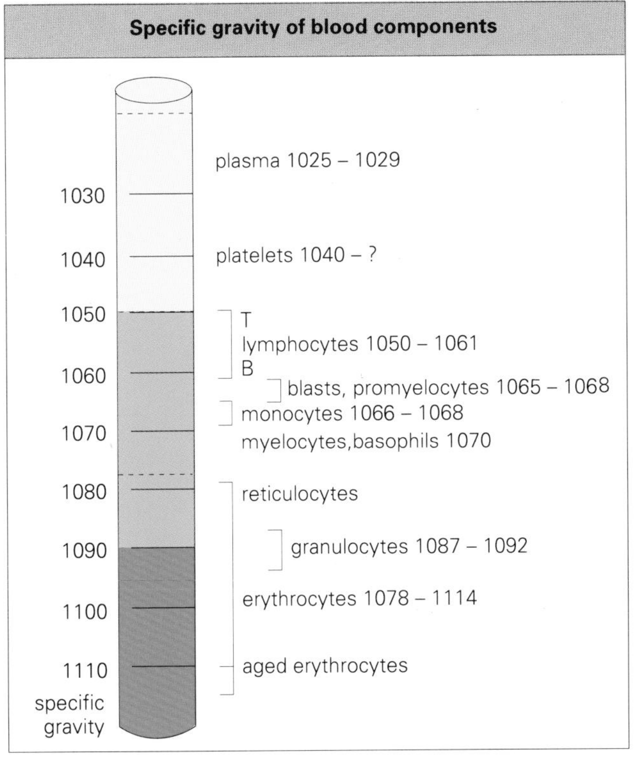

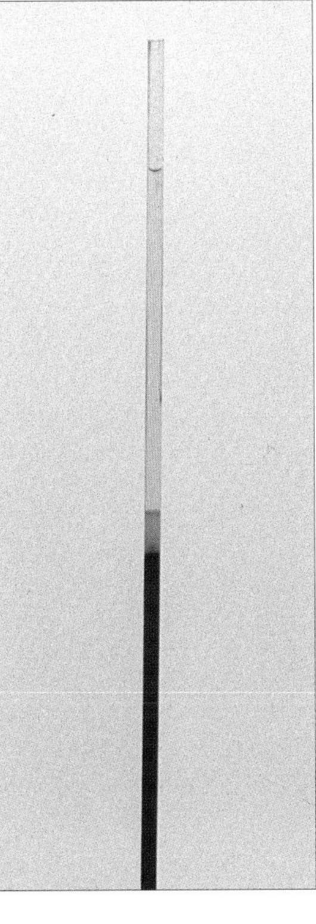

Fig 29.1 Separation of blood by specific gravity. Left: on centrifugation blood cells and plasma separate according to their respective specific gravities. Right: an exagerated buffy coat in a microhaematocrit tube following the centrifugation of blood from a patient with chronic lymphocytic leukaemia.

Discontinuous flow cell centrifuges

These machines have their origin in the Swedish dairy industry. Cohn's group at Harvard adapted a hand cranked De Laval E-19 cream separator to separate plasma from whole blood, and this machine was developed by Latham into subsequent generations of Haemonetics cell separators (Fig. 29.2). In principle, a large vessel is filled from the bottom while spinning. The blood components separate as the vessel is filled and the less dense components are collected from the top until the vessel is filled with red cells, which must then be returned to the patient together with replacement fluid before the cycle can be repeated. The volume of the bowl is 225ml and the maximum extracorporeal volume is appoximately 600ml; smaller bowls are available for paediatric use. The whole process may be repeated as many times as necessary.

Continuous flow cell centrifuges

The need to remove white cells from the leukaemic child of an IBM engineer led to a collaboration between the American National Cancer Institute and IBM to produce the first continuous flow cell centrifuge, which has since undergone a number of design modifications. In principle, blood is kept at a steady state of separation within the centrifuge by the balanced inflow of whole blood and outflow of components. The outflow of components is

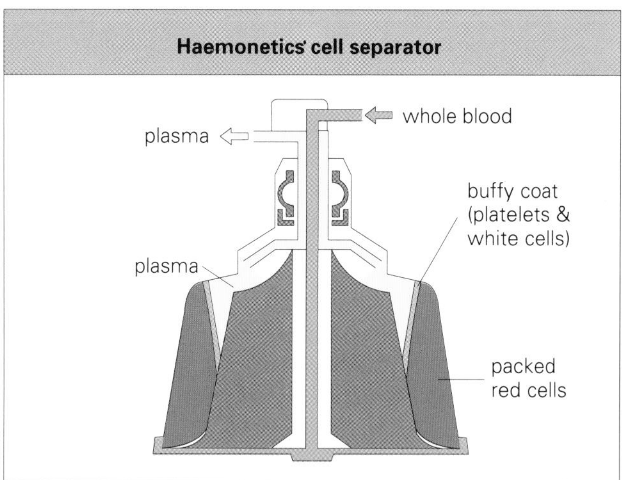

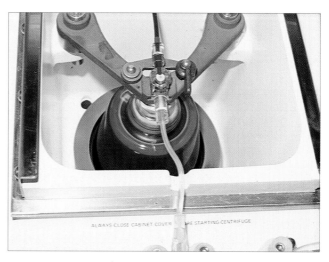

Fig. 29.2 Anti-coagulated blood is delivered through the central core, about which the bowl rotates. Blood enters the separation chamber at the bottom of the bowl and the supernatant leaves at the top. The sloping outer wall of the chamber causes the red cells which are sedimented against the wall to slide to the base of the bowl. A system of switches on the outflow line permit air, plasma, platelets and white cells to be collected in sequence. When the bowl is full of packed red cells, the centrifuge is stopped and the red cells returned to the patient as the bowl refills with sterile air.

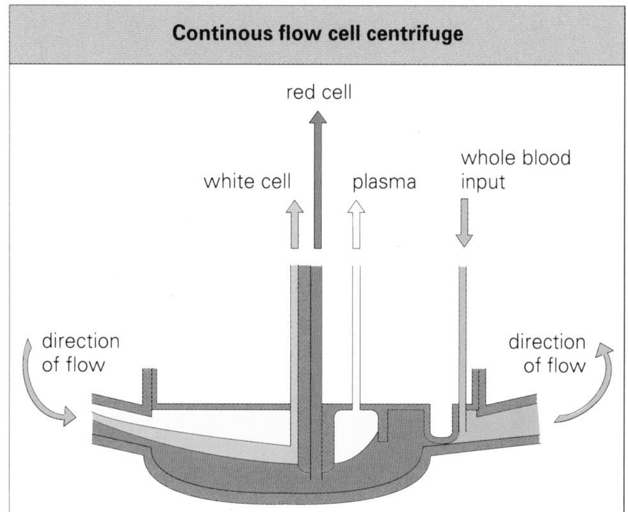

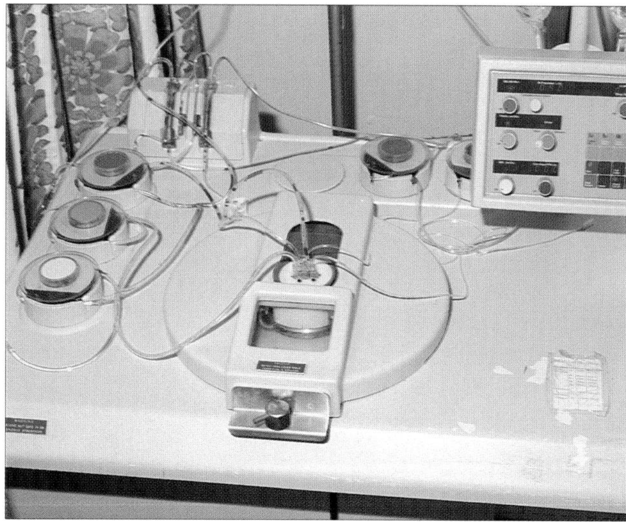

Fig. 29.3 Separation chamber of IBM continuous flow cell separator. Blood entering at the whole blood input port must travel in a circle in a rotating strap-like channel before entering the chamber. Within the chamber the centrifugal force forms interfaces between blood components according to their specific gravities. By altering the flow rates through the red cell and plasma ports the positions of the interfaces are altered.

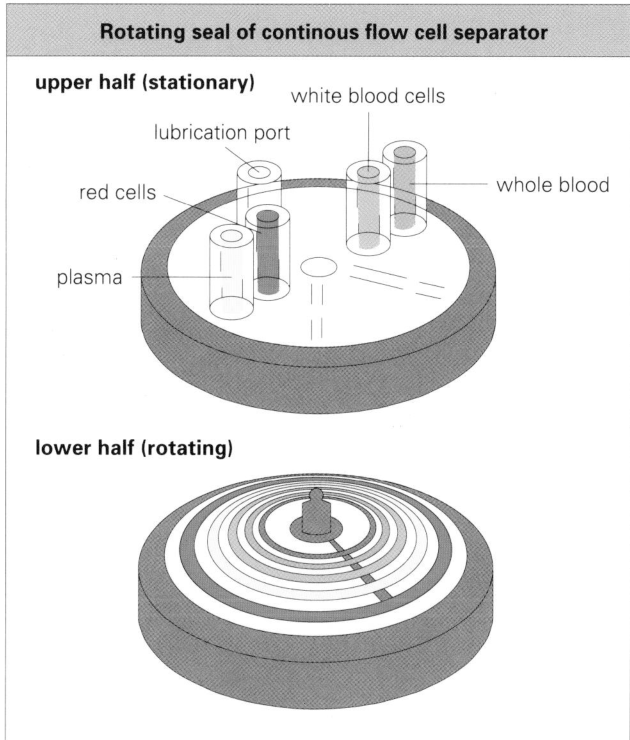

Fig. 29.4 The rotating seal allows a continuous sterile pathway through the cell separator for all blood components. The ceramic discs are lubricated by normal saline at high pressure which forms a barrier between the channels.

controlled by strategically placed outlet ports within the separation chamber (Fig. 29.3).

The major design problem was how to allow a separation chamber connected to a bundle of plastic tubes to rotate around the tubes without twisting them. This was solved by the use of a lubricated rotating seal consisting of two ceramic discs. The input ports in the upper stationary disc communicate with concentric circular channels in the lower rotating disc and these are connected to a corresponding set of tubes leaving the seal (Fig. 29.4).

The Fenwal CS 3000 solves the problem in a novel manner. In this design a bundle of flexible tubes is connected to the top of the centrifuge and loops around the outside to be connected to the stationary parts of the system. As the centrifuge rotates, the loop of tubes counter-rotates around the same axis at half the angular velocity, thus preventing the bundle from twisting (Fig. 29.5). The CS 3000 is further refined by continuous monitoring by microprocessor.

FILTRATION TECHNIQUES

Whereas cell centrifuges may be used to collect or remove any of the blood's components, filtration devices are used just to separate plasma from cells. The principle of separation is the application of blood under pressure to

Fenwal CS 3000

2ω

2ω

ω

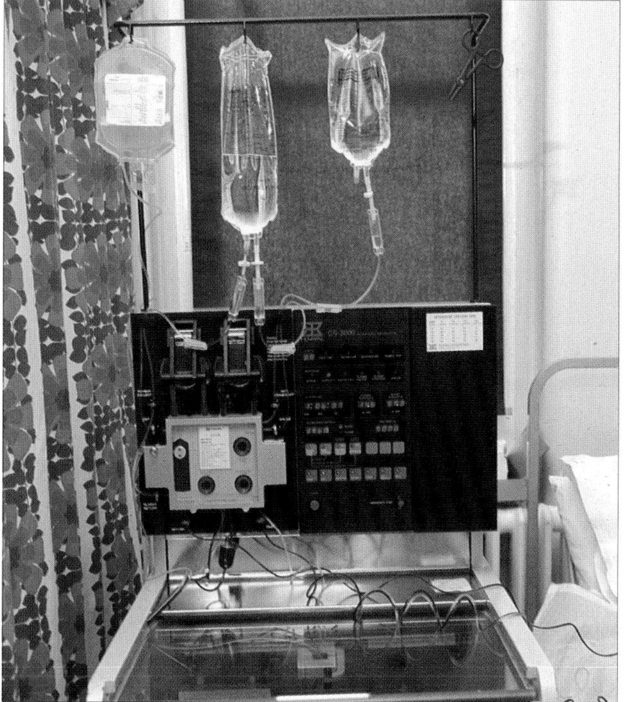

Fig. 29.5 Left: A bundle of tubes is connected to the centrifuge bowl at one end and tightly supported at the other end, forming a loop. The bowl rotates around a central axis at an angular velocity of 2ω, while the loop revolves around the same axis at ω and simultaneously untwists at ω thus preventing a tangle. Right: the Fenwall CS 3000 in use.

a thin plastic semi-porous membrane that permits the passage of plasma but not of cells. Devices are constructed in various configurations — usually as flat bed membranes (Fig. 29.6) or hollow fibres — with surface areas of 0.12–0.6m². The pore size is 0.1–0.5mm and the transmembrane pressure is 50mmHg or less. The major developmental problems have been in producing a membrane that does not activate complement or the clotting cascade and does not clog with protein or platelets.

SELECTIVE PLASMAPHERESIS

Where a specific plasma component has been identified as the principle cause of a disease, selective removal of that component would appear to be the ideal form of plasmapheresis. A number of methods for specifically depleting plasma components have been described (Figs 29.7–29.9). All involve an in-line device designed to absorb either whole Ig or specific antibody.

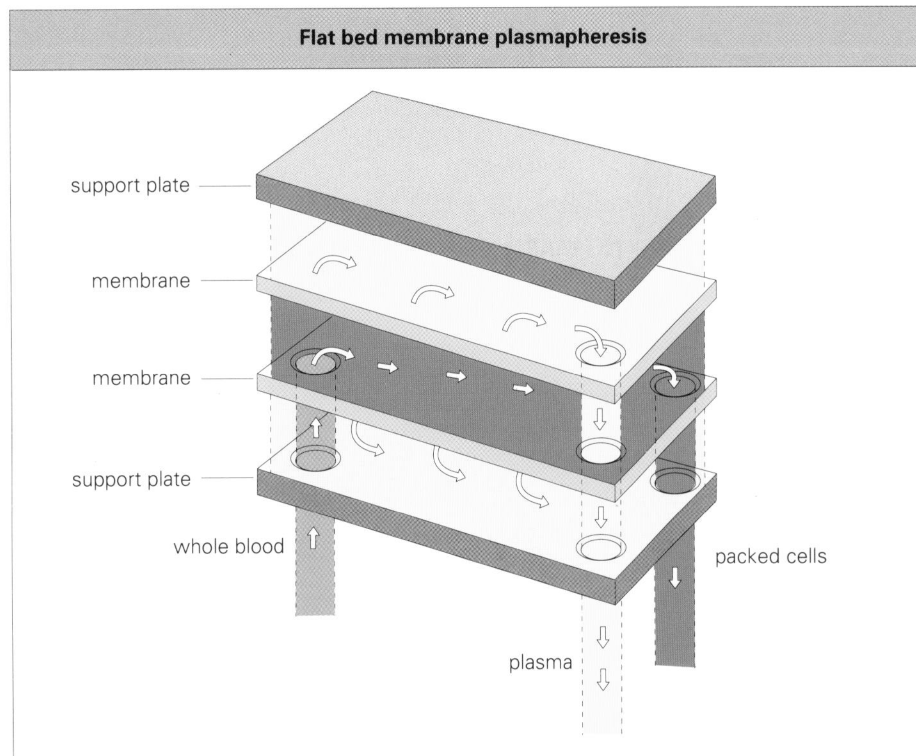

Fig. 29.6 Expanded view of flat bed membrane plasmapheresis. Blood under pressure is forced into the central channel. Plasma is able to pass through the semi-porous membranes into the two outer channels and packed red cells are collected from the central channel.

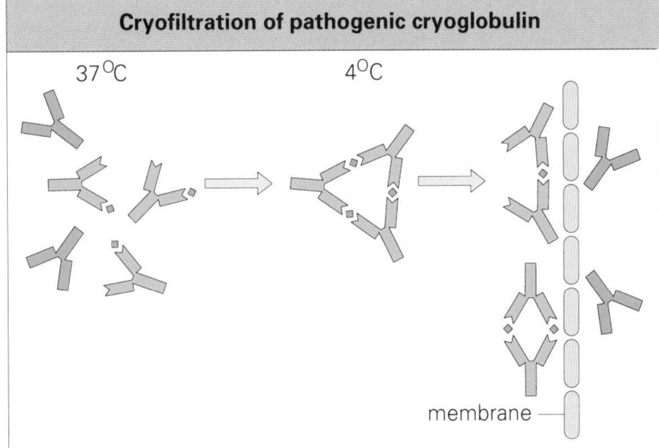

Fig. 29.7 As the temperature of the plasma is lowered, soluble immune complexes aggregate. A micropore membrane retains the aggregated immune complexes and allows free passage of other plasma components.

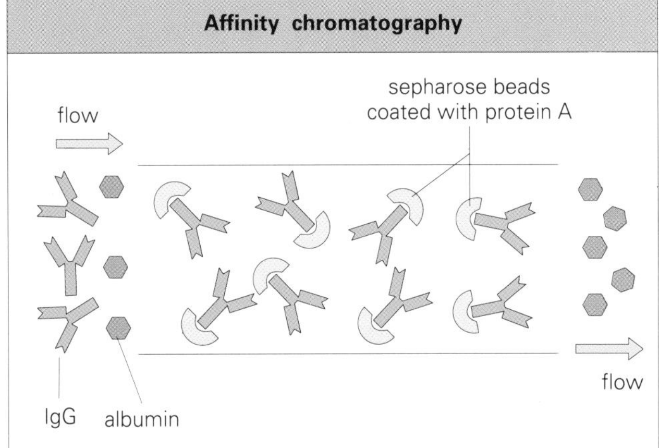

Fig. 29.8 Plasma flowing over sepharose beads linked to protein A is depleted of antibody (except IgG3 subclass). In certain circumstances antigen can be linked to beads and the method used to deplete specific antibody.

However, none of these methods has been shown to be more beneficial clinically than removal of whole plasma and replacement with albumin solution, and a decision on their use is heavily influenced by economic factors.

REPLACEMENT FLUID

When removing large volumes of plasma it is necessary to replace the fluid during the procedure to prevent circulatory collapse. Theoretically, the best replacement fluid would be the patient's own plasma with the offending toxin removed (see above). However, in most circumstances only the osmotic effect of the plasma needs to be replaced and therefore a 5% solution of human albumin obtained from donor blood is a safe and effective replacement. It is standard practice to add 2ml of KCl solution (1mmol/ml)and 2ml of 10% calcium gluconate solution to the albumin. Five percent human albumin solution (HAS) is slightly hyperosmotic and leads to an inflow of water into the circulation following plasma exchange. Most plasma exchange units replace every 2 litres of plasma removed with 1.5 litres of HAS and 0.5 litres of normal saline. Under certain circumstances, replacement of other plasma components is necessary for the full therapeutic effect. Sometimes, a specific component such as IgG is added to the HAS; fresh frozen plasma is an alternative, but this has associated hazards.

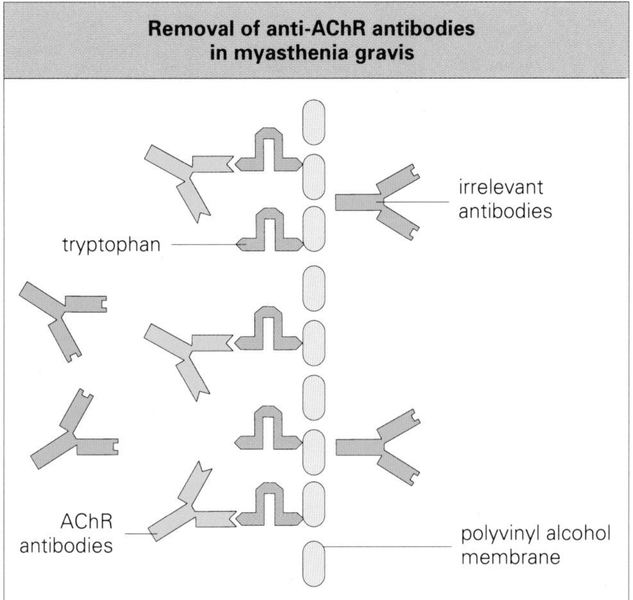

Fig. 29.9 A hydrophobic membrane consisting of a tryptophan-linked polyvinyl alcohol membrane has a particular affinity for anti-acetylcholine receptor (AChR) antibodies and has been used successfully to deplete these antibodies in myasthenia gravis. The reason for the specific affinity is not known.

EFFECT OF PLASMAPHERESIS ON PLASMA COMPONENTS

Anything that appears in plasma may be removed by plasma exchange. A simplified model of plasma exchange is shown in Fig. 29.10. If it is assumed that the time taken for plasma exchange is so short that values for synthesis, catabolism, trans-capillary escape and return rate are effectively zero, then the effect of plasma exchange on a particular component that is not present in the replacement fluid is expressed by the formula:

$$Y_t = Y_0 . e^{-X} \quad \text{(Fig. 29.11)}$$

where Y_t is the final concentration, Y_0 the initial concentration and x the number of plasma volumes exchanged.

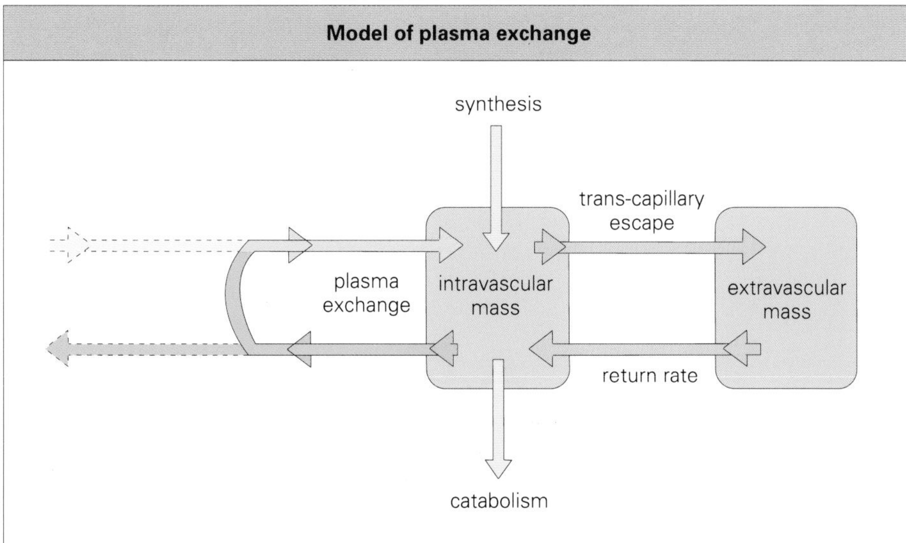

Fig. 29.10 Simplified model of plasma exchange. The intravascular mass of a particular compound is the product of the plasma concentration and the plasma volume. In the steady state, trans-capillary escape to the extravascular mass (which is related to the molecular weight of the substance) is balanced by the return rate, and synthesis is balanced by catabolism. Thus plasma exchange, by removing the offending compound from the intravascular mass, is forcing the equilibrium to the left.

This exponential function decrees that the greater the volume of plasma exchanged the more likely it is that the procedure will remove the replacement fluid rather than the offending substance. For this reason the procedure is usually halted after the exchange of a single plasma volume (approximately 3 litres for a 70kg man). This will remove 40–50% of a plasma component, while a 5 litre exchange would only remove another 10%. Re-equilibration between the intravascular and extravascular spaces takes about a day for IgG, so that daily plasma exchange is both physiologically sound and clinically convenient.

A special case exists for certain high molecular weight proteins and polymers. These compounds are hyperviscous and hyperoncotic so that, when present in large amounts, they give rise to the hyperviscosity syndrome (see below), producing a greatly expanded plasma volume due to the inflow of crystalloid into the intravascular space. Removal of these substances by plasma exchange may lead to rapid reduction in the oncotic pressure, outflow of water from the intravascular space, and a less than expected reduction of serum concentration of the particular component.

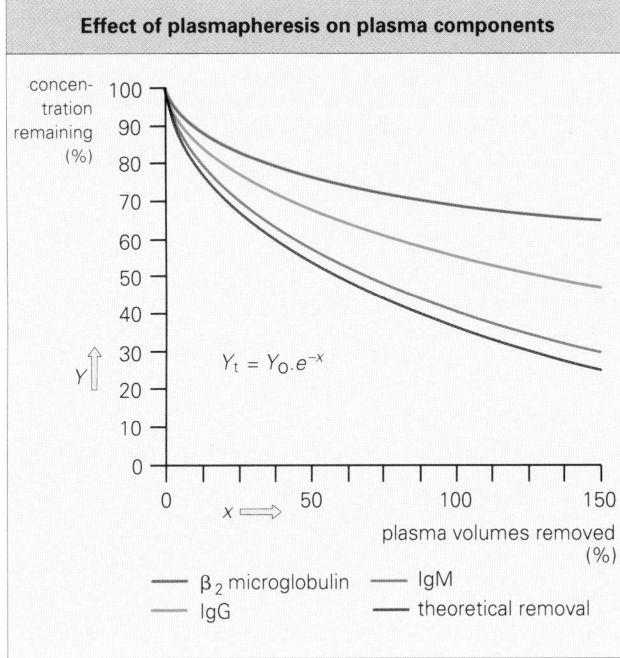

Fig. 29.11 For substances which are mostly intravascular and which have slow re-equilibration with the extravascular space, the disappearance curve approximates to the formula shown. However, lower molecular weight substances that equilibrate freely with the extravascular space have a smaller reduction in the plasma concentration.

EFFECT ON IMMUNOGLOBULIN CATABOLISM

The fractional catabolic rates of IgA, IgM and IgG3 are independent of serum levels and therefore unaffected by plasma exchange. However, for other subclasses of IgG the fractional catabolic rate is proportional to the serum level (Fig. 29.12). For very low levels of IgG it is about 2% per day and for very high levels, for example in myeloma, it is as much as 18% per day. Thus, as IgG levels are reduced, plasma exchange becomes progressively less efficient at removing the antibody. Since it is generally not IgG as a whole but a specific antibody within the IgG fraction that must be depleted, adding non-specific IgG to the replacement fluid surmounts this difficulty.

The catabolism of circulating immune complexes is a function of macrophages in the spleen and elswhere. In diseases associated with circulating immune complexes, such as SLE and rapidly progressive glomerulonephritis, this function appears to be inhibited. It can be measured by estimating the half-clearance time of radio-labelled heat-damaged red cells, which in immune complex diseases is increased and explained by the fact that circulating monocytes have diminished bacterial killing activity and reduced acid hydrolase levels. Following plasma exchange all of these measurements return to normal. It

Metabolic characteristics of some plasma proteins

	IgG*	IgA	IgM	IgD	IgE	Albumin	C3
mean serum concentration (g/litre)	12.1	2.6	0.9	0.02	0.003	42	1.5
half life (days)	22.5	5.8	5.1	2.8	2.5	5	1
mol wt (kDa)	150	160	950	175	195	66	180
% intravascular	45	42	76	75	41	40	53
fractional catabolic rate (% intravascular mass/day)	6.7	25	18	37	89	10	56
changes in FCR with concentration	↓	0	0	↑	↑	↓	?

* (excluding IgG3)

Fig. 29.12 Metabolic characteristics, including fractional catabolic rate (FCR), of certain plasma proteins.

has long been recognized that in immune complex diseases even low-volume plasmapheresis is capable of reducing circulating immune complex levels by a far greater degree than could be accounted for by the quantity of complexes in the removed plasma. The presumed explanation for this is the relief of a blockaded mononuclear phagocytic (MP) system (Fig. 29.13).

EFFECT ON IMMUNOGLOBULIN SYNTHESIS

The synthetic rate of immunoglobulins is independent of the serum concentration of immunoglobulins as a whole, or even of a specific class of immunoglobulins. However, synthesis of individual antibodies is subject to feedback inhibition by the serum level of that particular antibody. Thus, particularly during a primary response, removal of specific antibody leads to increased synthesis and a rebound rise and overshoot of the antibody level. Such an effect may also be observed during a secondary response, but this depends on continued antigenic stimulation. Removal of antibody persisting after a bankrupt immune response will not generate a rebound in antibody levels (Fig. 29.14). Autoantibodies have the characteristics of secondary responses continually fuelled by antigenic stimulation, and rebound with overshoot is the rule following the removal of specific autoantibodies.

Experimentally, antibody rebound may be of great value in helping to generate the maximum amount of antibody in response to a scarce antigen. However, clinically it is the major restriction on the use of therapeutic plasma exchange and dictates that in most circumstances it is necessary to take separate measures to inhibit antibody synthesis, usually with immunosuppressive drugs.

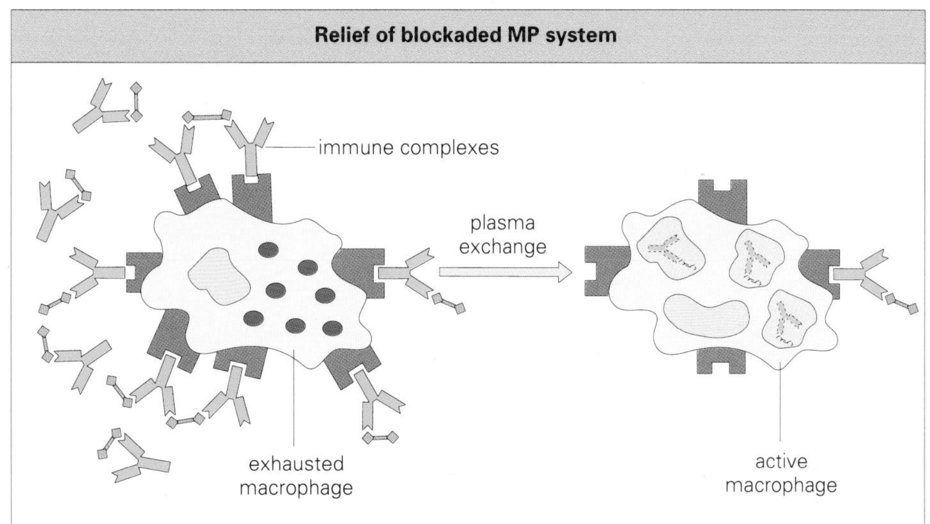

Fig. 29.13 An 'exhausted' macrophage is blockaded by circulating immune complexes and is unable to pinocytose and digest complexes bound to Fc receptors. Plasma exchange 'lifts the seige' and restores macrophages to health and vigour.

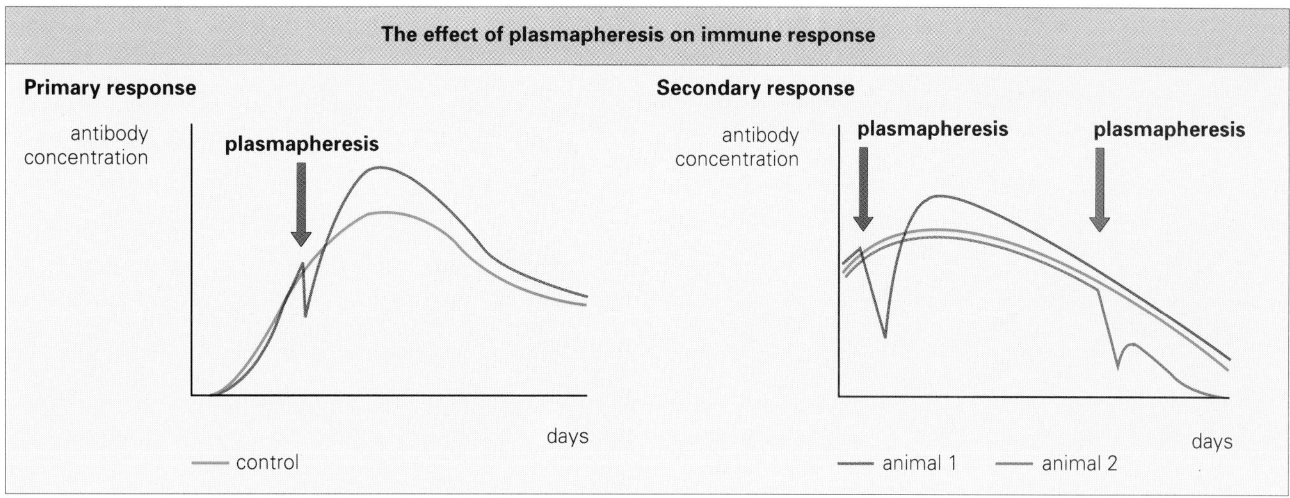

Fig. 29.14 Animal 1 shows a fall with rebound and overshoot of antibody production following plasmapheresis soon after immunization in both primary and secondary responses. Animal 2 shows no overshoot after late plasmapheresis, as antigenic stimulation has ceased.

SYNERGY WITH IMMUNOSUPPRESSIVE DRUGS

It has been suggested that removal of antibody may synchronize the proliferation and division of the lymphoid cells responsible for the immune response, rendering them especially susceptible to a pulse of cytotoxic drugs (Fig. 29.15). Although there is some evidence for this in experimental systems, any benefits from such synergy with the kind of immunosuppressive regimens available to the clinician have been too small to observe. Nevertheless, there have been numerous anecdotal reports in which the addition of plasma exchange to an immunosuppressive protocol has been sufficient to tip the balance in favour of disease control.

EFFECT ON INFLAMMATORY MEDIATORS

It has been suggested that part of the benefit of plasma exchange derives from the removal of inflammatory mediators, particularly complement components, fibrinogen and fibronectin. However, all of these components have short half-lives and are rapidly replaced following plasma exchange. Moreover, what evidence there is points to slightly greater benefits from the use of fresh frozen plasma rather than albumin as a replacement fluid for plasma exchange in the treatment of inflammatory disease; it is thought that this is because of the ability of complement to solubilize immune complexes.

EFFECT OF PLASMAPHERESIS ON CELLULAR IMMUNITY

Plasmapheresis appears to have no effect on the cellular immune function of normal donors. Numerous authors have reported changes in T cell, B cell and mononuclear phagocytic function following plasma exchange in patients with autoimmune disease or cancer. Most of the changes were, in effect, a restoration of previously impaired function towards normal levels, implying that in these patients, there are circulating factors which impair the cellular immune response.

COMPLICATIONS

Plasmapheresis performed in a unit with experienced staff is an extremely safe procedure. However, a long list of complications has been recognized including over 50 deaths attributed to the procedure. The complications may be broken down as follows:

- Related to vascular access. Complications include poor flow due to inadequate or thrombosed veins, thrombosed or infected shunts and fistulae, and amputation (very rare).
- Related to anti-coagulant. Citrate toxicity can lead to circumoral parasthesiae, muscle twitching, vomiting, chills and syncope, all of which are common. Tetany and cardiac arrhythmias are rare, and bleeding occurs only with heparin.
- Related to apparatus. Complications may be caused by clotting or leaking within the machine, or air emboli (very rare).
- Related to replacement fluid. Anaphylaxis, acute respiratory distress syndrome or death may occur, mainly with fresh frozen plasma. Pyrexia and bradycardia may follow administration of some human albumin solutions due to the presence of prekallikrein activator.
- Related to removal of blood components.Thrombocytopenia may occur but is significant only if the patient is already deficient. Anaemia and fainting are further possible complications. Infection is rarely due to reduced immunoglobulin levels but is more likely to be caused by associated immunosuppressive drugs. Bleeding is unlikely to be caused by removing clotting factors but thrombosis may follow removal of anti-thrombin III.

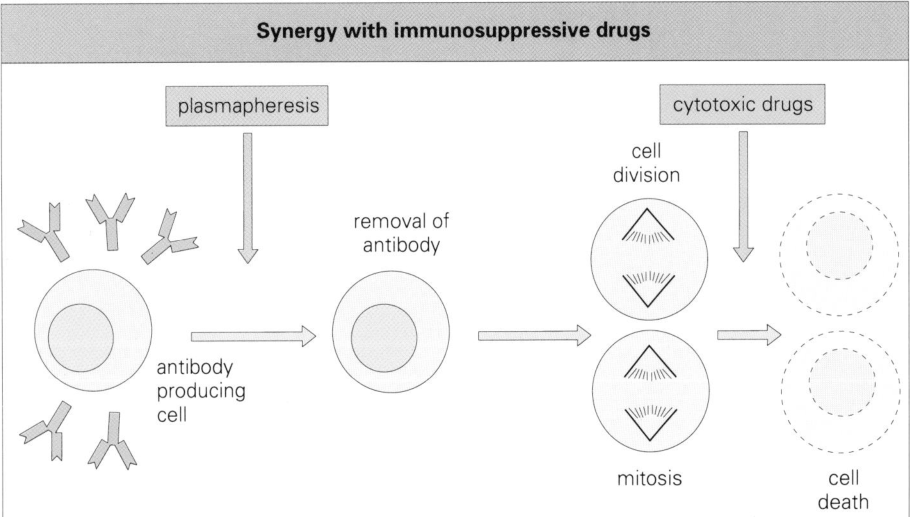

Fig. 29.15 Removal of antibody leads to multiplication of antibody-producing cells, leaving them susceptible to cycle-specific cytotoxic drugs.

CLINICAL APPLICATIONS

Plasmapheresis has been used in over 200 different conditions, but in most there is either no clear evidence of any benefit, or no evidence of any advantage over less costly conventional treatments. However, in a small number of conditions this treatment does have an established role in therapy.

HYPERVISCOSITY SYNDROME

The association between highly viscous serum and macroglobulinaemia was first noticed by Jan Waldenström in 1944, and the presence of a monoclonal IgM paraprotein remains the most common cause of the syndrome. Monoclonal IgG and IgA paraproteins are less common causes of hyperviscosity, which may also be associated with polyclonal immune complexes in certain connective tissue disorders.

Characteristically, the syndrome presents with visual disturbances ranging from minor problems with focusing to complete blindness. This is accompanied by abnormal bleeding from skin, mucous membranes and surgical wounds, neurological symptoms, including headache, dizziness, vertigo, somnolence, deafness and coma, and cardiovascular symptoms including breathlessness and oedema. The physical signs include the characteristic fundoscopic appearance (Fig. 29.16), confluent dependent purpura, and the signs of heart failure. A dilutional anaemia is common. Clinical features are unlikely to occur with a relative viscosity of less than 4.

Plasmapheresis leads to rapid amelioration of symptoms and signs although the procedure may be complicated by low blood flow rates. Some patients are controlled by regular plasmapheresis, but others require control of the underlying lymphoplasmacytoid malignancy with cytotoxic drugs.

ANTIBODY MEDIATED DISEASES

Alloantibodies

Rh haemolytic disease. Damage to the fetal red cells is caused by the transfer across the placenta of maternal antibody generated in response to a previous Rh-positive pregnancy or blood transfusion. In most cases the immune response is fuelled by a feto-maternal leak of red cells at delivery, but passive anti-D antibody given to the mother within 72 hours of delivery prevents the development of anti-Rh antibodies. Despite every effort, however, a small

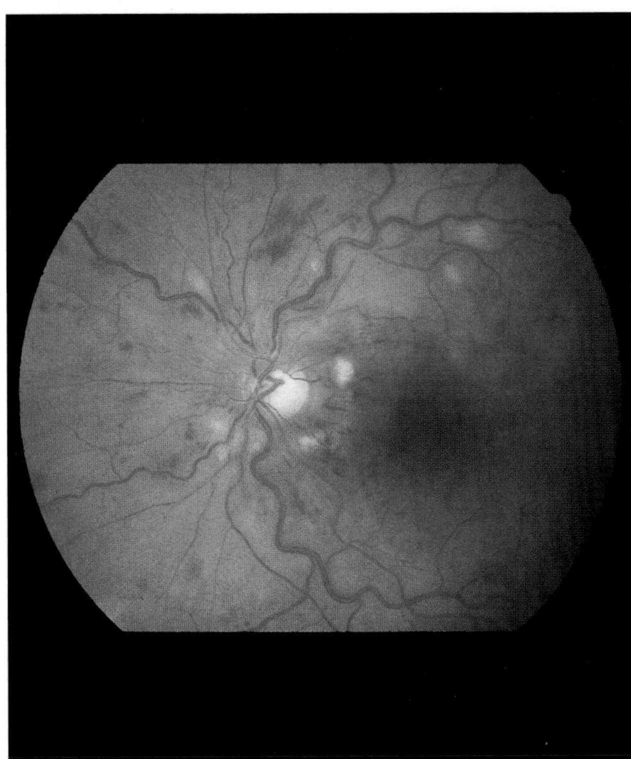

Fig. 29.16 Fundoscopic appearance in hyperviscosity syndrome. Venous dilatation, with the 'string of sausages' appearance, haemorrhages and microaneurysms are evident. Papilloedema and retinal vein thrombosis may occur.

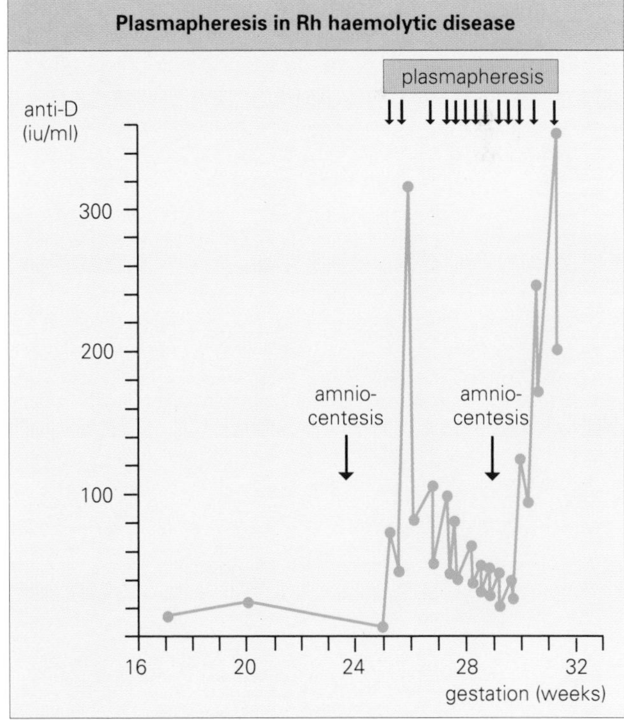

Fig. 29.17 Although plasmapheresis causes a fall in anti-D titres any refuelling of the immune response by fresh antigenic stimulation, such as that which occurs after amniocentesis, can lead to a rapid increase in antibody titre at a rate beyond the counteractive capacity of plasma exchange.

number of patients continue to be affected. Although no controlled trial has been performed, plasmapheresis during pregnancy demonstrably lowers the antibody concentration in the mother and this has led to the delivery of live babies who were expected by historical criteria to die. It appears that amniocentesis is dangerous in such pregnancies since it makes a new materno-fetal leak and thus increases the likelihood of refuelling the immune response (Fig. 29.17).

Haemophilia. The inhibitors which arise in 10% of patients severely affected by haemophilia are alloantibodies against the coagulant portion of the Factor VIII molecule, which is seen as a foreign protein in the patient. In some cases the inhibitor may be bypassed or overcome by increasing doses of Factor VIII concentrate, but in a minority of patients plasmapheresis provides the means of removing antibody. It is usually reserved for life threatening haemorrhage.

Autoantibodies

Many diseases are marked by the presence of autoantibodies in the serum but only in a minority has the autoantibody been shown to be responsible for the pathological change. Although plasmapheresis has been demonstrated to be effective in the management of diseases mediated by autoantibodies, in almost every case it has been necessary to use steroids and cytotoxic drugs in combination to gain full control of the disease. In some cases these drugs alone seem to be able to suppress the disease and one should consider whether plasmapheresis adds anything to the treatment. Although there is speculation that plasmapheresis and cytotoxic drugs act synergistically, the major benefit from the former is probably speed of response.

Goodpasture's syndrome. Antibodies against glomerular basement membrane, which produce the characteristic linear pattern on immunofluorescent staining (see chapter 8) lead to an acute inflammatory glomerulonephritis which, unchecked, gives rise to irreversible renal failure. In smokers especially, the antibody, which cross-reacts with pulmonary alveolar basement membrane, causes lung haemorrhage which is frequently fatal. The grave prognosis of this disease has been ameliorated by an aggressive immunosuppressive regimen introduced by Lockwood, comprising prednisolone 60mg/day, cyclophosphamide 3mg/kg/day, azathioprine 1mg/kg/day and daily 4 litre plasma exchanges. With this treatment lung haemorrhage is abated and renal function is restored so long as the patient is not already oliguric. The anuric kidney cannot be saved. The progression of the disease is so rapid, and the damage to the end organ so final that the speed with which plasmapheresis lowers the antibody level is an essential part of the treatment.

Myasthenia gravis. In this condition, antibodies against the acetylcholine receptor at the muscle motor end plate lead to complement-mediated lysis of the post-synaptic membrane and to antigenic modulation and pinocytosis of the acetylcholine receptor (see chapter 9). If the antibody is removed the receptor is re-expressed. In patients who are failing to respond to anti-cholinesterase drugs, treatment with immunosuppressive drugs is effective, but there is a lag period during which the patient may need to be managed on a respirator. Short-term, speedy relief is obtained with plasma exchange before the drugs have time to work.

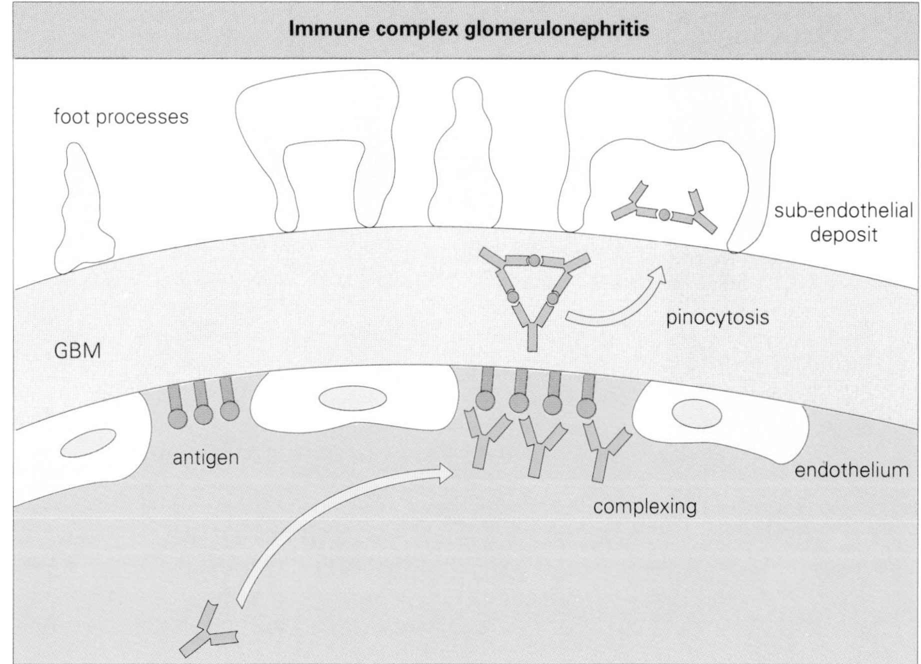

Fig. 29.18 In some cases immune complexes form with antigen which is either intrinsic to the glomerular basement membrane (GBM) or bound to it. Modulation and pinocytosis carry the complex across the membrane to form a sub-endothelial deposit which leads to fusion of foot processes.

Guillain-Barré syndrome. In this condition the ascending paralysis is apparently mediated by a serum factor able to transfer a nerve conduction blockade into experimental animals. The serum factor is probably related to one of the autoantibodies to nerve antigens which have been demonstrated by immunofluorescence. A large, American, multicentre, controlled trial has conclusively demonstrated the beneficial effect of plasmapheresis during the first week. The benefit is less apparent during the second week of the illness and not demonstrable thereafter, thus illustrating the need to rapidly remove the toxic factors before end organ damage is irreversible.

IMMUNE COMPLEX MEDIATED DISEASES

Circulating immune complexes are even more difficult to relate to specific diseases than are circulating autoantibodies. Plasmapheresis has a two-fold effect on circulating complexes:

- it unblocks the mononuclear phagocytic system to allow the normal clearance of complexes;
- it acts as part of an immunosuppressive regimen.

For the former even small-volume plasma exchanges will suffice, but the benefit is usually transitory. For the latter, an intensive immunosuppressive regimen similar to that used in Goodpasture's syndrome is probably required.

There is undoubtedly some confusion about the nature of the immune complexes demonstrated in the glomerulus by immunofluorescence as characteristic granular deposits. Recent evidence suggests that they are formed *in situ* by the combination of circulating antibody with extrinsic antigens bound to the glomerular basement membrane (Fig. 29.18). The patchy appearance is probably caused by antigenic modulation.

Controlled studies in immune complex diseases are rare. A study of plasma exchange in patients with rapidly progressive glomerulonephritis associated with Wegener's granulomatosus or microscopic polyarteritis, or of unknown cause, demonstrated that plasma exchange added nothing of benefit to a regimen comprising cyclophosphamide, azathioprine and prednisolone, except in patients who were already oliguric, whose renal function could only be restored when plasma exchange formed part of the treatment.

On the other hand, despite numerous anecdotal reports of response to plasma exchange in systemic lupus erythematosus, a recent American study shows that in lupus glomerulonephritis plasma exchange confers no benefit to an adequate immunosuppressive regimen.

Other presumed immune complex diseases that respond to plasma exchange are shown in Fig. 29.19.

Immune complex diseases that respond to PE	
Disease	**Indication for plasma exchange**
SLE	no advantage over steroids & cytotoxic drugs except in cerebral lupus
rapidly progressive glomerulonephritis	as above except in oliguric patients
rheumatoid arthritis	no benefit except in rheumatoid vasculitis
systemic vasculitis	indicated
mixed connective tissue disease	sometimes effective not evaluated against other treatments
Sjögren's syndrome	as above
Raynaud's phenomenon	effective against digital ulceration
cryoglobulinaemia	treatment of choice

Fig. 29.19 Some presumed immune complex diseases that respond to treatment with plasma exchange.

FURTHER READING

Berkman EM, Umlas J, eds. *Therapeutic haemapheresis.* Arlington VA: American Association of Blood Banks, 1981.

Hamblin TJ. *Plasmapheresis and plasma exchange.* Quebec: Eden Press, 1979.

Pattern E. Therapeutic plasmapheresis and plasma exchange. *Crit Rev Clin Lab Sci* 1986;**23**:147–175.

Shumak KH, Rock GA. Therapeutic plasma exchange. *N Engl J Med* 1984:**310**:762–772.

30

Laboratory Investigations

INTRODUCTION

Laboratory investigations are used to aid the diagnosis and management of patients with disorders of the immune system. The techniques often involve the use of immunological reagents of high specificity and sensitivity. These tools are also used by other laboratory disciplines (for example clinical chemistry, microbiology and haematology) to define and measure microbial antigens, hormones, biochemical analytes, cell types and many other substances of interest to workers in those fields.

When considering involvement of the immune system in a disease process the following questions need to be answered:

- is the immune system involved?
- are its constituent parts functioning properly?
- is it reacting against autoantigens?
- is it reacting against non-replicating environmental substances?
- are the immune reactions themselves producing tissue damage?
- are the control mechanisms of the various cellular and humoral systems functioning properly?
- has neoplastic change occurred in any of the cells of the system?
- are the abnormalities primary or secondary to some other disease process?

Investigations are often requested on an empirical basis, depending on the history, physical examination and other clinical features of the case. Some tests have been found to be positive in certain diseases and are good diagnostic or prognostic markers, without necessarily revealing the underlying pathological mechanism. Clinical immunology, like other disciplines, makes use of empirical observations in addition to applying basic theory in the management of patients.

Important antigens in clinical immunology		
Extrinsic antigens	derived from pathogenic & saprophytic micro-organisms non-invasive plant & animal products drugs & simple chemicals (acting as haptens) alloantigens	
Intrinsic antigens	autoantigens	organ-specific non-organ-specific

Fig. 30.1 Non-replicating, non-invasive environmental substances can provoke an abnormal immunological response which may, on subsequent exposure, lead to allergic reactions in the host.

ASSESSMENT OF ANTIGENS

There are numerous clinically important antigens which can be extrinsic or intrinsic (Fig. 30.1).

Micro-organisms

The presence of microbial antigens in tissues or body fluids is indicative of an established infection, but some infections can be diagnosed by immunological detection or measurement of the products of the invading organisms (Fig. 30.2).

Allergens

Inert antigens are generally referred to as allergens, and include a wide variety of macromolecular plant and animal products, foods and pharmaceutical agents which may be harmful in sensitive subjects. However, the clinical question is not whether the substances are present in an individual patient (or in their environment), but whether the individual's immune response could produce the observed clinical effects. Hence there are usually no

Common infections diagnosed by immunological detection of microbial products	
Viruses	respiratory syncytial virus — immunofluorescence of tracheal/bronchial washings hepatitis B virus — radioimmunoassay of plasma & other body fluids
Bacteria	*Mycobacterium tuberculosis*— immunofluorescence of sputum/CSF debris pneumococcus — counter-current electrophoresis of serum and/or CSF
Parasites	schistosomal infections — radioimmunoassay of soluble egg antigen in plasma

Fig. 30.2 Immunological identification of organisms is more rapid than culture techniques and can lead to more rapid initiation of treatment.

clinical requirements to identify these antigens — only to evaluate the immunological response to them.

Alloantigens

These antigens are present in the blood and tissues of other individuals of the same species. They may gain entry during pregnancy, blood transfusion or organ grafting procedures and may cause a variety of immunologically mediated clinical disorders, such as Rhesus haemolytic disease of the newborn, transfusion reactions, allograft rejection or graft-versus-host disease.

The antigens involved include blood group substances, HLA antigens and the various allotypes of plasma proteins. They are evaluated using largely serological techniques which are performed mainly in Blood Transfusion Departments, and are seldom part of routine clinical immunology, at least in the UK.

ASSESSMENT OF SPECIFIC ANTIBODIES

Specific antibodies may be directed against extrinsic or intrinsic antigens.

ANTIBODIES TO EXTRINSIC ANTIGENS

These are either antibodies to antigens derived from pathogenic micro-organisms, or antibodies directed against non-replicating environmental antigens that cause disease because they provoke an allergic response in susceptible subjects (Fig. 30.3).

Antibodies to extrinsic antigens	
To microbial products	
	Disease association
Wasserman & Kahn antibodies	syphilis
S. typhi agglutinins	typhoid
streptolysin-O	] streptococcal infections
DNA-ase B	] streptococcal infections
staphylococcal toxin	staphylococcal infections
Brucella agglutinins	brucellosis
To non-replicating environmental antigens	
grass pollen	] allergic rhinitis & asthma
house dust mite	] allergic rhinitis & asthma
bird droppings	extrinsic allergic alveolitis
bee venom	severe reaction to bee stings

Fig. 30.3 Antibodies to pathogenic micro-organisms are used by microbiologists to diagnose infectious disease, and these tests represent some of the earliest applications of
30.2 immunological concepts in clinical medicine.

Allergy

Antibodies to non-replicating environmental antigen are associated with allergic symptoms (see chapter 17). The mere possession of antibodies to extrinsic allergens (IgG or IgE) is necessary to establish a diagnosis of allergy. However, this alone is not sufficient for diagnosis as many individuals who possess such antibodies do not show any allergic symptoms on exposure to the allergen. Specific IgE antibodies are more likely to be clinically relevant as are precipitating antibodies, for example to *Aspergillus* which, when found in a patient with extrinsic allergic alveolitis, strongly suggest immunopathology. Acute allergic symptoms due to IgE-mediated reactions form the bulk of the practice of allergy and the sensible use of specific IgE antibody tests (Fig. 30.4) will allow triggering factors to be identified in many patients.

Type III reactions

Other types of antibody mediated allergic reaction are usually due to IgG antibodies directed against allergens bound to cells, or against soluble antigens which cause immune complex disease. Detection of the antibodies may not be sufficient for diagnosis, and *in vivo* challenge (either intradermal or organ provocation) may be necessary. In the extrinsic allergic alveolitis of bird fancier's lung, antibodies to bird droppings are diagnostic (Fig. 30.5).

Type IV reactions

Contact dermatitis is an example of allergy caused by cell-mediated immune mechanisms (see chapter 14), in which chronic lymphokine production results in the local induration and inflammation which characterizes this condition (Fig. 30.6).

Drug hypersensitivity

Reactions to pharmacological drugs are a common clinical problem mediated by a variety of hypersensitivity mechanisms (see chapter 19). For example, penicillamine nephropathy may result from immune complex deposition in the glomeruli (see chapter 8), but other types of acute IgE-mediated reactions and contact sensitivity can also occur with the same agent. Laboratory tests are of limited value in such situations.

ANTIBODIES TO INTRINSIC ANTIGENS (AUTOANTIBODIES)

Although the direct pathogenetic role of the autoantibodies is often uncertain, they do indicate likely immunopathological effects and are often useful in the diagnosis of disease, and in some cases in monitoring therapy. In many diseases autoantibodies are detected by indirect immunofluorescence, the principle of which is shown in Fig. 30.7.

Use of specific IgE antibody tests	
Measure total serum IgE — if low (<50 K U/litre in adults, 10 K U/litre in children) positive results very unlikely — if very low (<25 in adults, <5 in children) test contra-indicated	
If IgE high, normal or elevated, assess symptoms:	Test for antibodies to:
respiratory symptoms (rhinitis/asthma)	house dust mite, animal danders, pollens, moulds (or identified allergens)
gastro-intestinal symptoms (oral oedema, vomiting, diarrhoea)	peanut, egg albumin, milk protein, wheat, fish (or identified foods, if any)
urticaria/angioedema	common foods (or identified allergens)
eczema, especially if IgE very high (>1000 K U/litre)	respiratory & food allergens (or identified allergens)
stinging insect sensitivity	bee & wasp venom

Fig. 30.4 While most patients with symptomatic allergy have raised total IgE levels, this is not invariable, and with isolated drug hypersensitivity or insect venom sensitivity the total IgE is often within the normal range. Nevertheless, a total IgE level may be helpful where there are no clear precipitating factors in the patients' history.

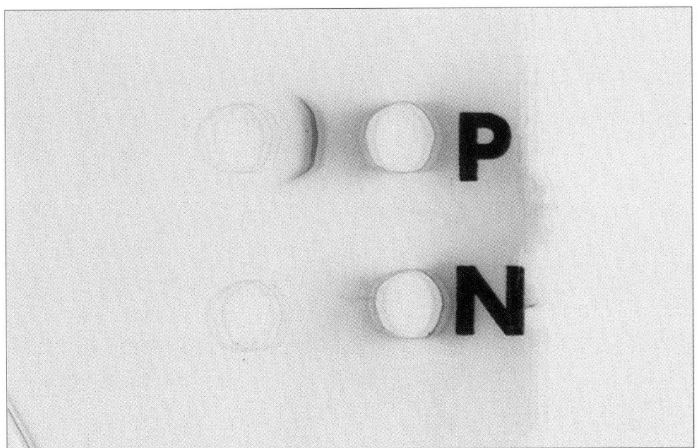

Fig. 30.5 Countercurrent electrophoresis to show precipitins to pigeon droppings in a patient with pigeon fancier's lung. P = patient's serum; N = normal serum. The anode is to the right.

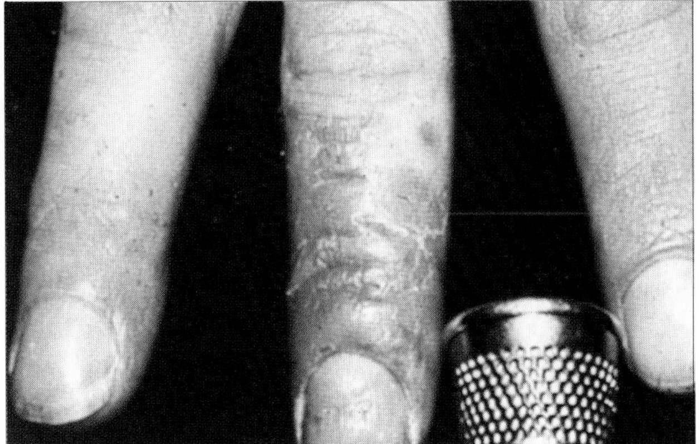

Fig. 30.6 The effects of hypersensitivity to nickel.

Thyroid autoantibodies

These were amongst the first autoantibodies to be described and are still widely used in the diagnosis of thyroid disease. The most commonly recognized antibodies are directed against thyroglobulin and thyroid microsomal antigens, and are found in more than 95% of patients with Hashimoto's thyroiditis and 50–70% of patients with Graves' disease, as well as in primary myxoedema. They are detected by passive haemagglutination or indirect immunofluorescence (Fig. 30.8). They are not found in simple goitre, and therefore the investigation is essential in any patient with a diffuse goitre in whom surgery is contemplated. A full discussion of the clinical value of thyroid autoauntibodies can be found in chapter 7.

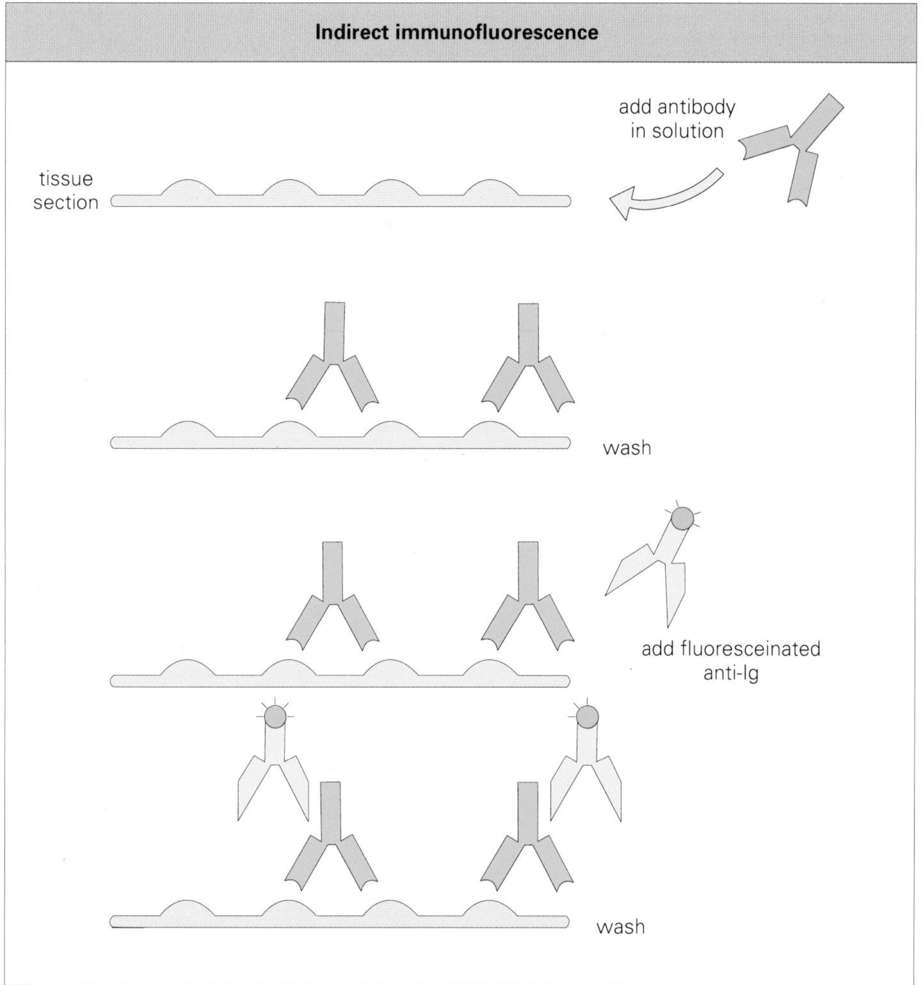

Fig. 30.7 Indirect immunofluorescence is performed using cryostat sections from frozen tissue blocks. This ensures that labile antigens are not damaged by fixatives. The test solution of antibody is added, incubated and washed off. Fluoresceinated anti-immunoglobulin is then added, and that which binds will fluoresce green when UV light is directed onto the section.

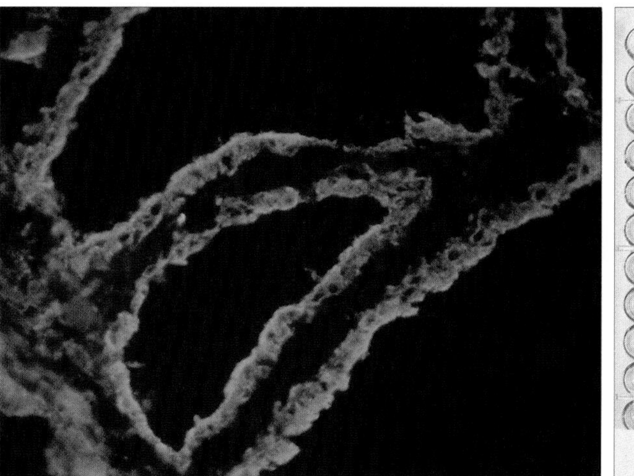

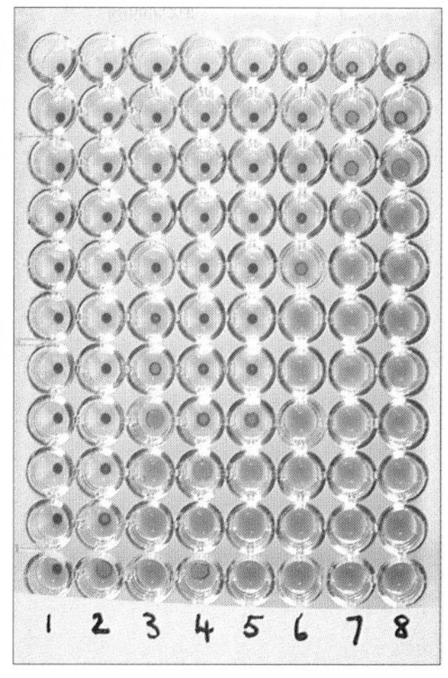

Fig. 30.8 Indirect immunofluorescence of thyroid microsomal antibodies (left) and passive haemagglutination of thyroglobulin-coated red cells in microtitre plate (right). Rows 2–8 contain positive sera (doubling dilutions), and row 1 negative serum.

Gastric autoantibodies

These classically occur in patients with pernicious anaemia (PA). They consist of antibodies to gastric parietal cells (GPC) and are usually detected by indirect immunofluorescence (see chapter 10). Intrinsic factor (IF)
30.4 antibodies are detected by the ability of the patient's serum to inhibit the binding of free, isotopically labelled B_{12} to a human intrinsic factor preparation (Fig. 30.9). This is the basis of the most commonly used test, but there are also antibodies which block the uptake of the IF–B_{12} complex by gastric mucosa.

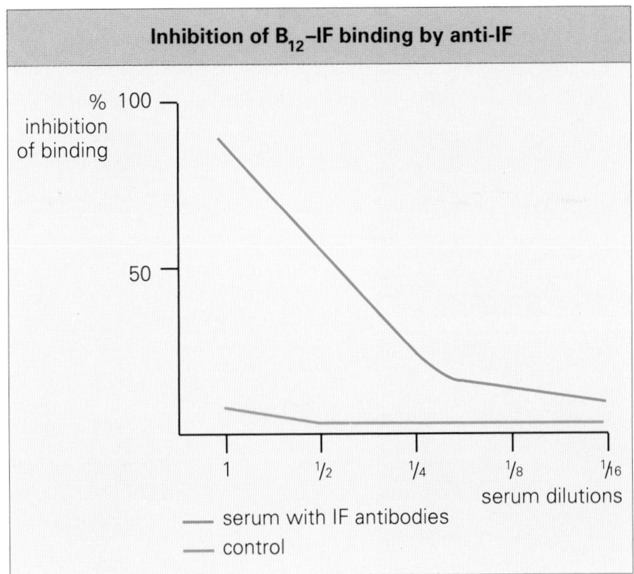

Fig. 30.9 ^{57}[Co]-labelled B_{12} is mixed with serial dilutions of a patient's serum containing intrinsic factor (IF) antibodies, and with a control serum. The anti-IF antibodies cause almost 90% inhibition of binding when the serum is undiluted.

Adrenal antibodies

These occur in about 50% of patients with idiopathic hypoadrenalism (Addison's disease), and are detected by indirect immunofluorescence, (see chapter 7). They are not used to diagnose hypoadrenalism — only to indicate its likely cause, since the antibodies are absent in tuberculous and neoplastic destruction of the adrenal gland.

Pancreatic islet cell antibodies

Antibodies to the β cells of the islets of Langerhans are a diagnostic feature of type I, or insulin dependent diabetes mellitus (IDDM). They occur in the early stages of the disease, and are associated with active insulitis. They then frequently decline and may be absent in treated diabetics. They are not found in type II, or non-insulin dependent diabetes (NIDDM). The antibodies are detected by indirect immunofluorescence using normal human pancreas as substrate (see chapter 7). They are often of low titre and those which fix complement are usually of greater pathogenetic significance. The test is used mainly to survey families of diabetics and in research, although in recent studies of the use of cyclosporin to treat early IDDM, they have been used to monitor the effectiveness of treatment.

Skeletal muscle antibodies

Antibodies to skeletal muscle characteristically occur in myasthenia gravis (MG). They are detected by indirect immunofluorescence (Fig. 30.10 upper) in one-third of non-thymomatous MG patients, but are present in 95% of those with thymomatous myasthenia. This test is not specific and may be positive in some patients with hepatitis, acute viral infections and polymyositis, where it is probably due to cross-reactions with antibodies to actin. A more specific test, positive in over 80% of patients, is for antibodies to the acetylcholine receptor (Fig. 30.10 lower). Some patients with ocular myasthenia have very low levels of antibodies and, while the absolute antibody level does not correlate with the clinical severity of the disease, serial estimations in an individual patient undergoing plasma exchange or intensive immunosuppression may be helpful in monitoring disease activity (see chapter 9).

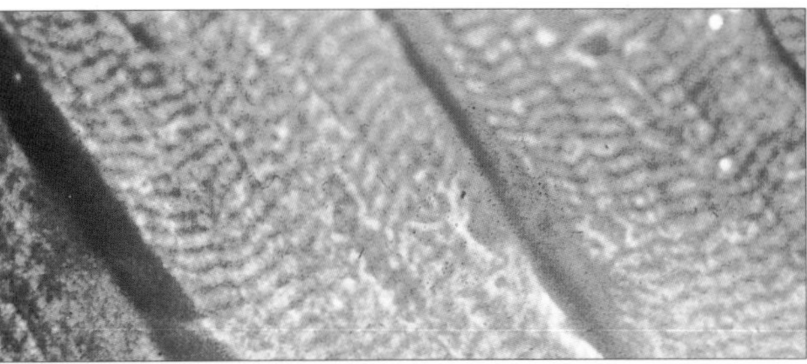

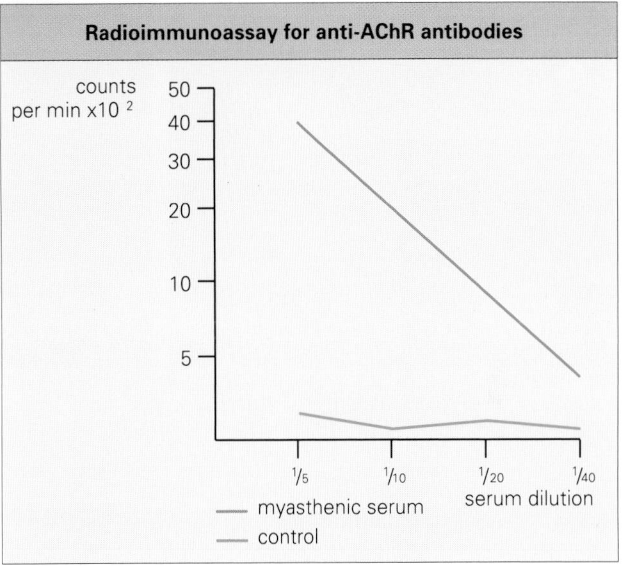

Fig. 30.10 Skeletal muscle antibodies. Upper: indirect immunofluorescence of rat skeletal muscle to show skeletal muscle antibodies reacting with the A-bands. Lower: radioactively labelled bungarotoxin, a snake venom, is specific for the acetylcholine receptor (AChR) and binds avidly to receptor preparations. The patient's antibodies also bind to the receptor–toxin complex and can be precipitated by polyethylene glycol or heterospecific anti-human immunoglobulin antibodies, as in this case. A high radioactive count in the precipitate indicates the presence of these antibodies.

Epidermal antibodies

Antibodies to elements of the epidermis occur in patients with bullous skin diseases, in particular bullous pemphigoid and pemphigus vulgaris. Antibodies to the epidermal basement membrane are seen in bullous pemphigoid, and to the epidermal intercellular substance in pemphigus. They are involved in the pathogenesis of the lesions and are best detected by direct immunofluorescence of skin biopsy specimens, obtained from unaffected juxtalesional skin (see chapter 14).

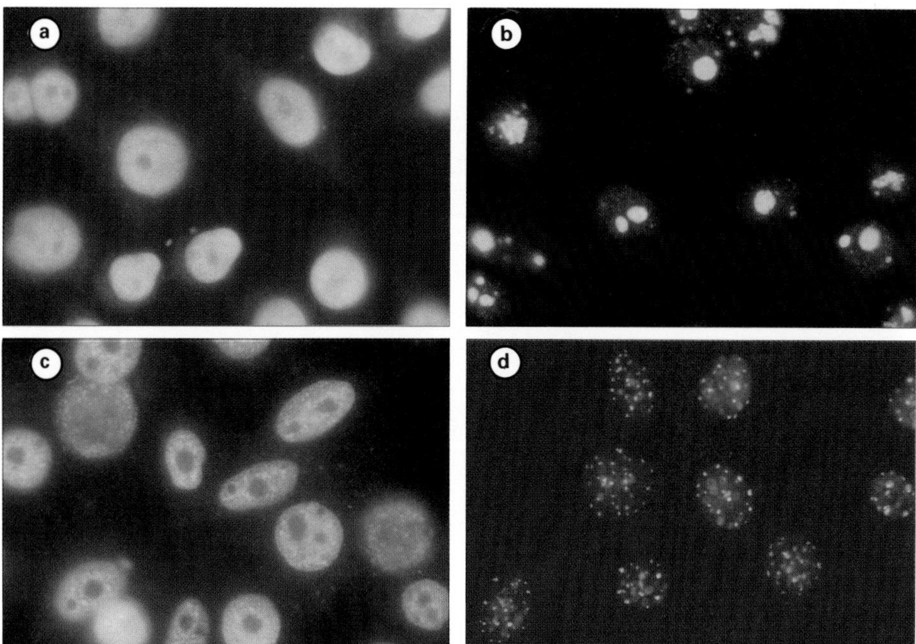

Fig. 30.11 Different patterns of anti-nuclear antibodies seen by indirect immunofluorescence on HEP2 cells. a) homogeneous; b) nucleolar; c) coarse speckled; d) centromere.

Anti-nuclear antibodies (ANA)

Recently, there has been a considerable increase in awareness of the range of nuclear and related antigens to which antibodies can arise in the connective tissue diseases, and of the clinical significance of different antibody patterns. ANA are the hallmark of systemic lupus erythematosus (SLE), occurring in 95% of cases, often with a high titre and a homogeneous pattern on indirect immunofluorescence (see chapter 6). Although the pattern of nuclear staining is not of major diagnostic importance, certain characteristic patterns often occur (Fig. 30.11). In patients with mixed connective tissue disease a speckled pattern is often seen, while in scleroderma RNA antibodies in high titre frequently give a nucleolar pattern, and in the CREST syndrome (calcinosis, Raynaud's phenomenon, (o)esophagitis, scleroderma and telangiectasis) antibodies to centromere antigens occur.

Antibodies to isolated nuclear antigens, and the application of techniques such as countercurrent electrophoresis, ELISA and radioimmunoassay have enhanced the ability to discriminate between a variety of related conditions (Fig. 30.12).

Mitochondrial antibodies

The most characteristic is the so-called M2 anti-mitochondrial antibody (Fig. 30.13 left), found in high titre in 95% of patients with primary biliary cirrhosis. The antigen is a lipoprotein of the inner mitochondrial membrane and, whilst present in all mitochondria, it is most heavily expressed in those of brown fat cells, distal renal tubules and in salivary, pancreatic and thyroid acinar cells. The presence of strongly positive mitochondrial antibodies makes assessment by indirect immunofluorescence of many other types of anti-cytoplasmic autoantibodies (for example gastric parietal cell antibodies) invalid.

Other mitochondrial-type antibodies (or antibodies to small cytoplasmic particles) are seen in other conditions. The so-called M3 or liver-kidney-microsomal antibody (Fig. 30.13 right) is seen as staining of coarse larger granules in proximal renal tubules and in hepatocytes. This antibody is said to occur principally in patients with chronic active hepatitis.

Smooth muscle antibodies

These are mainly directed against actin, and are best seen in cells in the media of arterioles, in the muscularis mucosa and in the muscle cells of the intergastric glands of the gastric mucosa (Fig. 30.14). They are characteristic of chronic active hepatitis (CAH), both the autoimmune type and that associated with chronic hepatitis B infection, where they are usually found in high titre (>1/100). However, patients with this condition may also have ANA, and in some patients with the autoimmune type a high titre ANA (usually with anti-ssDNA) may be the only significant autoantibody present. Thus anti-smooth muscle antibodies are not diagnostic of CAH, nor is their presence essential for this diagnosis.

They are found in low titre and low frequency in normal subjects, but are more common after acute infections, especially acute virus infections, such as hepatitis A and glandular fever, where they may decline and disappear during convalescence.

Reticulin antibodies

These antibodies are directed at fibrillary structures found in connective tissue and applied to the basement membrane of epithelial cell layers. Although they are referred to as reticulin antibodies, the nature of the antigen is often unclear. The most characteristic type I antibodies are found in about 30–50% of patients with coeliac disease

Anti-nuclear and related antibodies		
Antigen	**Test**	**Specificity**
ds (native) DNA	RIA, ELISA, IIF	70% SLE 10% RA, CAH (in low titre)
ss (denatured) DNA	ELISA	>90% SLE, 60% CAH, 40% RA, other connective tissue diseases
RNP (ribonucleo-protein)	CC, ELISA	50% SLE, 95% MCTD
Sm	CC, ELISA	30% SLE
Histones	IIF	90% drug induced LE, up to 70% SLE, 20% RA
Scl70	CC, ELISA	30% scleroderma
Jo-1	CC, ELISA	30% polymyositis
Centromere	IIF	70% CREST syndrome
Ro/SS-A	CC, ELISA	40% SLE, 30% Sjögren's syndrome
La/SS-B	CC, ELISA	15% SLE, 50% Sjögren's syndrome
Cardiolipin	ELISA	40% SLE, venous thrombosis (also all stages of syphilis)

Fig. 30.12 Anti-nuclear antibody specificities. IIF = indirect immunofluorescence; RIA = radioimmunoassay; CC = counter-current electrophoresis; ELISA = enzyme-linked immunosorbent assay; CREST = calcinosis, Raynaud's, (o)esophagitis, sclero-derma, telangiectasia; MCTD = mixed connective tissue disease; CAH = chronic active hepatitis.

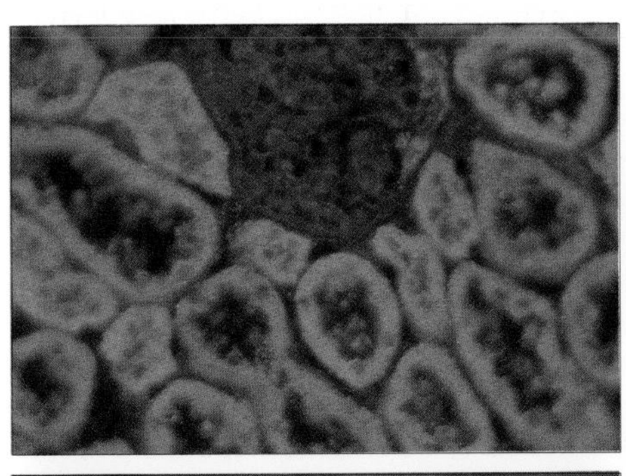
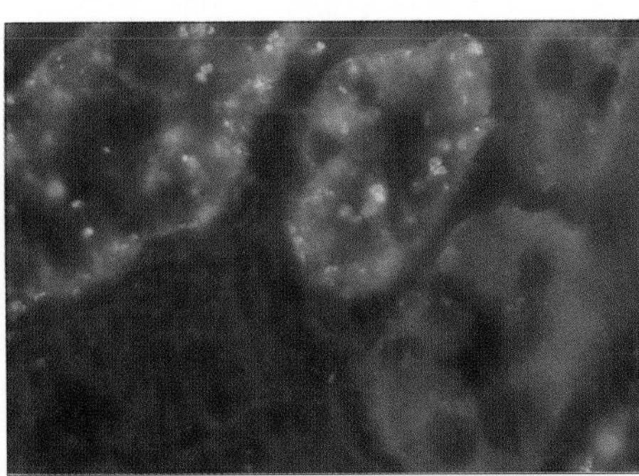

Fig. 30.13 Mitochondrial antibodies. Left: indirect immunofluorescence of rat kidney to show anti-mitochondrial antibody M2 in primary biliary cirrhosis. Right: M3 or liver-kidney-microsomal antibody.

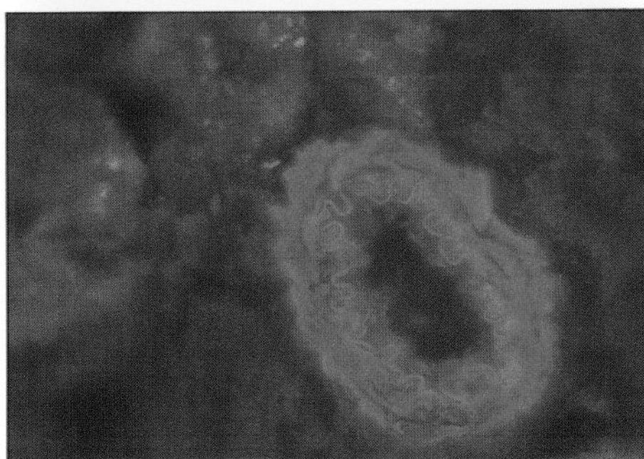
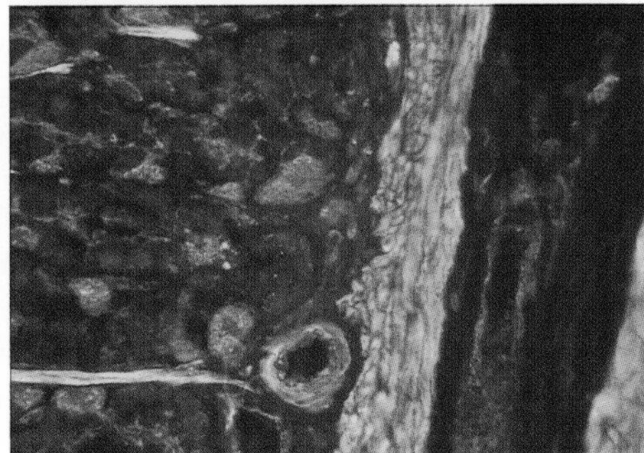

Fig. 30.14 Smooth muscle antibodies. Left: indirect immunofluorescence of rat tissues to show smooth muscle antibodies in arteriolar walls. Right: smooth muscle antibodies in the muscularis mucosa and intergastric gland muscle fibres.

(see chapter 10); they are seen more commonly in children with this condition who often also have IgA anti-reticulin antibodies. They are also found in about one-third of patients with other gut diseases, such as Crohn's disease and occasionally ulcerative colitis. The type I reticulin antibody gives fluorescence around kidney tubules and in the gastric mucosa. Other types of reticulin antibody react with supporting tissue in arterioles and muscle and in the lining of hepatic sinusoids. Very often the clinical significance of these antibodies is unclear.

Neutrophil leucocyte cytoplasmic antibodies

In 1984 Woude and colleagues described antibodies in the sera of patients with Wegener's granulomatosis which react with cytoplasmic constituents in human peripheral blood neutrophils (Fig. 30.15). The antigen appears to be

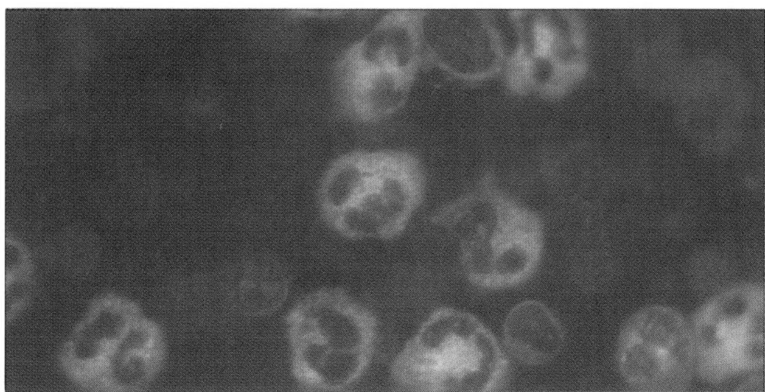

Fig. 30.15 Indirect immunofluorescence of a preparation of human neutrophils to show anti-neutrophil cytoplasmic antibodies (ANCA) in the serum of a patient with Wegener's granulomatosis.

associated with a 29 kDa serine protease in the primary granules in the cytosol, but these and other antibodies occur in other small vessel vasculitides. However, it is a very useful test in Wegener's, for which there was previously no serological test of any diagnostic significance. In remission the level of antibody activity frequently declines and the test may become negative, but it is not entirely reliable as a guide to therapy. Human neutrophils prepared for use as substrate ingest variable amounts of normal human IgG, which may confuse the interpretation. A common false positive result also occurs with many sera, including normal subjects, which give a rim of perinuclear staining. For these reasons, the interpretation of this test requires experience.

Autoantibodies to plasma proteins

The main plasma proteins which give rise to clinically significant autoantibodies are IgG, complement components, (especially C3), and clotting factor VIII.

Anti-IgG antibodies. The best characterized are those that act as rheumatoid factor (RF). They are found in the three main classes of immunoglobulin. It is the IgM rheumatoid factors which are detected in most of the RF tests, and which have most clinical significance in the diagnosis of rheumatoid arthritis (RA), occurring in over 90% of patients with this condition (see chapter 5). Tests which use rabbit IgG as the target antigen (for example the Rose-Waaler test) have a lower sensitivity but greater specificity. While only positive in 70% of RA patients, they are seldom positive in other conditions, except in those associated with chronic antigen challenge, such as subacute bacterial endocarditis, kala-azar, leprosy and chronic liver disease. The latex agglutination test which uses human IgG as the target antigen is more sensitive, being positive in 95% of RA patients, but it is also positive in a range of acute inflammatory conditions. Tests for RF are useful diagnostic markers but of little value in monitoring treatment, although the factor usually declines and sometimes becomes negative in patients who respond to gold or penicillamine treatment.

Other types of anti-IgG antibodies include those which react with allotypic markers (Gm), found sometimes after pregnancy or transfusion, and anti-idiotypic antibodies which are directed against variable region determinants of antibody molecules. Neither of these types of autoantibody generally have clinical significance, except that antibodies which react against the idiotypes of anti-hormone antibodies may then cross-react with the hormone receptor site on the cell surface and have the potential to act as pathological autoantibodies. This has been shown in some diabetic patients on insulin therapy who develop anti-insulin antibodies, and the anti-idiotypes of these act as antibodies to the insulin receptor on the patients' cells.

Antibodies to complement proteins. These are termed immunoconglutinins and are mainly IgM; they react with determinants on bound complement components revealed after activation. Although they increase in bacterial infections and other complement-consuming illnesses, their measurement has little place in routine clinical immunological practice.

C3 nephritic factor reacts with the C3 convertase of the alternative pathway and stabilizes the convertase, with the resulting progression of C3 activation and very low circulating C3 levels. It was first described in patients with chronic membranoproliferative glomerulonephritis (see chapter 8) but is also found in partial lipodystrophy, and in occasional individuals with a tendency to infections. It can be a cause of secondary immunodeficiency due to hypocomplementaemia, although this is rare. Measurement of C3 nephritic factor is indicated in patients with a very low C3 titre, with or without nephritis, as its presence may indicate an increased risk of subsequent renal damage even in those without evidence of renal disease.

Anti-factor VIII antibodies. These occur in patients with haemophilia treated with factor VIII preparations and may cause relative resistance to therapy. The antibodies may occur spontaneously in patients with lymphoma or SLE, and may antedate by years the other associated clinical features of the disease but they may be associated with thrombotic rather than haemorrhagic clinical problems. They always cause a prolonged bleeding time and a prolonged cephalin cholesterol clotting time.

EVALUATION OF HUMORAL IMMUNODEFICIENCY

Most normal individuals develop a range of antibodies to common environmental antigens as they mature. These arise from clinical infections or sub-clinical contact with common micro-organisms. Tests for such antibodies are important in the evaluation of patients with putative immunodeficiency. They should include tests for thymus dependent antigens (for example tetanus and diphtheria toxoids) and for thymus independent antigens (for example *E. coli* or pneumococcal polysaccharides). Determination of the IgG subclass of the antibodies may be particularly helpful, since protective antibodies to bacterial capsular polysaccharides are of the IgG2 subclass.

Leucocyte surface antigens (CD nomenclature)		
Lymphocytes		
CD number	**previous associations**	**cell type**
1	OKT6	cortical thymocytes
2	OKT11, Leu 5 sheep E receptor	mature & immature T cells
3	OKT3, Leu 4 UCHT1	mature T cells
4	OKT4, Leu 3a	helper/inducer T cells
5	OKT1, Leu 1	mature & immature T cells; small subset B cells
8	OKT8, Leu 2a	suppressor/cytotoxic T cells
10	CALLA	immature B cells common acute lymphoid leukaemia
22		mature B cells (also by surface Ig)
Monocytes/granulocytes		
11b/18	OK M1, MAC-1	monocytes; macrophages granulocytes
16	Fc receptor-III	NK cells, granulocytes
11a/18	LFA-1	granulocytes, monocytes NK cells, lymphocytes

Fig. 30.16 Leucocyte surface antigens (CD nomenclature). Some of these antigens are also expressed on other tissue cells.

LYMPHOCYTE TESTS

CD antigens

Tests to determine peripheral blood lymphocyte phenotypes and their *in vitro* functional ability are most often employed in the assessment of presumed immunodeficiency, and in lymphoid malignancy. The determination of cell phenotypes is now carried out mainly using monoclonal antibodies which detect antigenic determinants of the surface structural glycoproteins that are characteristic of particular stages of differentiation or functional capabilities of the lymphocytes. These determinants have been the subject of much international collaborative research, and a system of classification has been evolved which has assigned CD (clusters of differentiation) numbers to these antigens, some of which are listed in Fig. 30.16.

The cells bearing these antigens can be detected by indirect immunofluorescence using mouse monoclonal antibodies, followed by fluorescein-labelled anti-mouse immunoglobulin, or by direct rosetting using particles (usually sheep or ox red cells) coated with the particular monoclonal reagent (Fig. 30.17 left). The results are given as the percentage of cells positive for the particular CD number. Fluorescein-labelled cells can also be conveniently analysed by the fluorescence-activated cell sorter which plots in graphic form the proportion of cells which have a light emission beyond a certain pre-set level (Fig. 30.17 right). By knowing the total lymphocyte count, the number bearing a particular CD antigen can be determined.

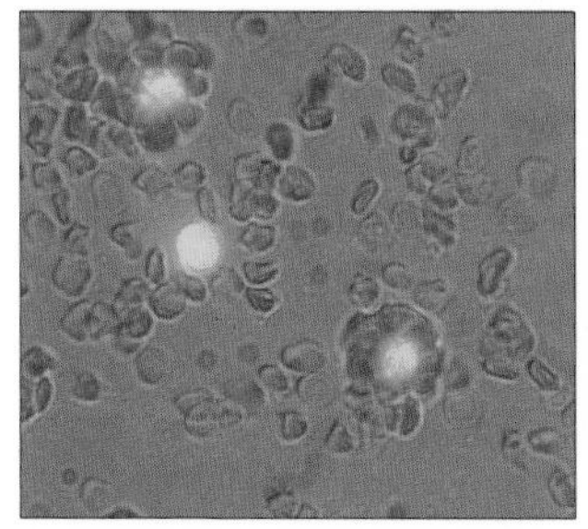

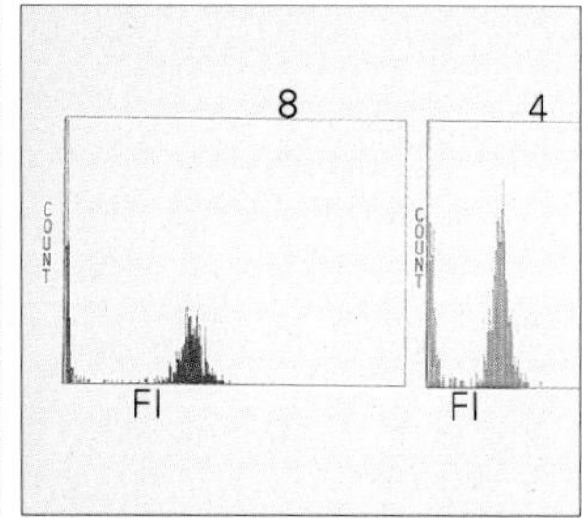

Fig. 30.17 Detection of CD-bearing cells. Left: lymphocytes stained with acricidine orange rosetting with anti-CD3 coated erythrocytes. Notice the two positive and one negative cell. Right: fluorescence emission pattern of peripheral blood lymphocytes stained for CD4 and CD8. FI = fluorescence intensity.

Peripheral blood lymphocyte phenotypes					
Total lymphocyte	**CD3**	**CD4**	**CD8**	**B cells**	**Disease association**
↓↓	↓	↓	↓	↓	severe combined immunodeficiency (SCID) severe immunosuppression due to drugs, X-rays or gut loss
N	↓	↓	↓	N or ↑	B cell SCID
N	N	N	N	↓↓	X-linked hypogammaglobulinaemia
↑	↑	N or ↑	↑↑	N	acute viral infection
N	N	N	↑	N	chronic viral infection
↓	N or ↓	↓	N or ↑	N or ↑	symptomatic HIV infection

Fig. 30.18 Peripheral blood lymphocyte marker patterns in disease. None of the patterns are absolutely diagnostic of any particular disease as considerable variation exists.

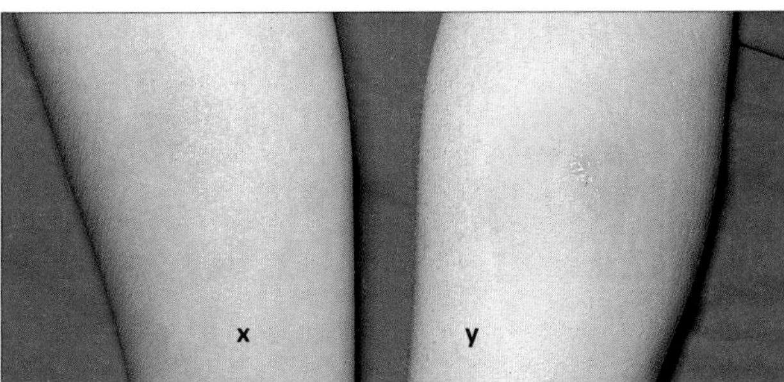

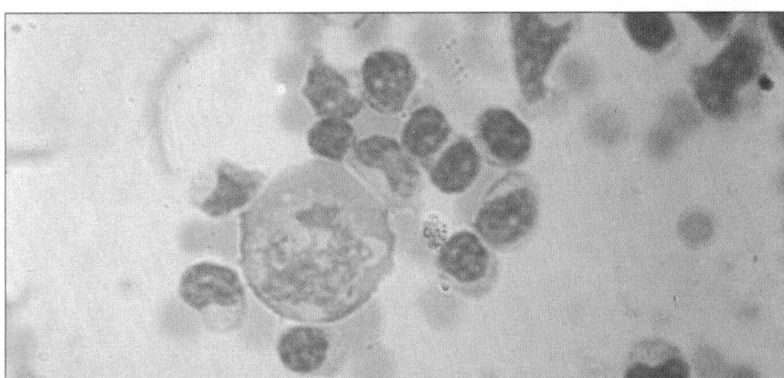

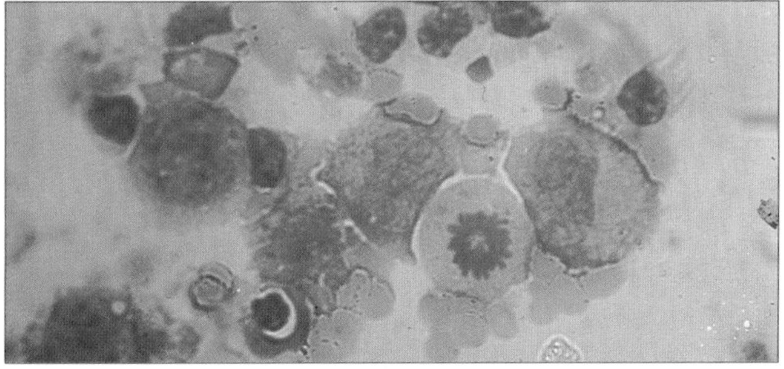

Fig. 30.19 Measurement of blast transformation. Upper: delayed hypersensitivity response to PPD in a normal subject (X) and a patient with primary tuberculosis (Y). Middle: lymphocytes from subject X cultured for 7 days in 5μg of PPD. Lower: lymphocytes from subject Y cultured for 7 days in 5μg PPD — note the large numbers of blast cells and mitotic figures.

Certain diseases are associated with abnormal peripheral blood lymphocyte phenotype patterns (Fig. 30.18).

Functional studies

Assessment of *in vitro* lymphocyte function is by short term lymphocyte culture in the presence of mitogens (usually derived from plants) and specific antigens. These agents cause the cells to undergo differentiation and cell division, a process referred to as blast transformation. Blast transformation can be measured by the incorporation into the cells' DNA of radioactively labelled precursor, ^{3}[H]-thymidine, the level of incorporation usually being proportional to the concentration of the stimulating agent. The cell-mediated response to antigens is classically determined by the delayed hypersensitivity skin test, which can be mirrored by the blast transformation response to the antigen concerned (Fig. 30.19).

Lymphocyte transformation. The results of this test must be interpreted with caution because it shows considerable day-to-day variation and is subject to technical artefacts. Nevertheless, in good hands, consistent results can be achieved. Poor responses to mitogens may indicate primary or secondary cellular immunodeficiency, but this state can be transient in any illness or after operation, when it is of little clinical significance. Depressed mitogen responses may also be found after trauma, in pregnancy, or in certain chronic inflammatory states. In such patients this can be caused by factors in the patients' serum which depress these non-specific responses. Failure to respond to a specific antigen may be because the patient has not been exposed to the relevant antigen (for example in the neonate), or it may be a non-specific manifestation, as indicated above. However in patients with clinical cellular immune deficiency, indicated by poor clinical responses to one or more specific infective agents, impaired lymphocyte transformation to specific antigens may be the most sensitive indicator of disordered function.

Malignancy

In lymphoid malignancy, in addition to characteristic CD markers and often poor *in vitro* lymphocyte transformation to mitogens and antigens, the cells develop evidence of restricted clonality; this is indicated by gene rearrangement of the V-D-J segments of the immunoglobulin heavy chain genes for B cell malignancy, or of the T cell receptor genes (for T cell malignancy) (see chapter 21). These can be detected by appropriate DNA probes, which are usually the most sensitive method of determining whether apparently abnormal cells represent clonal expansion of B or T cells.

In most malignant lymphoid states there is an increased turnover of lymphoid cells. This results in an increased turnover of HLA antigens, including the non-polymorphic 12kDa polypeptide chain associated with class I antigens (β_2-microglobulin). Levels of this protein increase in malignant states, for example multiple myeloma and non-Hodgkin's lymphoma, and can be used in the monitoring of therapy.

Lymphocytes in tissue fluids

Immunohistological techniques employing monoclonal antibodies have allowed considerable additional information to be gained by the examination of lymphoid tissue obtained at biopsy or autopsy (Fig. 30.20). This technique is now essential in the histological diagnosis of lymphoid malignancy, and is being extended to the histological analysis of disorders, particularly malignant disorders, of many other systems.

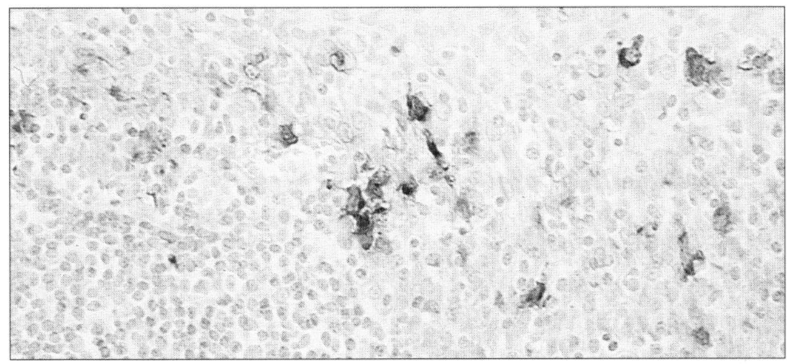

Fig. 30.20 Lymph node stained with a monoclonal antibody to protein S-100 to show dendritic cells; counterstained with haematoxylin.

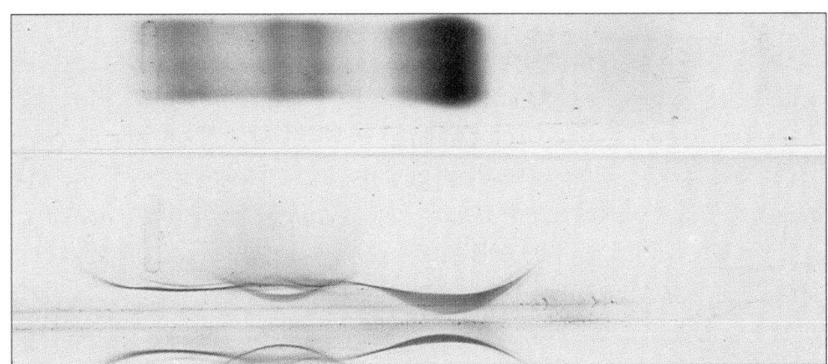

Fig. 30.21 Comparison of serum electrophoresis followed by protein staining (upper pattern) with immunoelectrophoresis of same sample (anode is to the right).

IMMUNOGLOBULIN ANALYSIS

A crude but rapid assessment of the humoral immune system can also be made by analysis of the serum immunoglobulins. These form the beta-gamma bands on protein electrophoresis, but with specific antisera their character and quantity can be more accurately determined (Fig. 30.21).

Monoclonal immunoglobulins

One important application of this test is the detection of the immunoglobulin product of an expanded clone of B cells. This shows as a dense gamma band, or serum monoclonal protein, which can be detected and analysed by immunofixation using specific antisera (Fig. 30.22). These 'paraproteins' are the hallmarks of multiple myeloma, but they may also be found in other B lymphoid cell malignancies such as Waldenström's macroglobulinaemia, non-Hodgkin's lymphoma and chronic lymphocytic leukaemia, and sometimes occur in individuals without evidence of disease, the so-called benign monoclonal gammopathies. The technique of iso-electrofocusing has been shown to be more sensitive in detection of such paraproteins (Fig. 30.23), but the determination of their significance still requires further clinical, laboratory and radiological investigations.

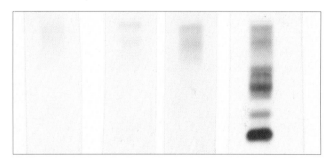

Fig. 30.22 Electrophoresis of serum containing two monoclonal bands, stained for protein (far right), or (from right to left) immunofixed with anti-ɣ heavy chain, anti-λ light chain, and anti-κ light chain antisera. The monoclonal proteins are both IgG-λ.

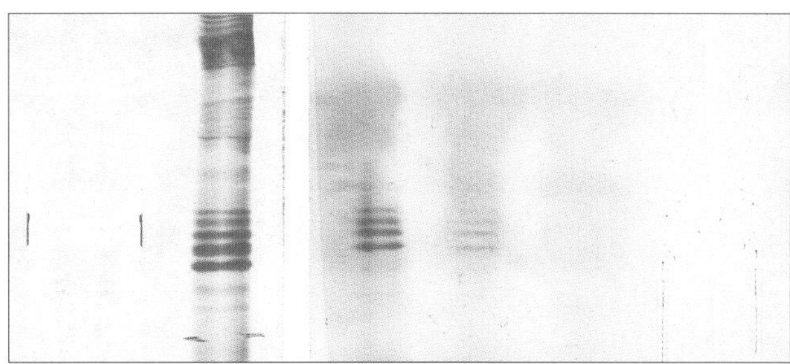

Fig. 30.23 Isoimmunoelectrofixation of a serum monoclonal IgG fixed in acid alcohol and stained with Coomassie blue (far left), and immunofixed (from left to right) with anti-ɣ heavy chain, anti-κ light chain and anti-λ light chain antisera. Note the characteristic multiple banding pattern of monoclonal immunoglobulins by this method.

Examination of the urine for Bence-Jones protein (BJP) (Fig. 30.24) is an important ancillary examination in such cases. These are the free monoclonal light chains produced in excess by the abnormal cells. The presence of BJP in the urine increases the likelihood that the clonal expansion is malignant, and it is found in around 70% of cases of myelomatosis.

Serum immunoglobulins

Quantitation of serum immunoglobulins can be performed using a number of techniques, the most simple being single radial diffusion, but nowadays most laboratories employ fluid phase turbidometric or nephelometric methods, which are susceptible to automation and which yield results more rapidly.

Interpretation of the results usually requires experience and understanding of the working of the immune system and the catabolism of these proteins, as well as a knowledge of other immune parameters. For these reasons such tests are best carried out in immunology departments, or at least, if the measurements are made in another laboratory, then the results should be interpreted by an immunologist. Some abnormal serum immunoglobulin patterns are associated with certain diseases (Fig. 30.25). However the range of variation of immunoglobulin levels is considerable and no pattern, apart from that of the antibody deficiency syndrome (hypogammaglobulinaemia), is diagnostic.

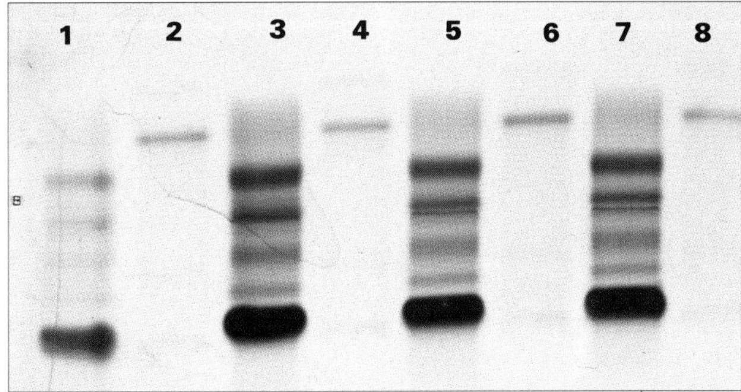

Fig. 30.24 Replicate electrophoreses of the serum (odd number tracks) and concentrated urine (even number tracks) from a patient with a monoclonal immunglobulin and a urinary Bence-Jones protein (free monoclonal light chains). Note the difference in electrophoretic mobility between the whole molecule in the serum and the free light chains in the urine.

Common immunoglobulin patterns in disease			
Disease	**IgG**	**IgA**	**IgM**
Antibody deficiency syndromes	↓↓	↓↓	↓or N
Lymphoid malignancy	N	N	↓or N
Coeliac disease	N	↑	↓or N
SLE/Chronic active hepatitis	↑or↑↑	N	N
Alcoholic cirrhosis/ Chronic sino-pulmonary infection	↑	↑↑	N
Primary biliary cirrhosis	N	N	↑
Obstructive jaundice	N	↑	N
Nephrotic syndrome	↓	N	N
Chronic pyogenic infection	↑	↑	↑

30.12 **Fig. 30.25** Common immunoglobulin patterns in disease.

IgG subclasses

With new monoclonal reagents which are specific for the subclasses of IgG, these proteins can now be confidently measured in serum and other body fluids. Patterns of clinically relevant deficiencies of these subclasses in serum are emerging. A true deficiency is probably only present when the level is barely detectable. Levels just below the normal range are of doubtful clinical significance. It is also doubtful if isolated IgG4 deficiency is a clinical entity, since in 15–20% of healthy subjects this protein may be very low, that is below the limits of detection of immunoprecipitation systems.

Immunoglobulins in other body fluids

Immunoglobulins can be measured in other body fluids. A low level of IgA in saliva may indicate a propensity to increased upper respiratory infections. Increased IgG in the cerebrospinal fluid may indicate local synthesis, which is characteristic of demyelinating diseases. This can be detected by comparing the CSF–serum IgG ratio with CSF–serum albumin ratio (Fig. 30.26). Such locally synthesized IgG is often oligoclonal (Fig. 30.27), and this test is very useful in the diagnosis of multiple sclerosis, particularly where the total CSF protein is normal or only slightly elevated.

COMPLEMENT

These proteins form part of the humoral effector system of the body (see chapter 1). Following trauma or inflammation their synthesis increases and the serum levels consequently rise. Chronic complement activation or acute massive activation may lead to lowering of the serum levels, which, in some chronic states may also be due to impaired synthesis.

C3 convertase

The activation of components of the complement system results in the formation of C3 cleaving enzymes, called C3 convertases. There are two systems of proteins, the classical

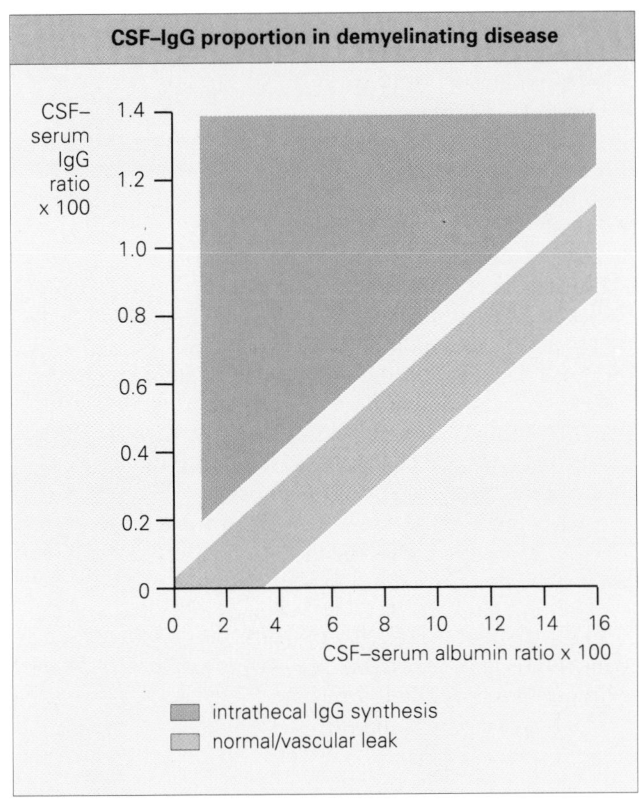

Fig. 30.26 Values lying on the grey area suggest meningitis and a leak in the CSF. Values in the blue area suggest intrathecal production of IgG and demyelinating disease.

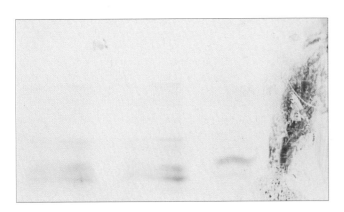

Fig. 30.27 Isoelectrofocusing of unconcentrated CSF followed by immunofixation with anti-IgG antiserum. Note the multiple bands in the two tracks on the left from a patient with multiple sclerosis, compared to that on the right from a patient with a stroke.

and alternative pathways (see chapter 1), each generating a separate C3 convertase, which cleaves and activates C3, the major constituent of the system. The major biological effects of complement occur at or around this stage; one of these is the activation of C5 and the formation of the membrane attack complex (C5b–9) which, if formed on the surface of a cell, renders it susceptible to lysis. This lytic action of complement on antibody-sensitized sheep red cells has been the method for analysing complement for most of this century, but it is only one of the biological roles of the system.

Complement component levels in disease

disease	C3	C4
Acute glomerulonephritis	↓	N
Membranoproliferative glomerulonephritis	↓or↓↓	N
Proliferative glomerulonephritis	N	↑
Henoch-Schönlein nephritis, Hypertensive nephropathy, etc.	N or↑	N or↑
Trauma/acute infections	↑	↑
Severe infections	↓	↓
SLE (or immune complex nephritis)	↓	↓
Cryoglobulinaemia	N or↓	↓or↓↓
Hereditary angioedema	N	↓

Fig. 30.28 Complement component levels in disease.

Involvement of complement in disease

The involvement of complement in disease is either due to activation by antibody in infection and hypersensitivity states, or activation via the alternative pathway in the absence of antibody. It may also be a consequence of a genetic or acquired deficiency of one of the components or inhibitors of the system.

Low complement levels are usually more clinically relevant than high levels. C3 and C4 components are commonly measured as part of the routine analysis of complement, and certain patterns are seen in clinical practice (Fig. 30.28). Even if the levels of complement are normal, *in vivo* utilization may be evident by measuring breakdown or activation products of the system in fresh EDTA plasma:

- C1r/C1s complex
- C4a
- C3a, C3dg
- C5a
- (C5b–9) complex

Elevated levels of these components have been reported in different diseases, including SLE, RA and haemolytic uraemic syndrome. Low levels of C1 esterase inhibitor or the presence of a dysfunctional protein is characteristic of hereditary angioedema. This can be primary or secondary to neoplastic disease.

IMMUNE COMPLEXES

Tests for circulating immune complexes have been developed over the last 15 years or so. Immune complex deposition is a feature of many disease states, such as post-streptococcal glomerulonephritis, SLE, hepatitis B-associated chronic active hepatitis and serum sickness.

Physiological immune complexes

Immune complexes may occur in the circulation during physiological states, for example after eating or pregnancy, or during infective episodes, and are not necessarily associated with separate immunopathological effects. The factors which determine the immunopathological potential of immune complexes are uncertain, but are concerned with the nature of the antigen, the antigen–antibody ratio, the affinity of the antibody and its secondary biological function, such as ability to fix complement.

Basis of tests for immune complexes

The tests for circulating immune complexes are mainly non-antigen-specific. That is, they depend on some change in physico-chemical or biological properties of antibody after it combines with antigen. Such tests include:

- anti-complement activity
- polyethylene glycol precipitation
- C1q binding
- conglutinin binding
- inhibition of rheumatoid factor binding
- inhibition of macrophage binding
- Raji cell binding
- platelet aggregation

These tests vary in their sensitivity, as measured by ability to detect heat-aggregated IgG, which takes on the physico-chemical and biological properties of immune complexes. When performing the tests, care must be taken to avoid artefacts which give false positive or falsely high immune complex levels. Some methods, such as inhibition of agglutination, or the use of binding to living cells, have additional problems of false positivity.

Thus, the detection and measurement of serum immune complexes has become less popular than it was 5–10 years ago. Nevertheless increased levels of immune complexes are characteristically found in the active stages of certain diseases (Fig. 30.29) and, although seldom of diagnostic value, they may be useful in monitoring the response to therapy.

The IUIS/WHO standardization committee on immune complexes recommend the C1q binding (Fc) and conglutinin binding (iC3b) methods as the most reliable and clinically useful of those available.

Immunofluorescence

Definite evidence of the involvement of immune complexes in disease also comes from studying biopsy specimens from affected organs or tissues by direct immunofluorescence. This may show immunoglobulin deposition

Some diseases associated with immune complex deposition

	Isotype involved	Circulating complex
Acute glomerulonephritis	IgG, IgM	often
Membranous glomerulonephritis	IgG	no
IgA nephropathy	IgA	no
SLE	IgG, IgM, IgA	yes
Rheumatoid arthritis	IgG, IgM	often
Crohn's disease	IgG, IgA	sometimes
Coeliac disease	IgG, IgA	sometimes
Subacute bacterial endocarditis	IgG, IgM	often

30.14

Fig. 30.29 The frequency of positive tests for immune complexes in any disease depends on its stage of activity and the nature of the test employed.

and/or complement in an irregular granular manner in and around vessel walls or along basement membranes of the affected tissue.

POLYMORPH TESTS

The neutrophil polymorphs act as the scavengers of the body, and their functions can be assessed in a number of ways (Fig. 30.30). The most frequently employed tests are those which measure the respiratory burst:

- NBT reduction
- chemi-luminescence
- O_2 consumption/CO_2 production
- oxygen radical generation
- polymorph protein iodination

The energy which is generated in the process of phagocytosis and microbial killing is another method of assessing function. Sometimes this is measured by the ability to kill test organisms (usually *Staphylococcus aureus*).

These tests may be abnormal for a number of reasons, most often secondary to other diseases. However some disorders represent primary defects of polymorphs, often on a genetic basis (Fig. 30.31). These are generally very rare conditions.

Chronic granulomatous disease. In this condition, the lack of ability to generate a respiratory burst is due to a missing cytochrome. The most applicable test for this is the nitro blue tetrazolium (NBT) reduction test in which the faintly yellow NBT is reduced to insoluble blue-black formazan granules during phagocytosis, and these can be seen within neutrophils (see chapter 23).

Chemotaxis. Cell movement or chemotaxis can be abnormal and is measured by movement of cells through millipore membranes. The filter is then incubated, fixed and stained, and the distance that the leading front of cells has moved towards the chemoattractant is measured with an appropriate microscope. Here again the defects are most often partial, and secondary to other diseases. Many affected patients have high IgE levels. In its most severe form, known as the hyper-IgE syndrome, patients have very high IgE levels (>2000 IU/litre) and may also have other abnormalities of lymphocyte function, suggesting a disorder of immunoregulation.

MACROPHAGE TESTS

Disorders of macrophages are less well recognized since the tests of macrophage function are less well developed and less widely employed:

- migration through millipore filters
- *Candida* killing
- ability to promote lymphocyte proliferative response to antigens
- IL-1 production by endotoxin

Defects mostly lead to increased risk of infection with fungi and parasites and are probably secondary to defects in lymphocyte function. However, a recent familial disorder of macrophage function has been described (defective IL-1 synthesis), in which the affected individuals suffered from repeated mucocutaneous and systemic fungal infections.

Methods of assessing neutrophil polymorph function

function	test
Mobilization from marrow stores	↑ blood WBC with adrenalin or steroids
Possession of LFA-1/CR3/gp150/90 antigens	monoclonal antibody markers
Adherence	adherence to glass wool columns
Directional migration	chemotaxis through filters
Ingestion of organisms	phagocytic index
Respiratory burst	NBT reduction
Intracellular killing	microbicidal tests

Fig. 30.30 Methods of assessing polymorph function.

Recognized primary abnormalities of polymorphs

syndrome	functional defect
Chediak-Higashi syndrome	bacterial killing (chemotaxis)
chronic granulomatous disease	bacterial killing (NBT)
myeloperoxidase deficiency	bacterial killing (MP)
complete G6-P-D deficiency	bacterial killing
'lazy leucocyte' syndrome (Job's syndrome, defective chemotaxis with ↑IgE)	chemotaxis

Fig. 30.31 Recognized primary abnormalities of polymorphs.

FURTHER READING

Thompson RA, ed. *Techniques in clinical immunology (2E).* Oxford: Blackwell Scientific Publications, 1981.

Stites DP, Stobo JD, Fudenberg HH, Wells JU. *Basic and clinical immunology (5E).* Los Altos, California: Lange Medical Publications, 1984.

Rose NR, Friedman H, Fahey JL, eds. *Manual of clinical laboratory immunology.* Washington, DC: American Society for Microbiology, 1986.

Thompson RA, ed. *Laboratory investigations of immunological disorders. Clinical immunology and allergy. Vol 5, no 3.* London, Philadelphia: WB Saunders, 1985.

IUIS/WHO report. Laboratory investigations in clinical immunology: Methods, pitfalls and clinical indications. *Clin Exp Immunol.* 1988; **74**: 494–503.

Hudson L, Hay FC. *Practical immunology (3E).* Oxford: Blackwell Scientific Publications, 1989.

Gooi HC, Chapel H. *Clinical immunology: A practical approach.* Oxford: Blackwell Scientific Publications, 1990.

Sheehan C. *Clinical immunology: Principles and laboratory diagnosis.* Philadelphia: JB Lippincott, 1990.

INDEX

In this index, fig. refers to the page number on which an illustration appears.

A

E

F

G

H

I

N

O

P

U

V

W

Y

Z